Brain Acetylcholine and Neuropsychiatric Disease

Brain Acetylcholine and Neuropsychiatric Disease

Edited by
Kenneth L. Davis
and
Philip A. Berger

Veterans Administration Hospital
Palo Alto, California
and
Stanford University School of Medicine
Stanford, California

Plenum Press · New York and London

Library of Congress Cataloging in Publication Data

Main entry under title:

Brain acetylcholine and neuropsychiatric disease.

Includes index.
1. Neuropsychiatry. 2. Acetylcholine — Physiological effect. 3. Choline —
Therapeutic use. 4. Brain chemistry. 5. Parasympathomimetic agents — Testing.
I. Davis, Kenneth L. II. Berger, Philip A.

RC343.B664	615'.78	79-862

ISBN-13: 978-1-4613-2936-7   e-ISBN-13: 978-1-4613-2934-3
DOI: 10. 1007/978-1-4613-2934-3

©1979 Plenum Press, New York
Softcover reprint of the hardcover 1st edition 1979

A Divsion of Plenum Publishing Corporation
227 West 17th Street, New York, N.Y. 10011

To Our Families

PREFACE

Recent years have witnessed a resurgence of interest in the possible role of brain acetylcholine in neuropsychiatric disease. Research in this area has involved the renewed investigation of the cholinomimetics physostigmine and arecoline, and has been facilitated by the development of new potential cholinomimetics such as dimethylaminoethanol (Deanol) and choline chloride. Current investigators also have taken advantage of new approaches to neurochemical studies. Increasingly sensitive assay techniques such as gas chromatography/mass spectrometry have allowed investigators to measure low concentrations of choline and acetylcholine in brain tissues. Improved neuroanatomical procedures such as immunohistochemical staining and the use of microelectrodes and micropipets have enabled skilled investigators to begin to map central acetylcholine pathways and to dissect the component parts of the complex interactions between brain acetylcholine and other neurotransmitters. The convergence of data from both clinical and basic studies now suggest that brain acetylcholine may be involved in affective illness, several movement disorders, and some cognitive disturbances.

The purpose of this book is to summarize recent clinical and pre-clinical investigations on the possible role of brain acetylcholine in several neurological and psychiatric disorders. The volume is divided into six major sections: (1) Brain Acetylcholine and Psychiatric Disorders; (2) Brain Acetylcholine and Movement Disorders; (3) Brain Acetylcholine and Cognitive Function; (4) The Electrophysiology of Cholinergic Agents; (5) Interactions of Brain Acetylcholine and Other Neurotransmitters; (6) Biochemical and Pharmacological Aspects of Cholinergic Treatment Strategies. The first three sections concentrate on the results of clinical trials with cholinergic agents. The final three sections present the basic studies which attempt to provide a theoretical framework for understanding the actions of cholinergic agents in clinical studies.

The relationship between acetylcholine and psychiatric disease is examined in discussions of the anti-manic properties of physostigmine, the depressant action of choline and deanol, red cell choline and affective disease, the interaction between lithium and acetylcholine, acetylcholinesterase activity in various psychotic disorders, and the results of clinical trials of cholinomimetics in schizophrenia. A detailed examination of the possible relationship between central cholinergic activity and Huntington's disease and tardive dyskinesia is also presented. This examination includes a summary of clinical trials of deanol, choline chloride, and both intravenous and oral physostigmine on the abnormal involuntary movements of these neurological diseases. Data on the status of muscarinic cholinergic receptors in Huntington's disease is described and evidence for two striatal dopamine receptors is presented.

Human and animal cognitive studies as well as neurochemical investigations have led to a cholinergic deficiency hypothesis of senile dementia. The implications of this theory are explored in a series of chapters dealing with the effects of physostigmine and choline chloride on human memory. A possible relationship between carbohydrate metabolism and acetylcholine synthesis is examined; this relationship could prove to have broad clinical implications.

The latter three sections of the volume examine the electrophysiology of cholinergic agents, the interaction between acetylcholine and dopamine, and the effect of choline on brain cholinergic activity. These chapters describe the scientific bases which have stimulated clinical studies of brain acetylcholine. Some of the basic data presented has important implications for the use of cholinomimetics in the treatment of neuropsychiatric disease.

The editors wish to express their deep appreciation to Barbara Harlow, Meredith Stuckey and Jo Ann Magliozzi for their skillful organization and preparation of this manuscript, and to the Kate Pande Memorial Fund for continued support. In addition, we would like to give special thanks to Drs. Leo E. Hollister and Jack D. Barchas for their continued guidance and support. Finally, we are grateful to the many investigators whose pioneering work has heavily influenced our own thinking.

Kenneth L. Davis, M.D.
Philip A. Berger, M.D.
Palo Alto, California, 1978

CONTRIBUTORS

ALAN ABRAMS
Department of Psychiatry
University of California at San Diego
School of Medicine
La Jolla, California 92093

JACK D. BARCHAS
Nancy Friend Pritzker Laboratory
  of Behavioral Neurochemistry;
Department of Psychiatry and
  Behavioral Sciences
Stanford University School of
  Medicine
Stanford, California 94305

LOUIS A. BARKER
Department of Pharmacology
Mt. Sinai School of Medicine
City University of New York
New York, New York 10029

PHILIP A. BERGER
Veterans Administration Hospital
Palo Alto, California 94304
Department of Psychiatry and
  Behavioral Sciences
Stanford University School of
  Medicine
Stanford, California 94305

JOHN P. BLASS
Department of Neurology
Division of Chronic and Degenerative
  Disease
Cornell University Medical Center
  and Dementia Research Center
Burke Rehabilitation Center
White Plains, New York 10605

DANIEL E. CASEY
Departments of Medical Research and
  Psychiatry
Veterans Administration Hospital
Portland, Oregon 97207
Department of Psychiatry
University of Oregon Health Sciences
  Center
Portland, Oregon 97207

CYNTHIA L. COULTER
Veterans Administration Hospital
Palo Alto, California 94304

BONNIE M. DAVIS
Veterans Administration Hospital
Palo Alto, California 94304

JOHN M. DAVIS
Department of Psychiatry
University of California at San Diego
  School of Medicine
La Jolla, California 92093

KENNETH L. DAVIS
Veterans Administration Hospital
Palo Alto, California 94304
Department of Psychiatry and
  Behavioral Sciences
Stanford University School of
  Medicine
Stanford, California 94305

J. ANTHONY DEUTSCH
Department of Psychology
University of California at San Diego
La Jolla, California 92093

JEFFERSON R. DoAMARAL
Nancy Friend Pritzker Laboratory
    of Behavioral Neurochemistry;
Department of Psychiatry and
    Behavioral Sciences
Stanford University School of
    Medicine
Stanford, California 94305

EDWARD F. DOMINO
Department of Pharmacology
University of Michigan
Ann Arbor, Michigan 48109
Laboratory of Pharmacology
    Lafayette Clinic
Detroit, Michigan 48207

KYM F. FAULL
Nancy Friend Pritzker Laboratory
    of Behavioral Neurochemistry;
Department of Psychiatry and
    Behavioral Sciences
Stanford University School of
    Medicine
Stanford, California 94305

GARY E. GIBSON
Department of Neurology
Division of Chronic and Degenerative
    Disease
Cornell University Medical Center
    and Dementia Research Center
Burke Rehabilitation Center
White Plains, New York 10605

J. CHRISTIAN GILLIN
Biological Psychiatry Branch
The National Institute of Mental
    Health, NIH
Bethesda, Maryland 20014
Laboratory of Clinical
    Psychopharmacology
The National Institute of Mental
    Health
St. Elizabeth's Hospital
Washington, D.C. 20032

GEOFFREY GROOM
Department of Psychiatry
University of California at San Diego
    School of Medicine
La Jolla, California 92093

JOHN H. GROWDON
Laboratory of Neuroendocrine Regulation
Department of Nutrition and Food
    Science
Massachusetts Institute of Technology
Cambridge, Massachusetts 02139
Department of Neurology
Tufts University Medical School
Boston, Massachusetts 02111

ISRAEL HANIN
Department of Psychiatry
Western Psychiatric Institute and Clinic
University of Pittsburgh School of
    Medicine
Pittsburgh, Pennsylvania 15261

ANA HITRI
Department of Neurological Sciences
Rush Presbyterian St. Luke's Medical
    Center
Chicago, Illinois 60612

LEO E. HOLLISTER
Veterans Administration Hospital
Palo Alto, California 94304
Department of Psychiatry and
    Behavioral Sciences
Stanford University School of
    Medicine
Stanford, California 94305

ROBERT E. HRUSKA
Department of Pharmacology
College of Medicine
The University of Arizona Health
    Sciences Center
Tucson, Arizona 85724

DAVID S. JANOWSKY
Department of Psychiatry
University of California at San Diego
    School of Medicine
La Jolla, California 92093

DONALD J. JENDEN
Department of Pharmacology
School of Medicine and The Brain
  Research Institute
University of California
Los Angeles, California 90024

LEWIS L. JUDD
Department of Psychiatry
University of California at San Diego
  School of Medicine
La Jolla, California 92093

ALEXANDER G. KARCZMAR
Department of Pharmacology
Loyola University Stritch School
  of Medicine
Maywood, Illinois 60153

R. A. PIETER KARK
Department of Neurology
UCLA School of Medicine
Los Angeles, California 90024

HAROLD L. KLAWANS
Department of Neurological Sciences
Rush Presbyterian St. Luke's Medical
  Center
Chicago, Illinois 60612

BERT S. KOPELL
Veterans Administration Hospital
Palo Alto, California 94304
Department of Psychiatry and
  Behavioral Sciences
Stanford University School of
  Medicine
Stanford, California 94305

JOHN LIVESEY
Veterans Administration Hospital
Palo Alto, California 94304
Department of Psychiatry and
  Behavioral Sciences
Stanford University School of
  Medicine
Stanford, California 94305

STANLEY McCUNNEY
Department of Psychiatry
University of California at San Diego
  School of Medicine
La Jolla, California 92093

RICHARD C. MOHS
Veterans Administration Hospital
Palo Alto, California 94304
Department of Psychiatry and
  Behavioral Sciences
Stanford University School of
  Medicine
Stanford, California 94305

PAUL A. NAUSIEDA
Department of Neurological Sciences
Rush Presbyterian St. Luke's Medical
  Center
Chicago, Illinois 60612

ADOLF PFEFFERBAUM
Veterans Administration Hospital
Palo Alto, California 94304
Department of Psychiatry and
  Behavioral Sciences
Stanford University School of
  Medicine
Stanford, California 94305

MARIA RODRIGUEZ-BUDELLI
Department of Neurology
UCLA School of Medicine
Los Angeles, California 90024

JOSEPH B. ROGERS
Department of Psychology
University of California at San Diego
La Jolla, California 92093

SUSAN C. SIMONTON
Veterans Administration Hospital
Palo Alto, California 94304

NATRAJ SITARAM
Biological Psychiatry Branch
The National Institute of Mental
  Health, NIH
Bethesda, Maryland 20014

M. ANNE SPENCE
Departments of Psychiatry and
    Biomathematics
UCLA School of Medicine
Los Angeles, California 90024

DANIEL TARSY
Veterans Administration Hospital
Boston, Massachusetts 02130
Department of Neurology
Boston University School of
    Medicine
Boston, Massachusetts 02130
Division of Neurology
Department of Medicine
Harvard Medical School
Boston, Massachusetts 02115

JARED R. TINKLENBERG
Veterans Administration Hospital
Palo Alto, California 94304
Department of Psychiatry and
    Behavioral Sciences
Stanford University School of
    Medicine
Stanford, California 94305

MELVIN H. VAN WOERT
Departments of Pharmacology and
    Neurology
Mt. Sinai School of Medicine
City University of New York
New York, New York 10029

ADELA L. VENTO
Veterans Administration Hospital
Palo Alto, California 94304

GREGORY J. WASTEK
Department of Pharmacology
College of Medicine
The University of Arizona Health
    Sciences Center
Tucson, Arizona 85724

WILLIAM J. WEINER
Department of Neurological Sciences
Rush Presbyterian St. Luke's Medical
    Center
Chicago, Illinois 60612

RICHARD J. WURTMAN
Laboratory of Neuroendocrine Regulation
Department of Nutrition and Food
    Science
Massachusetts Institute of Technology
Cambridge, Massachusetts 02139

HENRY I. YAMAMURA
Department of Pharmacology
College of Medicine
The University of Arizona Health
    Sciences Center
Tucson, Arizona 85724

JEROME A. YESAVAGE
Veterans Administration Hospital
Palo Alto, California 94304
Department of Psychiatry and
    Behavioral Sciences
Stanford University School of
    Medicine
Stanford, California 94305

CONTENTS

BRAIN ACETYLCHOLINE AND PSYCHIATRIC DISORDERS

BRAIN ACETYLCHOLINE AND MOVEMENT DISORDERS

BRAIN ACETYLCHOLINE AND COGNITIVE FUNCTION

THE ELECTROPHYSIOLOGY OF CHOLINERGIC AGENTS

INTERACTIONS OF BRAIN ACETYLCHOLINE AND OTHER NEUROTRANSMITTERS

BIOCHEMICAL AND PHARMACOLOGICAL ASPECTS OF CHOLINERGIC TREATMENT STRATEGIES

BRAIN ACETYLCHOLINE AND PSYCHIATRIC DISORDERS

PSYCHOLOGICAL EFFECTS OF CHOLINOMIMETIC AGENTS

D. S. Janowsky and J. M. Davis

Department of Psychiatry, University of California at San Diego,
School of Medicine, La Jolla, California 92093

INTRODUCTION

Janowsky, Davis and colleagues began in 1972 to explore the possibility that the affective disorders, mania and depression, might be due to a complex balance, or inter-action, between adrenergic and cholinergic factors (Janowsky *et al.*, 1972a). Proposed most simply, mania was hypothesized to be a syndrome due to relatively diminished central acetylcholine (ACh) activity, compared to normal or increased noradrenergic and/or dopaminergic activity; and depression was proposed to be the converse (Janowsky *et al.*, 1972b).

The most obvious analogy to this hypothesis lies in the adrenergic-cholinergic control of peripheral autonomic functions, such as heart rate, bronchial diameter, or pupillary size, in which sympathetic and parasympathetic activation cause opposite effects (Goodman and Gilman, 1970). As reviewed by J.M. Davis *et al.*, (1976), a more sophisticated analogy may be the relationship of adrenergic-cholinergic balance to parkinsonian symptoms. Here, diminished dopaminergic activity and relatively increased cholinergic activity co-exist in the extrapyramidal system. In the case of parkinsonian symptoms, this situation may occur if cholinergic function is intact and either dopaminergic neurons are destroyed, or pharmacologic blockade or pharmacologic depletion of extrapyramidal dopaminergic neurons occurs. Pre-existing parkinsonian symptoms intensify if cholinergic activity is increased, but increased cholinergic activity alone does not usually cause parkinsonian symptoms if central dopaminergic activity is normal. Conversely, increased or normal central ACh activity is a necessary precondition for the development of parkinsonian symptoms, assuming dopaminergic activity is decreased.

In this chapter, we will present our observations concerning the possible role of cholinergic factors in the etiology and/or regulation of affective and schizophrenic symptoms. We will focus on the role of ACh in these disorders, being fully aware that ACh may well be involved in only one of a series of complex, multiple neurotransmitter interactions regulating affective and cognitive processes.

CHOLINERGIC-ANTICHOLINERGIC EFFECTS OF PSYCHOACTIVE DRUGS

Although much recent literature has focused on the adrenergic and anti-adrenergic effects of psychoactive drugs in the regulation of affect (Schildkraut, 1965; Davis, 1970), a cogent argument can be made for consideration of the cholinergic-anticholinergic effects of these drugs. Indeed, as reviewed by Janowsky et al., (1972b), most somatic antidepressant therapies are associated with decreased cholinergic activity, as well as increased adrenergic activity. These somatic antidepressant therapies include: electroconvulsive therapy, the tricyclic antidepressants, the monoamine oxidase inhibitors, and the short-term effects of the psychostimulants. Conversely, anti-adrenergic drugs, including reserpine, propranolol, and alpha-methyldopa, have prominent central and peripheral cholinergic side effects, including nausea, vomiting, diarrhea, bradycardia, and anergy. These three anti-adrenergic drugs can also precipitate depression in predisposed individuals. Similarly, guanethidine, which is reported not to cross the blood brain barrier, has prominent peripheral cholinergic side effects, in addition to anti-adrenergic effects. It does not cause depression.

EARLY STUDIES USING CHOLINOMIMETIC DRUGS

Acetylcholinesterase inhibitors have served as valuable tools in the study of the behavioral effects of ACh. Generally, as reviewed below, they have been found to increase depression and antagonize mania. Gershon (1961) reported several cases of individuals, poisoned with cholinesterase-inhibitor insecticides, who developed depression and peripheral parasympathetic toxicity. He also noted that the incidence of depression may be higher in orchidists who use cholinesterase inhibitor insecticides. Rowntree et al., (1950) administered the irreversible cholinesterase inhibitor, diisopropylfluorophosphonate (DFP) to ten normal and nine manic-depressive patients. Normal subjects developed irritability, lassitude, depression, apathy, and slowness or poverty of thoughts which appeared before the onset of peripheral cholinergic symptoms. Two manic-depressive patients, tested while in remission, showed mental changes like the normals, and two hypomanic patients improved with DFP and continued to be euthymic after its administration. One other hypomanic patient became less manic and was minimally depressed after each of two courses of DFP, but relapsed upon DFP withdrawal. One nearly remitted hypomanic patient became floridly manic upon DFP withdrawal. One depressed patient showed a considerable increase in depression during DFP administration. In addition, Bowers et al., (1964) noted that the irreversible cholinesterase inhibitor, EA01701, caused depressed mood, decreased energy, decreased enthusiasm, lethargy, and decreased friendliness in normal volunteers.

STUDIES USING PHYSOSTIGMINE

We have (Janowsky et al., 1973a, 1973b) used intravenous physostigmine (a reversible cholinesterase inhibitor which is centrally-acting) and neostigmine (a similar cholinesterase inhibitor which does not cross the blood brain barrier; Goodwin and Gilman, 1970) to study central cholinergic mechanisms in mania and depression.

General Effects of Physostigmine and Neostigmine

Physostigmine, in contrast to neostigmine, rapidly caused a series of behavioral effects in virtually all subjects who received it. This syndrome, which can be labeled the "physostigmine inhibitory state" (Janowsky, 1973a, 1973b), was characterized by anergy, lethargy, feelings of tiredness, psychomotor retardation, the perception of having no thoughts or decreased thoughts, a desire to be left alone, and social withdrawal. Subjects receiving neostigmine exhibited no such symptoms, and, if anything, tended to feel slightly more relaxed. The inhibitory effects of physostigmine occurred within 10-15 min of its administration, lasted between 30 and 90 min, and were rapidly antagonized by small doses of atropine, scopolamine, or methylphenidate. The physostigmine inhibitory state often preceded sensations of nausea and episodes of vomiting, which were selectively antagonized by centrally acting anticholinergic agents (i.e. atropine) – suggesting that they were a central, rather than a peripheral, phenomena.

Antimanic Effects of Physostigmine

In contrast to neostigmine, physostigmine caused significant antimanic effects in hypomanic and manic patients. We have studied 11-manic or hypomanic patients who gave informed consent for the administration of physostigmine and neostigmine (Janowsky et al., 1973a). Administration of physostigmine to these manic patients in most cases resulted in a dramatic reduction of manic symptoms, whereas placebo and neostigmine produced no changes. Initially, these patients exhibited typical manic symptoms, such as rapidity of thought and speech, grandiose ideation, punning and rhyming. Physostigmine converted the manic symptoms to those consistent with a psychomotor retarded depression, with patients appearing lethargic, slower in their movements and speech. They were less euphoric, talkative, active, cheerful, friendly, happy, grandiose, and had a decrease in flight of ideas, as rated by the Beigel-Murphy scale for mania (Beigel and Murphy, 1971). Patients also reported "inhibitory symptoms", such as feeling drained, becoming apathetic, and having "no thoughts". Less consistently, the manic patients' responses to physostigmine included the onset of depression, with crying and other signs of depressed affect. Examples of the effects of physostigmine on manic symptoms are illustrated by the following cases:

Case 1

A 43-year-old white woman with a history of bipolar manic-depressive illness showed hypomanic symptoms including moderate talkativeness, flight of ideas, grandiosity, and cheerfulness during the placebo-baseline phase. She was energetic, friendly, and showed increased interactions, as well as occasional hostility. Administration of a total of 1.75 mg IV physostigmine caused the patient to show a marked decrease in her interactions, talkativeness, grandiosity, cheerfulness, and flight of ideas. She became withdrawn, wanted to be left alone, was lethargic, stated that she lacked thoughts and was somewhat depressed. She complained of nausea five minutes after the onset of the above syndrome.

Case 2

A 34-year-old white female bipolar manic-depressive patient demonstrated marked flight of ideas, increased talkativeness, rapid fluctuations from cheerfulness and euphoria to anger and argumentativeness, as well as manipulative behavior toward staff members. Administration of placebo caused no change in the patient's clinical state. Administration of IV physostigmine caused the patient to rapidly become more passive, quiet, and reflective, and her anger dissipated. She said that she felt sad and scared, but on an "even keel", and that she felt warm towards the staff. She showed decreased talkativeness and decreased flight of ideas. She was neither confused, lethargic, nor disoriented. After receiving a total of 2.0 mg of physostigmine, about 20 min after the onset of the more subdued behavior, the patient became nauseated and vomited. One milligram of atropine, administered intravenously, partially reversed the "antimanic" state and the vomiting.

The observation that physostigmine decreases manic symptoms has been partially confirmed by others. Modestin (1973a) noted that two of four manic patients studied showed a lessening of mania following physostigmine administration; and more recently, Davis *et al.*, (1978) have reported that physostigmine has antimanic effects.

However, some controversy (Carroll *et al.*, 1973; Shopsin *et al.*, 1975) has existed as to whether or not the "antimanic" effects of physostigmine are truly "antimanic", or whether they are "nonspecific". Carroll *et al.*, (1973) and Shopsin *et al.*, (1975) found that while physostigmine caused a decrease in manic hyperactivity and talkativeness, no change in mood or "thought disorder" occurred. As outlined by J.M. Davis *et al.*, (1976), the key to whether or not, in the opinion of a given investigator, physostigmine alleviates mania may rest with how an investigator clinically diagnoses mania. If mania is primarily considered to be the cognitive aspects of the syndrome – i.e. the grandiosity and paranoia – then physostigmine would seem to exert relatively weak or nonspecific effects, since it does not dramatically decrease manic patients' grandiose or paranoid delusions. If mania is considered to be primarily a disturbance of rate – i.e. increased talkativeness, cheerfulness, hyperactivity, and thoughts – then physostigmine is obviously effective as an antimanic agent. In any case, it is important to note that the "decrease in rate" caused by physostigmine in manics and others is not just sedation. Barbiturates and sedative hypnotics, in contrast to physostigmine, are not particularly effective in controlling mania. A patient can be markedly sedated with these agents – i.e. sleepy, dysarthric, and ataxic – and still display a very high level of mania. In contrast, physostigmine causes only slight sedation, and does not cause sleep, yet is dramatic in antagonizing many manic symptoms.

"Rebound" Effects Following Physostigmine Administration

Shopsin and Gershon, in collaboration with ourselves (Shopsin *et al.*, 1975), studied the effects of physostigmine on three manic patients at Bellvue Psychiatric Hospital in New York. These patients were given intravenous doses of physostigmine up to 6 mg. All developed the "physostigmine inhibitory syndrome", in addition to a decrease in certain manic symptoms (activity, cheerfulness, flight of ideas, tangentiality, pressure of speech, talkativeness, etc.). Manic grandiosity was at best equivocally decreased. However, most impressively in two subjects, a rebound into a "hypermanic state" occurred. This "rebound" was noted approximately two hr following physostigmine administration and lasted up to four hr. In the two patients in whom "rebound" was noted, a marked exacerbation and intensification beyond baseline of the manic state occurred, with observation for the first time of obvious primary process behavior.

The "rebound" phenomena following physostigmine administration may parallel the effects of physostigmine noted in rats by Fibiger *et al.*, (1971). In these studies, physostigmine initially caused behavioral inhibition, followed several hours later by a rebound increase over baseline in locomotor activity. This rebound into hyperactivity was prevented by administration of scopolamine prior to physostigmine administration, and augmented by scopolamine administration early in the rebound phase. Fibiger *et al.*, (1971) suggest that the rebound phenomena may be due to an unmasking of compensatory adrenergic activity, as physostigmine activity decreases over time.

Mood Depressant Effects of Physostigmine

In addition to its nonspecific inhibitory-anergic effects and its antimanic effects, physostigmine is capable of inducing a depressed mood in certain individuals (Janowsky *et al.*, 1973a, 1973b). Physostigmine can cause a mild depressed mood, consisting of such symptoms as sadness, tearfulness, feelings of worthlessness, futility, hopelessness, uselessness, and intensification of suicidal feelings in subjects who have pre-existing symptoms of an affective disorder. Thus, depressed mood, as contrasted with the more pervasive nonspecific anergic-inhibitory effects of physostigmine, can occur in actively depressed schizo-affective patients, manics, and depressed patients following physostigmine infusion. This depressant effect contrasts with that caused by physostigmine in schizophrenic patients without an affective component to their illness where only the physostigmine inhibitory syndrome develops (Janowsky *et al.*, 1973b). The following case example is illustrative of the ability of physostigmine to precipitate depression in patients with pre-existing affective disorder.

Case 1

A 48-year-old woman showing mild psychomotor retardation, depressed mood, feelings of hopelessness, pessimism, and worthlessness, received 1 mg of physostigmine IV. Her psychomotor retardation markedly increased and she stated that she felt drained, apathetic, and withdrawn. She also claimed that she felt substantially more depressed, hopeless and worthless, and very pessimistic. She noted that this was similar to a time when her depression was more severe. Administration of 1 mg atropine IV restored the patient to a baseline state of mild psychomotor depression.

More recently, K.L. Davis *et al.*, (1976) administered physostigmine to 23 normal volunteers. Although a physostigmine inhibitory syndrome occurred frequently, depression was noted in only two subjects, one who was marijuana intoxicated and one who had a history of premenstrual depression. In contrast, K.L. Davis *et al.*, (1978) noted frequent occurrence of depressed mood in manic patients following physostigmine infusion. Thus, there is evidence from the work of K.L. Davis *et al.*, (1976, 1978), and Janowsky *et al.*, (1973b) to support the suggestion that physostigmine may selectively cause a depressed mood in subjects with pre-existing affective disorder, in contrast to normals or non-affective disorder patients.

Furthermore, it is also possible that physostigmine may selectively induce a depressed mood in patients who are euthymic, but have a history of affective disorder. In support of this possibility, Robert Belmaker (personal communication, 1977) has reported that euthymic manic-depressive patients receiving lithium become moderately depressed when given intravenous physostigmine.

Modestin and his co-workers (1973a, 1973b) have added considerably to our knowledge concerning physostigmine's effect on depressed patients. After pretreatment with methscopolamine, these investigators administered 1.25 to 1.5 mg of physostigmine and neostigmine (IV), using a double-blind, crossover design. One drug was administered in the morning and the other in the afternoon. Random assignment was used to determine which drug was administered first. These authors used the Cutler-Kurland depressive rating scale (1961), and a self-rating scale to quantitate changes in the depressive symptomatology produced by physostigmine. In the sample of 24 depressed patients, four manic patients, and 40 nonpsychotic, nondepressive control patients, physostigmine produced a substantial overall increase in depressive symptomatology ($p < 0.01$).

Modestin et al., (1973a, 1973b) noted that after physostigmine infusion, some patient controls experienced a fair degree of depression, and others experienced only minimal depression. Unfortunately, these authors did not divide their patients into those with pre-existing affective symptomatology and those without such symptoms, so that a comparison between physostigmine's effects in subjects having and not having affective symptoms was not possible.

Data from Modestin et al., (1973a, 1973b) are also helpful in clarifying whether or not the depressive symptoms noted following physostigmine infusion are secondary to physostigmine's physical side effects, such as nausea and vomiting. If physostigmine-induced depressive symptoms are a consequence of physical symptomatology, one would expect a good correlation between the intensity of depressive symptoms and physical symptoms. When the results of the studies of Modestin et al., are summarized (1973a, 1973b), there is no correlation between depressive symptomatology and the observed somatic symptoms. Also, it has been our observation that physostigmine's anergic-depressant effects precede, rather than follow its emetic and nausea inducing effects. Thus, it is likely that physostigmine induced depression is not merely due to the effects of feeling nauseous and physically ill.

Depressant Effects of Physostigmine Plus Marijuana

Preliminary evidence exists that marijuana intoxication may grossly intensify physostigmine's mood depressing effects. In a pilot study, involving two normal, non-depressed volunteers, (El-Yousef et al., 1973), the effects of a social dose of marijuana were initially antagonized by a low dose of physostigmine. However, within minutes, both subjects were observed to become profoundly depressed. These two cases are described below.

Case 1

A female patient arrived apparently intoxicated on marijuana. She was garrulous, cheerful, full of hilarity, showing flight of ideas, talkativeness, and inability to remember three 2-digit numbers for 30 sec. Pulse rate was elevated to 120 and her conjunctiva were red. Five minutes after receiving a total of 0.25 mg physostigmine, the patient stated that she was no longer "high", that her thoughts were slowed down and that she didn't feel euphoric. By the time the patient had received 1.25 mg physostigmine, her clinical state had progressed until she reported and appeared to be lethargic, felt drained, sad, extremely depressed, hopeless, useless and worthless. She sobbed and cried and manifested extreme psychomotor retardation and reported having no thoughts. Pulse rate at this time was 96. She stated that she had never been so depressed in her life, yet could offer no explanations for her feelings. She stated that she would have committed suicide had she not known that the syndrome was due to a drug. She appeared to be as depressed as any patient the authors had ever observed. Within one minute after atropine administration the patient commented that she felt better and improvement progressed over the next half hour.

Case 2

A male patient arrived stating that he was "high". He showed increased talkativeness, friendliness, and interactions. He was slightly euphoric, but somewhat apprehensive and anxious about the experiment. He stated that this was his normal "high" and that he was at as "high" a level as he usually reached. His pulse rate was 120. Administration of a total of 0.75 mg of physostigmine caused the patient to report that his thoughts had slowed down and that he no longer felt "high". His pulse rate was 105. With administration of an additional 0.25 mg of physostigmine, this progressed into a profound depression, similar to that of the female patient. The patient exhibited extreme psychomotor retardation, was sad, dejected, drained, apathetic, weak, and depressed. He spontaneously said he felt useless, worthless and hopeless and that he wished he could die. He stated that he felt he could understand how depressed people felt and wondered why they all didn't kill themselves. He claimed to have virtually no thoughts and spent time with eyes closed, moaning weakly, "Oh, oh." Administration of atropine caused noticeable improvement in symptoms within one minute, which progressed over the next hour.

Similar to the above cases, K.L. Davis, *et al.*, (1976) parenthetically noted that one of two normal volunteers out of 23 who became depressed following physostigmine infusion had been marijuana intoxicated prior to the experiment. The subject's depression was described as severe for him and lasted for several days.

Animal studies also support the possibility that marijuana, or its active ingredient, Δ9-tetrahydrocannabinol, significantly increases the effects of physostigmine. Rosenblatt *et al.*, (1972) noted that the lethality of physostigmine was increased by Δ9-tetrahydrocannabinol administration, an effect prevented by prior administration of atropine or methscopolamine.

How marijuana augments the effects of physostigmine is uncertain. Generally, marijunana exerts effects which appear anticholinergic (Brown, 1971). Possibly, marijuana increases receptor sensitivity or inhibits feedback mechanisms which would usually antagonize cholinomimetic effects. In any event, the fact that this drug-drug interaction occurs supports the notion that increasing central ACh activity may lead to depression.

DEPRESSANT EFFECTS OF ACETYLCHOLINE PRECURSORS

Consistent with the mood depressant effects of physostigmine plus marijuana and of physostigmine alone, several anecdotal reports suggest that the ACh precursors, deanol and choline, may, in some cases, cause depressed mood. Tamminga *et al.*, (1976) reported that choline administration caused an atropine reversible severe depressed mood in two of four tardive dyskinesia patients to whom it was given. Furthermore, Casey and Denney (1977) have observed depressed mood as a side effect in four of six tardive dyskinesia patients who developed affective symptoms after high dose deanol administration. However, two of their other subjects became agitated and had manic symptoms after deanol administration.

ANTAGONISTIC EFFECTS OF METHYLPHENIDATE AND PHYSOSTIGMINE

Methylphenidate, presumably a central norepinephrine and dopamine releasing agent, and physostigmine appear to exert opposite effects on animals (Janowsky et al., 1972c) and in man, (Janowsky et al., 1973c). Thus, methylphenidate causes increases in locomotion and stereotypy in rats, causes increases in thoughts, talkativeness, interactions in normal human subjects and increases manic symptoms in manic patients, including flight of ideas, talkativeness, elation, and grandiosity. Thus, there is evidence that an adrenergic agent and a cholinergic agent exert opposite effects in a given subject.

A pharmacologic model for naturally occurring adrenergic and cholinergic central nervous system interactions may be found in the interaction of the effects of physostigmine and methylphenidate. We have noted (Janowsky, 1972c) that methylphenidate-induced psychostimulation in rats (gnawing behavior) and in various types of psychiatric patients (1973c) can be antagonized by physostigmine, but not by neostigmine. Conversely, the inhibitory syndrome caused by physostigmine in rats and in man can be antagonized by methylphenidate. Thus, in this pharmacologic model, there is evidence that the balance or interaction of central adrenergic and cholinergic factors determines the relative degree of psychostimulation versus behavioral inhibition.

THE ROLE OF ADRENERGIC-CHOLINERGIC BALANCE IN SCHIZOPHRENIA

Although this chapter has focused on the possible regulation of affect by adrenergic-cholinergic interactions, the possibility that such a balance regulates schizophrenic symptoms has been proposed (Janowsky, 1972b). Indeed, it is true that antipsychotic agents, including reserpine, decrease central catecholamine activity and increase central ACh turnover. Conversely, at least one report alleges that central anticholinergic agents increase psychotic symptoms, when added to an antipsychotic drug regime. However, we (Janowsky et al., 1973b) and Modestin et al., (1973b), found that, while physostigmine induced anergy in schizophrenic subjects, it exerted no qualitative effects on such symptoms as delusions and hallucinations. However, we (Janowsky et al., 1973c) did note that the activation of psychotic symptoms by methylphenidate was effectively antagonized by physostigmine. This suggests that adrenergic-cholinergic balance may determine the floridness of schizophrenic symptoms, but not the quality of these symptoms.

DISCUSSION

In the above paragraphs we have presented considerable pharmacologic evidence suggesting that shifting central adrenergic-cholinergic balance regulates affect in man. It is worthwhile to point out some of the limitations of the evidence supporting this hypothesis.

First, it is important to note that the evidence supporting a role for cholinergic, as well as adrenergic factors in the regulation of affect, is based primarily on pharmacologic evidence. Thus, as yet there is no direct evidence that cholinergic mechanisms are abnormal in naturally occurring affective states. Most of the evidence supporting a role for acetylcholine in the regulation of affective disorders involves the artificial increase of central cholinergic activity by a cholinesterase inhibitor, or an acetylcholine precursor. Simplistically, we infer that if ACh is artificially elevated and mood changes occur, ACh must be involved in the regulation of affect. However, it is entirely possible that artificially changing central ACh alters the relationships of other neurotransmitters or neuroregulators which may actually be the regulators of affect (Davis *et al.*, 1977). These compounds might vary normally, independent of ACh activity. Thus, we may be seeing a pharmacologic effect which has little to do with the regulation of endogenous affective changes.

Some evidence not supporting a role for ACh in naturally occurring mood regulation does exist. Anticholinergic agents alone are not particularly effective antidepressant agents (Safer and Allan, 1971; Meduna and Abood, 1959), and there appears no obvious relationship between the degree of central anticholinergic activity of a given tricyclic antidepressant and its clinical efficacy or potency (Snyder and Yamamura, 1977).

The observation that cholinergic agents increase depression in patients with pre-existing affective disorders, but not in subjects without affective illness suggests that increasing central ACh is not by itself adequate to cause depression. Although it is possible that enough cholinesterase inhibition would cause depression in anyone, it is also possible that vulnerability in the affective disorder patient is a necessary pre-condition for ACh to exert its mood depressant effects. Perhaps, patients with affective disorder have a lack of compensatory biochemical mechanisms (as there may be in the parkinsonian patient), which cause them to become depressed following cholinergic stimulation. Alternatively, it is possible that patients with affective disorder have learned that decreased thinking and behavioral inhibition is synonymous with depression. Thus their response to cholinomimetic drugs may be essentially conditioned or learned.

It is also important to refine the concept of adrenergic-cholinergic balance. Such a concept infers a "teeter-totter phenomenon", in which increasing the weight or influence of one chemical outweighs the effect of another. There is much evidence to suggest that cholinergic and adrenergic neurotransmitters are in dynamic equilibrium, and exert mutual feedback on each other. For example, blocking dopaminergic receptors with neuroleptics leads to an increase in acetylcholine turnover, (Stadler *et al.*, 1973; Trabucchi *et al.*, 1975), as does depletion of monoamines with reserpine (Sulser *et al.*; 1964). Conversely, there is evidence that apomorphine, L-DOPA, and amphetamine, presumably by increasing dopaminergic activity, at least acutely decrease ACh turnover and output (Trabucchi *et al.*, 1975). Similar effects have been observed after norepinephrine infusion (Gorney *et al.*, 1976). Thus, adrenergic and cholinergic influences may mutually inhibit each other, at least acutely, and "adrenergic-cholinergic balance" may be more a matter of adrenergic and cholinergic influences on each other.

Furthermore, there is evidence that, over time, compensatory adrenergic hyper-activity may occur following cholinergic stimulation, and similarly the converse may occur following adrenergic activation (Mandell and Knapp, 1971). Thus, the role of a disordered compensatory mechanism in patients with affective disorder is possible, and deserves exploration.

SUMMARY

In summary, considerable pharmacologic evidence supports the concept that cholinergic influences may affect the regulation of mood and activation, and that these influences may interact with corresponding adrenergic and/or serotonergic influences. In man, increasing cholinergic activity causes anergy and inhibition and causes depression in predisposed or marijuana pretreated individuals. Increasing cholinergic activity causes decreased mania in manic patients and antagonism of psychostimulation in methylphenidate intoxicated subjects. The nature of the above interactions is probably complex, rather than simple, and possibly involves a number of chemical systems, defined and still to be defined. Whether the above pharmacologic evidence reflects endogenous events occurring in patients with affective disorders remains an open question, a subject of conjecture, worthy of continuing investigation.

ACKNOWLEDGEMENTS

This work was supported in part from the Medical Research Service of the Veterans Administration Hospital, San Diego, (MRIS #4576) and NIMH Grant #1 P50 MH 30914-01; Department of Psychiatry, University of Chicago, Illinois State Psychiatric Institute, Chicago, Illinois.

REFERENCES

Beigel, A., and Murphy, D.L., 1971, Assessing clinical characteristics of the manic state, *Am. J. Psychiatry 128:*688.

Bowers, M.B., Goodman, E., and Sim, V.M., 1964, Some behavioral changes in man following anticholinesterase administration, *J. Nerv. Ment. Dis. 138:*383.

Brown, H., 1971, Some anticholinergic-like behavioral effects of trans (-) – Δ8-tetrahydrocannabinol, *Psychopharmacologia 21:*294.

Carroll, B.J., Frazer, A., Schless, A., and Mendels, A., 1973, Cholinergic reversal of manic symptoms, *Lancet I:*427.

Casey, D.E., and Denney, D., 1977, Pharmacological characterization of tardive dyskinesia, *Psychopharmacology 54:*1.

Cutler, R.P., and Kurland, H.D., 1961, Clinical quantification of depressive reactions, *Arch. Gen. Psychiatry 5:*88.

Davis, J.M., 1970, Theories of the biological etiology of affective disorders, *Int. Rev. Neurobiol. 12:*145.

Davis, J.M., Janowsky, D.S., Tamminga, C., and Smith, R.C., 1976, *Cholinergic Mechanisms and Psychopharmacology* (D.J. Jenden, ed.), Plenum Publishing Corporation, New York.

Davis, K.L., Hollister, L.E., Overall, J., Johnson, A., and Train, K., 1976, Physostigmine: effects on cognition and affect in normal subjects, *Psychopharmacology 51:*23.

Davis, K.L., Hollister, L.E., Goodwin, F.K., and Gordon, E.K., 1977, Neurotransmitter metabolites in the cerebrospinal fluid of man following physostigmine, *Life Sci. 21:*933.

Davis, K.L., Berger, P.A., Hollister, L.E., and Defraites, E., 1978, Physostigmine in mania, *Arch. Gen. Psychiatry 35(1):*119.

El-Yousef, M.K., Janowsky, D.S., Davis, J.M., and Rosenblatt, J.R., 1973, Induction of severe depression by physostigmine in marijuana intoxicated individuals, *Br. J. Addict. 68:*321.

Fibiger, J.D., Lynch, G.S., and Cooper, H.P., 1971, A biphasic action of central cholinergic stimulation on behavioral arousal in the rat, *Psychopharmacologia 20:*366.

Gershon, S., and Shaw, F.H., 1961, Psychiatric sequelae of chronic exposure to organophosphorous insecticides, *Lancet I:*1371.

Goodman, L.S., and Gilman, A., (eds.), 1970, *"The Pharmacological Basis of Therapeutics, 4th Ed.,"* Collier-MacMillan, Toronto, Canada.

Gorny, D., Billewicz-Stankiewicz, J., Zajqczkowska, M., and Kutarski, A., 1976, Effect of noradrenaline on the content, synthesis and catabolism of acetylcholine in the brain, *Acta Physiol. Pol 27:*55.

Janowsky, D.S., El-Yousef, M.K., Davis, J.M., Sekerke, H.J., and Hubbard, B.J., 1972a, Cholinergic antagonism of manic symptoms, *Lancet I:*1236.

Janowsky, D.S., El-Yousef, M.K., Davis, J.M., and Sekerke, H.J., 1972b, A cholinergic-adrenergic hypothesis of mania and depression, *Lancet II:*632.

Janowsky, D.S., El-Yousef, M.K., Davis, J.M., Sekerke, H.J., 1972c, Cholinergic antagonism of methylphenidate-induced stereotyped behavior, *Psychopharmacologia 27:*295.

Janowsky, D.S., El-Yousef, M.K., Davis, J.M., and Sekerke, H.J., 1973a, Parasympathetic suppression of manic symptoms by physostigmine, *Arch. Gen. Psychiatry 28:*542.

Janowsky, D.S., Davis, J.M., El-Yousef, M.K., and Sekerke, H.J., 1973b, Acetylcholine and depression, *Psychosom. Med. 35(5):*568.

Janowsky, D.S., El-Yousef, M.K., and Sekerke, H.J., 1973c, Antagonistic effects of physostigmine and methylphenidate in man, *Am. J. Psychiatry 130:*1370.

Mandell, A.J., and Knapp, S., 1971, The effects of chronic administration of some cholinergic and adrenergic drugs on the activity of choline acetyltransferase in the optic lobe of the chick brain, *Neuropharmacology 10:*513.

Meduna, L.J., and Abood, L.G., 1959, Studies of a new drug (DITRAN) in depressive states, *J. Neuropsychiatry 1:*20.

Modestin, J.J., Hunger, R.B., and Schwartz, R.B., 1973a, Uber die depressogene Wirkung von Physostigmin, *Arch. Psychiatr. Nervenkr. 218:*67.

Modestin, J.J., Schwartz, R.B., and Hunger, J., 1973b, Zur frage der beeinflussung schizophrener symptome physostigmin, *Pharmakopsychiatrie 9:*300.

Rosenblatt, J.E., Janowsky, D.S., Davis, J.M., and El-Yousef, M.K., 1972, The augmentation of physostigmine toxicity in the rat by $\Delta 9$-tetrahydrocannabinol, *Res. Commun. Chem. Pathol. Pharmacol. 3(3):*479.

Rowntree, D.W., Neven, S., and Wilson, A., 1950, The effects of diisopropylfluorophosphonate in schizophrenic and manic depressive psychosis, *J. Neurol. Neurosurg. Psychiatry 13:*47.

Safer, D.J., and Allen, R.P., 1971, The central effects of scopolamine in man, *Biol. Psychiatry 3:*347.

Schildkraut, J.J., 1965, The catecholamine hypothesis of affective disorders: a review of supporting evidence, *Am. J. Psychiatry 122:*509.

Shopsin, B., Janowsky, D.S., Davis, J.M., and Gershon, S., 1975, Rebound phenomena in manic patients following physostigmine, *Neuropsychobiology 1:*180.

Snyder, S.H., and Yamamura, H.I., 1977, Antidepressants and the muscarinic acetylcholine receptor, *Arch. Gen. Psychiatry 34:*236.

Stadler, H., Lloyd, K.G., Gadea-Cira, M., and Bartholini, G., 1973, Enhanced striatal acetylcholine release by chlorpromazine and its reversal by apomorphine, *Brain Res. 55:*476.

Sulser, F., Bickel, M.H., and Brodie, B.B., 1964, The action of desmethylimipramine in counteracting sedation and cholinergic effects of reserpine-like drugs, *J. Pharmacol. Exp. Ther. 144:*321.

Tamminga, C., Smith, R.C., Chang, S., Haraszti, J.S., and Davis, J.M., 1976, Depression associated with oral choline, *Lancet II:*905.

Trabucchi, M., Cheney, D.L., Racagni, G., and Costa, E., 1975, *In vivo* inhibition of striatal acetylcholine turnover by L-DOPA, apomorphine and (+) -amphetamine, *Brain Res. 85:*130.

PHARMACOLOGICAL INVESTIGATIONS OF CHOLINERGIC MECHANISMS IN SCHIZOPHRENIA AND MANIC PSYCHOSIS

P. A. Berger[1,2], K.L. Davis [1,2] and L.E. Hollister[1,2]

[1]Veterans Administration Hospital, 3801 Miranda Avenue,
Palo Alto, California 94304

[2]Department of Psychiatry and Behavioral Sciences, Stanford University
School of Medicine, Stanford, California 94305

INTRODUCTION

During the past twenty years the biological investigation of major emotional disorders has focused on possible disturbances of central neurotransmission. The possible roles of serotonin, norepinephrine and dopamine have been reviewed recently (Schildkraut, 1974; Shopin et al., 1974; Goodwin and Murphy, 1974; Matthysse and Lipinski, 1975; Baldessarini, 1975; Berger, 1977; Berger et al., 1978). Other recent reviews have considered the possible role of alterations in the balance between neurotransmitters (Janowsky et al., 1972b; Friedhoff and Alpert, 1973; Davis et al., 1975). This chapter will focus on the possible role of cholinergic mechanisms in the pathophysiology of schizophrenia and the affective disorders.

SCHIZOPHRENIA

A number of pharmacological and metabolic investigations have pointed to the possible involvement of cholinergic mechanisms in schizophrenia. An early suggestion that increasing central cholinergic activity might improve schizophrenic symptoms came from the report that arecoline, a cholinomimetic, produced a brief period of lucidity in patients with catatonic schizophrenia (Pfeiffer and Jenny, 1957). This transient action of arecoline was reported to be similar to the "lucid interval" produced by amobarbital (Fulcher et al., 1957). Oxotremorine, another central muscarinic agonist, was also reported to produce lucid periods in otherwise withdrawn chronic schizophrenics (Collard et al., 1965). However, neither arecoline nor oxotremorine produced more than brief remissions in schizophrenic patients. A longer remission in chronic schizophrenic patients refractory to traditional antipsychotics was reported following the combination of neuroleptics and oral doses of the reversible acetylcholinesterase inhibitor, physostigmine. However, these patients seemed to develop tolerance to this combination and returned in a few days to their prephysostigmine levels of psychopathology (Rosenthal and Bigelow, 1973). Evidence from one pharmacological investigation suggests that the beneficial actions of physostigmine on schizophrenia may involve acetylcholine and dopamine (Janowsky et al., 1973a). Intravenously administered methylphenidate, a dopamine agonist, exacerbates the symptoms of schizophrenia. This methylphenidate induced worsening is reversed by the intravenous administration of physostigmine (Janowsky et al., 1973a).

Thus, there is some pharmacological support for the suggestion that increasing central cholinergic activity may improve schizophrenic symptoms. However, there is also some contradictory evidence. The non-competitive cholinesterase inhibitor diisopropyl-fluorophosphonate (DFP) either exacerbated or had no acute effects on schizophrenic symptoms in one study (Rowntree et al., 1957). These results are consistent with the report that intravenous physostigmine did not improve schizophrenic symptoms (Modestin et al., 1973b).

The converse situation, exacerbation of schizophrenic symptoms by anticholinergics, would also lend some support to the idea that cholinergic mechanisms were important in the disorder. The potent central anticholinergic Ditran has been used to deliberately aggravate symptoms of schizophrenia in treatment-resistant patients. The hypothesis was that by desynchronizing the hypersynchronous EEG of these patients they might then better respond to subsequent treatment with antipsychotics. Only scanty evidence was produced to support this hypothesis and true aggravation of schizophrenia could be questioned because Ditran produces a transient psychotic organic brain syndrome due to its powerful deliriant effects (Itil et al., 1969).

It has been reported that concomitant use of anticholinergic antiparkinson drugs may reduce the efficacy of antipsychotic drug therapy (Singh and Smith, 1973; Singh and Kay, 1975a; 1975b; 1975c). Some of the changes reported were cognitive and these could represent direct anticholinergic effects rather than a true aggravation of schizophrenia. In addition, antiparkinsonian and anticholinergic drugs may also sharply reduce prevailing plasma levels of chlorpromazine (Rivera-Calimlin et al., 1973; Gautier et al., 1977). Clinical experience does not indicate that antiparkinson anticholinergic treatment diminishes the efficacy of antipsychotic agents. Further, neuroleptics with strong anticholinergic activity, such as thioridazine and clozapine, are effective antipsychotic agents. Thus the evidence that anticholinergics aggravate schizophrenia is confounded by a number of problems, but suggests further investigation.

Traditional antipsychotics are hypothesized to act by blocking dopamine receptors in the central nervous system (Matthysse and Lipinski, 1975; Berger et al., 1978; Carlsen, 1978). Three major dopamine pathways have been delineated in the brain: the nigro-striatal dopamine pathway has cell bodies in the substantia nigra (A-9) which project to the ipsilateral caudate-putamen (corpus striatum); the tuberoinfundibular pathway originates in the arcuate nucleus and terminates in the median eminence; the mesolimbic pathway, which is implicated in schizophrenic symptoms, has cell bodies in the midbrain medial to the substantia nigra (A-10) and terminal projections in the limbic system, including the nucleus accumbens, the olfactory tubercle, the bed nucleus of the stria terminalis and the septal region. Cell bodies from A-9 and A-10 may also project at cortical areas (Ungerstedt, 1971; Stevens, 1973; Lindvall et al., 1974). Cholinergic-dopaminergic relationships are best described for the nigrostriatal dopamine pathway.

These include anatomical, biochemical and pharmacological relationships (Klawans, 1970; Klawans and Rubovits, 1974). The successful treatment of Parkinson's disease by both anticholinergic agents and levodopa is presumably based on this dopamine-acetylcholine relationship in the nigrostriatal pathway.

Successful cholinomimetic treatments of schizophrenia are based on the hypothesis of an analogous cholinergic-dopaminergic relationship in the mesolimbic dopamine pathways where neuroleptics are presumed to have their antipsychotic dopamine blocking action. In the rat brain, cholinomimetics increased homovanillic acid (HVA) in both the corpus striatum and in the limbic system (Anden, 1974). However, anticholinergic agents decreased the neuroleptic induced rise in HVA to a greater extent in the corpus striatum than in the limbic system (Anden, 1972; Anden, 1974). In the corpus striatum, dopamine has a tonic inhibitory effect on acetylcholine release. This effect has not been demonstrated in the limbic system (Bartholini et al., 1976). Thus the evidence for a cholinergic-dopaminergic interaction in the mesolimbic dopamine pathways is not as strong as the evidence for such an interaction in nigrostriatal pathways.

Animal stereotyped behaviors caused by apomorphine or amphetamine are proposed to be caused by increased central dopaminergic activity (Randrup and Munkvad, 1974). Reversal of this stereotypy has been used as a screening test for neuroleptic drugs. Most investigators find that stereotypy is abolished by corpus striatum destruction and this suggests that stereotypy reflects nigrostriatal dopamine activity (Randrup and Munkvad, 1974; Naylor and Olley, 1972). However, one investigator reported that destruction of the nucleus accumbens prevented stereotypy while caudate-putamen destruction did not (McKenzie, 1972). Three studies have shown that cholinomimetics including physostigmine and oxotremorine block stereotypy, a pharmacological action similar to most neuroleptics (Klawans et al., 1972; Davis et al., 1978; Janowsky et al., 1972a). However, neuroleptics with strong antimuscarinic activity, such as thioridazine and clozapine, are less active in blocking stereotypy than their antipsychotic potency would predict (Snyder et al., 1974; Burki et al., 1975). Thus, blockade of stereotypy does not always correlate with antipsychotic activity.

Injection of dopamine or amphetamine into the limbic system of rats produces an increase in the locomotor activity. Reversal of this increased activity by neuroleptics may be a better reflection of their mesolimbic and hence antipsychotic activity (Pijnenburg et al., 1975; Pijnenburg et al., 1976). Most neuroleptics reverse dopamine-induced increased locomotor activity with a potency consistent with their antipsychotic activity (Costall and Naylor, 1976; Pijnenburg et al., 1975). However clozapine does not significantly reduce the effects of dopamine on locomotor activity (Pijnenburg et al., 1976). Furthermore, the cholinomimetic, carbachol, like dopamine, increased locomotor activity when injected into the nucleus accumbens. Thus, in this test system one cholinomimetic has pharmacological activity that is opposite from most antipsychotics. Further testing of the effect of pharmacological agents on dopamine-induced increases in locomotor activity will be required to determine whether activity in this test predicts antipsychotic activity.

AFFECTIVE DISORDERS

Cholinergic underactivity may also play a role in manic psychosis (Janowsky et al., 1972b; Davis et al., 1975). More than 25 years ago it was reported that the irreversible cholinesterase inhibitor diisopropylfluorophosphonate (DFP) depressed the mood of four of six hypomanic patients (Rowntree et al., 1957). However, each of these patients also experienced anorexia, nausea, and vomiting. More recently, intravenous physostigmine was reported to transiently reverse manic symptoms in eight patients (Janowsky et al., 1973b). Other investigators suggest these results can be explained by the somatic effects of cholinesterase inhibition (Carroll et al., 1973). Two manic patients and one patient with manic symptoms following exogenous corticosteroid administration had no change in manic thought content or mood following intravenous physostigmine. All three patients had an anergic syndrome, characterized by decreased speech and physical activity that was suggested as easily misinterpreted as a true improvement in manic thought content (Carroll et al., 1973).

In another study four patients with mania participated in eight crossover trials of physostigmine and neostigmine. Only in two trials, in two different patients, did physostigmine diminish manic symptoms significantly more than neostigmine. In the other six trials there was no significant difference between physostigmine and neostigmine on manic symptoms (Modestin et al., 1973a). In this study only 1.25-1.50 mg of physostigmine was given while doses of 2.5-6.0 mg have been used by investigators who report a reversal of manic symptoms by physostigmine.

Some patients exposed to irreversible organophosphate cholinesterase inhibitors have been reported to develop depressive symptoms. Acute administration of DFP produced a marked depression in four of six hypomanic patients (Rowntree et al., 1957). In the same study ten normal subjects developed depression, lassitude, irritability, and apathy without disturbance of such cognitive functions as memory, orientation or intellectual ability. Atropine in doses of 1-5 mg was found to partially counteract this depressant action of DFP. Another group of investigators evaluated 16 people chronically exposed to organophosphate anticholinesterase insecticides (Gershon and Shaw, 1961). The period of exposure in these subjects ranged from 1-10 years. Seven of the 16 patients developed depression, in two of these individuals the depression was described as severe. Five patients developed schizophrenic-like reactions without a major depressive component. All 16 subjects had impaired memory and concentration. In another study, normal subjects were given a potent percutaneous cholinesterase inhibitor (Bowers et al., 1964). Subjects with blood cholinesterase activity 40% below control values were reported to be significantly more depressed, more anxious, more confused and less energetic when compared to those subjects whose cholinesterase activity was not decreased to 40% of control values.

The reversible cholinesterase inhibitor, physostigmine, has also been reported to cause depression in some individuals. One investigator administered 1.25-1.50 mg of physostigmine to 40 nonpsychotic, nondepressed subjects with the diagnoses of either drug addiction, alcoholism, psychopathy or neurosis (Modestin et al., 1973a). A significant increase in depressive symptoms was reported. The depressive symptoms did not seem to correlate with the somatic disturbances caused by physostigmine. The same investigator also reported that physostigmine caused depression in schizophrenic subjects (Modestin et al., 1973b). In another study, two patients who were intermittant users of marijuana received 1.25 mg of intravenous physostigmine after smoking marijuana (El-Yousef et al., 1973). These two patients developed a depressive syndrome characterized by sadness, apathy, hopelessness, decreased thoughts, suicidal ideation and psychomotor retardation. These symptoms were terminated by 1 mg of intravenous atropine. This interaction between marijuana and physostigmine is consistent with the report that a daily user of marijuana became severely depressed for several days following 3 mg of intravenous physostigmine (Davis *et al.*, 1976b). In the same study 12 additional subjects received the 3 mg of intravenous physostigmine. All subjects developed an anergic syndrome characterized by decreased verbalization, slowed thoughts, mild sedation, and nausea. Only one of these 12 subjects became tearful and expressed depressive thought content during the infusion of physostigmine. This subject was unique in having a history of repeated episodes of depression during the premenstrual period.

Other evidence suggestive of a cholinergic mechanism in depression comes from the clinical and pharmacological actions of reserpine and tricyclic antidepressants. Reserpine depletes indoleamines and catecholamines and has central cholinomimetic properties. Reserpine has been reported to cause depression in some patients (Fries, 1954). In addition to their enhancement of central biogenic amine activity, tricyclic antidepressants are all potent anticholinergic agents (Snyder and Yamamura, 1977). Thus, central cholinergic blockade may add to their efficacy in depression (Berger, 1977).

Human trials with choline chloride in movement disorders, including tardive dyskinesia and Huntington's disease, have produced depression only sporadically. The effects of choline chloride on tardive dyskinesia and Huntington's disease are similar to the transient effects of physostigmine on these movements (Davis *et al.*, 1977). However, only one of eleven patients given 20 gm of choline chloride per day became depressed in our studies. In contrast, it has been reported that two patients given 9 gm choline chloride for tardive dyskinesia became severely depressed (Tamminga *et al.*, 1976). One patient developed feelings of worthlessness and agitation and made a suicide attempt. This patient's depression was relieved by 2.4 mg of atropine given over 30 min and remitted in 4-5 days when choline was discontinued.

RATIONALE FOR PHARMACOLOGICAL INVESTIGATIONS

These earlier studies on the possible role of cholinergic mechanisms in schizophrenia and affective disorders suggest two hypotheses which led to the pharmacological investigations described in this chapter. The first hypothesis is that relative cholinergic underactivity contributes to schizophrenic symptoms; the second hypothesis is that cholinergic underactivity is involved in the symptoms of mania. These hypotheses suggest that an increase in central cholinergic activity might ameliorate the symptoms of manic or schizophrenic psychosis.

In our pharmacological studies intravenous physostigmine and oral choline chloride were used in an attempt to increase central cholinergic activity. Intravenous physostigmine has been used in earlier investigations, but an important goal of these studies was to use a method of physostigmine infusion and clinical rating that could distinguish between the somatic effects of physostigmine and any possible effects of physostigmine on the symptoms of schizophrenia and mania.

In addition to the transient action of physostigmine, we sought an agent that might more chronically increase central cholinergic activity. Some recent animal studies suggested that choline chloride might increase cholinergic activity in the central nervous system. Two groups of investigators reported that rat brain acetylcholine was increased after the parenteral administration of choline chloride (Haubrich *et al.*, 1975; Cohen and Wurtman, 1975). Dietary addition of choline chloride was also reported to raise rat brain acetylcholine (Cohen and Wurtman, 1975). In human studies, a dose dependent increase in plasma choline has been reported following oral choline administration (Aquilonius and Eckernas, 1975; Davis *et al.*, 1976a). In addition it has been shown in a double-blind study that physostigmine and choline chloride both decrease the movements of some patients with tardive dyskinesia and Huntington's disease, suggesting parallel pharmacological activity (Davis *et al.*, 1976a). A more detailed discussion of the evidence that choline chloride increases central cholinergic activity is found in Jenden's chapter in this book. Thus, choline chloride, like physostigmine, might be a useful pharmacological tool for evaluating cholinergic mechanisms in schizophrenia and mania.

METHODS

Subjects

Eight men and one woman with the diagnosis of manic depressive illness between the ages of 25 and 52 gave informed consent to participate in the study. All patients met diagnostic criteria for primary affective disorder, mania (Feighner *et al.*, 1972). Chloral hydrate was the only psychoactive medication six patients received for 2 days prior to the physostigmine infusion. Two other patients were drug free for 2 days, but were given 10 mg of prochlorperazine 60 min prior to the physostigmine infusion in an attempt to minimize nausea and vomiting. One patient had been given 40-60 mg of fluphenazine daily for 7 days in an unsuccessful attempt to control manic behavior. Fluphenazine was discontinued 12 hr prior to this patient's physostigmine infusion.

Seven male patients with a diagnosis of schizophrenia between the ages of 25 and 34 gave their informed consent to participate in this study. All seven met diagnostic criteria for schizophrenia (Feighner *et al.*, 1972). The schizophrenic patients received no psychoactive medications for at least seven days before the physostigmine infusion.

Physostigmine Infusion Procedure

Prior to the physostigmine infusion all patients received 0.5 mg of methscopolamine bromide subcutaneously. An additional 0.5 mg of subcutaneous methscopolamine was given to patients whose heart rate remained below 100 after 20 min. When the heart rate reached 100 the intravenous physostigmine was started.

Patients were given 4.0 mg of physostigmine in 200 cc of normal saline by constant infusion over 60 min. Heart rate and rhythm were continuously monitored by electrocardiogram.

Thirty minutes prior to the infusion, schizophrenic patients were rated on the Brief Psychiatric Rating Scale (BPRS) following a structured interview by a psychiatrist and a nurse (Overall, 1974). Both knew the patient was to receive physostigmine. The patient was also told that an investigational drug was being administered. However, the patient was not told what psychological effects to expect from the drug. The BPRS was again completed after a structured interview 5-30 min and three hours after the 60 min infusion ended. Thirty minutes prior to the infusion and every 30 min thereafter for 4 hr, schizophrenic patients were asked to rate the intensity of their auditory hallucinations, if these were present, by placing a mark on a 100 millimeter line, a visual analogue scale. One end of the line was labeled "the worst you have ever been", while the other end read "not present."

Thirty minutes prior to the infusion and every 30 min thereafter for 4 hr, manic patients were asked to report on their mood by marking a 100 millimeter line. One end of this line was labeled "the saddest I have ever felt", the other end read "the happiest I have ever felt." Patients were asked to record their mood and to attempt to separate their mood from any gastrointestinal discomfort they might be experiencing. A psychiatrist and a nurse, who knew the patient was receiving physostigmine, completed the Petterson Mania Scale after a structured interview 30 min prior to the physostigmine infusion, at the end of the infusion and 3 hr after the infusion. The mania scale rates seven components of mania: motor activity, pressure of speech, flight of ideas, noisiness, aggressiveness, orientation and elevated mood (Petterson et al., 1973). All items are rated on a five step scale except orientation which is assessed on a three step scale. The mania scale also provides a global assessment and an item that evaluates the patients global state compared to previous rating (Petterson et al., 1973). Manic patients knew that physostigmine was being administered, but the patients were not told what psychological changes to expect.

Choline Chloride Administration

Eight schizophrenic patients and one manic patient received choline chloride. The drug is dissolved in distilled water to a concentration of 0.5 gm per milliliter and is flavored with strawberry syrup. Patients started with a dose of 1 gm four times per day. This was increased by 1 gm four times a day every 2-3 days until a total daily dose of 20 gm per day was reached. Subjects were maintained on the maximum dose for 3-4 weeks and then switched to placebo. The placebo had a color and taste that were similar to choline. All eight schizophrenic patients and the one manic attempted a 4 week placebo period, but if their behavior became unmanageable they were started on neuroleptics and placebo was discontinued. Schizophrenic and manic patients completing the placebo period were placed on psychotropic agents if indicated. Patients were not told when they were receiving choline chloride or placebo.

The BPRS was used to record the clinical status of choline chloride in schizophrenia and mania. Patients were rated once just before starting choline chloride and at weekly intervals thereafter for the duration of the study. The Petterson Mania Scale and 100 millimeter visual analogue mood line described above were also used to follow the course of the manic patient. Ratings on the manic and schizophrenic patients were recorded by a psychiatrist and a nurse after a structured interview with both raters participating. When possible the same two raters assessed a patient throughout the study. Raters knew when patients were receiving choline chloride or placebo.

RESULTS

Physostigmine Infusion

Mania

Eight patients with a diagnosis of mania received at least 4.0 mg of physostigmine. One patient (K.C.) asked that the infusion be discontinued after 2.5 mg because she was feeling severely depressed. Scores on the visual analogue scale for all nine patients demonstrated significantly more depression at the end of the infusion when compared to predrug and 3 hr post drug scores combined ($p < .005$ t-test for unpaired data). Figure 1 displays the data from the 100 mm visual analogue mood line. Each patient's course is represented by a set of three bars. From left to right these are the predrug, end of infusion and 3 hr post infusion scores. Despite instructions to separate feelings of physical discomfort from mood changes this proved difficult for many subjects. Scores on the first seven items of the Petterson Scale are depicted in Figure 2. This figure uses the same format for depicting predrug, end of infusion and 3 hr postinfusion scores that was used in Figure 1. Mean scores on these seven items for all nine patients combined were significantly less at the end of the infusion when compared to predrug scores ($p < .05$ t-test for unpaired data) or when compared to predrug and 3 hr post drug combined ($p < .05$). Differences recorded on the Petterson Scale were not as great as on the 100 mm visual analogue line. For example, according to the Petterson scores H.K. was not changed by physostigmine, and K.C. did not return to a manic state. The Petterson scores are closer to our clinical impressions than the mood line scores. Interestingly, K.C. was the only manic patient infused on the switch day from depression to mania.

Figure 3 presents the combined scores for the three items on the Petterson Scale that most accurately measure manic thought content and mood in manic patients whose dominant symptom is euphoria. These scales reflect elevated mood, pressure of speech, and flight of ideas. The mean scores for these items for all nine patients combined at the end of the infusion were significantly less than before and 3 hr after the infusion ($p < .005$ t-test, unpaired data).

Three manic patients H.K., R.R. and E.O. had irritability rather than euphoria as a dominant symptom. The aggressiveness item on the Petterson Scale best describes their clinical course, and is depicted in Figure 4. All three irritable manics were more aggressive at the end of the infusion than before physostigmine. No other patients had increased aggressiveness. The responses to physostigmine in these three patients whose affect was predominantly irritable are complex. Although two of these patients had a decrease in total Petterson score, both became more irritable as the infusion progressed.

K.C., D.J., and M.D. cried during or at the end of the infusion. F.B., R.E., E.L., K.C., D.J. and M.D. demonstrated depressive thought content. These patients discussed such feelings as failure, self-doubt and they talked of such things as divorces, bad business deals, the sad plight of hospitalized psychiatric patients and K.C. even said she wanted "to die."

Four of the nine manic patients became nauseated, and three actually vomited. M.B. and R.R., the patients who received prochlorperazine, and D.J. who had been taking fluphenazine until 12 hr prior to the infusion experienced no gastrointestinal distress.

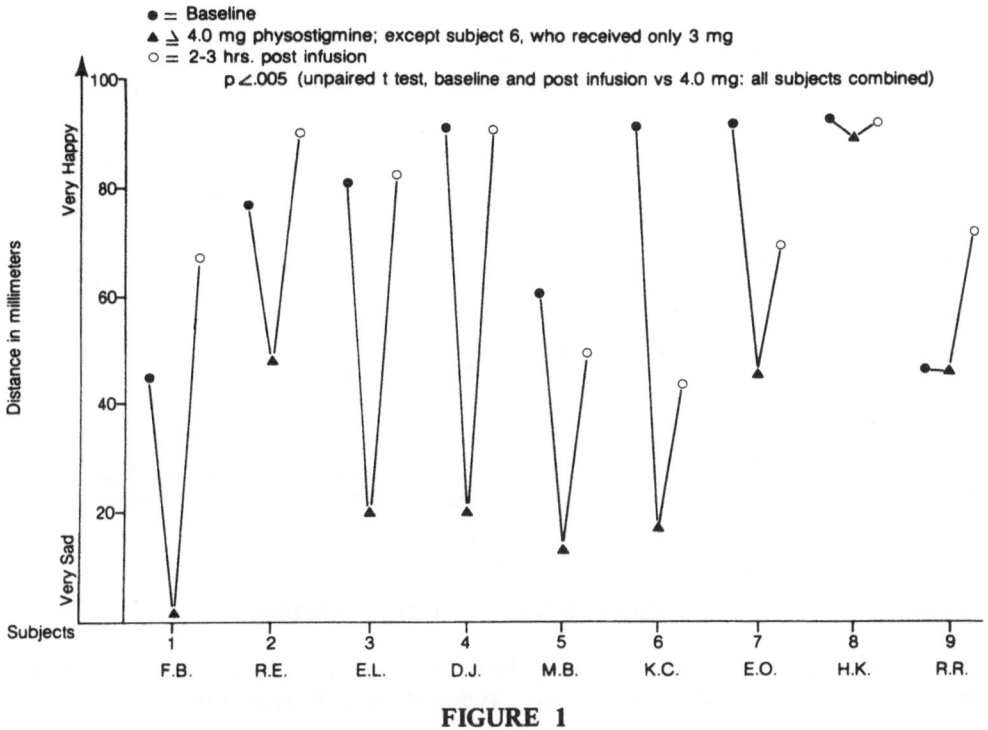

FIGURE 1

Physostigmine in Manics — 100 mm Mood Lines

Each patient's score is represented by 3 points. From left to right these are predrug, end of infusion and post 3 hr scores on the 100 mm mood lines.

Schizophrenia

Three patients with the diagnosis of schizophrenia received physostigmine. Comparison of predrug, 5-30 min postdrug, and 3 hr postdrug BPRS scores reveals no significant changes. Intensity of auditory hallucinations, as measured by a 100 mm visual analogue scale, was also unchanged.

Choline Chloride Administration

Schizophrenia

Eight patients received choline chloride. Only two of them, G.H. and M.B., also had received physostigmine, and neither had improved on this drug. For six patients there is no indication that their condition was improved by choline chloride administration compared to the placebo period. Two patients could not complete the full 4 week placebo period and required neuroleptic medication due to disruptive behavior.

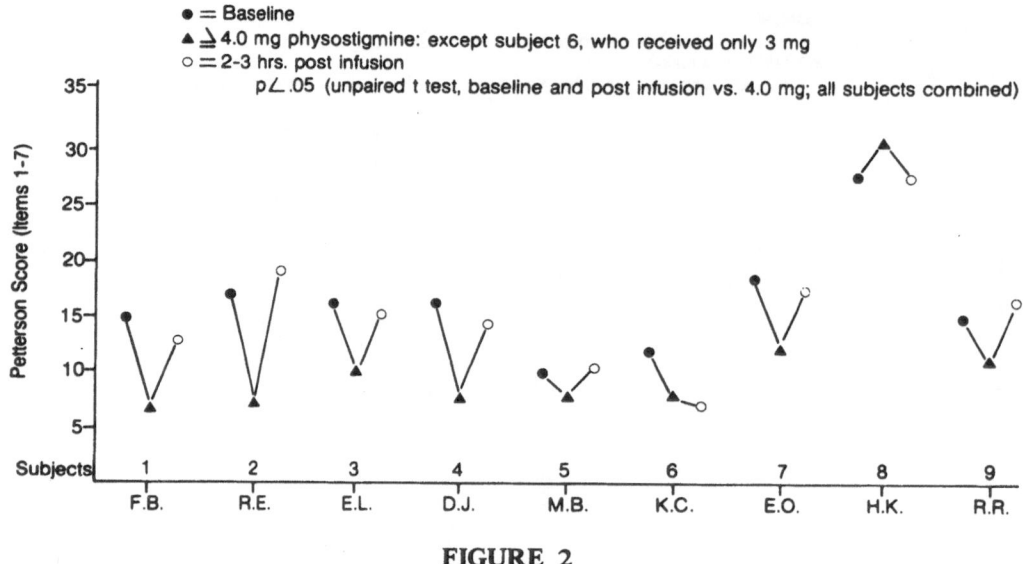

FIGURE 2

Physostigmine in Manics — Petterson Scores

Each patient's score is represented by 3 points. From left to right these are predrug, end of infusion and post 3 hr scores on the first 7 items of the Petterson scale.

Five other patients were given neuroleptics after a 4 week placebo period. Four of these five subjects had a greater improvement on neuroleptics than during choline chloride administration. One patient was not improved by either choline chloride or neuroleptics. Four patients, M.B., B.V., T.O. and R.B. had lower BPRS scores at the end of the choline chloride period than before receiving choline. This apparent remission persisted throughout placebo administration. These data are summarized in Figure 5.

Mania

One manic patient (R.E.) received choline chloride. All other manic patients refused to give informed consent, or could not be managed on an open ward for the time required to complete the protocol. According to his family, R.E. returned to his premorbid level of functioning by the end of the choline period. His remission persisted throughout the placebo period. Petterson and BPRS scores are presented in Figure 6. They demonstrate a trend toward improvement while on choline chloride.

DISCUSSION

These investigations are preliminary attempts to evaluate the role of cholinergic mechanisms in mania and schizophrenia. The investigation of the contribution of cholinergic underactivity to manic symptoms focused on the issue of whether increased central cholinergic activity truly changed the mood and thought content of manic patients.

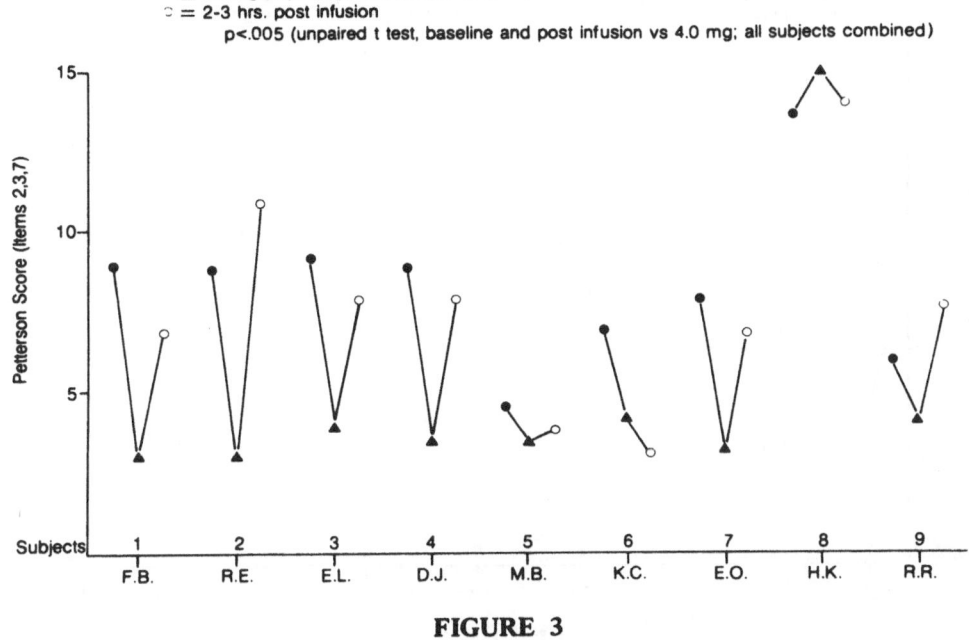

FIGURE 3

Physostigmine in Manics
Petterson Scores for Items 2,3,7
(Pressure of Speech, Flight of Ideas, Elevated Mood)

Each patient's score is represented by 3 points. From left to right these are predrug, end of infusion and post 3 hr scores on items 2, 3 and 7 of the Petterson scale.

One group of investigators has suggested that physostigmine makes manic patients so sedated and nauseated that they simply do not demonstrate the symptoms of mania (Carroll *et al.*, 1973). In our study, the patients' subjective reports, their spontaneous statements and Petterson Scale scores indicate that some manic patients whose dominant symptom is euphoria are significantly less manic in mood and thought content and more depressed after physostigmine infusion. The manic patients whose dominant symptom is irritability improved on some rating scales, but also became more aggressive after the physostigmine infusion. These irritable manic patients did not have the major component of their manic symptomatology significantly altered by physostigmine.

These results were obtained using a method of physostigmine infusion that differs from the procedures used in other studies with manic patients. A slower infusion of physostigmine allowed a more gradual evolution of the drug's effects. Premedication of two patients with prochlorperazine and one with fluphenazine minimized nausea to a point where it was less of a compounding factor. These results suggest that long acting oral cholinomimetics might be a useful treatment for the acute symptoms of some

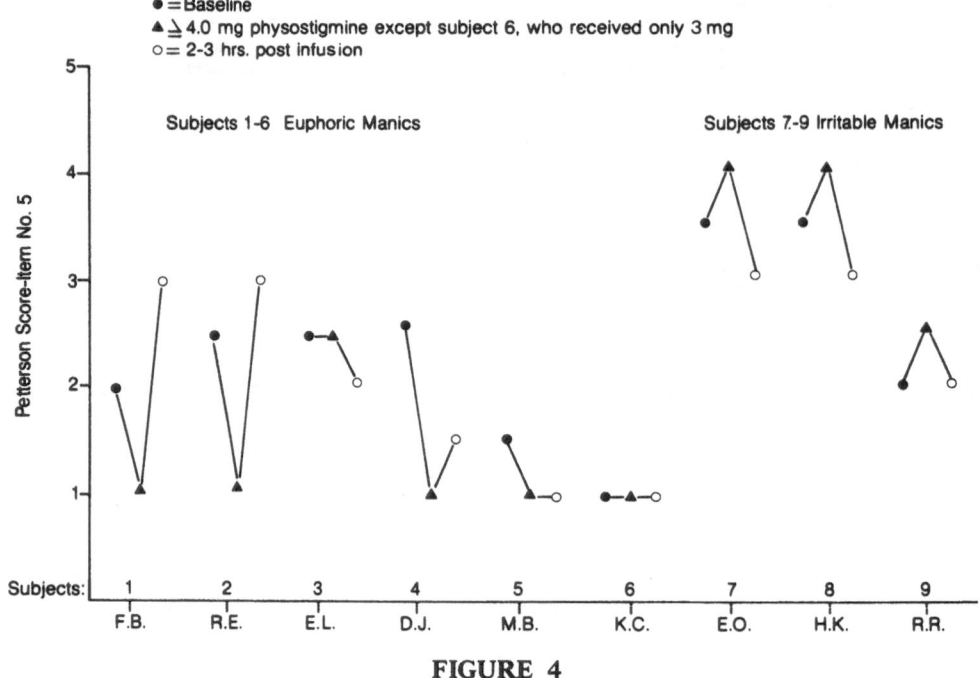

● = Baseline
▲ ≧ 4.0 mg physostigmine except subject 6, who received only 3 mg
○ = 2-3 hrs. post infusion

Subjects 1-6 Euphoric Manics   Subjects 7-9 Irritable Manics

Petterson Score-Item No. 5

Subjects: 1   2   3   4   5   6   7   8   9
          F.B.   R.E.   E.L.   D.J.   M.B.   K.C.   E.O.   H.K.   R.R.

FIGURE 4

**Physostigmine in Manics
Petterson Score — Item No. 5**

Physostigmine in Mania, Aggressiveness Scores from Petterson Scale. Each patient's score is represented by 3 points. From left to right these are predrug, end of infusion and post 3 hr scores on the aggressiveness item of the Petterson scale.

patients with mania. The initial response of the first manic patient to receive choline chloride supports this suggestion. Further studies of choline chloride or other cholino-mimetics in patients with mania will be important.

The possible role of cholinergic mechanisms in schizophrenia was also studied. The negative results with physostigmine and the generally negative results with choline chloride do not support the hypothesis that increasing central cholinergic activity is an effective treatment for patients with a diagnosis of schizophrenia. In all these trials only one patient on choline chloride dramatically improved compared to the placebo period. The improvement compared to baseline of five patients could have been a spontaneous remission. Six schizophrenic patients did better on neuroleptics than on choline chloride. However, the response of these eight schizophrenic patients to neuroleptics was also not dramatic. These patients were generally chronic schizophrenics. A further trial of cholino-

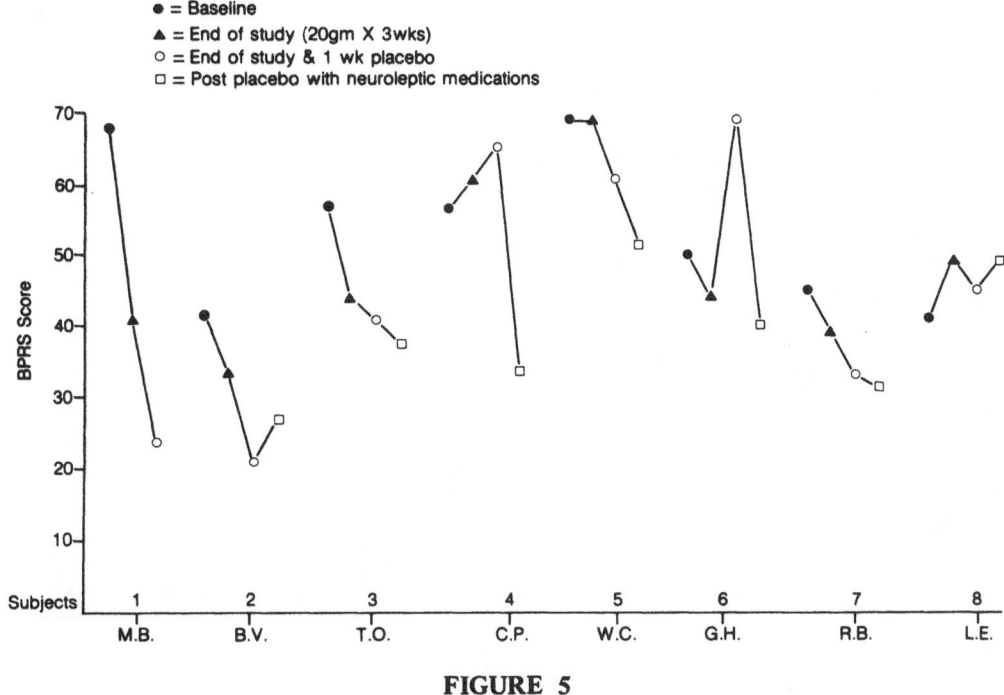

FIGURE 5

Choline Chloride in Schizophrenics

BPRS Scores in Schizophrenic Patients on Choline Chloride. Each patient's score is represented by a set of 3 or 4 points. From left to right these are before choline, end of choline, after one week of placebo, and after ten days of an antipsychotic medication.

mimetics in acute schizophrenics who prove to be dramatically improved by neuroleptics is needed before the hypotheses of the role of cholinergic mechanisms in some schizophrenics or in some schizophrenic symptoms can be rejected.

The investigation of neurotransmitter imbalance hypotheses has added a new dimension to research in biological psychiatry. Studies with physostigmine have implicated cholinergic mechanisms in diseases that were previously suggested to result from abnormalities in biogenic amines. The investigation of the possible role of cholinergic mechanisms in mania and schizophrenia is a relatively new direction for research in these psychiatric disorders. The use of physostigmine to produce a transient increase in central cholinergic activity is an important tool in this research. Studies with cholinomimetics such as choline chloride which cause more chronic increases in central cholinergic activity may not only help test cholinergic activity but could also lead to new treatment approaches for such disabling conditions as mania.

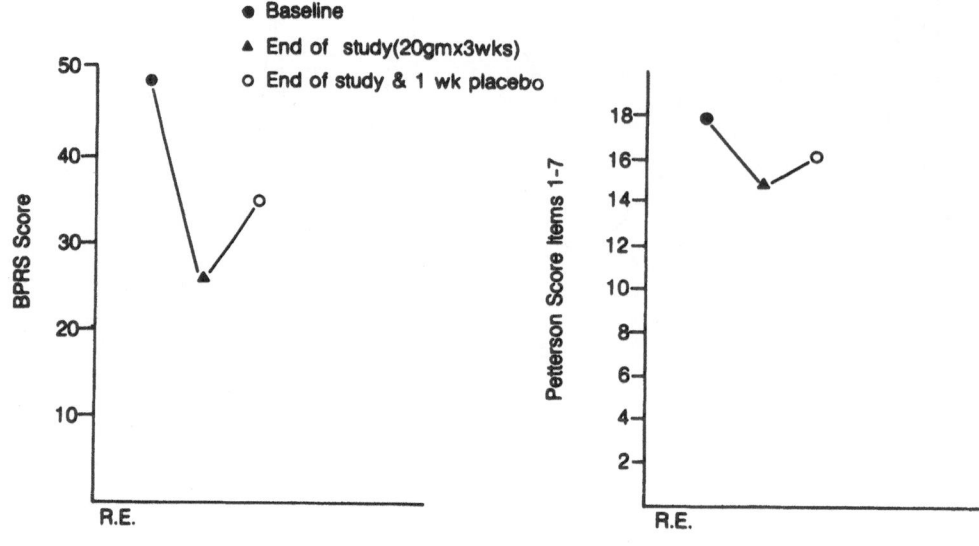

FIGURE 6

Choline Chloride in Manics

BPRS and Petterson Scores in a Manic Patient on Choline Chloride. RE's scores are expressed for both BPRS and Petterson scales in two sets of 3 points. From left to right these bars represent before choline, end of choline, and one week of placebo scores.

ACKNOWLEDGEMENTS

This research was supported in part by the Medical Research Service of the Veterans Administration and by National Institute of Mental Health Grants MH-30854, MH-03030 and MH-23861.

REFERENCES

Anden, N.E., 1972, Dopamine turnover in the corpus striatum and the limbic system after treatment with neuroleptic and anti-acetylcholine drugs, *J. Pharm. Pharmacol. 24:*905.

Anden, N.E., 1974, Effects of oxotremorine and physostigmine on the turnover of dopamine in the corpus striatum and the limbic system, *J. Pharmacol. 26:*738.

Aquilonius, S.M., and Eckernas, S.A., 1975, Plasma concentration of free choline in patients with Huntington's chorea on high doses of choline chloride, *N. Engl. J. Med. 293:*1105.

Baldessarini, R.J., 1975, The basis for the amine hypothesis in affective disorders, *Arch. Gen. Psychiatry 32:*1087.

Bartholini, G., Stadler, H., Gadeo-Ciria, M., and Lloyd, K.G., 1976, The use of the push-pull cannula to estimate the dynamics of acetylcholine and catecholamines within various brain areas, *Neuropharmacology 15:*515.

Berger, P.A., 1977, Neurotransmitters and affective disorders, in *"Neurotransmitter Function"* (W. Fields, ed.), pp. 305-335, Stratton, New York.

Berger, P.A., Elliott, G.R., and Barchas, J.D., 1978, Neuroregulators and schizophrenia, in *"Psychopharmacology: A Generation of Progress"* (M. Lipton, A. Dimascio and K. Killam eds.), pp. 1071-1083, Raven Press, New York.

Bowers, M.B., Goodman, E., and Sim, V.M., 1964, Some behavioral changes in man following anticholinesterase administration, *J. Nerv. Ment. Dis. 138:*383.

Burki, H.R., Eichenberger, E., Sayers, A.C., and White, T.C., 1975, Clozapine and the dopamine hypothesis of schizophrenia: a critical appraisal, *Pharmakopsychiatry 8:*115.

Carlsen, A., 1978, Antipsychotic drugs, neurotransmitters and schizophrenia, *Am. J. Psychiatry 135:*164.

Carroll, B.J., Frazer, A., Schless, A., and Mendels, J., 1973, Cholinergic reversal of manic symptoms, *Lancet I:*427.

Cohen, E.L., and Wurtman, R.J., 1975, Brain acetylcholine: increase after systematic choline administration, *Life Sci. 16(7):*1095.

Collard, J., Lecoq, R., and Demaret, A., 1965, Un essai de therapeutique pathogenique de la schizophrenic par un acetylcholinique: l'oxotremorine, *Acta. Neurol. Belg. 65:*122.

Costall, B., and Naylor, R.J., 1976, Antagonism of the hyperactivity induced by dopamine applied intracerebrally to the nucleus accumbens septi by typical neuroleptics and by clozapine, sulpiride and thioridazine, *Eur. J. Pharmacol. 35:*161.

Davis, K.L., Hollister, L.E., Berger, P.A., and Barchas, J.D., 1975, A cholinergic imbalance hypothesis of psychoses and movement disorders: strategies for evaluation, *Psychopharmacology Comm. 1:*533.

Davis, K.L., Hollister, L.E., Barchas, J.D., and Berger, P.A., 1976a, Choline in tardive dyskinesia and Huntington's disease, *Life Sci. 19:*1507.

Davis, K.L., Hollister, L.E., Overall, J.A., Johnson, A., and Train, K., 1976b, Physostigmine: effects on cognition and affect in normal subjects, *Psychopharmacology 51:*23.

Davis, K.L., Berger, P.A., and Hollister, L.E., 1977, Cholinergic mechanisms in tardive dyskinesia and Huntington's chorea, in *"Neurotransmitter Function"* (W. Fields ed.), pp. 247-262, Stratton, New York.

Davis, K.L., Hollister, L.E., and Tepper, J., 1978, Cholinergic inhibition of methylphenidate induced stereotypy with oxotremorine, *Psychopharmacology 56:*1.

El-Yousef, M.K., Janowsky, D.S., Davis, J.M., and Rosenblatt, J.E., 1973, Induction
of severe depression by physostigmine in marijuana intoxicated individuals, *Br. J.
Addict. 68:*321.

Feighner, J.P., Robins, R., Guze, S.B., Woodruff, R.A., Winokur G., and Munoz, R.,
1972, Diagnostic criteria for use in psychiatric research, *Arch. Gen. Psychiatry 26:*57.

Friedhoff, A.J., and Alpert, M., 1973, A dopaminergic-cholinergic mechanism in production of psychotic symptoms, *Biol. Psychiatry 6:*165.

Fries, E.D., 1954, Mental depression in hypertensive patients treated for long periods
with large doses of reserpine, *N. Engl. J. Med. 251:*1006.

Fulcher, J.H., Gallagher, W.J., and Pfeiffer, C.C., 1957, Comparative lucid intervals after
amobarbital, CO_2, and arecoline in the chronic schizophrenic, *AMA Arch. Neurol.
Psychiatry 78:*392.

Gautier, J., Jus, A., Villeneuve, A., Jus, K., Pires, P., and Villeneuve, R., 1977, Influence
of the antiparkinsonian drugs on the plasma level of neuroleptics, *Biol. Psychiatr. 12:*
389.

Gershon, S., and Shaw, F.H., 1961, Psychiatric sequelae of chronic exposure to organophosphorous insecticides, *Lancet I:*1371.

Goodwin, F.K., and Murphy, D.L., 1974, Biological factors in affective disorders and
schizophrenia, in *"Psychopharmacological Agents"* (M. Gordon, ed.), pp. 9-37,
Academic Press, New York.

Haubrich, D.R., Wang, P.F.L., Clody, D.E., and Wedeking, P.W., 1975, Increase in rat
brain acetylcholine induced by choline or deanol, *Life Sci. 17(6):*975.

Itil, T.M., Keskiner, A., and Holden, O.M.C., 1969, The use of LSD and ditran in the
treatment of therapy resistant schizophrenics (symptom provocation approach),
*Dis. Nerv. Syst. (Suppl.) 30:*93.

Janowsky, D.S., El-Yousef, M.K., Davis, J.M., and Sekerke, H.J., 1972a, Cholinergic
antagonism of methylphenidate-induced stereotyped behavior, *Psychopharmacologia
27:*295.

Janowsky, D.S., El-Yousef, M.K., Davis, J.M., and Sekerke, H.J., 1972b, A cholinergic
hypothesis of mania and depression, *Lancet II:*632.

Janowsky, D.S., El-Yousef, M.K., Davis, J.M., and Sekerke, H.J., 1973a, Antagonistic
effects of physostigmine and methylphenidate in man, *Am. J. Psychiatry 130:*1370.

Janowsky, D.S., El-Yousef, M.K., Davis, J.M., and Sekerke, H.J., 1973b, Parasympathetic
suppression of manic symptoms by physostigmine, *Arch. Gen. Psychiatry 28:*542.

Klawans, H.L., 1970, A pharmacological analysis of Huntington's chorea, *Eur. Neurol.
4:*148.

Klawans, H.L., and Rubovits, R., 1974, Effect of cholinergic and anticholinergic agents
on tardive dyskinesia, *J. Neurol. Neurosurg. Psychiatry 37:*941.

Klawans, H.L., Rubovits, R., Patel, B.C., and Weiner, W.J., 1972, Cholinergic and anticholinergic influences on amphetamine-induced stereotyped behavior, *J. Neurol.
Sci. 17:*303.

Lindvall, O., Bjorklund, A., and Moore, R.Y., 1974, Mesencephalic dopamine neurons
projecting to neocortex, *Brain Res. 81:*325.

Matthysse, S., and Lipinski, J., 1975, Biochemical aspects of schizophrenia, *Annu. Rev.
Med. 26:*551.

McKenzie, G.M., 1972, Role of the tuberculum olfactorium in stereotyped behavior
induced by apomorphine in the rat, *Psychopharmacologia 23:*212.

Modestin, J., Hunger, J., and Schwartz, R.B., 1973a, Uber die depressogene Wirkung von physostigmin, *Arch. Psychiatry Nervenkr. 218*:67.

Modestin, J., Schwartz, R.B., and Hunger, J., 1973b, Zur Frage beeinflussung schizophrener symptome durch physostigmin, *Pharmakopsychiatrie Neuropsychopharmakol 6*:300.

Naylor, R.J., and Olley, J.E., 1972, Modification of the behavioral changes induced by amphetamine in the rat by lesions in the caudate nucleus, the caudate putamen and globus pallidus, *Neuropharmacology 11*:91.

Overall, J.E., 1974, The brief psychiatric rating scale in psychopharmacology research, in *"Psychological Measurements In Modern Psychopharmacology: Mod. Probl. Pharmacopsychiat. Vol. 7"* (P. Pichot, ed.), pp. 67-78, Karger, Basel.

Petterson, U., Fyro, O.G., and Sedvall, G., 1973, A new scale for the longitudinal rating of manic states, *Acta. Psychiatr. Scand. 49*:248.

Pfeiffer, C.C., and Jenny, E.H., 1957, The inhibition of the conditioned response and the counteraction of schizophrenia by muscarinic stimulation of the brain, *Ann. N.Y. Acad. Sci. 66*:753.

Pijenenburg, A.J.J., Honig, W.M.M., and Van Rossum, J.M., 1975, Effects of antagonists upon locomotor stimulation induced by injection of dopamine and noradrenaline into the nucleus accumbens of nialimide-pretreated rats, *Psychopharmacologia 41*:174.

Pijnenburg, A.J.J., Honig, W.M.M., and Van der Heyden, J.A.M., 1976, Effects of chemical stimulation of the mesolimbic dopamine system upon locomotor activity, *Eur. J. Pharmacol 35*:45.

Randrup, A., and Munkvad, I., 1974, Pharmacology and physiology of stereotyped behavior, *J. Psychiatr. Res. 11*:1.

Rivera-Calimlin, L., Castaneda, L., and Lasagna, L., 1973, Effects of mode of management on plasma chlorpromazine in psychiatric patients, *Clin. Pharmacol. Ther. 14*: 978.

Rosenthal, R., and Bigelow, L.G., 1973, The effects of physostigmine in phenothiazine resistant chronic schizophrenic patients: preliminary observations, *Compr. Psychiatry 14*:489.

Rowntree, D.W., Nevin, S., and Wilson, 1957, The effects of diisopropylfluorophosphonate in schizophrenic and manic depressive psychosis, *J. Neuro. Neurosurg. Psychiatry 78*: 392.

Schildkraut, J.J., 1974, Biogenic amines and affective disorders, *Ann. Rev. Med. 25*:333.

Shopsin, B., Wilk, S., Sathananthan, G., Gershon, S., and Davis, K.L., 1974, Catecholamines and affective disorders revised: a critical assessment, *J. Nerv. Ment. Dis. 158*:369.

Singh, M.M., and Smith, J.M., 1973, Reversal of some therapeutic effects of an antipsychotic agent by an antiparkinsonism drug, *J. Nerv. Ment. Dis. 157*:50.

Singh, M.M., and Kay, S.R., 1975a, Therapeutic reversal with benztropine in schizophrenics, *J. Nerv. Ment. Dis. 160*:258.

Singh, M.M., and Kay, S.R., 1975b, A comparitive study of haloperidol and chlorpromazine in terms of clinical effects and therapeutic reversal with benztropine in schizophrenia. Theoretical implications for potency differences among neuroleptics, *Psychopharmacologia 43*:103.

Singh, M.M., and Kay, S.R., 1975c, A longitudinal comparison between two prototypic neuroleptics (haloperidol and chlorpromazine) in matched groups of schizophrenics. Non-therapeutic interactions with trihexyphenidyl. Theoretical implications for potency differences, *Psychopharmacologia 43*:115.

Snyder, S.H., and Yamamura, H.I., 1977, Antidepressants and the muscarinic acetylcholine receptor, *Arch. Gen. Psychiatry 34*:236.

Snyder, S.H., Greenburg, D., and Yamamura, H.I., 1974, Antischizophrenic drugs and brain cholinergic receptors, *Arch. Gen. Psychiatry 31:*58.

Stevens, J.R., 1973, An anatomy of schizophrenia? *Arch. Gen. Psychiatry 29:*177.

Tamminga, C., Smith, R.C., Chang, S., Harvuszti, J.S., and Davis, J.M., 1976, Depression associated with oral choline, *Lancet II:*905.

Ungerstedt, U., 1971, Stereotoxic mapping of the monoamine pathways in the rat brain, *Acta Physiol. Scand. (Suppl.) 367:*1.

AFFECTIVE CHANGES WITH DEANOL

D. E. Casey

Departments of Medical Research and Psychiatry, Portland VA Hospital, Portland, Oregon 97207

Department of Psychiatry, University of Oregon Health Sciences Center, Portland, Oregon 97201

INTRODUCTION

Depression and mania are most prominently characterized by alterations in mood which may be accompanied by changes in motor activity, cognitive abilities, sleep, and autonomic nervous system function. Depressed patients experience sadness, hopelessness, self-blame or guilt, decreased energy, poor concentration, insomnia or hypersomnia, anorexia, and decreased libido. Conversely, manic patients have exaggerated moods of gaiety, euphoria or anger, grandiosity, excess energy, pressured thought and speech, decreased need for sleep, and increased sexual interests. The idea that these contrasting disorders might evolve from a disruption of a single basic catecholamine system was hypothesized by Schildkraut (1965) and others (Bunney and Davis, 1965). In simplistic terms, this hypothesis states that depression results from a deficit of central nervous system catecholamine-mediated activity, while mania is secondary to an excess of these amines. Further research has made it clear, however, that a one-dimensional model of catecholaminergic disequilibrium cannot entirely explain the complex biochemical aspects of affective disorders (Baldessarini, 1975).

Recognizing that cholinergic influences may play a role in mood disorders, Janowsky *et al.* (1972) expanded upon the catecholamine hypothesis. They proposed that acetylcholinergic and catecholaminergic systems function reciprocally to modulate mood. Thus, a relative dominance of acetylcholinergic influences could produce the symptoms of depression while a relative dominance of catecholaminergic or serotonergic influences could lead to manic symptoms. This hypothesis is supported by a variety of clinical and pharmacological findings. In uncontrolled studies, synthetic anticholinergic agents and scopolamine have been considered to have mild antidepressant action (Safer and Allen, 1971; English, 1962). These drugs can also produce behavioral activation and euphoria, but their usefulness as tools for investigating affective disorders is limited by their tendency to produce a toxic delirium. The antidepressant effects of the tricyclic drugs may also be due to their potent anticholinergic action, in addition to their ability to increase the norepinephrine available in the synaptic cleft by inhibition of reuptake (Maas, 1975; Sulser *et al.*, 1964).

A relative excess of cholinergic function can affect mood as both long-acting (Gershon and Shaw, 1961; Rowntree *et al.*, 1950) and short-acting acetylcholinesterase inhibitors (Janowsky *et al.*, 1973a, 1973b) have produced depression. Although reserpine is generally thought to produce depression via presynaptic amine depletion, its cholino-mimetic effects (Bogdanski *et al.*, 1961) may also contribute to depression.

Increasing brain acetylcholine by loading the pathway for synthesis with putative precursors may also influence affective disorders. Choline has consistently raised brain acetylcholine in animals (Cohen and Wurtman, 1976; Cohen and Wurtman, 1975; Haubrich *et al.*, 1975) and produced psychotic depression in humans (Tamminga *et al.*, 1976). Deanol has been shown to raise brain acetylcholine in some studies (Haubrich *et al.*, 1975; Goldberg and Silbergeld, 1974; Danysz *et al.*, 1967) but not in others (Zahniser *et al.*, 1977; Pepeu *et al.*, 1960). The hypothesis that affective disorders result from an imbalance in cholinergic and adrenergic systems suggests that deanol, as a putative cholinergic precursor, may produce major alterations in affect.

OBSERVATIONS

Thirty-three patients with involuntary movement disorders received deanol in open, single-blind placebo-controlled, and double-blind placebo-controlled clinical trials. Twenty-eight patients had tardive dyskinesia, two patients had oromandibular dystonia, and one each had Huntington's disease, benign essential tremor, and spinocerebellar degeneration. The dosage range was 400-6000 mg/day, and the duration of treatment varied from 1 to 14 months. Maintenance medications were held constant throughout and consisted of 16 patients taking neuroleptics, 8 of whom were taking anticholinergic agents, 1 taking lithium carbonate, and 16 taking no other drugs. During deanol therapy the tardive dyskinesia improved in 11 patients, remained unchanged in 13, and worsened in 4 patients. The patients with oromandibular dystonia, benign essential tremor, and spinocerebellar degeneration showed modest improvement but the patient with Huntington's disease was unchanged while taking deanol. Eight of the 33 patients experienced a pronounced mood change; 5 became depressed and 3 became hypomanic. All the patients who experienced mood changes were taking deanol in the range of 1000-2499 mg/day (Table 1). These changes in mood occurred 5-7 days after deanol had been raised to the respective dose and the mood changes spontaneously resolved within 5-10 days after deanol was changed to placebo or discontinued.

The eight patients who developed mood changes had tardive dyskinesia and a psychiatric diagnosis, while none of the five patients with other movement disorders developed mood changes or had psychiatric diagnoses. Of the eight patients, seven had histories of prominent affective symptoms serious enough to merit psychiatric attention. Six of these seven patients had experienced clinical depressions and the other patient had a history of bipolar mood changes associated with the diagnosis of schizoaffective schizophrenia. Of the 25 patients who had no mood change during deanol therapy, only 1 had a history of affective symptoms serious enough to warrant past psychiatric hospitalization. This patient had bipolar manic-depressive illness and was receiving mainte-ance lithium carbonate (serum lithium level of 1.0 mEq/l). Figure 1 displays the highly

TABLE 1

Mood Change and Deanol Dose

Deanol Range mg/day	Number of Patients Taking Deanol*	Number of Patients With Mood Change
200-499	33	0
500-999	32	0
1000-1499	26	1
1500-1999	22	4
2000-2499	13	3
2500-6000	4	0

*Number of patients receiving deanol, starting with the original 33 patients and continuing with smaller subgroups of the original 33. Dosage level was increased for a given patient until the movement disorder stabilized, affective symptoms developed, or other side effects appeared.

significant relationship between a prior history of affective symptoms and the occurrence of mood changes during deanol. This relationship is statistically significant at the 0.00003 level using the Fisher Exact Probability Test.

The changes in mood were not related to the changes in tardive dyskinesia during deanol therapy. Of the five patients who became depressed, two experienced improvement in their tardive dyskinesia, two became worse, and one was unaffected. Of the three patients who became hypomanic, one showed improvement in tardive dyskinesia, and two were unaffected. In the remaining 20 patients, 8 showed decreased dyskinetic movements, 10 were unaffected, and 2 became worse. There was no observable relationship between maintenance medications and changes in mood while taking deanol.

Alcohol abuse became a serious problem in five of the eight patients with mood changes (three with depression and two with hypomania). These five patients had histories of episodic or chronic alcohol abuse, but had been free of alcohol from 6 months to 7 years. The episodes of intoxication coincided with the periods of marked mood changes and spontaneously stopped when deanol was changed to placebo. The three depressed patients reported having an irresistible craving for alcohol and explained their intoxication as a way of escaping the dysphoria of depression. Two of the remaining 20 patients with tardive dyskinesia had past histories of alcohol abuse, but did not use alcohol while taking deanol. None of the patients with other movement disorders had histories of alcohol abuse, nor did they abuse alcohol while taking deanol. The abuse of alcohol was not related to the change in tardive dyskinesia during deanol treatment, as the dyskinesia improved in three patients, was unaffected in one patient, and worsened in one patient.

Six case histories are presented to illustrate the nature of the affective changes seen in some patients taking deanol.

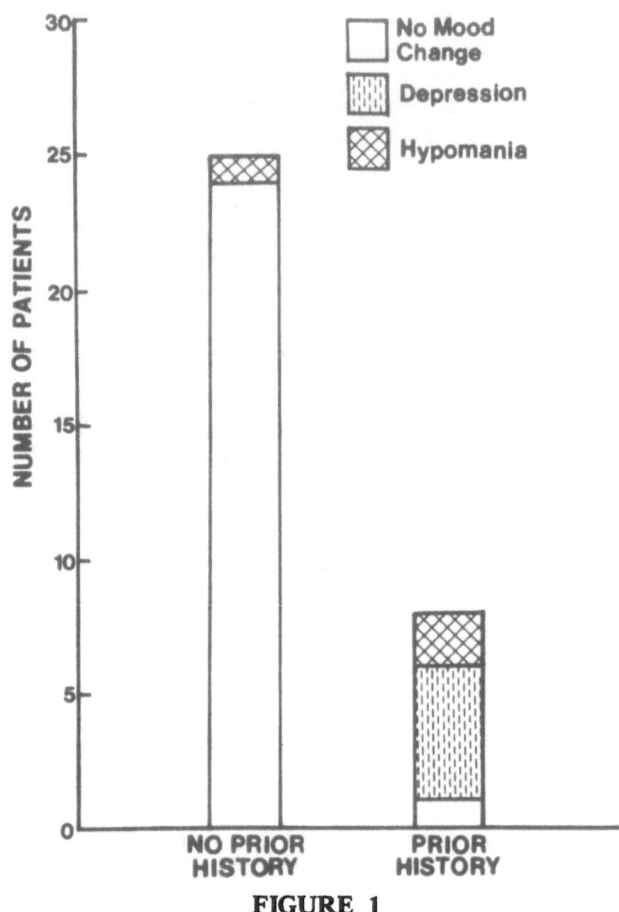

FIGURE 1

Mood Change During Deanol Therapy and Prior History of Affective Symptoms.

Case History 1

A 46-year-old man with a diagnosis of depressive neurosis had suffered from symptoms of chronic nonpsychotic depression, anxiety, insomnia, infrequent visual hallucinations of World War II battle scenes, and episodes of alcohol abuse. Since taking thioridazine 300 mg/day for the past 4 years, the patient had been doing well with a modest reduction of symptoms and no alcohol use. Signs of orofacial dyskinesias with finger and toe choreoathetosis had been present for the past 2 years.

Two weeks prior to starting deanol, the patient reported feeling depressed and felt like crying for about 4 hours after 1 mg of physostigmine I.V. Deanol, 800 mg/day, was given for 1 week without side effects. However, during the second week of deanol therapy of 1200 mg/day, the patient became tearful, reported somatic delusions about having cancer, felt that life had suddenly become hopeless, and began to make plans to purchase life insurance and then kill himself. He eloped from the hospital and became intoxicated for the first time in 4 years. His wife returned him to the hospital, saying she had never seen her husband so depressed. The deanol was discontinued; within 5 days the patient's mood returned to normal, and he sadly spoke about how depressed he had felt the week before. Deanol was restarted at 400 mg/day and gradually increased to a maintenance dose of 800 mg/day. The tardive dyskinesia improved without a recurrence of depression.

Case History 2

A 55-year-old man with a 30-year history of symptoms of social withdrawal, agitation, and auditory hallucinations commanding him to harm himself had been hospitalized for the past 18 months. He had made one serious suicide attempt 3 years prior by cutting both arms with a razor blade. His symptoms had been muted, but not fully controlled on thioridazine 1000 mg/day. Tardive dyskinesia, consisting of orofacial symptoms, increased blinking, truncal rocking, and choreoathetoid movements of hands and fingers had been evident for 3 years. The patient's dyskinesias increased while taking deanol, and at a dose of 2000 mg/day he became withdrawn, reported feeling depressed, and had many short uncontrollable crying spells. These symptoms resolved during the first week of placebo and the tardive dyskinesia returned to its pre-treatment level.

Case History 3

Episodes of withdrawal, violent outbursts against family members and property, nonpsychotic depression, and sprees of alcohol abuse were symptoms of this 52-year-old man's psychiatric disorder. Several trials with tricyclic antidepressants and anti-anxiety drugs were unsuccessful, but fluphenazine decanoate 25 mg I.M. q/14 days for the past 2 years had controlled the patient's symptoms. While taking deanol 1600 mg/day, he became withdrawn, depressed, cried easily, and said he felt compelled to abuse alcohol to escape depression. The patient subsequently became intoxicated three times, and then spontaneously stopped his alcohol abuse during the first week of deanol placebo. Within 1 week the depression resolved and his mood returned to normal. The tardive dyskinesia improved on deanol and gradually returned to its pre-treatment level at the end of 2 weeks of placebo.

Case History 4

A 52-year-old man with a diagnosis of chronic undifferentiated schizophrenia for 25 years had past psychotic symptoms of thought disorder, auditory hallucinations, paranoid delusions, and alcohol abuse during periods of active psychosis. These symptoms were controlled by trifluoperazine 10 mg/day and benztropine 2 mg/day, and the patient had remained out of the hospital for the past 9 years. Records documented neuroleptic use for the past 14 years. The patient reported mild tardive dyskinesia symptoms of tongue movements, tongue protrusion, and lip smacking movements for the past 3 years. Gradually increasing doses of deanol were added to the maintenance medications. During the fourth week of deanol, at 1600 mg/day, the patient reported a feeling of well-being, and a new level of energy. He began to sleep much less, developed pressured speech and a heightened affect, bought a car, and made plans to buy a new house. He also began to frequent bars and to express an interest in other women. Initially his wife was pleased to see her husband "happier than ever before" but a few days later she complained that she could not keep up with his energy level. Symptoms of thought disorder, auditory hallucinations, and paranoid delusions did not reappear.

During the first 10 days of placebo, the patient's euphoric mood diminished; he abandoned his plans for new purchases, stopped his alcohol consumption, and returned to his normal sleep pattern. The dyskinesias were almost completely suppressed while taking deanol and did not return during the ensuing 2 weeks of placebo.

Case History 5

A 40-year-old man with a diagnosis of schizoaffective schizophrenia for 15 years had demonstrated thought disorder, persecutory auditory hallucinations, grandiose and paranoid delusions, bipolar mood swings, and alcohol abuse during earlier periods of psychotic exacerbation. He had developed orofacial signs of tardive dyskinesia for the past 2 years while taking daily maintenance medications of haloperidol 15 mg and trihexyphenidyl 5 mg. After increasing deanol dosage to 1600 mg over a 4-week period, the patient became hyperactive, developed a euphoric affect, and insomnia. He left the hospital against advice, and became intoxicated on 2 consecutive days. These symptoms abated during the next 5 days following a switch to placebo. Neither deanol nor placebo had an effect on his movement disorder.

Case History 6

A 64-year-old man had been taking neuroleptic and anticholinergic drugs for the past 5 years for symptoms of social isolation, paranoid and somatic delusions, depression, and two suicide attempts. The medications were discontinued because they produced minimal improvement in the patient's depression and he was developing orofacial signs of tardive dyskinesia. Over the next 3 weeks the patient developed increased symptoms of tongue choreoathetosis and protrusions, respiratory grunting, truncal rocking, choreoathetosis of his hands and feet, and akathisia which had remained unchanged for 2 months before deanol was started. Modest improvement in his movement disorder occurred at 1200 mg/day, but a higher dosage was limited because late night insomnia developed. After 2 months, imipramine was added to treat persisting depressive symptoms of withdrawal, unkempt personal hygiene, and feelings of hopelessness. Over the ensuing 2 months imipramine was increased to 225 mg/day. There was no antidepressant effect, but it further aggravated all the movements, especially akathisia. Imipramine was discontinued and the patient signed himself out of the hosptial to live in a nursing home. Deanol 1200 mg/day was continued and the patient was followed at monthly intervals for the next 5 months without noticeable change in his dyskinesias or depression. Inadvertently the nursing home doubled the deanol dose to 2400 mg/day. At the next appointment, the patient was nicely dressed, had pressured speech, was euphoric, told of sleeping only 3-4 hours each night, had bought two automobiles, was now living in an apartment, and planned to start an automobile repair business. His tardive dyskinesia was unchanged, but he stated that he felt like his old self for the first time in 5 years. The deanol was discontinued, the hypomanic condition resolved, and the patient remained free of depression. The tardive dyskinesia has continued without change.

DISCUSSION

It has been proposed that counterbalancing cholinergic and adrenergic central nervous system influences modulates mood. Specifically, dominance by cholinergic influences results in depression, while dominance by noradrenergic influences results in mania (Janowsky *et al.*, 1972). The occurrence of depression during deanol therapy is consistent with this hypothesis, but further explanations may be necessary to account for the observations of elevated mood that are contrary to the specifically proposed etiological mechanisms of depression and mania.

Depression during deanol therapy is compatible with the hypothesis that depression results from a relative dominance of cholinergic influences. Deanol was first suggested as an acetylcholinergic precursor by Pfeiffer *et al.* (1957). Evidence supporting this proposal is suggestive, but not conclusive. Some studies have demonstrated a significant increase in whole brain acetylcholine following acute (Goldberg and Silbergeld, 1974) and long-term (Danysz *et al.*, 1967) deanol intake. Additionally, a significant increase in both striatal choline and acetylcholine was found following deanol administration (Haubrich *et al.*, 1975). However, other studies have not found these significant changes in brain acetylcholine (Zahniser *et al.*, 1977; Pepeu *et al.*, 1960). Clinical observations lend support to the notion that deanol may be a cholinergic precursor, as peripheral cholinergic symptoms of sweating, salivation, and bronchial constriction have been reported (Casey, 1977; Nesse and Carroll, 1976). Furthermore, deanol has produced variable clinical changes in patients with involuntary movement disorders thought to involve cholinergic mechanisms: tardive dyskinesia, Parkinsonism and levodopa-induced dyskinesias, and Huntington's disease (Casey, 1977). The occurrence of depression in one patient from both physostigmine and deanol also supports the notion that deanol may act through cholinergic mechanisms to produce depression.

Deanol-related depression is consistent with other findings that suggest an excess of central nervous system cholinergic activity may result in clinical depressive states. One study described an increased incidence of depression and parasympathetic toxicity in patients chronically exposed to organophosphate cholinesterase inhibitor insecticides (Gershon and Shaw, 1961), while other reports found depression commonly associated with drugs that inhibit acetylcholinesterase (Bowers *et al.*, 1964; Rowntree *et al.*, 1950). Additionally, physostigmine, a temporary acetylcholinesterase inhibitor, transiently reversed mania and produced depression in manic-depressive patients (Janowsky *et al.*, 1973a) and blocked the increased mood, activity, and talkativeness that followed the administration of methylphenidate (Janowsky *et al.*, 1973b). Two patients taking 9 grams/day of choline developed psychotic depression that resolved when the drug was discontinued (Tamminga *et al.*, 1976). Reserpine has also been implicated in depression. Although it is generally thought to reduce mood via amine depletion, its cholinomimetic actions may also contribute to causing depression (Bogdanski *et al.*, 1961).

Animal data using activity parameters as a model for depression also support the proposal that depression may result from a cholinergic excess. Self-stimulation (Domino and Olds, 1968) and locomotor activity (Fibiger *et al.*, 1971) in rats decreased when central cholinergic activity was increased.

Alternatively, deanol-related depressions could merely be manifestations of the cholinergic syndrome seen with physostigmine. This is usually characterized by lethargy, fatigue and mental dullness (Tamminga *et al.*, 1977; Davis *et al.*, 1976a). However, physostigmine has not produced the psychotic delusions, guilt, or self-disparagement that was seen in the patients receiving deanol in this report or choline (Tamminga *et al.*, 1976).

Although deanol might be expected to produce depression, hypomania during deanol therapy is seemingly inconsistent with the cholinergic-adrenergic balance concept of mood disorders. However, deanol may have properties other than as a putative cholinergic precursor. Initially it was classified as a stimulant because it enhanced the reticular activating system and produced EEG changes in animals and humans similar to amphetamines (Pfeiffer *et al.*, 1963; Murphree *et al.*, 1960). Many uncontrolled trials noted that deanol, in doses of 25-100 mg/day, relieved chronic fatigue and mild to moderate depression, and produced a mild increase in energy (Pfeiffer, 1959). Further clinical evidence supporting deanol's role as a stimulant comes from its beneficial effect in childhood hyperkinesis (Coleman *et al.*, 1976; Lewis and Young, 1964). Although there is very little biochemical data to support the contention that deanol is similar to dextroamphetamine, the fact that these drugs ameliorate some symptoms of hyperkinesis implies there may be some actions, perhaps catecholaminergic, common to both agents. In one patient who failed to benefit from 225 mg/day of imipramine, 2400 mg/day of deanol appeared to have antidepressant activity. This is supported by the temporal correlation of mood elevation after an increase in deanol, and the resolution of hypomania after stopping deanol. However, this must remain a curious observation since imipramine blood levels were not monitored and the change from depression to a brief period of hypomania may have occurred coincidentally.

Perhaps the heightened mood and increased level of energy are related to a compensatory adrenergic response. An increase in central nervous system acetylcholine produced by physostigmine initially led to a decrease in animal locomotion, but subsequently produced an increase in locomotion (Fibiger *et al.*, 1971). Although this phenomenon was demonstrated in animals given physostigmine acutely, it bears investigation as a possible explanation for deanol-related hypomania. While the idea of a compensatory rebound is speculatively interesting, the more compelling point is that virtually no information exists about the acute or long-term effects of deanol on central dopamine, norepinepherine, or serotonin. Preliminary investigations into the interactions of choline and adrenergic systems have shown that choline stimulates tyrosine hydroxylase (Ulus and Wurtman, 1976; Lewander *et al.*, 1975), and increases urinary catecholamine excretion (Scally *et al.*, 1977). Until information about the specific central nervous system interactions of cholinergic and aminergic influences becomes available, explanations regarding the actions of deanol and other proposed cholinergic precursors must be considered tentative and incomplete.

The significant finding that seven of the eight patients who developed a mood disorder during deanol therapy had a prior history of affective symptoms implies the existence of an underlying predisposition. Physostigmine produced a depression-like syndrome only in patients with prior affective symptoms and schizophrenics did not experience such affective changes (Janowsky *et al.*, 1973a). Also, physostigmine produced depression and crying in 2 of 17 normal controls who, on further questioning, related a history of mood changes with marijuana use or premenstrually (Davis *et al.*, 1976a).

Perhaps patients with histories of affective symptoms are more susceptible to drug-induced neurochemical imbalances because of a lower threshold or a reduced ability to modulate changes in brain chemistry. This is supported by the observation that affective symptoms did not occur until deanol was raised above 1000 mg/day, and resolved when the drug was reduced below the level which produced these symptoms. A similar phenomenon of increased sensitivity is seen in some manic-depressive patients who may become hypomanic while taking tricyclic antidepressants (Bunney et al., 1972), whereas patients without manic-depressive illness usually do not respond in this way to tricyclic drugs. Further evidence for the notion of an underlying predisposition comes from the finding that manic-depressive patients have significantly lower red blood cell cholinesterase activity than normal controls (Milstoc et al., 1975). While one patient with manic-depressive illness did not develop affective symptoms on 2000 mg/day of deanol, it might be argued that the maintenance lithium carbonate provided protection from deanol-related mood disorders. These findings suggest that caution should be used with deanol doses greater than 1000 mg/day in patients with prior histories of affective symptoms, as these patients may be more vulnerable to drugs which affect neurochemical systems regulating mood.

The absence of a relationship between the effect of deanol on mood and tardive dyskinesia raises interesting questions. It has been stated that more active patients with tardive dyskinesia tend to have higher scores on dyskinesia rating scales, while less active patients with tardive dyskinesia have lower scores (Tamminga et al., 1977). If this single parameter of activity was directly related to mood, patients who became depressed and withdrawn should have a reduction in their dyskinesias, while patients who became hypomanic would have an increase in their dyskinesias. However, no such relationship was seen. Any explanation of a relationship between affective disorders and tardive dyskinesia must take into account the pathophysiology of each disorder. Mood disorders are postulated to arise either from abnormalities in norepinephrine turnover (Bunney and Davis, 1965; Schildkraut, 1965), the interaction of cholinergic and adrenergic influences (Janowsky et al., 1972), or the balance between catecholaminergic and serotonergic influences (Asberg et al., 1975; Maas, 1975) in as yet undetermined neuroanatomical structures. Tardive dyskinesia is thought to involve hypersensitive dopamine receptors (Klawans, 1973) which interact with counterbalancing cholinergic influences in the striatum (Gerlach et al., 1974). A cholinergic role common to both affective disorders and tardive dyskinesia has been promulgated (Davis et al., 1976b), but the differences in neurochemistry, neuroanatomy, and receptor physiology suggest that any relationship between these two disorders will involve a complex interaction of variables.

It has been proposed that alcohol abuse may be a symptom of affective disorders (Barraclough et al., 1974; Winokur and Pitts, 1965). The interrelation of these two factors is supported by the finding that alcohol abuse occurred during the periods of most prominent mood disorder, and that the abuse subsided during placebo use. Since these patients had histories of alcohol abuse, it is likely that the mood disorder exacerbated an underlying symptom. Further evidence comes from the observation that 2 of the remaining 25 patients had histories of alcohol abuse, but did not develop mood changes or abuse alcohol while taking deanol. The reports that maintenance lithium carbonate reduced the alcohol abuse in patients with affective symptoms may be additional support for the proposed interaction of these two disorders (Merry et al., 1976).

SUMMARY

It has been proposed that mood disorders develop from an imbalance between cholinergic and adrenergic central nervous system influences. The observation that 8 of 33 patients taking deanol for involuntary movement disorders developed affective symptoms adds support to this concept. Deanol, a putative acetylcholine precursor, theoretically should produce depression; however, in this series of patients, five became depressed and three became hypomanic. A predisposition toward affective symptoms is suggested as seven of the eight patients who developed mood changes had prior histories of such symptoms, whereas only one patient with a history of mood disorder did not develop affective symptoms during deanol therapy. Since the effect of deanol on tardive dyskinesia and the development of affective symptoms were not related, these two disorders are not directly interactive, even though both disorders may involve disturbances in cholinergic function. Alcohol abuse became a clinical problem in five patients who developed affective symptoms and all had histories of alcohol abuse, suggesting that deanol-related mood disorders exacerbate the propensity toward alcohol abuse.

While the association of depression and cholinergic function is supported by these findings, there are the inconsistencies of some patients becoming hypomanic. Further research into the pharmacology of deanol and its effect on aminergic neurotransmitters is needed before the explanations of the observed phenomena can advance beyond the speculative stages. Toward this end, deanol could be a useful and unique tool for investigating some neurobiologic aspects of affective disorders.

ACKNOWLEDGEMENTS

The author wishes to acknowledge the expert technical assistance provided by Marian Karr. This work was supported in part by funds from the Portland Veterans Administration Hospital Research Committee, Portland, Oregon, MRIS #1314-01, and in part by funds from The Grass Foundation.

REFERENCES

Asberg, M., Thoren, P., Traskman, L., Bertilsson, L., and Ringberger, V., 1975, Serotonin depression — a biochemical subgroup within the affective disorders? *Science 191:*478.

Baldessarini, R.J., 1975, The basis for amine hypotheses in affective disorders, *Arch. Gen. Psychiatry 32:*1087.

Barraclough, B., Bunch, J., Nelson, B., and Sainsbury, P., 1974, A hundred cases of suicide: clinical aspects, *Br. J. Psychiatry 125:*355.

Bogdanski, D.F., Sulser, F., and Brodie, B.B., 1961, Comparative action of reserpine, tetrabenazine and chlorpromazine on central parasympathetic activity: effects on pupillary size and lacrimination in rabbit and on salivation in dog, *J. Pharmacol. Exp. Ther. 132:*176.

Bowers, M.B., Goodman, E., and Sim, V.M., 1964, Some behavioral changes in man following anticholinesterase administration, *J. Nerv. Ment. Dis. 138:*383.

Bunney, W.E., and Davis, J.M., 1965, Norepinephrine in depressive reactions, *Arch. Gen. Psychiatry 13:*483.

Bunney, W.E., Goodwin, F.K., and Murphy, D.L., 1972, The "switch process" in manic depressive illness, *Arch. Gen. Psychiatry 27:*312.

Casey, D.E., 1977, Deanol in the management of involuntary movement disorders: a review, *Dis. Nerv. Syst. 38:7.*

Cohen, E.L., and Wurtman, R.J., 1975, Brain acetylcholine: increase after systemic choline administration, *Life Sci. 16:*1095.

Cohen, E.L., and Wurtman, R.J., 1976, Brain acetylcholine: control by dietary choline, *Science 191:*561.

Coleman, N., Dexheimer, P., DiMascio, A., Redman, W., and Finnerty, R., 1976, Deanol in the treatment of hyperkinetic children, *Psychosomatics 17:*68.

Danysz, A., Kocmierska-Grodzka, D., Kostro, B., Polocki, B., and Kruszewska, J., 1967, Pharmacological properties of 2-dimethylaminoethanol (bimanol-DMAE), *Diss. Pharm. Pharmacol. 19:*469.

Davis, K.L., Hollister, L.E., Overall, J., Johnson, A., and Train, K., 1976a, Physostigmine: effects on cognition and affect in normal subjects, *Psychopharmacology 51:*23.

Davis, K.L., Berger, P.A., and Hollister, L.E., 1976b, Tardive dyskinesia and depressive illness, *Psychopharmacol. Comm. 2:*125.

Domino, E.F., and Olds, M.E., 1968, Cholinergic inhibition of self-stimulation behavior, *J. Pharm. Exp. Ther. 164:*202.

English, D.C., 1962, Reintegration of affect and psychic emergence with ditran, *J. Neuropsychiatry 3:*304.

Fibiger, H.D., Lynch, G.S., and Cooper, H.P., 1971, A biphasic action of central cholinergic stimulation on behavioral arousal in the rat, *Psychopharmacologia 20:*366.

Gerlach, J., Reisby, N., and Randrup, A., 1974, Dopaminergic hypersensitivity and cholinergic hypofunction in the pathophysiology of tardive dyskinesia, *Psychopharmacologia 34:*21.

Gershon, S., and Shaw, F.H., 1961, Psychiatric sequelae of chronic exposure to organophosphorus insecticides, *Lancet 7191(1):*1371.

Goldberg, A.M., and Silbergeld, E.K., 1974, Neurochemical aspects of lead-induced hyperactivity, *Trans. Amer. Soc. Neurochem. 5:*185.

Haubrich, D.R., Wang, P.F.L., Clody, D.E., and Wedeking, P.W., 1975, Increase in rat brain acetylcholine induced by choline or deanol, *Life Sci. 17:*975.

Janowsky, D.S., Davis, J.M., El-Yousef, M.K., and Sekerke, H.J., 1972, A cholinergic-adrenergic hypothesis of mania and depression, *Lancet 7778(2):*632.

Janowsky, D.S., El-Yousef, M.K., Davis, J.M., and Sekerke, H.J., 1973a, Parasympathetic suppression of manic symptoms by physostigmine, *Arch. Gen. Psychiatry 28:*542.

Janowsky, D.S., El-Yousef, M.K., Davis, J.M., and Sekerke, H.J., 1973b, Antagonistic effects of physostigmine and methylphenidate in man, *Am. J. Psychiatry 130:*1370.

Klawans, H.L., 1973, The pharmacology of tardive dyskinesia, *Am. J. Psychiatry 130:*82.

Lewander, T., Joh, T.H., and Reis, D.J., 1975, Prolonged activation of tyrosine hydroxylase in noradrenergic neurones of rat brain by cholinergic stimulation, *Nature 258:* 440.

Lewis, J.A., and Young, R., 1974, Deanol in learning disorders, *Clin. Pharmacol. Ther. 15(2):*210.

Maas, J.W., 1975, Biogenic amines and depression, *Arch. Gen. Psychiatry 32:*1357.

Merry, J., Reynolds, C.M., Bailey, J., and Coppen, A., 1976, Prophylactic treatment of alcoholism by lithium carbonate, *Lancet 7984(2):*481.

Milstoc, M., Teodoru, C.V., Fieve, R.R., and Kumbaraci, T., 1975, Cholinesterase activity and the manic depressive patients, *Dis. Nerv. Syst. 36:*197.

Murphree, H.B., Jr., Pfeiffer, C.C., and Backerman, I.A., 1960, The stimulant effect of 2-dimethylaminoethanol (deanol) in human volunteer subjects, *Clin. Pharmacol. Ther. 1(3):*303.

Nesse, R., Carroll, B.J., 1976, Cholinergic side-effects associated with deanol, *Lancet 7975(2):*50.

Pepeu, G., Freedman, D.X., Giarman, N.J., 1960, Biochemical and pharmacological studies of dimethylaminoethanol (deanol), *J. Pharmacol. Exp. Ther. 129:*291.

Pfeiffer, C.C., 1959, Parasympathetic neurohumors, possible precursors and effect on behavior, in *International Review of Neurobiology* (C.C. Pfeiffer and J.R. Smythies, eds.), pp. 195-244, Academic Press, New York.

Pfeiffer, C.C., Jenney, E.H., Gallacher, W., Smith, R.P., Bevan, J., Killam, K.F., Killam, E.K., and Blackmore, W., 1957, Stimulant effect of 2-dimethylaminoethanol — possible precursor of brain acetylcholine, *Science 126:*610.

Pfeiffer, C.C., Goldstein, L., Munoz, C., Murphree, H.B., and Jenney, E.H., 1963, Quantitative comparisons of the electroencephalographic stimulant effects of deanol, choline, and amphetamine, *Clin, Pharmacol. Ther. 4(4):*461.

Rowntree, D.W., Nevin, S., and Wilson, A., 1950, The effects of diisopropylfluorophosphonate in schizophrenia and manic depressive psychosis, *J. Neurol. Neurosurg. Psychiatry 13:*47.

Safer, D.J., and Allen, R.P., 1971, The central effects of scopolamine in man, *Biol. Psychiatry 3:*437.

Scally, M.C., Ulus, I.H., and Wurtman, R.J., 1977, Choline administration increases urinary catecholamine excretion in the rat, (Abstract), *The Pharmacologist 19:*526.

Schildkraut, J.J., 1965, The catecholamine hypothesis of affective disorders: a review of supporting evidence, *Am. J. Psychiatry 122:*509.

Sulser, F., Bickel, M.H., and Brodie, B.B., 1964, The action of desmethylimipramine in counteracting sedation and cholinergic effects of reserpine-like drugs, *J. Pharmacol. Exp. Ther. 144:*321.

Tamminga, C., Smith, R.C., Chang, S., Haraszti, J.S., and Davis, J.M., 1976, Depression associated with oral choline, *Lancet 7991(2):*905.

Tamminga, C., Smith, R.C., Ericksen, S.E., Chang, S., and Davis, J.M., 1977, Cholinergic influences in tardive dyskinesia, *Am. J. Psychiatry 134:*769.

Ulus, I.H., and Wurtman, R.J., 1976, Choline administration: activation of tyrosine hydroxylase in dopaminergic neurons of rat brain, *Science 194:*1060.

Winokur, G., and Pitts, F.N., Jr., 1965, Affective disorder: VI. A family history study of prevalence, sex differences and possible genetic factors, *J. Psychiatry Res. 3:*113.

Zahniser, N.R., Chou, D., and Hanin, I., 1977, Is 2-dimethylaminoethanol (deanol) indeed a precursor of brain acetylcholine? A gas chromatographic evaluation, *J. Pharmacol. Exp. Ther. 200:*545.

LITHIUM AND ACETYLCHOLINE INTERACTIONS

D. S. Janowsky, A. Abrams, S. McCunney, G. Groom and L. L. Judd

Department of Psychiatry, University of California at San Diego, School of Medicine, La Jolla, California 92093

INTRODUCTION

It has been proposed that affective disorders may be regulated by a complex balance between adrenergic and cholinergic factors, with depression being a disease of cholinergic predominance and mania being the converse (Janowsky et al., 1972a). As reviewed elsewhere (Janowsky et al., 1972a), much psychopharmacologic information supports this possibility, including the observation that effective antidepressant treatments such as the tricyclic antidepressants and ECT generally increase adrenergic activity and decrease cholinergic activity. Conversely, two effective antimanic agents, reserpine and haloperidol, increase cholinergic activity, and drugs which cause depression, such as reserpine and propranolol, have cholinergic, as well as antiadrenergic properties.

As an effective agent in the treatment of mania, the prevention of manic and depressive episodes, and in the possible treatment of some depressions (Gershon and Shopsin, 1973), lithium carbonate has received considerable investigative attention. Theories as to its mode of action have usually focused either on its ionic-membrane effects or its antiadrenergic properties. However, several studies have explored the effects of lithium on cholinergic mechanisms. It is the purpose of this chapter to review the work of others, and to present some preliminary behavioral data suggesting that lithium may effect the cholinergic, as well as the adrenergic nervous system.

A number of *in vitro* studies have suggested that lithium ion inhibits both presynaptic and postsynaptic acetylcholine (ACh) activity. Waziri (1968) found sodium-free seawater with 10-20 mEq/1 of lithium ion added reduced inhibitory postsynaptic potentials by 50% in an aplysia cholinergic interneuron, an effect they attributed to inhibition of presynaptic ACh release. Similarly, Onodera and Yamakawa (1966), using frog sciatic nerve-sartorius muscle preparations, found decreased resting end plate potentials and reduced posttetanic end plate potentials in preparations bathed in Ringer's solution in which lithium ion replaced sodium ion, although Branisteanu and Volle (1975) reported opposite findings.

45

Bjegovic and Randic (1971), sampling ACh from cat cerebral cortex perfused with Ringer-Locke solution in which lithium ion entirely replaced sodium ion, found no difference in the passive release of ACh. However, when a contralateral peripheral nerve was stimulated, ACh release was blocked in the presence of lithium ion. Vizi et al., (1972), using rat cortex slices, bathed in Krebs solution in which lithium ion replaced sodium, initially found increased resting ACh release, followed later by blockade of potassium stimulated ACh release. They also found that lithium blocked ACh synthesis in cortex slices. These authors proposed that decreased synthesis, decreased ion gradient across the cellular membrane, and reduced vesicular storage of ACh all contribute to a reduction in stimulated ACh output.

Lithium ion also may inhibit postsynaptic cholinergic mechanisms. Pappano and Volle (1967) reported that when cat superior cervical ganglion was perfused with Locke's solution in which lithium ion replaced sodium, ganglionic transmission and ACh induced depolarization of the ganglion decreased. These investigators concluded that lithium caused ganglionic blockade by depressing the postsynaptic activation of ganglion cells by ACh. However, Haas and Ryall (1974) found an increase in synaptic discharge after micro-electrophoretic administration of lithium to cholinergic spinal interneurons in the cat.

Also, there is some in vivo information suggesting that lithium may exert effects on the cholinergic nervous system. Neil et al., (1976) reported that myasthenia gravis is intensified in patients receiving lithium carbonate, presumably due to a decrease in the availability of neuromuscular acetylcholine. In contrast to data suggesting that lithium ion decreases cholinergic activity, Samples et al., (1977) recently noted that pretreatment with lithium chloride 100 mg/kg and 200 mg/kg i.p. of Simonsen rats for periods up to 4.5 days caused an increase in the lethal effects of the cholinesterase inhibitor, physo-stigmine. These results, shown in Table 1, suggest that lithium may indeed increase peripheral cholinergic effects, since lithium itself does not appear to alter cholinesterase activity (Simpson 1974).

TABLE 1

Lithium Chloride and Physostigmine Salicylate Lethality in Adult Male Rats

N=	Drugs	Lethality
15	Physostigmine 1 mg/kg	0%
10	LiCl 200 mg/kg (5 days)	0%
20	LiCl 200 mg/kg (4.5 days) + Physostigmine 1 mg/kg	80%
10	LiCl 200 mg/kg (1 day) + Physostigmine 1 mg/kg	40%
10	LiCl 100 mg/kg (4.5 days) + Physostigmine 1 mg/kg	40%
10	LiCl 200 mg/kg (4.5 days) + Scopolamine 1 mg/kg + Physostigmine 1 mg/kg	0%

To date, no studies of lithium's possible influence on ACh's behavioral effects have been reported. However, ACh activation causes profound behavioral effects (De Feudis, 1974; Arnfred and Randrup, 1968; Janowsky, *et al.*, 1972b) which could be influenced by lithium. In animals, as reviewed elsewhere (Janowsky *et al.*, 1972a), increasing central cholinergic activity induces behavioral inhibition, decreases intracranial self-stimulation, and causes alterations in operant behavior (Arnfred and Randrup, 1968). Recently, Janowsky *et al.*, (1972b) have found that physostigmine (a centrally active acetyl-cholinesterase inhibitor) given 10 min before methylphenidate injection, effectively prevents methylphenidate induced stereotyped gnawing behavior for a period of about 30 min, presumably by shifting dopaminergic-cholinergic balance to a cholinergic pre-dominance. The purpose of the experiment reported below is to determine *in vivo* whether acutely administered lithium influences the ability of physostigmine to prevent methylphenidate induced stereotyped gnawing behavior. If lithium indeed does affect the methylphenidate-physostigmine behavioral interaction, clues might be gained con-cerning lithium's antimanic and/or antidepressant effects.

METHODS

Adult mature male Sprague-Dawley rats (Simonsen Laboratories), weighing 200-350 g, housed under standard conditions with ad lib access to food and water, regulated on a 12 hr day-night cycle, were divided into four experimental groups of 39 rats each. For seven days prior to the experiment: 1) two groups received lithium chloride 100 mg/kg/day in drinking water, and two groups received tap water. 2) on the day of the experiment, one lithium pretreated group and one saline pretreated group received physo-stigmine salicylate 0.2 mg/kg s.q. in 0.2 ml saline: the other lithium pretreated and saline pretreated groups received saline 0.2 ml (0.9%) s.q. 3) ten minutes later, all groups received methylphenidate hydrochloride 57.8 mg/kg i.p. Thus, 1) one group received saline, followed by saline, followed by methylphenidate; 2) one group received lithium, followed by saline, followed by methylphenidate; 3) one group received saline, followed by physostigmine, followed by methylphenidate; and 4) one group received lithium, followed by physostigmine, followed by methylphenidate. Rats were then rated by a trained observer, blind to the drug treatments, every five min for 20 min. Rats were rated for 1) the presence or absence of stereotyped gnawing behavior; and 2) the strength of methylphenidate induced stereotyped gnawing behavior, using a scale in which gnawing behavior was rated from 1 to 5 (1 = not at all, 5 = continuous and intense). Experimental groups were then compared for the degree of methylphenidate induced stereotyped gnawing behavior using an analysis of variance for repeated measures, and for presence or absence of gnawing behavior using a chi square analysis.

RESULTS

Table 2 shows the percentage of rats showing stereotyped gnawing behavior during the 20 min observation phase under the various experimental conditions. Physostigmine alone significantly decreased the incidence of methylphenidate induced gnawing behavior when compared to the saline pretreated rats, the lithium pretreated rats, and the rats receiving a combination of physostigmine and lithium. Thus, pretreatment with lithium chloride significantly reversed the ability of physostigmine to inhibit methylphenidate induced stereotyped gnawing behavior. Analysis of variance similarly demonstrated a significant physostigmine-lithium interaction ($p < .05$).

TABLE 2

Effects of Physostigmine Salicylate*, Lithium Chloride,
and Saline Alone and in Combination
on Methylphenidate Hydrochloride Induced Stereotyped Gnawing
Behavior in Sprague-Dawley Rats

Group	Drugs Given	Number of Rats Gnawing	% Rats Gnawing
1	Saline + Saline + Methylphenidate	29/38	76%
2	Lithium + Saline + Methylphenidate	33/39	85%
3	Saline + Physostigmine + Methylphenidate	12/39	31%
4	Lithium + Physostigmine + Methylphenidate	27/39	69%

* physostigmine salicylate = 0.2 mg/kg sq; lithium chloride = 100 mg/kg p.o. x 7 days; methylphenidate hydrochloride = 58 mg/kg i.p.; saline = normal saline p.o. x 7 days.

** $p < .001$ = comparison of difference between physostigmine + methylphenidate (Group 3) and other experimental groups. No other experimental groups differed significantly from each other.

DISCUSSION

The results of this preliminary experiment indicate that the administration of lithium chloride for seven days reversed physostigmine's antagonism of methylphenidate induced stereotyped gnawing behavior. This effect is consistent with most neurophysiologic and biochemical observations indicating that administration of lithium ion decreases ACh activity (i.e., turnover, etc.). Thus, our results parallel the majority of neurochemical studies of lithium's effects on cholinergic transmission. Our results are not consistent with those of Samples *et al.*, (1977), who demonstrated that chronic lithium chloride administration increased the toxicity of both neostigmine and physostigmine, thus suggesting a facilitation of ACh activity. Possibly, chronic lithium treatment, by decreasing ACh activity, causes ACh receptor hypersensitivity, leading to hyper-responsiveness in the peripheral nervous system. Alternatively, the central and peripheral effects of lithium on the cholinergic nervous system may differ.

Before proceeding to discuss the theoretical implications of our results, a number of qualifications are indicated. It is important to note that our observed antagonism of physostigmine's effects occurred using one methylphenidate, one lithium, and one physostigmine dose, given at single points in time (i.e. after seven days of lithium). Alteration of any of these variables might have changed our findings. Indeed, in replications of the above experiment, results occurred most consistently when a dose of physostigmine sufficient to cause almost complete suppression of methylphenidate induced gnawing behavior was given. When low doses of physostigmine, capable of causing only minimal suppression of methylphenidate's effects were utilized, less consistent results occurred. Thus, although lithium appears to antagonize physostigmine induced behavioral effects, the exact nature of this interaction and its complexities will require further study.

In spite of the above reservations, our results may have important theoretical implications. Evidence has accumulated suggesting that adrenergic-cholinergic balance may play a role in affective disorders (Janowsky et al., 1972a), with depression being a disease of relatively increased central ACh activity and mania being a disease of relatively increased adrenergic (i.e. noradrenergic or dopaminergic) activity. Support for this hypothesis includes the observations that: 1) physostigmine, a cholinesterase inhibitor, antagonizes manic symptoms (Janowsky et al., 1972a); 2) induces depression in patients with an affective component to their illness (Janowsky et al., 1974); 3) induces severe depression in marijuana-intoxicated normal volunteers (El-Yousef et al., 1973; Davis et al., 1976); and 4) rapidly antagonizes methylphenidate-induced psychostimulation and euphoria (Janowsky et al., 1973). Furthermore, choline, an ACh precursor, has been reported to induce severe depression in several psychiatric patients with tardive dyskinesia (Tamminga et al., 1976). Conversely, L-DOPA and methylphenidate activate mania, and methylphenidate antagonizes physostigmine induced depression and anergy. Thus, it is at least possible that methylphenidate's and physostigmine's effects on rat gnawing behavior may be an animal model for mania and depression respectively (Janowsky et al., 1972b), since these agents activate mania, cause depression and antagonize each other respectively in man (Janowsky et al., 1973).

Lithium carbonate has been noted to alleviate mania, alleviate depression, and to be prophylactic against recurrent episodes of depression and mania (Gershon and Shopsin, 1973). To date, no entirely satisfactory mechanistic explanation of lithium's effects on both mania and depression has been proposed. As reviewed by Flemenbaum (1977), and others (Katz et al., 1968), lithium has been noted to decrease adrenergic activity and to antagonize d-amphetamine, methylphenidate and apomorphine induced psychostimulation in animals, and these findings have been used to support an antiadrenergic hypothesis of lithium's action. Although our results suggest that, if anything, lithium may actually exaggerate stereotyped gnawing behavior (presumably a dopaminergic phenomenon), our results also demonstrate that lithium may, at least in rats, antagonize the cholinergic effects of physostigmine, an effect which could be an animal model of lithium's effects on depression. Thus, lithium could be postulated to have a bidirectional effect on presumptive animal models of both mania and depression, based on its effects on adrenergic and cholinergic mechanisms respectively. If the assertions of others concerning lithium's antiadrenergic effects are correct, lithium could "normalize" the adrenergic and cholinergic nervous system of patients with affective disorder, antagonizing both adrenergic activity, and thus alleviating mania; and simultaneously decreasing cholinergic activity, and thus decreasing or preventing depression. Although such speculations are at present most tentative, the further study of the effects of lithium on behavioral cholinergic mechanisms, both in animals and in man, would seem to be indicated.

ACKNOWLEDGEMENTS

This work was supported in part from the Medical Research Service of the Veterans Administration Hospital, San Diego, (MRIS #4576) and NIMH Grant #1 P50 MH 30914-01.

REFERENCES

Arnfred, T., and Randrup, A., 1968, Cholinergic mechanisms in brain inhibiting amphetamine-induced stereotyped behavior, *Acta Pharmacol. Et. Toxicol. 26:*384.

Bjegonic, M., and Randic, M., 1971, Effect of lithium ions on the release of acetylcholine from the cerebral cortex, *Nature 230:*487.

Branisteanu, D.D., and Volle, R.L., 1975, Modification by lithium of transmitter release at the neuromuscular junction, *J. Pharmacol. Exp. Ther. 194:*362.

Davis, K.L., Hollister, L.E., Overall, J., Johnson, L., and Train, K., 1976, Physostigmine: effects on cognition and affect in normal subjects, *Psychopharmacologia (Berl.) 51:*23.

DeFeudis, F.U., 1974, *"Central Cholinergic Systems and Behavior,"* Academic Press, New York.

El-Yousef, M.K., Janowsky, D.S., Davis, J.M., and Rosenblatt, J.E., 1973, Induction of severe depression by physostigmine in marijuana intoxicated individuals, *Br. J. Addict. 68:*321.

Flemenbaum, A., 1977, Lithium inhibition of norepinephrine and dopamine receptors, *Biol. Psychiatry 12:*563.

Gershon, S., and Shopsin, B., 1973, *"Lithium: Its Role in Psychiatric Research and Treatment,"* Plenum Press, New York.

Haas, H.L., and Ryall, R.W., 1974, Proceedings: a selective excitatory effect of lithium on cholinoceptive neurones in the spinal cord and brain of cats and rats: a possible significance in manic-depression, *Br. J. Pharmacol. 52:*444P.

Janowsky, D.S., El-Yousef, M.K., Davis, J.M., and Sekerke, H.J., 1972a, A cholinergic-adrenergic hypothesis of mania and depression, *Lancet 2:*632.

Janowsky, D.S., El-Yousef, M.K., Davis, J.M., and Sekerke, H.J., 1972b, Cholinergic antagonism of methylphenidate-induced stereotyped behavior, *Psychopharmacologia (Berl.) 27:*295.

Janowsky, D.S., El-Yousef, M.K., Davis, J.M., and Sekerke, H.J., 1973, Antagonistic effects of physostigmine and methylphenidate in man, *Am. J. Psychiatry 130:*1370.

Janowsky, D.S., El-Yousef, M.K., and Davis, J.M., 1974, Acetylcholine and depression, *Psychosom. Med. 36:*248.

Katz, R., Chase, N., and Kopin, I.J., 1968, Evoked release of norepinephrine and serotonin from brain slices: inhibition by lithium, *Science 162:*466.

Neil, F., Himmelhoch, J.J., and Licata, S.M., 1976, Emergence of myasthenia gravis during treatment with lithium carbonate, *Arch. Gen. Psychiatry 33:*1090.

Onodera, K., and Yamakawa, K., 1966, The effects of lithium on the neuromuscular junction of the frog, *Jpn. J. Physiol. 16:*541.

Pappano, A.J., Volle, R.L., 1967, Actions of lithium ions in mammalian sympathetic ganglia, *J. Pharmacol. Exp. Ther. 157:*346.

Samples, J., Janowsky, D.S., Pechnick, R., and Judd, L.L., 1977, Lethal effects of physostigmine plus lithium in rats, *Psychopharmacologia (Berl.) 52:*307.

Simpson, L.L., 1974, The effects of lithium and physostigmine on rat brain acetylcholinesterase activity, *Psychopharmacologia (Berl.) 38:*145.

Tamminga, C., Smith, R.C., Chang, S., Haraszti, J.S., and Davis, J.M., 1976, Depression associated with oral choline, *Lancet 2:*905.

Vizi, E.S., Illes, A., Ranai, A., and Knoll, J., 1972, Effect of lithium ions on the release of acetylcholine from the cerebral cortex, *Neuropharmacology 11:*521.

Waziri, R., 1968, Presynaptic effects of lithium on cholinergic synaptic transmission in aplysia neurons, *Life Sci. 7:*865.

CEREBROSPINAL FLUID ACETYLCHOLINESTERASE IN PSYCHOSIS AND MOVEMENT DISORDERS

K. L. Davis[1,2], J. Livesey[1], L. E. Hollister[1,2] and P. A. Berger[1,2]

[1]Veterans Administration Hospital, 3801 Miranda Avenue,
Palo Alto, California 94304

[2]Department of Psychiatry and Behavioral Sciences, Stanford University
School of Medicine, Stanford, California 94305

INTRODUCTION

Acetylcholinesterase (AChE) has been identified in cerebrospinal fluid (CSF) (Kalsbeek *et al.*, 1950; Svensmark, 1961; Johnson and Domino, 1971; Yaksh *et al.*, 1974). The majority of CSF AChE has been shown to derive from the brain with little if any contribution from the plasma (Yaksh *et al.*, 1975). The possibility of a large contribution to CSF AChE from the spinal cord is unlikely as histochemical studies of spinal tracts have failed to demonstrate appreciable staining for AChE (Koelle, 1963). The caudate nucleus contains the highest concentrations of AChE (Yaksh *et al.*, 1975). Its proximity to the lateral ventricles suggests that this structure makes a sizeable contribution to total CSF AChE.

Brain AChE can be either membrane bound or in a soluble form (Hollunger and Niklasson, 1973; Wenthold *et al.*, 1974). Under normal conditions the origin of CSF AChE is presumed to be the soluble fraction (Yaksh *et al.*, 1975). The physiological role of soluble AChE is not clear, complicating any interpretation of the pathophysiological importance of CSF AChE. In patients suffering from degenerative brain diseases membrane bound AChE could conceivably enter the CSF.

Thus, existing data indicates that CSF AChE is derived from the brain, with the basal ganglia being a major source. However, of total brain AChE, only a small part gets into the CSF, and this is probably from the soluble fraction. The relationship between the activity of brain AChE and CSF AChE is not determined. However, abnormalities in central cholinergic activity have been postulated to underlie a number of neuropsychiatric disorders (Davis *et al.*, 1975). Conceivably, cholinergic abnormalities in patients with some of these conditions could be reflected in CSF AChE.

This study investigated CSF AChE in normal subjects and in patients with Huntington's disease, depression and schizophrenia. In addition, the effects of the drugs physostigmine and probenecid on CSF AChE activity were determined.

METHODS

Subjects

Twenty-five male subjects between the ages of 21 and 60 gave their informed consent to participate in this study and undergo a lumbar puncture (LP).

Huntington's Disease

Five patients had a diagnosis of Huntington's disease. All these patients had a family history of Huntington's disease for at least one previous generation, and all displayed typical choreiform movements. These patients had from one to four lumbar punctures. The first LP was done at 8:00 a.m. The following day at 3:00 p.m. some patients had a second LP after receiving 100 mg/kg of probenecid in divided doses. Approximately 2 months later this double LP procedure was repeated, if possible. Not all patients participated in the entire study. Four of the five subjects were receiving neuroleptics at the time of their LPs. All subjects who had a second pair of LPs were also receiving 20 gm of choline chloride daily.

Depression

Four patients met diagnostic criteria for primary affective disorder, depression (Feighner *et al.*, 1972). One of these patients had a prior history of mania. These patients had two LPs at 8:00 a.m. on 2 consecutive days. Patients were drug free for a minimum of 2 weeks before the LPs. Prior to the second LP patients received 100 mg/kg of probenecid in divided doses.

Schizophrenia

Seven patients met diagnostic criteria for schizophrenia (Feighner *et al.*, 1972). Four patients were given the diagnosis of chronic undifferentiated schizophrenia, two patients the diagnosis of schizoaffective, and one patient the diagnosis of paranoid schizophrenia according to DSM II (Committee on Nomenclature and Statistics of the American Psychiatric Association, 1968). Four patients underwent two LPs separated by 24 hours, both performed at 8:00 a.m. Three patients only participated in one LP. All patients received no neuroleptics for at least 2 weeks before the LPs. In all cases the second LP was preceded by a 24-hr period in which patients received 100 mg/kg of probenecid. One patient who underwent a single LP also was given 100 mg/kg of probenecid in divided doses.

Mania

One patient met diagnostic criteria for primary affective disorder, mania. He underwent a single LP at 8:00 a.m. preceded by the administration of probenecid in a dose of 100 mg/kg. He was also taking 20 gm of choline chloride per day.

TABLE 1

Diagnosis, Drug Administration, and Time of Lumbar Puncture

Patient	Diagnosis	Time of L.P.	Probenecid	Neuroleptics	ChCl
H.S.	Schizophrenia	8			
		4	X		
O.M.	Huntington's	8		X	X
	Chorea	8		X	
		8	X	X	
J.H.	Huntington's	8			X
	Chorea	8	X		X
		8			
		8	X		
J.C.	Huntington's Chorea	4	X		
J.E.H.	Schizophrenia	8			
		8	X		
M.B.	Schizophrenia	2			
		2	X		
S.C.	Schizophrenia	8			
G.B.	Huntington's	8		X	
	Chorea	8	X	X	
T.O.	Schizophrenia	8			
G.H.	Schizophrenia	8			
		3	X		
M.J.B.	Mania	8	X		X
J.R.	Depression	8			
		8	X		
R.L.	Depression	8			
		8	X		
L.S.	Depression	8			
		8	X		
L.O.	Depression	8			
		8	X		
K.S.	Huntington's	8			
	Chorea	3	X		

Normals

Eight subjects were without an immediate or family history of psychiatric illness. These subjects underwent two LPs separated by a 1 week interval. LPs were performed at 2:00 p.m. For 18 hr before the LPs all subjects received 100 mg/kg of probenecid in divided doses. Four and one-half hours prior to one of their LPs subjects received 2.0 mg of physostigmine by a constant infusion over a 60-min period. Prior to their other LP, subjects received a saline infusion, between 9:30 am and 10:30 am. The order of saline and physostigmine infusions were randomized. Patients, drugs, diagnosis and time of LP are summarized in Table 1.

RESULTS

All results are reported in terms of true AChE activity per mg protein in CSF. However, statistical analyses based on activity per mg glucose in CSF or activity per ml CSF yielded the same degree of statistical significance as activity per mg protein.

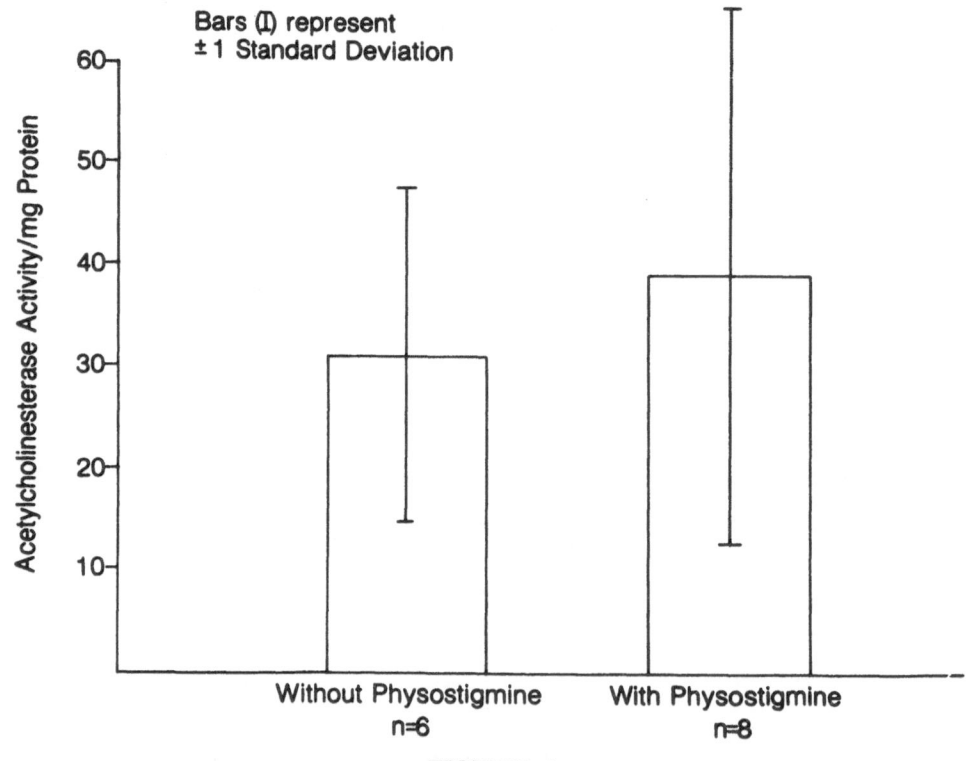

FIGURE 1

Acetylcholinesterase Activity: Effect of Physostigmine

Physostigmine

The differences between CSF AChE activity on days when normal subjects received physostigmine and days when the same subjects receive saline were not significant. These results are presented in Figure 1.

Probenecid

CSF AChE activity was compared in patients who received probenecid before their second LP with CSF AChE activity from their first LP. No significant effect of probenecid on CSF AChE activity was found, as summarized in Figure 2.

Diurnal Variations

Diurnal variations in CSF AChE activities from all lumbar taps performed at 8:00 am were compared with AChE activity from 2:00-4:00 pm. No significant differences were found. These results are presented in Figure 3. Similarly no diagnostic subgroup had a significant diurnal rhythm of AChE activity. Although probenecid and physo-

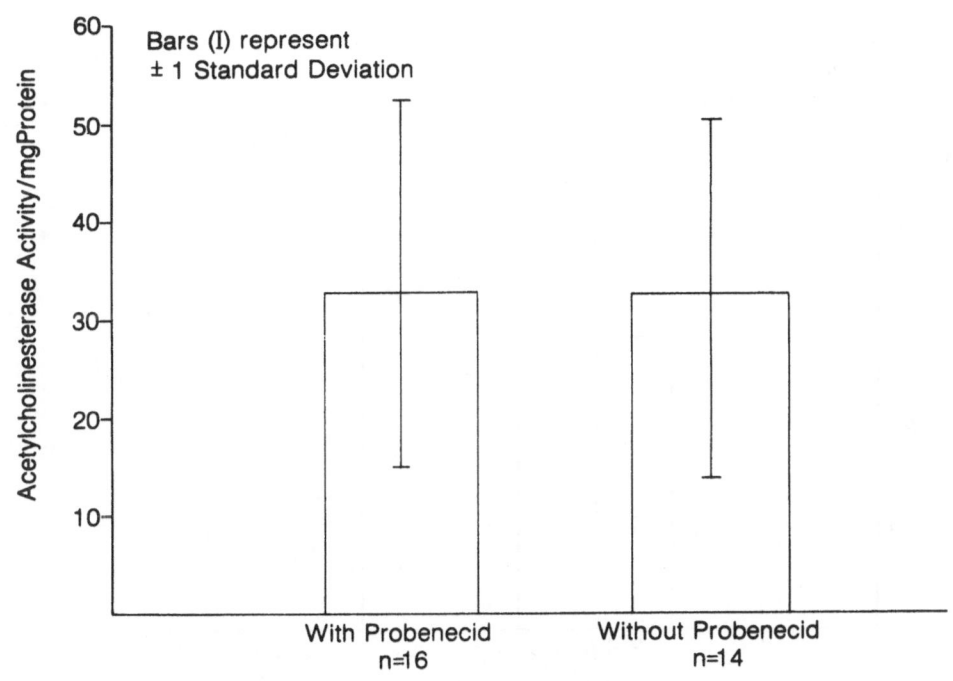

FIGURE 2

Acetylcholinesterase Activity: Effect of Probenecid

stigmine were not shown to have a significant effect on CSF AChE, separate analyses were conducted to eliminate any effect these drugs might be having on possible diurnal variations. Only LPs from patients or normal subjects in which probenecid was administered, and those from normal subjects who did not receive physostigmine were compared. Still there was no significant difference between 8:00 am and 2:00 pm to 4:00 pm LPs.

Choline

Comparison of CSF AChE activity in 4 patients, who received choline chloride was compared to CSF AChE activity in 11 patients who had not received choline chloride, but whose LPs were at the same time of day. As Figure 4 illustrates, choline chloride treatment had no effect on CSF AChE.

DISCUSSION

AChE activity has been measured in the red blood cell, plasma and brain of patients with a number of neurological and psychiatric disease (Domino *et al.*, 1973; Milstoc *et al.*, 1975; Whittaker and Barry, 1977). Euthymic manic-depressive patients are reported to have decreased mean red blood cell true cholinesterase activity, although there is some

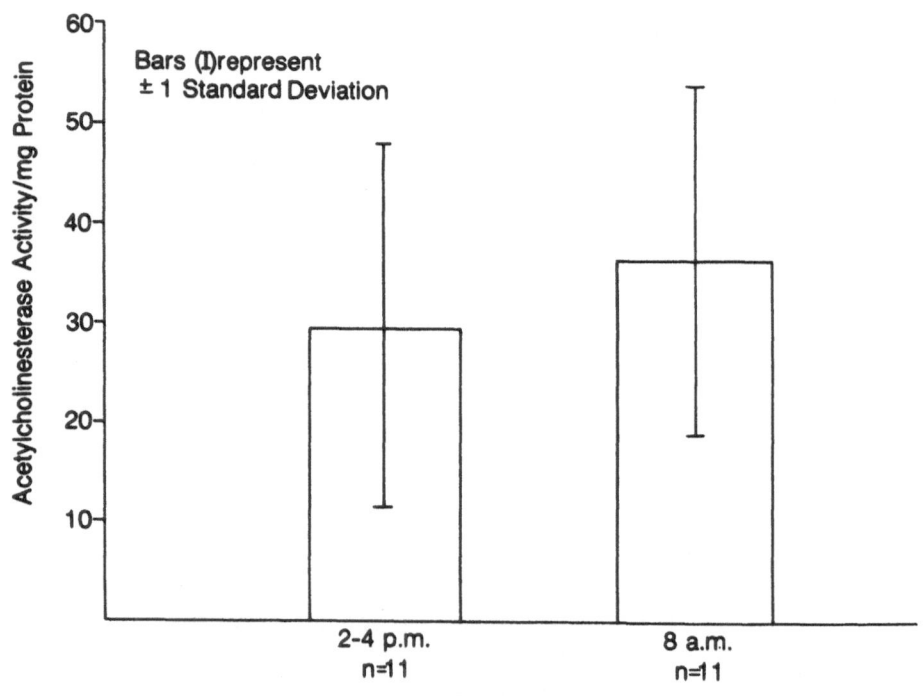

FIGURE 3

Acetylcholinesterase Activity: Effect of Time

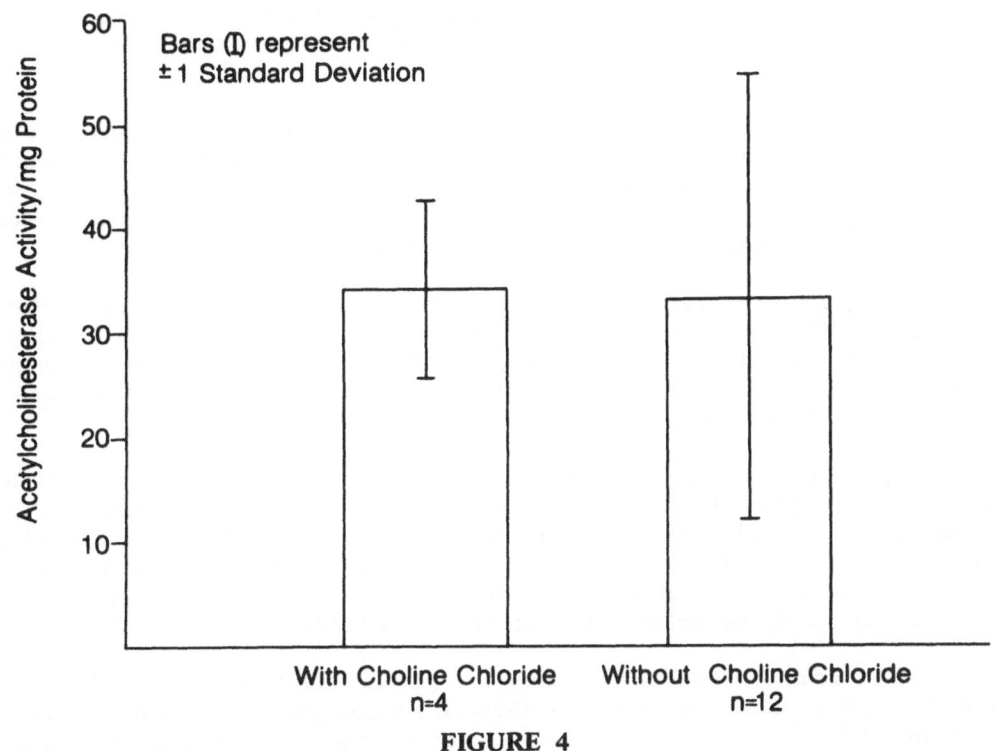

FIGURE 4

Acetylcholinesterase Activity: Effect of Choline Chloride

overlap between patients and controls. Patients and controls did not differ in plasma true cholinesterase activity (Milstoc *et al.*, 1975). In contrast, two groups have reported elevated plasma total cholinesterase activities in a mixed group of psychotic patients compared to healthy controls (Tod and Jones, 1937; Richter and Lee, 1942a; 1942b). There is further disagreement as to the activity of plasma cholinesterase in patients with a diagnosis of schizophrenia. Both increased and decreased total plasma cholinesterase activity have been reported (Antebi and King, 1962; Domino *et al.*, 1975).

Electrophoretic analysis has been used to help determine plasma total cholinesterase phenotypes in patients with various neuropsychiatric disease. These procedures have determined that patients with psychosis and Huntington's chorea are significantly more likely to have an unusual phenotypic variant of plasma total cholinesterase than the normal population. However, the plasma total cholinesterase activity of these patients did not differ from normals (Whittaker and Barry, 1977).

A study conducted on brains obtained at autopsy investigated total cholinesterase, AChE and pseudocholinesterase along the human visual systems. Patients dying with a diagnosis of chronic schizophrenia and organic brain syndrome were compared to patients without neuropsychiatric illness. The schizophrenic group had significantly higher total cholinesterase activity in the superior colliculus and lateral geniculate than the other groups.

Although no significant differences in CSF AChE were noted in this study, some of the negative findings are of interest. Despite striatal degeneration in patients with Huntington's disease, true AChE activity in these patients was almost identical to CSF true AChE activity in normal subjects. In contrast, CSF choline activity has been reported to be low in patients with Huntington's disease (Aquilonius *et al.*, 1972).

CSF true AChE of patients with a diagnosis of affective disease or schizophrenia also did not differ from normal controls. This could indicate no real effect of those disorders on true AChE. However, this negative result could be an artifact of the origin of CSF true AChE, which might in large part derive from brain areas that are unaffected by these psychiatric disorders.

Physostigmine, a drug known to be both a central and peripheral total AChE inhibitor, also had no effect on CSF true AChE. Since physostigmine was administered over a one-hour period, 3½-4½ hr before the lumbar puncture, and physostigmine has a relatively short half-life, it seems likely that the effects of physostigmine were no longer present by the time of the lumbar puncture. During the physostigmine infusion all of the subjects experienced central effects of AChE inhibition.

Choline administration has been shown to increase brain levels of ACh (Haubrich *et al.*, 1964; 1975; Cohen and Wurtman, 1976). It has been presumed that elevated brain acetylcholine levels occur through increased availability of precursor. However, choline is also a breakdown product of ACh. If AChE is subject to negative feedback inhibition by choline, it is possible that patients receiving large doses of choline would alter CSF true AChE. This was not found in the patients in this study despite the fact that the oral ingestion of 20 gm per day of choline chloride has been reported to increase CSF choline (Growdon *et al.*, 1977). This is a preliminary study, and additional investigation will be required to verify and extend these findings. Further important information regarding central cholinergic function would be derived from simultaneous determinations of CAT and AChE.

ACKNOWLEDGEMENTS

This research was supported by the Medical Research Service of the Veterans Administration, National Institute of Mental Health Specialized Research Center Grant MH-30854, U.S. Public Health Service Grant MH-03030, and the Kate Pande Memorial Research Fund.

REFERENCES

Antebi, R.N., and King, J., 1962, Serum enzyme activity in chronic schizophrenia, *J. Ment. Sci. 108:*75.

Aquilonius, S.M., Nystrom, B., Schuberth, J., and Sundwall, A., 1972, Cerebrospinal fluid choline in extrapyramidal disorders, *J. Neurol. Neurosurg. Psychiatry 35:*720.

Davis, K.L., Hollister, L.E., Berger, P.A., and Barchas, J.D., 1975, Cholinergic imbalance hypotheses of psychoses and movement disorders: Strategies for evaluation, *Psychopharmacol. Comm. 1(5):*533.

Cohen, E.L., and Wurtman, R.J., 1976, Brain acetylcholine control by dietary choline, *Science 191:*561.

Committee on Nomenclature and Statistics of the American Psychiatric Association, 1968, *"Diagnostic and Statistical Manual of Mental Disorders,"* American Psychiatric Association, Washington, D.C.

Domino, E.F., Krause, R.R., and Bowers, J., 1973, Regional distribution of some enzymes involved with putative neurotransmitters in the human visual system, *Brain Res. 58:* 179.

Domino, E.F., Thiessen, M.M., and Batsakis, J.D., 1975, Blood protein fraction comparisons of normal and schizophrenic patients, *Arch. Gen. Psychiatry 32:*717.

Feighner, J.P., Robins, R., Guze, S.B., Woodruff, R.A., Winokur, G., and Munoz, R., 1972, Diagnostic criteria for use in psychiatric research, *Arch. Gen. Psychiatry 26:*57.

Growdon, J.H., Cohen, E.L., and Wurtman, R.J., 1977, Effects of oral choline administration on serum and CSF choline levels in patients with Huntington's disease, *J. Neurochem. 28:*229.

Haubrich, D.R., Wedeking, P.W., and Wang, P.F.L., 1964, Role of choline in biosynthesis of acetylcholine, *Fed. Proc. 33:*477.

Haubrich, D.R., Wang, P.F.L., Clody, D.E., and Wedeking, P.W., 1975, Increase in rat brain acetylcholine induced by choline or deanol, *Life Sci. 17:*975.

Hollunger, E.G., and Niklasson, B.H., 1973, The release and molecular state of mammalian brain acetylcholinesterase, *J. Neurochem. 20:*821.

Johnson, S., and Domino, E.F., 1971, Cholinergic enzymatic activity of cerebrospinal fluid of patients with various neurological disease, *Clin. Chim. Acta. 35:*421.

Kalsbeek, S., Cohen, J.A., and Bovens, B.R., 1950, Cholinesterase in cerebrospinal fluid, *Biochem. Biophys. Acta 5:*548.

Koelle, G., 1963, Cytological distribution and physiological functions of cholinesterase, in *"Handbuch der Experimentellen Pharmakologie"* (O. Eichler and A. Farah, eds.), pp. 243-245, Springler-Verlag, Berlin.

Milstoc, M., Teodoru, C.V., Fieve, R.R., and Kumbaraci, T., 1975, Cholinesterase activity and the manic depressive patient, *Dis. Nerv. Syst. 36:*197.

Richter, D., and Lee, M., 1942a, Serum cholinesterase and anxiety, *J. Ment. Sci. 88:* 428.

Richter, D., and Lee, M., 1942b, Serum cholinesterase and depression, *J. Ment. Sci. 88:* 435.

Svensmark, O., 1961, Cholinesterases in human spinal fluid and brain, *Acta Physiol. Scand. 52:*372.

Tod, H., and Jones, M.S., 1937, A study of the cholinesterase activity in nervous and mental disorders, *Q. J. Med. 6:*1.

Wenthold, R.J., Mahler, H.R., and Moore, W.J., 1974, Properties of acetylcholinesterase from rat brain, *J. Neurochem. 22:*945.

Whittaker, M., and Barry, M., 1977, The plasma cholinesterase variants in mentally ill patients, *Br. J. Psychiatry 130:*397.

Yaksh, T.L., Fedele, C.A., and Yamamura, H.I., 1974, Recovery of cholinesterase activity in cerebrospinal fluid, brain stem and plasma of the unanesthetized cat after irreversible cholinesterase inhibition. *Experientia 30:*38.

Yaksh, T.L., Filbert, M.G., Harris, L.W., and Yamamura, H.I., 1975, Acetylcholinesterase turnover in brain, cerebrospinal fluid and plasma, *J. Neurochem. 25:*853.

BRAIN CHOLINERGIC ENZYMES IN SCHIZOPHRENIA

E. F. Domino

Department of Pharmacology, University of Michigan,
Ann Arbor, Michigan 48109

Laboratory of Pharmacology, Lafayette Clinic,
Detroit, Michigan 48207

INTRODUCTION

It is a fact that acetylcholine (ACh) is involved in many aspects of animal and human behavior (Karczmar and Dun, 1978). It is natural that the cholinergic system be investigated for possible abnormalities in mental disease including the schizophrenias. The enzymes of obvious interest are those which synthesize and hydrolyze ACh. In addition, the levels of the two substrates acetylcoenzyme A and choline are of great importance, as well as the turnover of both substrates and their product ACh. In human autopsy material the cholinergic brain enzymes and receptors are the only substances that can be measured reliably. Hence, this review will concentrate on these enzymes in schizophrenia.

These are two major forms of enzymes which hydrolyze ACh. One type found mainly in the human brain and red blood cells is acetylcholine acetylhydrolase (E.C. 3.1.1.7) commonly known as "true" or acetylcholinesterase (AChE). The other type, found mainly in blood plasma but also in the brain, is acetylcholine acetylhydrolase (E.C. 3.1.1.8) commonly known as "pseudo" or butyrylcholinesterase (BChE). When the terms AChE or BChE are used then one is specifically referring to these enzymes. On the other hand, if the general term cholinesterase (ChE) is used, either or both enzymes may be referred to. Hence, ChE does not specify exactly what is being measured except enzymes which hydrolyze ACh. Some chemical assays measure both AChE and BChE, hence total cholinesterase (TChE). When TChE is measured then this term is used instead of ChE. The term ChE is reserved for those times when the specific enzymes described are not clear or when it is purposely meant to be more general.

Among the important chemical variables which influence ChE activity are: 1. The source of the enzyme such as red cell, plasma, cerebrospinal fluid, brain, etc. 2. The substrate used such as ACh, methacholine (MCh), butyrylcholine (BCh), benzolylcholine, acetylthiocholine, etc. 3. The temperature and pH of the reaction mixture as well as other methodological variables. 4. Clinical variables including psychiatric diagnosis, age, sex, diurnal rhythm, time of menstrual cycle, nutritional status, type of medication, dosage, duration of therapy, etc. 5. Genetic factors related to genotype and phenotype of the cholinesterase activity being measured. Thus, there is little wonder why there has been a large number of conflicting reports in this field. Inasmuch as the activity of the enzymes in non-brain tissues such as blood does not necessarily reflect what is happening in the brain, this review will concentrate on the evidence that the cholinergic system in the brain is altered in the schizophrenias.

In 1971 we reviewed the literature regarding cholinesterase activity in the blood, cerebrospinal fluid and brain in mental disease (Domino and Krause, 1971). We concluded that stress and psychiatric conditions with marked autonomic discharge increase plasma BChE activity. Some chronic schizophrenic patients have decreased plasma or serum BChE activity, suggesting a possible metabolic, liver, nutritional, or genetic deficiency. The AChE activity of red cells of chronic schizophrenics generally is within normal limits.

The predominant form of human cerebrospinal fluid (CSF) cholinesterase is AChE. The activity of AChE and BChE in CSF vary independently from each other and from that in red cells and plasma. There is some evidence of an increase in CSF cholinesterase activity in chronic schizophrenics.

The predominant form of brain cholinesterase is AChE. Frontal cortical AChE activity may be increased in some chronic schizophrenic patients. Further research is needed on the relationship of mental illness and cholinesterase activity in blood and especially CSF and brain. Since 1971 a number of studies have appeared on the cholinergic enzyme activity of deceased chronic schizophrenic patients. As background material the reader would do well to refer to the recent chapters by Jenden (1977), J. Davis *et al.* (1977) and K. Davis *et al.* (1977) in the recent book by Usdin *et al.* (1977) and by Berger *et al.* (1978) in the book by Lipton *et al.* (1978).

Especially relevant is the observation of J. Davis *et al.* (1977) that physostigmine in doses of 1.25 to 1.5 mg i.v. does not alter the psychotic thinking of schizophrenic patients but does induce psychomotor depression and increased symptoms of depression. These authors suggested a behavioral antagonism between the cholinergic and dopaminergic system in a variety of behavioral states. Evidence for this hypothesis is the fact that physostigmine effectively antagonizes the psychosis activation of methylphenidate in schizophrenic patients (Janowsky *et al.*, 1973).

As pointed out by K. Davis *et al.* (1977), there is both animal and human evidence that altered central cholinergic activity may have an etiological role in schizophrenia, especially in the context of an enhanced dopaminergic and reduced cholinergic system model (Friedhoff and Alpert, 1973). Pfeiffer and Jenney (1957) suggested that arecoline, a predominant muscarinic cholinergic agonist, caused a transient lucid interval in schizophrenic patients. A similar observation has been made with the reversible cholinesterase inhibitor physostigmine given to catatonic patients (Van Andel, 1959). Both arecoline and physostigmine readily penetrate the blood brain barrier and hence act both centrally and peripherally. Rosenthal and Bigelow (1973) reported some very exciting preliminary observations that patients who were therapy resistant to dopamine antagonists improved dramatically in 2 to 17 days when oral physostigmine was combined with the neuroleptic. However, tolerance developed and produced a return in a few weeks to their previous psychopathology. The beneficial effects of combined cholinergic agonist-dopaminergic antagonist therapy must be verified, for the theoretical implications of such therapy are enormous. It should be pointed out that there is "soft" evidence that anticholinergic drugs that penetrate blood-brain barrier may reduce the therapeutic effectiveness of neuroleptics in patients (Singh and Smith, 1973) and in animals (Hanson *et al.* 1970). However, the reduced therapeutic effectiveness of such drug combinations has not been observed generally. When given alone to schizophrenic patients, the muscarinic anticholinergic Ditran activates psychotic symptoms in addition to producing memory loss (Gershon and Olariu, 1960). What does not fit are the observations that chronic administration of cholinesterase inhibitors that penetrate the blood-brain barrier intensify schizophrenic symptoms (Rowntree *et al.*, 1950; Gershon and Shaw, 1961). These data would be compatible with a hypothesis of deficient ACh only if there is an excess of ACh producing "depolarization" blockade and hence decreased functional ACh activity.

In summary, most of the clinical psychopharmacological evidence would suggest that there is decreased central cholinergic function in schizophrenic patients. A related model is that of Huntington's chorea in which there appears to be a functional cholinergic deficit, although other neurotransmitters like GABA are also involved in this neurological disease.

BRAIN CHOLINESTERASE

Brain ChE activity has been measured in mental patients since 1941. Both AChE and BChE are found in the central nervous system but AChE predominates (Augustinsson, 1963). Birkhauser (1941b) determined gross regional brain TChE activity using ACh as the substrate in six female and five male schizophrenics from 9 to 40 hours postmortem. The brain areas studied were the neocortex, thalamus and basal ganglia including the caudate, putamen and pallidum. As might be expected from animal data, the basal ganglia showed the greatest TChE activity and the cortex the least. A total of 15 to 23 brains of mentally healthy patients who died of physical diseases served as controls. No difference in TChE activity was noted between the various brain areas of schizophrenics and those of mentally normal subjects.

Pope *et al.* (1949) studied the histochemical distribution of TChE and acid phosphatase in prefrontal cortex obtained by biopsy at the time of neurosurgery of both psychotics and non-psychotics. These investigators used ACh as the substrate. In a limited number of patients they found that enhanced TChE activity was correlated with clinical diagnosis. Five of the seven patients with deteriorated schizophrenia showed an increase in cortical (area 9) TChE activity exceeding the range found in patients with intractable pain and psychoneurosis.

These investigators also studied the quantitative cytotechtonic distribution of ChE and showed the amount to be relatively great in layer I in the II-III junction, in the midzones of III and of V, and in VIB. These are the cortical layers of rich axonal plexuses. For example, the acellular plexiform layer is layer I and the probable zone of thalamic afferents is layer IIIB. There was a greater tendency for the histochemical reaction to be reduced in the deteriorated schizophrenics (8 of 12) than among the chronic pain and psychoneurotic patients (1 of 4), although these may represent normal variations. It was of special interest that the brain biopsies showed insignificant deviations histologically despite the presence of a quantitative increase in ChE activity. One of the problems of interpreting these data was that two of the control patients with intractable pain were on a morphine regimen for some time. Morphine is a known but variable inhibitor of ChE, depending on enzyme source (Long, 1963). However, the other two chronic patients were neurotics and actually had even lower ChE activity.

In a subsequent report, Pope *et al.* (1952) described the architectonic distribution of AChE in the frontal isocortex (area 9 of Bronmann, FDm of von Economo, IEfs of Bailey and von Bonin) in a larger series of patients. The AChE activity of psychotics showed a much greater range than that of the non-psychotics. In this larger series of psychotics not matched for age and clinical status, the cortical AChE activity was not significantly different from that of controls. However, when the patients were separated into more homogeneous clinical groups the elevation in AChE activity was statistically significant (p <.05). Thiopental anesthesia was ruled out as a critical variable by Pope *et al.* (1952) inasmuch as rats killed by excessive doses showed no difference in brain AChE in comparison to unanesthetized rats.

Similarly, Schutz (1943) has shown that single anesthetizing doses of barbiturates do not alter guinea pig brain ChE activity. However, chronic administration of barbiturates to guinea pigs does lower ChE activity in muscle and spinal cord but not in cerebellum. Schutz (1944) also reported that serum BChE activity was reduced in epileptics given prolonged barbiturate medication.

In 1952 Sherwood injected a suspension of human red cell AChE with penicillin into the frontal horn of the lateral ventricle of a female schizophrenic. The patient collapsed after three hours and needed to be treated as a medical emergency. After a mild fever for three days, she became more lucid and alert. There was an amelioration of her psychotic state for at least seven weeks. Subsequently, a smaller amount of intraventricular red cell AChE injected with 10,000 U of penicillin caused a generalized convulsion with recovery and again some mental improvement. However, these changes were not long lasting. In another patient this treatment seemed of little value. There is no good rationale for the use of an intraventricular suspension of AChE in schizophrenia. Even if there was a documented deficiency of brain AChE, one could hardly expect the enzyme to distribute itself at suitable cholinergic synaptic sites in the brain. It would appear that the recovery of the first patient was due to a form of shock therapy and was not specifically related to the AChE administered.

Takahashi and Ogushi (1953) determined the TChE activity of areas 9 and 10 of the frontal lobe of 10 schizophrenic patients subjected to topectomy. ACh was used as substrate. One oligophrenic and three psychopathic patients were subjected to the same therapeutic procedure. In general, mean cortical TChE activity of the schizophrenics was similar to that of the psychopaths. The oligophrenic had the lowest TChE activity and a paranoid schizophrenic had the highest. Five hebephrenics tended to have lower and four catatonics had intermediate cerebral enzymatic activity. In view of the wide variation and small sample size, these investigators concluded that there was no significant difference in cortical TChE activity of schizophrenics compared to psychopaths.

We had an opportunity to study postmortem 15 different regional brain levels of various cholinergic enzymes in six mentally normal and eight chronic schizophrenic patients who died of various physical diseases (Domino et al., 1973; Domino, 1976). The mean ± SE age of the mentally normal group was 53.5 ± 9.9, that of the chronic schizophrenic patients was 62.2 ± 4.9 years. Using a group comparison t-test, the age difference between the normals and the chronic schizophrenics was not statistically significant. The concentration of protein/gm of wet brain tissue among the various brain areas was approximately 10%. There were no significant differences between the mentally normal and chronic schizophrenic patients.

Using ^{14}C-ACh as substrate, marked regional differences in TChE were found in the brain areas studied. The lowest activity was present in the frontal cortex and the highest activity in the body of the caudate nucleus. There were no significant regional brain differences between the mentally normal and chronic schizophrenics except that the septal area of chronic schizophrenics showed significantly less TChE ($p < .05$). These findings were also significant when the TChE was normalized by comparing each value to the rat brain standard run simultaneously.

Using the specific AChE inhibitor, BW 284c51, and subtracting residual ChE activity, an estimate of AChE activity was obtained. As has been described previously for brain tissue, we showed via this technique that the major cholinesterase activity is due to AChE. The qualitative distribution of AChE in the brain was similar to that of TChE with the frontal cortex showing the lowest and the caudate the highest activity in both the mentally normal and chronic schizophrenic groups. In addition to a significant decrease ($p < .05$) in AChE in the septal area, the head of the caudate of the chronic schizophrenics also showed significantly lower activity ($p < .05$). When the data was normalized by comparing each value to rat brain standard run simultaneously, only the difference in the septum remained significant ($p < .05$). BChE did not show as striking regional differences as seen with AChE. However, the relative activity, with cerebral cortex being lowest and caudate nucleus highest, still remained the same. Surprisingly, BChE was enhanced compared to the mentally normal group in the posterior hypothalamus, hippocampus, medial amygdala, cingulate gyrus, caudate nucleus (all portions), anterior cerebellum, pons and reticular formation of the chronic schizophrenic patients. These differences were significant ($p < .05$ to .01). When the data was normalized, that is, expressed as a fraction of the BChE standard for each assay, the differences were still statistically significant ($p < .05$ to .01).

Very recently, McGeer and McGeer (1977) measured a number of enzymes including AChE in a total of 50 regions in the brains of 11 chronic schizophrenic patients, 2 patients with senile dementia, one depressive patient and 18 mentally normal controls. They used a colorimetric method for measuring TChE using acetylthiocholine as the substrate. They refer to this as AChE activity throughout most of their studies.

In reality they are measuring TChE. They reported that the only statistically significant findings were abnormally high levels in the septal area and thalamus of the schizophrenic patients. Our own data (Domino et al., 1973; Domino, 1976) in which ^{14}C-ACh was used as the substrate to measure TChE activity indicated that the septal area showed statistically significant decreases. This diametrically opposite finding seems very strange indeed and can only be resolved with further research, especially with a better anatomical definition of what is meant by the septum (Domino, 1976). Thalamic TChE activity in our chronic schizophrenic patients was normal. Our findings that BChE activity was enhanced in most of the brain areas of the schizophrenic patients would be only in partial agreement with a measure of TChE activity. There is a great need in any neurochemical study of brain ChE to distinguish between AChE and BChE activity. For example, Op den Velde and Stam (1976) showed that AChE is reduced while BChE activity is increased in the temporal lobe of patients with Alzheimer's dementia. Such evidence suggests declining neuronal (AChE) and increasing glial (BChE) activity. Although both ChE enzymes are found in neurons, there is evidence that glial ChE activity is predominantly BChE. Davies (1977) has reported that both AChE and ChAc are decreased to less than 25% of normal in the hippocampus of patients with Alzheimer's disease. Surprisingly, McGeer and McGeer (1977) found no change in TChE in the hippocampus in their two cases of senile dementia. In our preliminary study of three patients with a senile organic brain syndrome, hippocampal TChE was 41% of normal, a figure in agreement with Davies (1977) for Alzheimer's disease. This strengthens our own conviction that as far as the schizophrenic brain is concerned BChE tends to be overactive, while AChE activity is essentially intact except in the septal area where it is low. Only more research will tell what is true. In any event, the ChE activity picture indicates that most areas of the schizophrenic brain can readily hydrolyze ACh. This is consistent with the recent clinical pharmacological observation that the cholinesterase inhibitor physostigmine does not make schizophrenics worse.

CEREBROSPINAL FLUID CHOLINESTERASE

Brain AChE is primarily in a bound non-soluble form. Nevertheless, both AChE and BChE are found in the CSF, presumably in equilibrium with brain pools of these enzymes. On the basis of this assumption, seven investigators have studied cholinesterase activity in the CSF of mental patients. Recently Chubb *et al.* (1976) raised the issue that AChE may be secreted from central neurons into the CSF.

Birkhauser (1941a,b) made a comparative study of brain, serum and CSF TChE activity using ACh as substrate. He was able to show, as was expected from animal studies, that much more TChE was present in the putamen of the brain than in serum or CSF. The TChE ratio of putamen: plasma: CSF was 3800:200:1. In 18 chronic schizophrenic patients CSF TChE activity was greater than that of normals. Since ACh was the substrate used, it was unclear whether AChE, BChE, or both were involved.

Subsequently, Reiss and Hemphill (1948) determined CSF cholinesterase activity using ACh, MCh and BCh as substrates. They studied a wide variety of psychotic patients with both organic and non-organic components. These investigators showed that AChE is the predominant form of ChE in human CSF. Marked individual variation in CSF ChE activity was observed but could not be correlated with any specific psychiatric diagnosis. The ratio of TChE activity in the CSF to that in the serum using ACh as substrate was 1:90 to 1:150. With MCh as substrate (to measure AChE) it was 1:8 to 1:40 and with BCh as substrate (for BChE) it was 1:125 to 1:300.

Early *et al.* (1949) also determined AChE and BChE activity in the CSF of various psychiatric patients. There was no difference in CSF ChE activity between old (mean age ± SE = 70.8 ± 6.3) psychotics and young (mean age ± SE = 25.3 ± 12.4) mental defectives using either ACh, MCh or BCh as substrates. No data were given on the CSF cholinesterase activity in psychotic patients compared to normals so that the findings of Birkhauser that CSF cholinesterase activity is elevated in schizophrenic patients was neither supported nor disproved. An interesting observation of Early *et al.* (1949) was that low serum or CSF ChE activity in mental defectives was not related to brain size. The major contribution of the study by Early *et al.* (1949) is that there is no correlation between ChE in serum and CSF in the same patient. CSF ChE activity, either AChE or BChE, could be the same whether serum AChE or BChE activity was high or low. The data of Early *et al.* (1949) on the independence of serum AChE and BChE are in agreement with that of Plum (1960). Our analysis of the published data of Early *et al.* (1949) showed that serum BChE and AChE activity in mental defectives is highly correlated ($r = +.793$, $p < .05$) but the activity of the enzymes is not correlated in the geriatric psychotics ($r = -.274$). In contrast, CSF AChE activity is significantly correlated with BChE activity ($r = +.626$, $p < .05$) in geriatric psychotics but not significantly correlated ($r = +.390$) in mental defectives. These data suggest an occasional relationship between AChE and BChE activity in serum or CSF. Their conclusion that AChE and BChE are independent enzymes from separate sources and compartments seems quite valid.

Birkhauser's data that CSF TChE activity is elevated in chronic schizophrenic patients is also of interest in view of the report of Rabassini and Chirillo (1957) of an increase in CSF glutamate pyruvate transaminase activity (GP-T) in schizophrenics. Antebi and King's (1962) report that serum GP-T is normal strengthens the conclusion that activity of an enzyme in the serum is unrelated to the activity of that enzyme in CSF.

An ACh-like substance is present in human CSF (Schain, 1960; Duvoison and Dettbarn, 1967) on the basis of bioassay. This substance occurs in very small concentrations apparently below the effective substrate concentration for either AChE or ChE. Another possibility is that it is protected by protein binding (Escalar and Galli, 1957). Nevertheless, it is of interest that Poloni (1951) found ACh-like activity in the CSF of 10 normals and many patients with neurological and neuropsychiatric conditions but only 2 of 50 schizophrenics had detectable CSF ACh. Poloni considered the absence of ACh in the CSF pathological. However, Turner and Mauss (1959) found ACh-like activity in the CSF in 4 of 12 schizophrenics, 5 of 8 epileptics and 21 of 41 other neurological patients. It would appear that there is not a specific absence of an ACh-like material in the CSF of schizophrenics but it may be reduced, a finding consistent with Birkhauser's data that CSF TChE activity is elevated.

Recently, B. Holmstedt (personal communication, 1977) has claimed that there is no ACh in human CSF, based on very sophisticated GC-MS techniques. Hence, the entire issue of what was bioassayed as an ACh-like material remains to be resolved in the future.

BRAIN CHOLINE ACETYLTRANSFERASE

Domino *et al.* (1973) and Domino (1976) also measured the activity of CAT in the same 15 brain areas of six mentally normal and eight chronic schizophrenic patients as described above. The distribution of CAT was qualitatively similar to that of TChE, AChE and BChE. In general, the lowest enzyme activity was in the cerebral cortex and the highest in the caudate nucleus. A similar pattern of distribution was seen in both the mentally normal and chronic schizophrenic patients. There was no significant difference between any of these groups except that the medial amygdala of the chronic schizophrenics showed twice the activity when compared to the normals (p < .05). This difference was still present when the data were normalized. Even when normalized there was no difference in septal CAT between these two groups, although there was a clear trend for a decrease in activity in the septum of the four schizophrenic patients measured. Of particular importance was the observation that the hippocampus of six chronic schizophrenic patients also showed no statistically significant change in CAT activity, although there was a tendency for CAT activity to be decreased but not as much as in the septal area. Obviously, the small number of subjects studied contributed to the lack of statistical significance observed. A slightly larger series of schizophrenic patients and mentally normal controls who subsequently died were studied by Wise *et al.* (1974) and Wise and Stein (1975). Although these investigators stressed a central noradrenergic deficiency in schizophrenia based on decreased brain dopamine *beta* hydroxylase activity, they also showed a statistically significant decrease in CAT activity in the pons-medulla, hippocampus and diencephalon of schizophrenic patients. Since the controls were younger and CAT activity correlated inversely with age (r = -0.67 in the diencephalon of the controls), these investigators matched both groups for age. After age matching, a statistically significant decrease in hippocampus ChAc activity was observed in the 14 schizophrenics compared to 9 controls (p < .05). These findings are in direct disagreement with those of McGeer and McGeer (1977) in which they reported that CAT activity was about three times higher in the hippocampus of the chronic schizophrenics. It should be noted that McGeer and McGeer (1977) found that hippocampal activity was normal in two patients with senile dementia, a finding which again disagrees with Davies (1977), Perry and Perry (1977) and Perry *et al.* (1977). All of these latter studies indicate a profound decrease in CAT in the hippocampus of patients with Alzheimer's presenile and senile dementia.

CHOLINERGIC RECEPTORS

Specific binding of a ligand to a receptor is an excellent method of quantifying receptors. In general, specific ligand binding must be saturable, of high affinity, usually membrane or particulate bound, and must show appropriate changes with pharmacological manipulation. Both agonists and antagonists of high specific activity have been used in various receptor studies. With regard to cholinergic receptors, the muscarinic antagonists atropine and 3-quinuclidinyl benzilate (QNB), and the nicotinic antagonist *alpha* bungarotoxin especially have been used. Since the brain contains a preponderance of muscarinic receptors, ^{3}H-QNB has been popular as a measure of ACh receptors in animal studies (Yamamura *et al.*, 1974; Kuhar and Yamamura, 1976). By assaying particularly the enzyme of synthesis of a transmitter and the number of its receptors, one can obtain evidence of selective vulnerability of a specific neurotransmitter in any brain disease. This approach has been used most successfully to prove the vulnerability of cholinergic neurons in Alzheimer's disease (Bowen and Davison, 1977). These investigators have shown that in this disease about one half of the nerve cells of the temporal lobe are lost. Markers of glial cells are unaffected. Markers of cholinergic neurons like CAT and high affinity binding of atropine, as a measure of muscarinic ACh receptor sites, indicate the specific vulnerability of cholinergic neurons in autopsy material from deceased schizophrenic patients. R.J. Wyatt and S. Snyder (personal communication, 1978) have observed that the number of QNB binding sites are normal in the brains of schizophrenic patients. Since ACh receptors are both pre- and postsynaptic, their studies would indicate that there is no specific cholinergic neuronal vulnerability in schizophrenia per se.

CONCLUSIONS

If one smells smoke, there probably is a fire nearby. By analogy, there is some evidence of a central cholinergic disturbance in schizophrenia. One smells "cholinergic" related smoke but has not found the fire. Although changes in cholinergic enzyme activity have been reported that differ from normal, their biologic significance is questionable. For example, it is well known that one can inhibit AChE up to 80 to 90% before functional impairment results. At what level increased cholinergic enzyme activity will result in functional alteration is not known.

The evidence for a cholinergic disturbance in schizophrenia is, at best, weak. Nevertheless, it would appear that further research to test the hypothesis of a functional disturbance of too much dopamine and too little ACh in some brain areas may lead to novel drug therapies for current neuroleptic resistant schizophrenic patients. We have so few leads as to the biological disturbances in the schizophrenias that it is incumbent that we pursue this one.

ACKNOWLEDGEMENTS

Supported in part by a grant from the Michigan State Legislature to the Lafayette Clinic for schizophrenia research.

REFERENCES

Antebi, R.N., and King, J., 1962, Serum enzyme activity in chronic schizophrenia, *J. Ment. Sci. 108:*75.

Augustinsson, K.B., 1963, Classification and comparative enzymology of the cholinesterases and methods for their determination, *"Handbuch der Experimentellen Pharmakologie, Vol. 15"* (G.B. Koelle, ed.), pp. 89-128, Springer-Verlag, Berlin.

Berger, P.A., Elliott, G.R., and Barchas, J.D., 1978, Neuroregulators and schizophrenia, in *"Psychopharmacology: A Generation of Progress"* (A. DiMascio, K.F. Killam, and M.A. Lipton, eds.), pp. 1071-1095, Raven Press, New York.

Birkhauser, H., 1941a, Cholinesterase im normalen und pathologischen Liquor cerebrospinalis des Menschen, *Schweiz. Arch. Neurol. Psychiatr. 46:*185.

Birkhauser, H., 1941b, Cholinesterase und Mono-Aminoxydase im zentralen Nervensystem, *Schweiz. Med. Wochenschr. 71:*750.

Bowen, D.M., and Davison, A.N., 1977, Selective vulnerability of neurons in Alzheimer's disease, *Br. J. Psychiatry 131:*319.

Chubb, I.W., Goodman, S., and Smith, A.D., 1976, Is AChE secreted from central neurons in the cerebral fluid? *Neurosci. 1:*57.

Davies, P., 1977, Cholinergic mechanisms in Alzheimer's disease, *Br. J. Psychiatry 131:*318.

Davis, J.M., Janowsky, D., and Casper, R.C., 1977, Acetylcholine and mental disease, in *"Neuroregulators and Psychiatric Disorders"* (E. Usdin, D.A. Hamburg, and J.D. Barchas, eds.), pp. 434-441, Oxford University Press, New York.

Davis, K.L., Hollister, L.E., and Berger, P.A., 1977, Cholinergic mechanisms in neurological and psychiatric disorders, in *"Neuroregulators and Psychiatric Disorders"* (E. Usdin, D.A. Hamburg, and J.D. Barchas, eds.), pp. 442-450, Oxford University Press, New York.

Domino, E.F., 1976, Cholinergic enzyme activity in the septum and related brain areas in deceased mentally normal, chronic schizophrenic and organic brain syndrome patients, in *"The Septal Nuclei"* (J.F. DeFrance, ed.), Plenum Press, New York.

Domino, E.F., and Krause, R.R., 1971, Cholinesterase activity and mental disease: a literature review, *Michigan Mental Health Research Bulletin 5:*3.

Domino, E.F., Krause, R.R., and Bowers, J., 1973, Various enzymes involved with putative neurotransmitters. Regional distribution in the brain of deceased mentally normal, chronic schizophrenics or organic brain syndrome patients, *Arch. Gen. Psychiatry 29:* 195.

Duvoison, R.C., and Dettbarn, W.D., 1967, Cerebrospinal fluid acetylcholine in man, *Neurology 17:*1077.

Early, D.F., Hemphill, R.E., Reiss, M., and Brummel, E., 1949, Investigations into cholinesterase levels in serum and cerebrospinal fluid of psychotic patients, *Biochem. J. 45:* 552.

Escalar, G., and Galli, G., 1957, Ricereche sul contenuto di acetilcolina "Libera", E. "Legata", in liquores normali e patologici, *Sist. Nerv. 5:*379.

Friedhoff, A.J., and Alpert, M., 1973, A dopaminergic-cholinergic mechanism in production of psychotic symptoms, *Biol. Psychiatry 6:*165.

Gershon, S., and Olariu, J., 1960, JB329 — a new psychotomimetic: its antagonism by tetrahydroaminacrin and its comparison with LSD, mescaline and sernyl, *J. Neuropsychiat. 1:*283.

Gershon, S., and Shaw, F.H., 1961, Psychiatric sequelae of chronic exposure to organophosphorus insecticides, *Lancet 1:*1371.

Hanson, H.M., Stone, C.A., and Witoslawski, 1970, Antagonism of the antiavoidance effects of various agents by anticholinergic drugs, *J. Pharm. Exp. Ther. 173:*117.

Janowsky, D.S., El-Yousef, M.K., Davis, J.M., and Sekerke, J.H., 1973, Antagonistic effects of physostigmine and methylphenidate in man, *Am. J. Psychiatry 130:*1370.

Jenden, D.J., 1977, Some recent developments in the biochemical pharmacology of cholinergic systems, in *"Neuroregulators and Psychiatric Disorders"* (E. Usdin, D.A. Hamburg, J.D. Barchas, eds.), pp. 425-433, Oxford University Press, New York.

Karczmar, A.G., and Dun, N.J., 1978, Cholinergic synapses: physiological, pharmacological and behavioral considerations, in *"Pharmacology: A Generation of Progress"* (M.A. Lipton, A. DiMascio, and K.F. Killam, eds.), pp. 293-305, Raven Press, New York.

Kuhar, M.J., and Yamamura, H.I., 1976, Localization of cholinergic muscarinic receptors in rat brain by light microscopic radioautography, *Brain Res. 110:*229.

Lipton, M.A., DiMascio, A., and Killam, K.F., 1978, *"Psychopharmacology: A Generation of Progress"* Raven Press, New York.

Long, J.P., 1963, Structure-activity relationships of the reversible anticholinesterase agents, in *"Handbuch der Experimentellen Pharmakologie, Vol. 15"* (G.B. Koelle, ed.), pp. 374-427, Springer-Verlag, Berlin.

McGeer, P.L., and McGeer, E.G., 1977, Possible changes in striatal and limbic cholinergic systems in schizophrenia, *Arch. Gen. Psychiatry 34:*1319.

Op den Velde, W., and Stam, F.C., 1976, Some cerebral proteins and enzyme systems in Alzheimer's presenile and senile dementia, *J. Am. Geriatr. Sco. 24:*12.

Perry, E.K., Gibson, P.H., Blessed, G., Perry, R.H., and Tomlinson, N.E., 1977, Neurotransmitter enzyme abnormalities in senile dementia. Choline acetyltransferase and glutamic acid decarboxylase activities in necropsy brain tissue. *J. Neurol. Sci. 34:*247.

Perry, E.K., and Perry, R.H., 1977, Cholinergic and GABA systems in dementia and normal old age, *Br. J. Psychiatry 131:*319.

Pfeiffer, C.C., and Jenney, E.H., 1957, The inhibition of the conditioned response and the counteraction of schizophrenia by muscarinic stimulation of the brain, *Ann. NY Acad. Sci. 66:*753.

Plum, C.M., 1960, Study of cholinesterase activity in nervous and mental disorders, *Clin. Chem. 6:*332.

Poloni, A., 1951, L'acetilcolini nel liquod dei malati di mento, *Cervello 27:*81.

Pope, A., Caveness, W., and Livingston, K.E., 1952, Architectonic distribution of acetylcholinesterase in the frontal isocortex of psychotic and nonpsychotic patients, *AMA Arch. Neurol. Psychiatry 68:*425.

Pope, A., Meath, Jr., J.A., Caveness, W.F., Livingston, K.E., and Thomson, R.H., 1949, Histochemical distribution of cholinesterase and acid phosphatase in the prefrontal cortex of psychotic and nonpsychotic patients, *Trans. Am. Neurol. Assoc. 74:*147.

Rabassini, A., and Chirillo, R., 1957, Le transaminasi liquorali nella schizofrenia, *Acta Vitaminol. 11:*197.

Reiss, M., and Hemphill, R.E., 1948, Cholinesterase activity in cerebrospinal fluid, *Nature 161:*18.

Rosenthal, R., and Bigelow, B., 1973, The effects of physostigmine in phenothiazine resistant chronic schizophrenic patients. Preliminary observations, *Comp. Psychiatry 14:*489.

Rowntree, D.W., Nevin, S., and Wilson, A., 1950, The effects of diisopropylfluorophosphonate in schizophrenia and manic depressive psychosis, *J. Neurol. Neurosurg. Psychiatry 13:*47.

Schain, R.J., 1960, Neurohumors and other pharmacologically active substances in cerebrospinal fluid: a review of the literature, *Yale J. Biol. Med. 33:*15.

Schutz, F., 1943, The effect of barbiturates on the cholinesterase in different tissues, *J. Physiol. 102:*269.

Schutz, F., 1944, Serum cholinesterase in barbiturate addiction and epilepsy, *Q. J. Exp. Physiol. 33:*35.

Sherwood, S.L., 1952, Intraventricular medication in catatonic stupor (preliminary communication), *Brain 75:*68.

Singh, M.M., and Smith, J.M., 1973, Reversal of some therapeutic effects of an antipsychotic agent by an antiparkinsonian drug, *J. Nerv. Ment. Dis. 157:*50.

Takahashi, Y., and Ogushi, T., 1953, On biochemical studies of schizophrenia. Report 1. An enzymological study on brain tissue and serum of schizophrenic patients. Cholinesterase, *Folia Psychiatr. Neurol. Jpn. 6:*244.

Turner, W.J., and Mauss, E.A., 1959, Serotonin (5-hydroxytryptamine) and acetylcholine in human ventricular and spinal fluids, *Arch. Gen. Psychiatry 1:*646.

Usdin, E., Hamburg, D., and Barchas, J., 1977, *"Neuroregulators and Psychiatric Disorders"*, Oxford University Press, New York.

Van Andel, H., 1959, Neuropharmacological studies on catatonic phenomena, in *"Neuropsychopharmacology"* (P.B. Bradley, P. Deniker, and C. Raduoco-Thomas, eds.), pp. 701-703, Elsevier, Amsterdam.

Wise, C.D., Baden, M.M., and Stein, L., 1974, Postmortem measurement of enzymes in human brain: evidence of a central noradrenergic deficit in schizophrenia, *J. Psychiatr. Res. 11:*185.

Wise, C.D., and Stein, L., 1975, Evidence of a central noradrenergic deficiency in schizophrenia, in *"Neurotransmitter Balances Regulating Behavior"* (E.F. Domino, and J.M. Davis, eds.), pp. 99-123, NPP Books, Ann Arbor.

Yamamura, H.I., Kuhar, M.J., and Snyder, S.H., 1974, *In vivo* identification of muscarinic cholinergic receptor binding in rat brain, *Brain Res. 80:*170.

RED CELL CHOLINE AND AFFECTIVE DISEASE

I. Hanin

Department of Psychiatry, Western Psychiatric Institute and Clinic,
University of Pittsburgh School of Medicine, Pittsburgh, PA 15261

INTRODUCTION

It is fascinating, from a historical point of view, to trace the progression of the clinical significance which has been attributed throughout the past 50 years to the role of acetylcholine (ACh) in a variety of centrally mediated disease states. The identity and involvement of ACh in neurotransmitter function have been known to investigators for over five decades. Nevertheless, a concrete understanding of the contribution of ACh to various central nervous system mediated disease states has been persistently elusive over this time span, although indirect evidence has accumulated which has implicated that activation of cholinergic mechanisms may generally be responsible for induction of behavioral suppression and reduction in affect (Rowntree et al., 1950; Pfeiffer and Jenney, 1957; Van Andel, 1959; Gershon and Shaw, 1961; Bowers et al., 1964; Collard et al., 1965; Modestin et al., 1973; Tamminga et al., 1976). Only recently, with the development of a number of other neurotransmitter-related hypotheses for psychiatric disease states, has there also been a serious attempt to implicate ACh in certain types of affective and neurologic disorders. Specifically, Janowsky and his coinvestigators, within the past several years, have been instrumental in directly promoting the concept that ACh may, indeed, play an important role in the etiology of affective disorders (Janowsky et al., 1972; 1974; See also Davis and Janowsky, and Janowsky et al., this book).

These earlier observations by Janowsky and his associates have been fortified as a result of recent observations accumulated by other investigators using experimental animals. Their findings are providing increased support for the concept that, in the case of the cholinergic system, there may be an "open-loop" system between blood and brain. This contention is supported by a number of interrelated observations. First, it is generally accepted that choline (Ch), the endogenous precursor of ACh, cannot be synthesized *de novo* in the brain (Bremer and Greenberg, 1961; Ansell and Spanner, 1967; 1968; Browning and Schulman, 1968; Zahniser et al., 1977; and others. However, note two opposing papers to this concept by Pfeiffer et al., 1957; and by Kewitz and Pleul, 1976). It has therefore been suggested that Ch involved in brain ACh synthesis

75

is supplied entirely from blood, both in free and lipid bound form (Duvigneaud *et al.*, 1941; Dross and Kewitz, 1966; 1972; Ansell and Spanner, 1968; Hoelzl and Frank, 1969; Illingworth and Portman, 1972; Hanin and Schuberth, 1974). Some of this Ch is used immediately in the synthesis of ACh (Dross and Kewitz, 1966; Schuberth *et al.*, 1969; 1970; Jenden *et al.*, 1974); the remainder of Ch for brain ACh synthesis is obtained from breakdown within the central nervous system of phospholipids, formed from the Ch supplied earlier from blood (Cooper and Webster, 1970; Browning, 1971; Collier *et al.*, 1972; Woelk *et al.*, 1974; see also review by Freeman and Jenden, 1976; and chapters by Jenden and by Barker in this book). Moreover, it has been shown that it is feasible to alter brain ACh and Ch levels in experimental animals by manipulating the amount of Ch supplied from the periphery, whether via injection or oral administration to these animals (Haubrich *et al.*, 1974; Cohen and Wurtman, 1975; 1976).

As a result of these developments, a variety of clinical studies has recently been initiated. These are already providing an ever increasing amount of evidence to consolidate the fact that ACh is also an important neurotransmitter to be considered when one is attempting to understand the etiology or the causes of certain mental disease states. In a number of cases of psychiatric/neurologic disorders in which a deficiency of central cholinergic activity has been implied, e.g., in L-DOPA-induced dyskinesia, in tardive dyskinesia, and in Huntington's chorea (review by Van woert, 1976), patients have been treated with partial success following administration of oral doses of large amounts (grams per day) of either dimethylaminoethanol (Deaner, Riker Laboratories, Inc., Northridge, California) or Ch. The rationale behind such treatment is inherent in the hypothesis that these compounds are endogenous precursors of ACh and would, therefore, be effective in the treatment of these dyskinesias via long-term elevation of ACh levels *in vivo*. Results at present, although encouraging, are still controversial, particularly with respect to the clinical efficacy of deanol. Representative publications on this subject include works of: Miller, 1974; Casey and Denney, 1975; 1977; Fann *et al.*, 1975; Klawans *et al.*, 1975; Davis *et al.*, 1975; 1976; 1977; Growdon *et al.*, 1977a; 1977b; Tamminga *et al.*, 1977, Aquilonius and Eckernas, 1977, and others. This subject is reviewed extensively in other chapters of this book.

RATIONALE

If an "open-loop" does exist between blood and brain for the cholinergic system, then one might assume that brain cholinergic activity would, in fact, be reflected to some extent by specific cholinergic parameters in blood. Recent observations conducted in our laboratories (Shih *et al.*, 1977) indicate that following chronic (two weeks) supplementation of tracer amounts of deuterium-labeled Ch in the diet of experimental mice, the specific activity of deuterium-labeled Ch in plasma is significantly correlated with the specific activity of deuterium-labeled Ch and ACh in brain. This correlation is long-lasting, and continues to exist even four weeks after discontinuation of feeding mice with the deuterium-labeled Ch supplement. In other words, blood Ch may, indeed, be studied as an index of brain Ch and, therefore, of brain ACh activity *in vivo*. If this is the case, one could conceivably monitor cholinergic phenomena in blood and obtain an indication of cholinergic occurrences in the brain. The value of eventually using such an approach for the analysis of central cholinergic mechanisms in humans, *in vivo*, is self-evident.

Parallel with our studies in experimental animals, we therefore sought to investigate this question by measuring levels of Ch in plasma and erythrocytes (RBC) of various psychiatric patients and normal controls, in an attempt to determine whether, in fact, one can observe differences in blood cholinergic parameters in individuals from different categories of affective disease states. We were encouraged by the initial observations of Janowsky and coinvestigators (1972, 1974) indicating that depression may be associated with elevated cholinergic activity in the central nervous system. Moreover, the incidence of anticholinergic side effects observed following administration to patients of a variety of tricyclic antidepressant agents commonly used in the clinic, and the fact that atropinic toxicity, often resulting from an overdose of such agents, can be eliminated via administration of physostigmine (Heiser and Wilbert, 1974; Snyder et al., 1974; Newton, 1975; Chin et al., 1976; also review by Weiss et al., 1976), all indicated that central cholinergic mechanisms might be very closely implicated either in the etiology or the consequence of affective disorders.

REVIEW OF EXPERIMENTAL OBSERVATIONS

The following is a review of studies which we have conducted during the past year, in an attempt to answer some of the questions alluded to in the previous section. Initially, experiments were designed to investigate basal conditions for the chemical analysis of levels of Ch and ACh in plasma and RBC samples. Conditions for extraction, isolation and derivatization of Ch were established based upon existing methodology utilizing gas chromatography/mass spectrometry for the analysis of Ch and ACh in tissue extracts (Jenden and Hanin, 1974; Hanin and Skinner, 1975). Levels of Ch in plasma and RBCs were found to be very stable once endogenous proteins were precipitated out of the tissue fluid, and if subsequently the samples were brought to a pH of 4 before freezing. Samples prepared in this manner are stable if frozen for months at a time (unpublished observations). We next established that Ch levels in plasma and RBCs are extremely resistant to osmotic dilution or treatment with a variety of acids. This indicated that Ch levels in plasma and RBC, which we measured under our established conditions, are not subject to artefactual changes, are highly reproducible, and therefore are remarkably reliable (Hanin et al., 1978).

The first interesting clinical observation to emerge from these experiments was that Ch levels in plasma provide a very different profile from that observed with RBCs. Whereas plasma Ch levels in a widespread, mixed, drug free population will vary over a very narrow range between individuals (4.6-12.7 nmoles/ml), RBC Ch levels are highly variable and can differ by over 40-fold between individuals (5.8-253.5 nmoles/ml) within this same population (Hanin et al., data in preparation). Based upon these observations, we have proposed that RBC Ch is a much more reliable index of interindividual variability of subjects than is plasma Ch.

Subsequent studies established that within each individual, levels of Ch in RBC and plasma are remarkably consistent over a long period of time, providing that the dietary input is consistent, and that the individual is not consuming drugs which may affect endogenous levels of Ch in his blood (Hanin et al., 1978). People thus appear to exhibit an individual profile of their plasma and RBC Ch levels. The question that arose from this finding was whether this profile could be used as an index or as a marker of a certain psychiatric disease state.

The intriguing fact is that there does appear to be a definitive difference in levels of RBC Ch in certain depressed psychiatric patients, when compared with levels of RBC Ch in a population of normal controls. In general, depressed individuals have a higher mean value of RBC Ch than do normal controls (Hanin *et al.*, 1978, and data in preparation). This is a challenging concept in view of the observation that cholinergic mechanisms in the central nervous system appear to be inextricably related to affective disease states. However, at this point in time, it is difficult to establish definitively whether changes in RBC Ch are indicative of either a drop or an elevation in brain Ch and ACh levels, or if blood cholinergic parameters provide an index at all of central cholinergic phenomena. Moreover, the relative effect of such high endogenous levels of Ch on subsequent improvement following treatment with appropriate medication is as yet an unstudied phenomenon. It will require parallel studies in humans and in experimental animals similar to those described earlier in this chapter, to begin to unravel some of these questions.

What about various drugs used in the psychiatric clinic and their effect on Ch levels in plasma and RBCs? To date, we have investigated on a longitudinal basis only two such compounds: amitriptyline (Elavil, Merck and Co., Inc., West Point, Pa.) and lithium carbonate (Eskalith, Smith Kline and French Laboratories, Philadelphia, Pa.). It is interesting to note that amitriptyline, a compound which is known to exert atropinic side effects, and is a potent muscarinic receptor antagonist (Snyder and Yamamura, 1977), does not appear to have any effect on either RBC or plasma Ch over a period of several weeks of chronic administration (Hanin *et al.*, data in preparation). Lithium, on the other hand, which does not exert any overt anticholinergic effects, does nevertheless induce a delayed, but steady increase in Ch levels in RBC. Moreover, this effect is delayed, occurs 24 hours after initial lithium administration, and appears to be long-lasting (Hanin *et al.*, data in preparation). Several theories can be proposed to explain this selective response of RBC Ch to lithium, based upon the known inhibitory effects of lithium on Ch transport across red cell membrance barriers (Lee *et al.*, 1974; Lingsch and Martin, 1976), and on ACh synthesis and release in general (Waziri, 1968; Bjegovic and Randic, 1971; Vizi *et al.*, 1972; Fieve *et al.*, 1976; Basuray and Harris, 1977). However, in the final analysis, one must establish experimentally each time a new drug is tested, whether the effect, or lack thereof, of any psychopharmacological agent on plasma and RBC Ch levels is exerted via its interaction with central cholinergic mechanisms, or as the result of a specific local (e.g., membrane) effect of the drug.

DISCUSSION AND SUMMARY

The concept of investigating cholinergic systems in blood and correlating them with clinical state is not new. Within the past decade, a number of papers have emerged in which it has been reported that blood levels of free and bound ACh, as well as cholinesterase activity, are subject to moderation as a result of a variety of physiological and pharmacologic conditions. For example, blood cholinergic activity is increased in patients with paroxysmal nocturnal hemoglobinuria and autoimmune cholinergic anemia (Savina *et al.*, 1973); changes during the different phases of tonic mesodiencephalic convulsive seizures (Sevostyanova and Tretyakova, 1970); and is subject to alterations by various brain traumas, following abstinence from alcohol, and during the various phases of pregnancy and birth (Kassil and Sokolinskaya, 1971). Blood cholinergic mechanisms have also been shown to vary during adaptation of individuals to stressful conditions of long-term isolation (Maslova, 1967). In addition, it has been reported that erythrocytes contain cholinergic receptors (Huestis, 1976); that there is a circadian variability in human plasma choline acetyltransferase activity (Massarelli et al., in press), that RBC, but not plasma, cholinesterase activity is significantly lower in patients with affective disorders as compared with normal controls (Milstoc et al., 1975); that lithium treatment will elevate RBC cholinesterase activity in bipolar female patients (Fieve et al., 1976), and that whole blood obtained from patients exhibits significantly higher levels of ACh in a group of depressive neurotics, and of Ch in unipolar depressives than does blood from normal controls, schizophrenics, or bipolar depressive patients (Stavinoha et al., 1977). All these reports imply that blood cholinergic phenomena may play a significant role in modulating and/or providing an index for the physiological function of brain ACh in vivo.

Our findings to date are consistent with this general notion. We have established that, in general, plasma and RBC Ch levels are extremely stable within the same individual over a long period of time. It is conceivable that alterations in dietary input would affect such levels, after ingestion of Ch-containing foods (Cohen and Wurtman, 1976; Wurtman et al., 1977; Eckernas and Aquilonius, in press). All the studies conducted in this report were, however, performed using blood obtained from individuals after an overnight fast, and therefore pertain to these specific dietary conditions. Plasma Ch levels have been shown to span a narrow range (up to a 3-fold variation), whereas RBC Ch levels exhibit over a 40-fold variation within a population of drug-free individuals. The first significant point which is to be gleaned from these findings, therefore, is that RBC rather than plasma levels might be a more sensitive index of individual variation of blood cholinergic parameters in human subjects.

The second important point from these experiments is to be obtained from our clinical studies, which have been reviewed in this chapter. These have demonstrated unequivocally that mean endogenous Ch levels in RBCs of drug-free patients with major depressive disorder are significantly higher than mean levels of RBC Ch measured in a population of normal controls (Hanin et al., 1978; and data in preparation). Consequently, based upon these findings and related observations of other investigators reported earlier in this chapter, we have proposed that RBC Ch might serve as a specific marker in the diagnosis of certain categories of mental illness.

Trials which we have conducted so far utilizing two commonly prescribed psychotherapeutic agents have at present yielded equivocal results. Chronically administered amitriptyline exerts no effect on either RBC or plasma Ch levels in depressed individuals, in spite of its documented central anticholinergic properties. Lithium, on the other hand, exerts a significant trophic effect on Ch levels in RBCs (but not in plasma), even after administration of a single dose of this salt. The apparent discrepancy may be due to the reported ability of lithium to irreversibly inhibit RBC membrane Ch transport (Lee et al., 1974; Lingsch and Martin, 1976).

Future studies obviously will have to be designed in such a manner as to allow one to distinguish between the ability of psychopharmacologic agents to control Ch levels in RBC and plasma through endogenous mechanisms, as opposed to local, membrane-specific effects of these agents. Subsequently, it would be essential to establish definitively whether there is any relationship between effective pharmacotherapy and changes in plasma and/or RBC Ch levels in psychiatric patients. The research summarized in this chapter is thus only at its early stages and requires a considerable amount of additional investigation. Particularly, it is essential that we first understand more about the physiological significance of RBC and plasma Ch levels, and their interrelationship with brain cholinergic mechanisms. Studies in our laboratories, utilizing mice and stable isotope dilution techniques are currently being conducted with that goal in mind, and with highly encouraging results (Shih *et al.*, 1977).

ACKNOWLEDGEMENTS

This work was supported by NIMH Grant MH 26320. The research studies summarized in this chapter have incorporated the significant efforts of a large number of individuals, including Ursula Kopp, Christina Nevar, Tsung-Ming Shih, David J. Kupfer, Duane G. Spiker, Elisabeth Koo, Rolland I. Poust, Jonathan M. Himmelhoch, John F. Neil, Alan G. Mallinger, Joan E. Mallinger, Nancy R. Zahniser and James R. Merikangas.

REFERENCES

Ansell, G.B., and Spanner, S., 1967, The metabolism of labelled ethanolamine in the brain of the rat *in vivo, J. Neurochem. 14:*873.

Ansell, G.B., and Spanner, S., 1968, The metabolism of [Me-^{14}C] choline in the brain of the rat *in vivo, Biochem. J. 110:*201.

Aquilonius, S.M., and Eckernas, S.A., 1977, Choline therapy in Huntington's chorea, *Neurology 27:*887.

Basuray, B.N., and Harris, C.A., 1977, Potentiation of d-Tubocurarine (d-Tc) neuromuscular blockade in cats by lithium chloride, *Eur. J. Pharmacol. 45:*79.

Bjegovic, M., and Randic, M., 1971, Effect of lithium ions on the release of acetylcholine from the cerebral cortex, *Nature 230:*587.

Bowers, M.B., Goodman, E., and Sim, O.M., 1964, Some behavioral changes in man following anticholinesterase administration, *J. Nerv. Ment. Dis. 138:*383.

Bremer, J., and Greenberg, D.M., 1961, Methyl transferring enzyme system of microsomes in the biosynthesis of lecithin (phosphatidylcholine), *Biochim. Biophys. Acta 46:*205.

Browning, E.T., 1971, Free choline formation by cerebral cortical slices from rat brain, *Biochem. Biophys. Res. Comm. 45:*1586.

Browning, E.T., and Schulman, M.P., 1968, [^{14}C] Acetylcholine synthesis by cortex slices of rat brain, *J. Neurochem. 15:*1391.

Casey, D.E., and Denney, D., 1975, Deanol in the treatment of tardive dyskinesia, *Am. J. Psychiatry 132:*864.

Casey, D.E., and Denney, D., 1977, Pharmacological characterization of tardive dyskinesia, *Psychopharmacology 54:*1.

Chin, L.S., Havill, J.H., Rothwell, R.P.G., and Bishop, B.G., 1976, Use of physostigmine in tricyclic antidepressant poisoning, *Anaesth. Intens. Care 4:*138.

Cohen, E.L., and Wurtman, R.J., 1975, Brain acetylcholine: increase after systemic choline administration, *Life Sci. 16:*1095.

Cohen, E.L., and Wurtman, R.J., 1976, Brain acetylcholine: control by dietary choline, *Science 191:*561.

Collard, J., Lecoq, R., and Demaret, A., 1965, Un essai de therapeutique pathogenique de la schizophrenia par un acetylcholinique: l'oxotremorine, *Acta Neurologica et Psychiatrica Belgica 65:*122.

Collier, B., Poon, P., and Salehmoghaddam, S., 1972, The formation of choline and of acetylcholine by brain *in vitro, J. Neurochem. 19:*59.

Cooper, M.F., and Webster, G.R., 1970, The differentiation of phospholipase A_1 and A_2 in rat and human nervous tissues, *J. Neurochem. 17:*1543.

Davis, K.L., Berger, P.A., and Hollister, L.E., 1975, Choline for tardive dyskinesia, *N. Engl. J. Med. 293:*152.

Davis, K.L., Hollister, L.E., Barchas, J.D., and Berger, P.A., 1976, Choline in tardive dyskinesia and Huntington's disease, *Life Sci. 19:*1507.

Davis, K.L., Berger, P.A., and Hollister, L.E., 1977, Deanol in tardive dyskinesia, *Am. J. Psychiatry 134:*807.

Dross, V.K., and Kewitz, H., 1966, Der einbau von i.v. zugefuhrtem cholin in das acetylcholin des gehirns (synthesis in brain of acetylcholine following i.v. administration of choline), *Naun. Schmied. Arch. Pharmakol. 255:*10.

Dross, V.K., and Kewitz, H., 1972, Concentration and origin of choline in the rat brain, *Naun. Schmied. Arch. Pharmakol. 274:*91.

Duvigneaud, V., Cohn, M., Chandler, J.P., Schenck, J.R., and Simmonds, S., 1941, The utilization of the methyl group of methionine in the biological synthesis of choline and creatine, *J. Biol. Chem. 140:*625.

Eckernas, S.A., and Aquilonius, S.M., (in press), Free choline in human plasma analyzed by a simple radio-enzymatic procedure: age distribution and effect of a meal, *Scand. J. Clin. Lab. Invest.*

Fann, W.E., Sullivan, J.L., III, Miller, R.D., and McKenzie, G.M., 1975, Deanol in tardive dyskinesia: a preliminary report, *Psychopharmacologia 42:*135.

Fieve, R.R., Milstoc, M., Kumbaraci, T., and Dunner, D.L., 1976, The effect of lithium on red blood cell cholinesterase activity in patients with affective disorders, *Dis. Nerv. Syst. 37:*240.

Freeman, J.J., and Jenden, D.J., 1976, Minireview: the source of choline for acetylcholine synthesis in brain, *Life Sci. 19:*949.

Gershon, S., and Shaw, F.H., 1961, Psychiatric sequelae of chronic exposure to organophosphorus insecticides, *Lancet 1:*1371.

Growdon, J.H., Cohen, E.L., and Wurtman, R.J., 1977a, Huntington's disease: Clinical and chemical effects of choline administration, *Ann. Neurol. 1:*418.

Growdon, J.H., Hirsch, M.J., Wurtman, R.J., and Wiener, W., 1977b, Oral choline administration to patients with tardive dyskinesia, *N. Engl. J. Med. 297:*524.

Hanin, I., and Schuberth, J., 1974, Labelling of acetylcholine in the brain of mice fed on a diet containing deuterium labelled choline: studies utilizing gas chromatography-mass spectrometry, *J. Neurochem. 23:*819.

Hanin, I., and Skinner, R.F., 1975, Analysis of microquantities of choline and its esters utilizing gas chromatography-chemical ionization mass spectrometry, *Anal. Biochem. 66:*568.

Hanin, I., Kopp, U., Zahniser, N.R., Shih, T.M., Spiker, D.G., Merikangas, J.R., Kupfer, D.J., and Foster, F.G., 1978, Acetylcholine and choline in human plasma and red blood cells: a gas chromatograph-mass spectrometric evaluation, in *"Cholinergic Mechanisms and Psychopharmacology"* (D.J. Jenden, ed.), pp. 181-195, Plenum Press, New York.

Haubrich, D.R., Wedeking, P.W., and Wang, P.F.L., 1974, Increase in tissue concentration of acetylcholine in guinea pigs *in vivo* induced by administration of choline, *Life Sci. 14:*921.

Heiser, J.F., and Wilbert, D.E., 1974, Reversal of delirium induced by tricyclic anti-depressant drugs with physostigmine, *Am. J. Psychiatry 131:*1275.

Hoelzl, J., and Franck, H.P., 1969, Incorporation of doubly labeled lecithin into the brain lipids at different developmental stages of rats, *Proc. Intl. Soc. Neurochem. Milan 1969:*219.

Huestis, W.H., 1976, Preliminary characterization of the acetylcholine receptor in human erythrocytes, *J. Supramol. Structure 4:*355.

Illingworth, D.R., and Portman, O.W., 1972, The uptake and metabolism of plasma lysophosphatidyl choline *in vivo* by the brain of squirrel monkeys, *Biochem. J. 130:*557.

Janowsky, D.S., El-Yousef, M.K., Davis, J.M., and Sekerke, H.J., 1972, A cholinergic-adrenergic hypothesis of mania and depression, *Lancet 2:*632.

Janowsky, D.S., El-Yousef, M.K., and Davis, J.M., 1974, Acetylcholine and depression, *Psychosom. Med. 36:*248.

Jenden, D.J., and Hanin, I., 1974, Gas chromatographic microestimation of choline and acetylcholine after N-demethylation by sodium benzenethiolate, in *"Choline and Acetylcholine: Handbook of Chemical Assay Methods"* (I. Hanin, ed.), pp. 135-150, Raven Press, New York.

Jenden, D.J., Choi, L., Silverman, R.W., Steinborn, J.A., Roch, M., and Booth, R.A., 1974, Acetylcholine turnover estimation in brain by gas chromatography-mass spectrometry, *Life Sci. 14:*55.

Kassil, G.N., and Sokolinskaya, R.A., 1971, Cholinergic activity of human blood associated with different states of the person, *Fiziol. Zh. SSSR, Imeni I.M. Sechenova 57:*248.

Kewitz, H., and Pleul, O., 1976, Synthesis of choline from ethanolamine in rat brain, *Proc. Natl. Acad. Sci. USA 73:*2181.

Klawans, H.L., Topel, J.L., and Bergen, D., 1975, Deanol in the treatment of levodopa-induced dyskinesias, *Neurology 25:*290.

Lee, G., Lingsch, C., Lyle, P.T., and Martin, K., 1974, Lithium treatment strongly inhibits choline transport in human erythrocytes, *Br. J. Clin. Pharmac. 1:*365.

Lingsch, C., and Martin, K., 1976, An irreversible effect of lithium administration to patients, *Br. J. Pharmac. 57:*323.

Maslova, A.F., 1967, On the participation of the sympatho-adrenaline system in the general reaction of adaptation, *Problemy Endokrinologii 13:*89.

Massarelli, R., Froissart, C., and Mandel, P., 1977, Diurnal oscillation of choline acetyl-transferase activity in human blood, *Neurosci. Lett. 5:*95.

Miller, E., 1974, Deanol in the treatment of levodopa-induced dyskinesias, *Neurology 24:*116.

Milstoc, M., Teodoru, C.V., Fieve, R.R., and Kumbaraci, T., 1975, Cholinesterase activity and the manic-depressive patient, *Dis. Nerv. Syst. 36:*197.

Modestin, J., Hunger, J., and Schwartz, R.B., 1973, Uber die depressogene wirkung von physostigmin, *Arch. Psychiat. Nervenkr. 218:*67.

Newton, R.W., 1975, Physostigmine salicylate in the treatment of tricyclic antidepressant overdosage, *JAMA 231:*941.

Pfeiffer, C.C., and Jenney, E.H., 1957, The inhibition of the conditioned response and the counteraction of schizophrenia by muscarinic stimulation of the brain, *Ann. N.Y. Acad. Sci. 66:*753.

Pfeiffer, C.C., Jenney, E.H., Gallacher, W., Smith, R.P., Bevan, J., Jr., Killam, K.F., Killam, E.K., and Blackmore, W., 1957, Stimulant effect of 2-dimethlaminoethanol — possible precursor of brain acetylcholine, *Science 126:*610.

Rowntree, D.W., Nevin, S., and Wilson, A., 1950, The effects of diisopropylfluoro-phosphonate in schizophrenia and manic depressive psychosis, *J. Neurol. Neurosurg. Psychiatry 13:*47.

Savina, L.S., Sokolinskaya, R.A., and Lobanova, N.A., 1973, Changes in cholinergic activity of blood in patients with paroxysmal nocturnal hemoglobinuria, *Probl. Gematol. Pereliev. Krovf. 20:*40.

Schuberth, J., Sparf, B., and Sundwall, A., 1969, A technique for the study of acetyl-choline turnover in mouse brain *in vivo, J. Neurochem. 16:*695.

Schuberth, J., Sparf, B., and Sundwall, A., 1970, On the turnover of acetylcholine in nerve endings of mouse brain *in vivo, J. Neurochem. 17:*461.

Sevostyanova, G.A., and Tretyakova, K.A., 1970, The state of the acetylcholine-cholinesterase system associated with tonic meso-diencephalic convulsive seizures, *Zhur. Nevropatol. Psikhiatr. Im. Korsakova 69:*1811.

Shih, T.M., Kopp, U., and Hanin, I., 1977, Choline in blood as a possible index of brain acetylcholine metabolism *in vivo, Neurosci. Abst. 3:*322.

Snyder, B.D., Blonde, L., and McWhirter, W.R., 1974, Reversal of amitriptyline intoxi-cation by physostigmine, *JAMA 230:*1433.

Snyder, S.H., and Yamamura, H.I., 1977, Antidepressants and the muscarinic acetyl-choline receptor, *Arch. Gen. Psychiatry 34:*236.

Stavinoha, W.B., Modak, A.T., and Bowden, C.L., 1977, Acetylcholine and choline in the blood of normal individuals and psychiatric patients, *Neurosci. Abstr. 3:*416.

Tamminga, C., Smith, R.C., Chang, S., Haraszti, J.S., and Davis, J.M., 1976, Depression associated with oral choline, *Lancet 2:*905.

Tamminga, C.A., Smith, R.C., Ericksen, S.E., Chang, S., and Davis, J.M., 1977, Cholinergic influences in tardive dyskinesia, *Am. J. Psychiatry 134:*769.

Van Andel, H., 1959, Neuropharmacological studies in catatonic phenomena, in *"Neuro-psychopharmacology"* (P.B. Bradley, P. Denicker, and C. Raduoco-Thomas, eds.), pp. 701-703, Elsevier Publ. Co., Amsterdam.

Van Woert, M.H., 1976, Parkinson's disease, tardive dyskinesia, and Huntington's chorea, in *"Biology of Cholinergic Function"* (A.M. Goldberg and I. Hanin, eds.), pp. 583-601, Raven Press, New York.

Vizi, E.S., Illes, P., Ronai, A., and Knoll, J., 1972, The effect of lithium on acetylcholine release and synthesis, *Neuropharmacology 11:*521.

Waziri, R., 1968, Presynaptic effects of lithium no cholinergic synaptic transmission in aplysia neurons, *Life Sci. 7:*865.

Weiss, B.L., Foster, F.G., and Kupfer, D.J., 1976, Cholinergic involvement in neuro-psychiatric syndromes, in *"Biology of Cholinergic Function"* (A.M. Goldberg and I. Hanin, eds.), pp. 603-617, Raven Press, New York.

Woelk, H., Ichikawa, K.P., Binaglia, L., Goracci, G., and Porcellati, G., 1974, Distribution and properties of phospholipases A_1 and A_2 in synaptosomes and synaptosomal fractions of rat brain, *Zeit. Physiol. Chem. 355:*1535.

Wurtman, R.J., Hirsch, M.J., and Growdon, J.H., 1977, Lecithin consumption raises serum-free-choline levels, *Lancet 2:*68.

Zahniser, N.R., Chou, D., and Hanin, I., 1977, Is 2-dimethylaminoethanol (deanol) indeed a precursor of brain acetylcholine (ACh)? A gas chromatographic evaluation, *J. Pharmacol. Exp. Ther. 200:*545.

BRAIN ACETYLCHOLINE AND MOVEMENT DISORDERS

TREATMENT OF HUNTINGTON'S DISEASE AND TARDIVE DYSKINESIA WITH CHOLINE CHLORIDE

K. L. Davis[1,2], L. E. Hollister[1,2] and P. A. Berger[1,2]

[1]Veterans Administration Hospital, 3801 Miranda Avenue,
Palo Alto, California 94304

[2]Department of Psychiatry and Behavioral Sciences, Stanford University
School of Medicine, Stanford, California 94305

INTRODUCTION

Reports that choline chloride increased brain acetylcholine in rats stimulated clinical trials of this drug in patients with Huntington's disease and tardive dyskinesia (Cohen and Wurtman, 1975; Haubrich et al., 1975; Davis et al., 1976; Aquilonius and Eckernas, 1977; Growdon et al., 1977a; Tamminga et al., 1977). The use of choline chloride in these movement disorders was based on previous investigations indicating that physostigmine, which increases central cholinergic activity, reduced the frequency of abnormal movements in some patients with Huntington's disease and tardive dyskinesia (Aquilonius and Sjostrom, 1971; Klawans and Rubovits, 1972; 1974; Gerlach et al., 1974). If choline chloride increases brain cholinergic activity, it would also be expected to improve the abnormal movements of patients with Huntington's disease and tardive dyskinesia in patients who were benefited by physostigmine.

The first patient with tardive dyskinesia to receive choline chloride had a significant reduction in the frequency of his abnormal movements while receiving 16 gm of the drug daily. When choline chloride was discontinued the frequency of his movements increased (Davis et al., 1975). Subsequently, the effect of choline chloride on four men with Huntington's disease, and four men with tardive dyskinesia was reported. All patients with tardive dyskinesia, and two of the patients with Huntington's disease had a significant improvement during treatment with choline chloride (Davis et al., 1976). These findings for patients with tardive dyskinesia have been confirmed. Two groups have reported that choline chloride significantly diminished buccal lingual masticatory movements in some of the patients they studied (Growdon et al., 1977a; Tamminga et al., 1977). The efficacy of choline chloride in the treatment of patients with Huntington's disease is unclear. In one series of five patients, two had a dose dependent decrease in the frequency of their choreic movements, and three patients were essentially unimproved (Aquilonius and

Eckernas, 1977). In another study of ten patients with Huntington's disease choline did not facilitate a consistent global improvement (Growdon *et al.*, 1977b). However, the interpretation of these findings is complicated by the fact that the dose of neuroleptics in four patients was lowered prior to starting choline therapy. Dose reduction of neuroleptics can exacerbate the choreic movements of patients with Huntington's disease. In addition, a relatively low dose of choline chloride was given to five patients (Growdon *et al.*, 1977b). Thus, additional work is necessary to determine if a subgroup of patients with Huntington's disease have the frequency of their choreiform movements decreased by treatment with choline chloride.

This paper reports the results of administering choline chloride to five patients with tardive dyskinesia and eight patients with Huntington's disease. Some of this data has been included in previous reports (Davis *et al.*, 1975; 1976).

METHODS

Subjects

Tardive Dyskinesia

Six male patients between the ages of 39 and 67 consented to participate in the study. Two other patients with tardive dyskinesia were eliminated from the study when it was determined that during the two week baseline period, their movements showed spontaneous improvement. Another patient was eliminated from the study because her chronic psychopathology made it difficult for her to participate in the investigation. Of those patients who completed the study, three had abnormal involuntary buccal lingual masticatory movements for 1-2 years that appeared after a decrease in dose or the discontinuation of neuroleptics. The fourth and fifth patients had exhibited abnormal movements for 3 months prior to the study. The sixth patient exhibited symptoms for only 2 months. No recent decrease in the frequency of abnormal movements in any of these patients had been noticed by the patients' referring physicians.

Three patients had been given the diagnosis of chronic undifferentiated schizophrenia; two were given the diagnosis of manic depressive illness, and one patient had been given the diagnosis of schizoaffective schizophrenia. One subject with the diagnosis of manic depressive illness was maintained on his regular dose of lithium carbonate throughout the study. Another patient with a diagnosis of chronic undifferentiated schizophrenia had been receiving 3 mg of haloperidol daily for 3 months prior to the study. He continued to receive this dose of haloperidol during the study.

Huntington's Disease

Eight male patients with Huntington's chorea consented to participate in this study. These patients were between the ages of 39 and 66. Seven patients had been disabled by the disease for at least 2 years, and a few had been disabled for as many as 7 years. One patient had been symptomatic for at least 10 years. All but one patient had a definite family history for the disease. Two patients were chronically hospitalized at the time of the study. The other patients, though living at home prior to the study, needed close supervision. Every subject was able to communicate reasonably well, although all exhibited speech difficulties. Three patients were confined to a wheelchair; two patients walked with some difficulty. Three patients had a moderately steady gait. Throughout the study, all patients received the dose of neuroleptics determined to be maximally effective by their referring physician. Chloral hydrate was the only other psychoactive drug patients received.

Physostigmine Infusion

Seven subjects were given a subcutaneous injection of 0.5 mg methscopolamine before the physostigmine infusion was begun. If after 20 min, a patient's heart rate remained below 100, a second subcutaneous injection of 0.5 mg methscopolamine was administered. When the patient's heart rate reached 100, an intravenous injection of physostigmine was begun. Three subjects with Huntington's disease and four of the tardive dyskinesia patients received 3.0 mg physostigmine in a 30 min period. This was administered gradually over the 30 min period in a vehicle of 0.25N saline. This procedure was altered for the remaining subjects as follows: 4.0 mg physostigmine dissolved in 200 cc of normal saline was infused at a constant rate during a 60 min period. Heart rate and rhythm were monitored during the infusion by an electrocardiogram.

To assess the effect of physostigmine, all patients were monitored by videotape prior to, during, and from 2 to 3 hr after the infusion. Patients, though aware that they were receiving physostigmine, did not know if the drug would improve or worsen their condition. Raters were blind to the study design. They counted each patient's most conspicuous and quantifiable abnormal movement by reviewing the videotapes. Movement frequencies were reported per 45 sec period.

Choline Chloride Administration

Dose Schedule

All eight patients with Huntington's disease and all five of the tardive dyskinesia patients received choline chloride. The concentration of choline chloride used in this study was 0.5 gm per milliliter of distilled water. The patients were given the drug in a flavored strawberry syrup. All patients were given an initial dose of 1 gm of choline chloride four times per day. This dose was increased by 1 gm four times per day every 2-3 days, and continued until the patient reached a total dose of 20 gm per day. The one exception to this was a tardive dyskinesia patient who only reached a maximum daily dose of 16 gm. This patient was maintained on 16 gm for 8 weeks and was then given a placebo. All other subjects continued receiving 20 gm a day for 2-4 weeks. Upon discontinuation of choline chloride, all subjects reveived a placebo that had a color and taste similar to choline. Seven of the eight patients with Huntington's disease received 4 weeks of placebo; the eighth subject received the placebo for only 3 weeks. This was followed by 3-4 weeks of a daily dose of 20 gm of choline. Four patients with tardive dyskinesia received 20 gm choline for 3-4 weeks, followed by 4 weeks of placebo. The other tardive dyskinesia patient was given placebo for only 2 weeks. Patients did not know if they were receiving choline chloride or placebo.

Clinical Assessment

All subjects were monitored by videotape prior to choline chloride administration and throughout the study. Each taping session lasted for about 5 min. The same general rating procedures were used for the choline chloride study and the physostigmine infusion. As in the physostigmine infusion, the most quantifiable abnormal movement was used by blind raters to assess the effect of choline. Movement frequencies were recorded per 45 sec period.

RESULTS

Tardive Dyskinesia

Figures 1 and 2 illustrate that all six patients with tardive dyskinesia had a statistically significant reduction in the frequency of their most quantifiable oral facial movement while on choline chloride compared to the baseline level. Furthermore, as Table 1 demonstrates, all of these patients who received physostigmine experienced a statistically significant reduction in their most quantifiable oral facial movement for a 30 min period 15-90 min after the conclusion of the physostigmine infusion compared to the baseline and 2½-24 hr post physostigmine periods combined. However, as is apparent from Figure 2, three of these patients did not have an exacerbation in the frequency of their abnormal buccal lingual movements when placebo was substituted for choline. Three patients, as depicted in Figure 1, did have an increase in the frequency of their abnormal movements upon substitution of placebo for choline chloride. However, in these patients it should be noted that the frequency of their involuntary movements was never reduced more than 40%.

Huntington's Disease

Figure 3 summarizes the course of five patients whose choreiform movements were not significantly reduced by choline chloride treatment. In Figure 4 the course of the remaining three patients is described. All of these patients had a significant reduction in the frequency of their most quantifiable choreiform movement during the last 2 weeks they received choline chloride compared to the last 2 weeks of the immediately preceding placebo period. Two of these three patients also had a significant reduction during their first treatment period with 16-20 gm of choline chloride. These three patients, and only these three patients, had a significant reduction in their most quantifiable choreiform movement for a 30 min period from 15-90 min after the conclusion of the physostigmine period compared to the baseline and 2½-24 hr post physostigmine periods. The effect of physostigmine on the patients with Huntington's disease is presented in Table 2.

DISCUSSION

All the patients with tardive dyskinesia were significantly improved by choline chloride. However, only two of these patients had an exacerbation in their movement frequency when placebo was substituted for choline, and the remaining three patients did not have an increase in the frequency of their abnormal movements when placebo was substituted for choline chloride. These results are consistent with the possibility

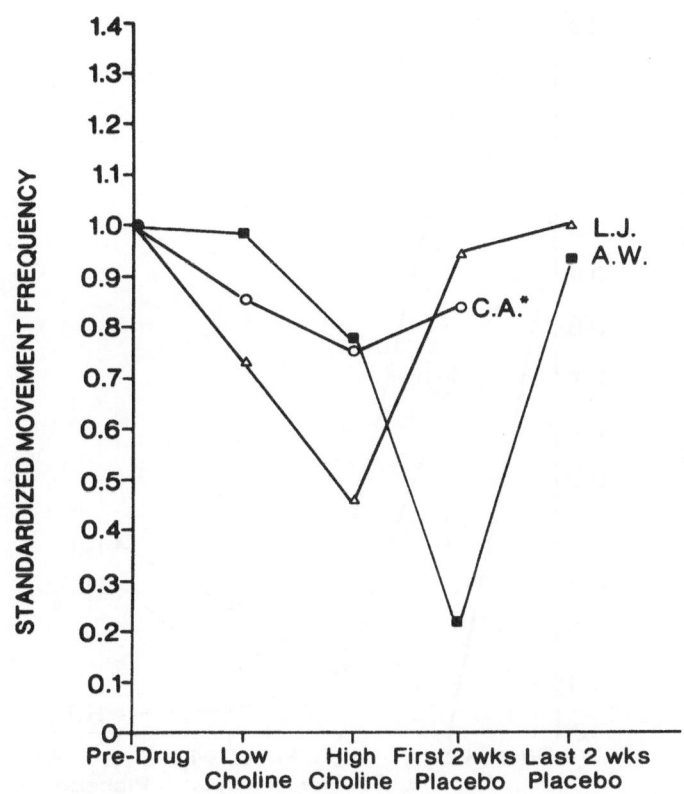

*Entire placebo period for 2 weeks only

FIGURE 1

Changes in Movement Frequencies During Choline Chloride and Placebo Treatment

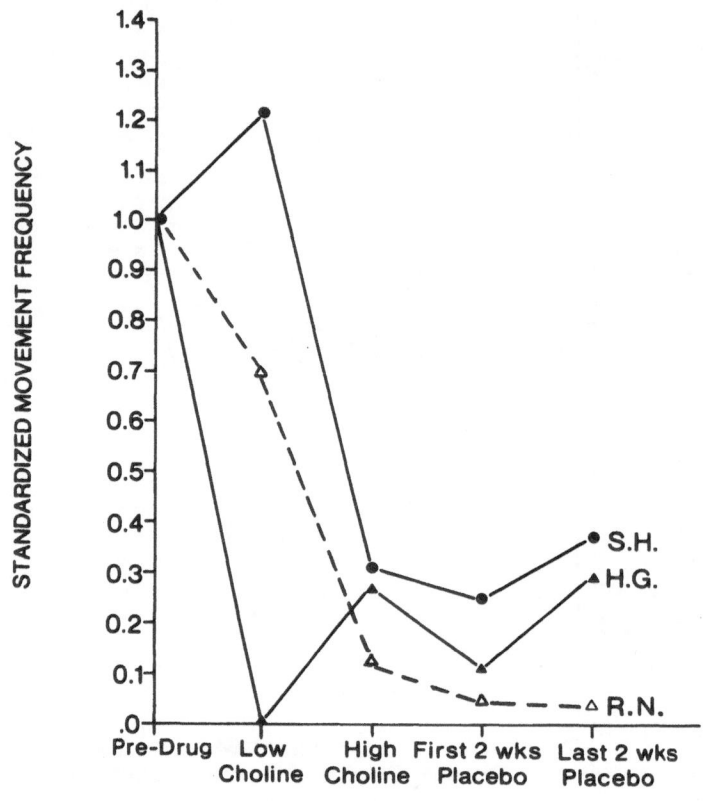

FIGURE 2

Changes in Movement Frequencies During Choline Chloride and Placebo Treatment

TABLE 1

Changes in Movement Frequency of Patients with Tardive Dyskinesia During Physostigmine Infusion

Patient	Pre-Infusion	15-90 min Post-Infusion	2½-24 hr Post-Infusion	P Value *
L.J.	7.0 ± 3.9	3.0 ± 1.0	7.3 ± 2.5	.02
C.A.	34.7 ± 1.5	16.7 ± 2.3	24.0 ± 3.8	.02
H.G.	5.3 ± 4.9	0.5 ± 0.5	5.5 ± 0.7	<.001
S.H.	2.7 ± 1.7	0.7 ± 1.6	1.8 ± 1.8	.05
R.N.	4.7 ± 6.5	0.8 ± 1.3	4.0 ± 3.8	.02

*p values are based on Mann-Whitney Rank Order test comparing data from 15-90 min post-infusion with pre-infusion and 2½-24 hr post-infusion.

NOTE: All figures represent abnormal movement frequencies during 45 sec epochs.

TABLE 2

Changes in Movement Frequency of Patients with Huntington's Disease During Physostigmine Infusion

Patient	Pre-Infusion	15-90 min Post-Infusion	2½-24 hr Post-Infusion	P Value *
J.M.	6.0 ± 3.2	0.7 ± 0.4	8.3 ± 3.4	.05
C.L.	2.7 ± 1.6	1.0 ± 0.5	1.6 ± 0.6	.03
O.M.	8.7 ± 5.6	2.7 ± 2.2	11.0 ± 5.4	.02
D.V.	2.7 ± 1.7	0.7 ± 0.8	0.7 ± 0.7	N.S.
J.H.	13.8 ± 3.7	8.7 ± 1.8	11.5 ± 0.7	N.S.
K.S.	26.1 ± 5.25	28.6 ± 5.69	26.5 ± 4.35	N.S.

*p values are based on Mann-Whitney Rank Order test comparing data from 15-90 min post-infusion with pre-infusion and 2½-24 hr post-infusion.

NOTE: All figures represent abnormal movement frequencies during 45 sec epochs.

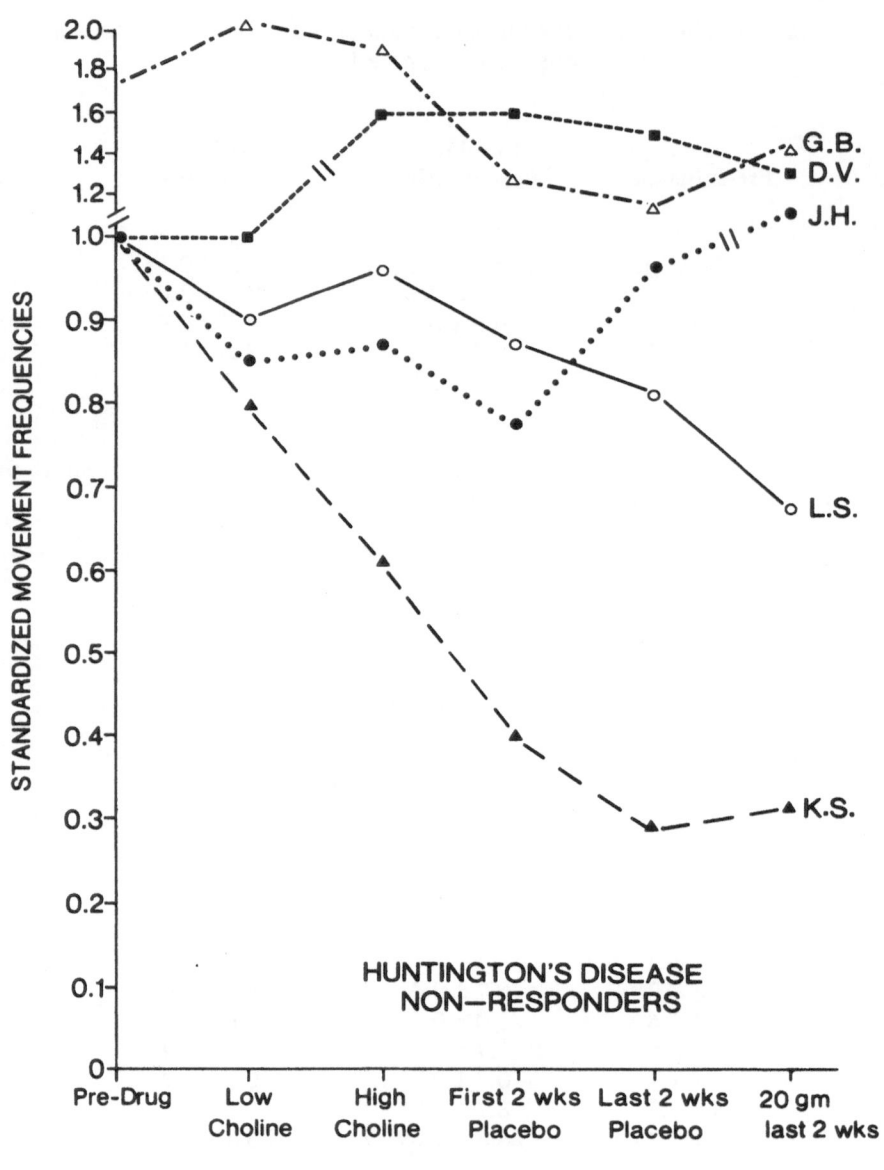

FIGURE 3

Changes in Movement Frequencies During Choline Chloride and Placebo Treatment

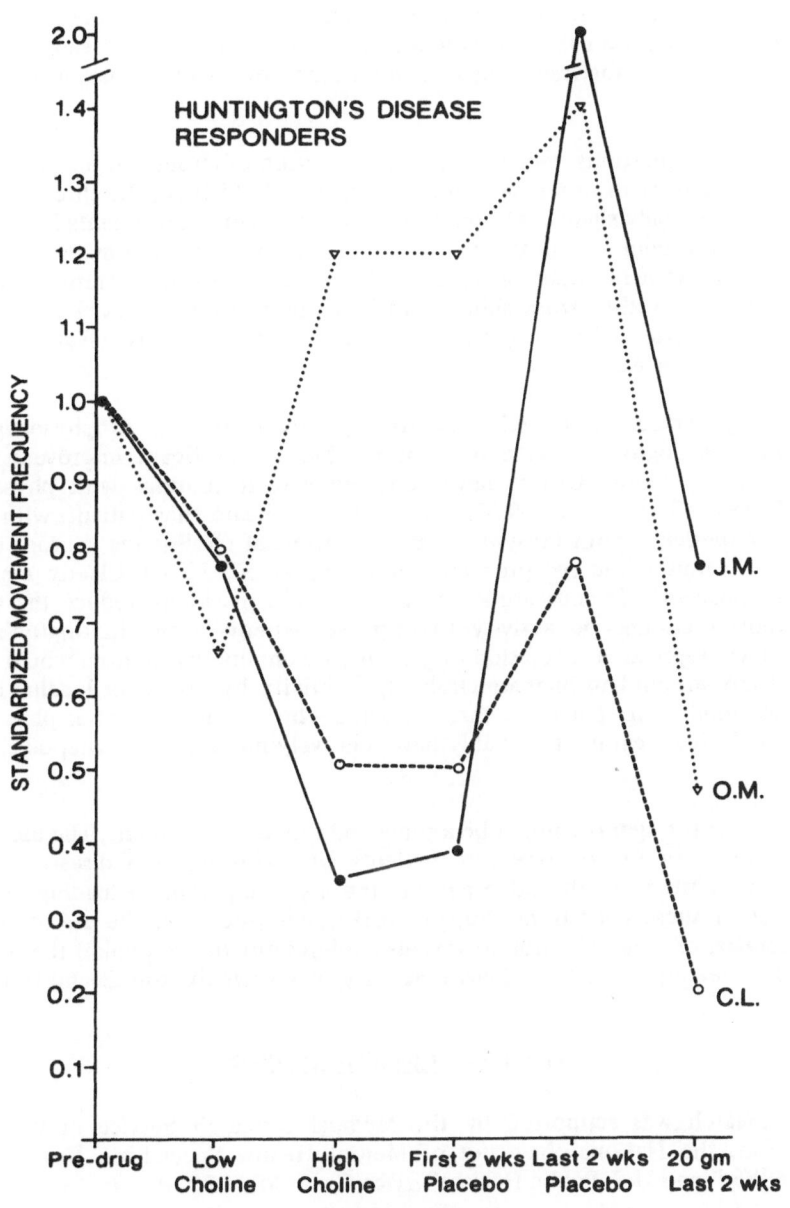

FIGURE 4

Changes in Movement Frequencies During Choline Chloride and Placebo Treatment

that the latter three patients had a slowly reversible tardive dyskinesia, and only the two patients whose movement disorder worsened on placebo had a relatively irreversible tardive dyskinesia. Thus, the three patients with a reversible dyskinesia may have gradually improved because they were no longer receiving neuroleptics. Furthermore, in those patients with a truely irreversible movement disorder, choline chloride treatment, although significantly diminishing the frequency of involuntary movements, by no means eliminated the condition.

A number of questions remain regarding the action of choline in the patients with a "reversible" movement disorder. According to a reliable history, the three patients had experienced no clinically significant change in their dyskinetic movements for 3-6 months before entering the choline study. The rather precipitous decrease in the frequency of their abnormal movements that was associated with choline administration need not be totally discounted. Further work should consider the possibility that choline treatment might produce a series of neurochemical changes that ultimately reverse neuroleptic induced receptor changes.

Increasing central cholinergic activity by administration of physostigmine to patients with Huntington's disease did not produce a significant improvement in the majority of our patients. Others have reported similar findings with physostigmine (Fann et al., 1973; Tarsy et al., 1974). Recent data indicate that patients with Huntington's disease experience both presynaptic degeneration of cholinergic neurons and a loss of postsynaptic muscarinic receptor binding (Enna et al., 1976). Clearly a significant reduction in postsynaptic muscarinic receptors would markedly reduce the ability of increased central cholinergic activity to improve patients with Huntington's disease. Furthermore, widespread degeneration of presynaptic cholinergic neurons would minimize the value of any attempt to increase cholinergic activity by precursor loading or acetylcholinesterase inhibition. Thus, the three patients who did improve after physostigmine and choline chloride treatment probably have relatively moderate presynaptic cholinergic degeneration.

Direct receptor agonists might be a preferred mode of treatment. The use of acetylcholine precursors in the treatment of patients with Huntington's disease and tardive dyskinesia has pointed out the value and limitations of a precursor loading strategy for the treatment of these conditions. Future work might focus on the use of cholinergic receptor agonists, or a combination of various cholinomimetics to exploit the therapeutic potential of increasing central cholinergic activity in tardive dyskinesia and Huntington's disease.

ACKNOWLEDGEMENTS

This research was supported by the Medical Research Service of the Veterans Administration, the National Institute of Mental Health Specialized Research Center Grant MH-30854, and U.S. Public Health Service Grant MH-03030.

REFERENCES

Aquilonius, S.M., and Eckernas, S.A., 1977, Choline therapy in Huntington's chorea, *Neurology 27:*887.

Aquilonius, S.M., and Sjostrom, R., 1971, Cholinergic and dopaminergic mechanisms in Huntington's chorea, *Life Sci. 10:*405.

Cohen, E.L., and Wurtman, R.J., 1975, Brain acetylcholine: increase after systemic choline administration, *Life Sci. 16:*1095.

Davis, K.L., Berger, P.A., and Hollister, L.E., 1975, Choline for tardive dyskinesia (a letter), *N. Engl. J. Med. 293:*152.

Davis, K.L., Hollister, L.E., Barchas, J.D., and Berger, P.A., 1976, Choline in tardive dyskinesia and Huntington's disease, *Life Sci. 19:*1507.

Enna, S.J., Bird, E.D., Bennet, J.P., Bylund, D.B., Yamamura, H.I., Iversen, L.L., and Synder, S.H., 1976, Huntington's chorea: changes in neurotransmitter receptors in the brain, *N. Engl. J. Med. 294:*1305.

Fann, W.E., Gerber, C.J., and McKenzie, G.M., 1973, Physostigmine in rigid Huntington's disease, *Confin. Neurol. 35:*312.

Gerlach, J., Reisby, N., and Randrup, A., 1974, Dopaminergic hypersensitivity and cholinergic hypofunction in the pathophysiology of tardive dyskinesia, *Psychopharmacologia 34:*21.

Growdon, J.H., Hirsch, M.J., Wurtman, R.J., and Weiner, W., 1977a, Oral choline administration to patients with tardive dyskinesia, *N. Engl. J. Med. 297:*524.

Growdon, J.H., Cohen, E.L., and Wurtman, R.J., 1977b, Huntington's disease: clinical and chemical effects of choline administration, *Ann. Neurol. 1:*418.

Haubrich, D.R., Wang, P.F.L., Wedeking, P.W., and Clody, D.E., 1975, Increase in rat brain acetylcholine induced by choline or deanol, *Life Sci. 17:*975.

Klawans, H.L., and Rubovits, R., 1972, Central cholinergic-anticholinergic antagonism in Huntington's chorea, *Neurology 22:*107.

Klawans, H.L., and Rubovits, R., 1974, Effect of cholinergic and anticholinergic agents on tardive dyskinesia, *J. Neurol. Neurosurg. Psychiatry 37:*941.

Tamminga, C.A., Smith, R.C., Ericksen, S.E., Chang, S., and Davis, J.M., 1977, Cholinergic influences in tardive dyskinesia, *Am. J. Psychiatry 134:*769.

Tarsy, D., Leopold, N., and Sax, D.S., 1974, Physostigmine in choreiform movement disorders, *Neurology 24:*28.

CHOLINE ADMINISTRATION TO PATIENTS WITH HUNTINGTON'S DISEASE OR TARDIVE DYSKINESIA

J. H. Growdon* and R. J. Wurtman

Laboratory of Neuroendocrine Regulation, Department of
Nutrition and Food Science, Massachusetts Institute of
Technology, Cambridge, Massachusetts 02139

*Department of Neurology, Tufts University Medical School,
Boston, Massachusetts 02111

INTRODUCTION

This chapter describes clinical trials of choline administration to patients with Huntington's disease (HD) or tardive dyskinesia (TD). The results illustrate a new mode of medical therapy whereby choline, a naturally occurring dietary constituent and precursor of the neurotransmitter acetylcholine (ACh), is used to treat non-nutritional brain diseases in which cholinergic activity may be deficient.

The use of choline in neuropsychiatric disease stems from two recent developments: 1) the finding that systemic administration of choline increased the levels of ACh in brains of rats and significantly increased choline levels in serum and cerebrospinal fluid of humans and 2) the publication of several independent reports describing pharmacologic testing or postmortem brain tissue analyses that indicated that ACh levels or release may be impaired in HD and TD. Investigators therefore attempted to treat these diseases by administering large doses of choline in an effort to increase ACh levels and release.

Choline has two major advantages over other cholinergic agonists, physostigmine and deanol, which have been used in the past. Deanol may be converted to choline in the liver, but its ability to increase brain ACh levels remains controversial; intravenous physostigmine does increase brain levels of ACh, but its side effects and requisite mode of administration make it an impractical form of therapy. In contrast, choline may be given orally and has few significant side effects. Choline salts, such as choline chloride, were used exclusively in the trials described here, but it is likely that numerous other choline-containing compounds will be tested in future studies. One of these, lecithin (the most common source of choline in the diet), elevates serum choline levels in human subjects more effectively than choline chloride and has even fewer side effects.

The studies reported in this chapter suggest that choline, or choline-containing compounds, may be useful in treating any disease in which only neurons that utilize ACh are involved. This may account for choline's ability to suppress the buccal-lingual-masticatory movements in some patients with TD. (This would be analogous to the beneficial effects of L-DOPA in patients with Parkinson's disease, in which dopaminergic neurons are primarily destroyed.) In contrast, choline precursor therapy may have much less value in diseases in which groups of neurons that contain ACh are only one of several underactive or degenerated neuronal populations. Thus, choline may not always help patients with HD, since several classes of neurons are often destroyed in this disease.

HUNTINGTON'S DISEASE

Huntington's disease (HD) is a chronic progressive neurologic disorder with an autosomal dominant pattern of inheritance. It is found throughout the world, and its incidence in the United States is approximately 5 per 100,000 (Bruyn, 1968). Many American patients with HD are descended from two half-brothers who immigrated from England in 1630. Their families settled in portions of the New England and mid-Atlantic states (Critchley, 1973) — some in East Hampton, Long Island, where young George Huntington saw them while making medical rounds with his physician father. In 1872, George Huntington presented his famous paper, "On Chorea," to the Meigs and Mason Academy of Medicine in Middleport, Ohio (Huntington, 1872). He described the choreics he had seen on Long Island and noted the hereditary nature of the illness, the tendency toward insanity and suicide, and the grave progressive course of the illness. He concluded that it was "one of the incurables."

Neurologic Features

Fifty percent of the children of HD patients may develop the disease. Although there are clinical variants (Juvenile, Westphal [Stevens, 1973]), the symptoms in the majority of cases begin during the third, fourth, or even fifth decades of life (Bruyn, 1968). The onset is often gradual. The first sign may be a personality change: a business-man who begins to insult his customers and forcibly ejects them from his store; a placid physician who becomes irritable and refuses to talk with or to see patients; a corporation executive who suddenly begins to make unexplained errors in judgment that are disastrous to his company. These changes are often accompanied by other signs of mental deterioration, including memory loss. As the disease progresses, patients lose interest in their surroundings; they discontinue watching television, reading, and seeing friends. They cannot recall what they have just seen or done, and become careless in dress and personal habits.

In some families, involuntary muscular contractions (chorea) signal the onset of the disease. Chorea is an abrupt involuntary movement, usually lasting 100-500 msec, that involves proximal as well as distal musculature. Unlike tremor, it is not rhythmically repetitive. When the movement is very fast it resembles the quick explosive muscular twitch of myoclonus; when chorea is slower it blends into the writhing movements of athetosis. Although these movements can usually be distinguished from chorea, many patients with HD show a range of involuntary movements that include all of these; in severe advanced stages, dystonia or fixed abnormal postures may also develop. In early or mild cases, both muscle tone (resistance to passive movement) and speed of movement are normal.

About 5-10% of patients with HD have a "rigid" form; tone is greatly increased, and akinesia may be so prominent that they superficially resemble patients with Parkinson's disease. Like patients with Parkinson's disease, those with HD have impaired postural reflexes and may fall over when tested on a tilt table. In general, however, patients with HD have neurologic deficits that are opposite from those seen in Parkinson's disease. In parkinsonism there is too little movement, as akinesia and rigidity are dominant features of the illness; in HD there is too much movement. Many patients with HD cannot stand or sit still and continuously shift their posture, fold their arms, and shuffle their feet in a perpetual dance.

Walking is often impaired, as the choreic twitches cause a lurching gait. Some patients cannot walk backwards; others either cannot run, or prance and gallop when they try to run. Speech is often affected, and both dysarthria and aphasia occur. When dysarthric, the speech is slow, slurred, and may have a jerky quality due to involuntary diaphragmatic contractions. In severely advanced cases, speech becomes dilapidated, and patients misname objects, make paraphasic errors, and may even lose verbal comprehension; some patients stop talking altogether.

Pathology

Postmortem examination shows decreased brain weight, widened cortical sulci, and shrunken cortical gyri, which attest to the general atrophic process (McMenemy, 1958). The most striking and characteristic changes, however, are in the basal ganglia, where the caudate nucleus is greatly shriveled. Normally, the head of the caudate nucleus bulges into the lateral ventricle and forms its lateral wall. In HD, caudate atrophy may be apparent on simple inspection; the convex bulge appears concave and accentuates further the hydrocephalic appearance of the brain. Microscopically, the small Golgi type II interneurons in the striatum are preferentially affected and simply disappear; there is a marked increase in the number of glial cells. The severity of the clinical signs roughly parallels the extent of cortical and caudate atrophy.

Evidence of Neurotransmitter Involvement

Phenobarbital was one of the first drugs used to treat HD and was successful in suppressing chorea to the extent that it produced sedation. Chorea, like most movement disorders, ceases during sleep, and minor tranquilizers, including the benzodiazepines, are still a useful treatment. In the 1950's, reserpine was given to patients with HD (again, as a sedative), and it also decreased the chorea somewhat. It is now known that reserpine depletes monoamine levels in the brain and that this action probably accounts for its effect on chorea.

More recently, neuroleptic drugs have been used to suppress choreic movements in patients with HD, and the more potent phenothiazines and haloperidol remain the principal modes of therapy (Whittier and Koreny, 1968). Although neuroleptics have multiple actions, they presumably suppress chorea by blocking dopamine (DA) receptors. HD is thus pharmacologically opposite from Parkinson's disease, in which the level of DA in the striatum is reduced as a result of degenerating cells in the pars compacta of the substantia nigra (Hornykiewicz, 1973). Attempts to increase DA concentrations by administering its biochemical precursor, L-DOPA, often result in clinical improvement of Parkinson's disease (Cotzias et al., 1969), whereas drugs that block DA receptors (neuroleptics) often worsen parkinsonism. In contrast, L-DOPA often exacerbates chorea, and was even used as a diagnostic "stress test" to identify subjects with HD prior to clinical manifestations (Klawans, 1972).

These pharmacologic data suggest that chorea is associated with excess DA in the basal ganglia, either in absolute level or in relation to other neurotransmitters, even though its turnover is not increased (Chase, 1973). Thus, by 1972, 100 years after George Huntington's report, drugs administered to block DA synaptic effects were the standard treatment for patients with HD (Fahn, 1972).

Even the most potent neuroleptics, however, failed to suppress chorea completely and had no effect at all on mental deterioration; it thus seemed unlikely that newer drugs of this class would provide much additional benefit. Evidence of other neurotransmitter involvement came in 1973, when Perry et al., (1973) reported that levels of glutamic acid decarboxylase (GAD), an important enzyme in the synthesis of gamma-aminobutyric acid (GABA), were reduced in brains of patients who died with HD. This was quickly confirmed, and it was also discovered that levels of choline acetyltransferase (CAT), the enzyme that catalyzes the conversion of choline to ACh, were also reduced, whereas levels of other synthetic enzymes, such as tyrosine hydroxylase (TH), were normal (Bird and Iversen, 1974; McGeer et al., 1973; Stahl and Swanson, 1974). These new observations indicated that neurons using ACh and GABA were also involved in HD and suggested new therapeutic strategies that are just now being tested. These data are also consistent with the histopathology in the caudate nucleus, since the small interneurons that atrophy are precisely the neurons that contain ACh or GABA (McGeer and McGeer, 1975; McGeer et al., 1971). Arregui et al., (1977) recently reported that levels of angiotensin-converting enzyme are greatly reduced in the globus pallidus in HD; the importance of this finding depends on whether or not angiotensin turns out to be a peptide neurotransmitter.

GABA is considered an inhibitory neurotransmitter in the central nervous system. It is synthesized according to the following reaction:

$$\text{glutamine} \xrightarrow[\text{NH}_3]{} \text{glutamic acid} \xrightarrow[\text{CO}_2]{\text{GAD}} \text{GABA} \xrightarrow{\text{GABA-T}} \text{succinic semialdehyde}$$

where GAD catalyzes the conversion of glutamic acid to GABA, which is then transaminated by GABA-transaminase (GABA-T) to succinic semialdehyde; this in turn may re-enter the Krebs cycle. Since levels of the synthetic enzyme GAD are low, levels of GABA may be low as well, and therapeutic attempts to raise them have included giving both GABA itself and its precursor, glutamate. Both are relatively excluded from the central nervous system by the blood-brain barrier, however, and their administration does not raise the levels of GABA in brain. Other strategies were used to inhibit GABA-transaminase, and thereby prolong the synaptic action of whatever GABA may be released. Dipropylacetic acid is an anticonvulsant drug that may inhibit GABA-T and thus elevate GABA levels; in one clinical trial, however, it did not suppress chorea (Shoulson et al., 1976). Other compounds that inhibit GABA-T more effectively may prove to be more useful (Perry *et al.*, 1977; Schwarcz *et al.*, 1977). Finally, imidazole-4-acetic acid, a putative GABA-receptor agonist, did not suppress chorea in patients with HD (Shoulson *et al.*, 1975).

An alternative strategy would be to increase the amount of ACh released in the striatum, since CAT levels are also reduced. Preliminary studies were consistent with this theory: antimuscarinic drugs (benztropine) increased the chorea, whereas physostigmine, a centrally active anticholinesterase, suppressed it in some instances (Davis *et al.*, 1976; Klawans and Rubovits, 1972). Physostigmine administered by intravenous infusion crosses the blood-brain barrier, and prolongs the intrasynaptic effects of ACh by inhibiting its degradation by acetylcholinesterase (AChE); the effects on the central nervous system begin within 15 min and subside after 1 hr or so. In theory, intravenous infusion of physostigmine can be a useful diagnostic test, but this mode of administration is not suitable for chronic therapy. Deanol is often described as an ACh precursor; it may be methylated to choline in the liver, but its ability to increase brain ACh levels after systemic administration is controversial (Zahniser *et al.*, 1977), and its utility in HD remains unconfirmed (Walker *et al.*, 1973). Deanol may also diminish brain ACh synthesis by competing with circulating choline for transport across the blood-brain barrier (Millington *et al.*, submitted). Thus, before choline was shown to increase brain levels of ACh, it was not possible to test the long-term clinical effects of increased cholinergic tone in patients with HD.

Choline is the physiologic precursor of ACh (Schuberth and Jenden, 1975; Schuberth *et al.*, 1969), and the amount of ACh synthesized depends on the amount of choline available in the brain (Cohen and Wurtman, 1975). The brain cannot make choline *de novo* (Ansell and Spanner, 1967) but extracts it from the systemic circulation by an unsaturated low-affinity uptake mechanism (Freeman *et al.*, 1975). Brain choline levels therefore depend on blood choline levels; treatments that increase blood choline also increase brain choline and thereby increase ACh synthesis (Cohen and Wurtman, 1976). Blood choline derives from two sources: synthesis in the liver and from the diet (Bjornsted and Bremer, 1966). In humans, the amount of choline (either as free choline or lecithin-bound choline) in the diet determines the amount of choline in the blood that is delivered to the brain (Hirsch *et al.*, in press). These data form the scientific basis for giving choline to patients with diseases, such as HD, that are associated with deficient cholinergic tone.

Clinical Trials with Choline Chloride

Experimental Design

Three clinical trials of choline chloride in patients with HD have been reported (Table 1). Each study sought to increase caudate levels of ACh by the administration of its precursor, choline. The patients in the series described by Davis *et al.*, (1976) consumed increasing amounts of choline chloride and also took a placebo; those in the studies reported by Growdon *et al.*, (1977b) and by Aquilonius and Eckernas (1977) took choline as a single open-label drug. Before choline ingestion, eight patients (three of four in the report by Davis *et al.*; five of 10 in the studies by Growdon *et al.*) received physostigmine salicylate (1.0-3.0 mg, intravenously) after pretreatment with antimuscarinic drugs that do not cross the blood-brain barrier. These patients were observed over the next hour for changes in their choreic movements. (Memory, intellectual ability, and personality were not formally graded in any of the series.)

TABLE 1

Effects of Choline Administration to Patients with HD: A Review of Three Series

Study	Number of HD Patients	Beneficial Response to Physostigmine	Choline Chloride Dose Range (g/day)	Clinical Improvement
Davis *et al.* (1976)	4	2/3	12-20	2/4
Growdon *et al.* (1977b)	10	0/5	8-20	0/10
Aquilonius and Eckernas (1977)	5	–	3-15	0/5

All three sets of investigators counted choreic movements from either videotape (Davis *et al.*, 1976; Aquilonius and Eckernas, 1977) or movies (Growdon *et al.*, 1977b). Growdon *et al.*, also counted the movements during periodic clinical examinations and used electrophysiologic techniques (Shahani and Young, 1976) to quantify the effect of choline objectively.

Patients took 3-25 g of choline chloride (except three patients in the study by Growdon *et al.*, who took an equivalent amount of choline bitartrate) in divided oral doses for between 1 week and 4 months. Growdon *et al.*, (1977b) and Aquilonius and Eckernas (1975, 1977) measured serum choline levels both before and during the period of choline ingestion, and Growdon *et al.*, (1977a) also measured choline levels in the cerebrospinal fluid. Neuroleptic medications were continued in cases where they had been previously prescribed (four of four subjects in the study by Davis *et al.*, seven of 10 subjects in the report by Growdon *et al.*, and one of five subjects in the series by Aquilonius and Eckernas).

Results

Davis *et al.*, (1976) treated four HD patients with choline chloride and reported that chorea decreased significantly in two, both of whom had improved transiently during physostigmine infusion.

Growdon *et al.*, (1977b) treated ten HD patients with choline. Prior to choline administration, five of the ten received physostigmine, and none improved. During choline ingestion, balance and gait improved in five patients, but this effect was transient and did not persist beyond two weeks despite continued choline administration. Thus, Growdon *et al.*, found that choline did not suppress chorea in any of the ten patients; the number of choreic movements actually increased in two patients during choline administration but returned to a pretreatment level once the choline was discontinued.

Aquilonius and Eckernas (1977) treated five patients. They also reported minor changes in chorea during choline ingestion, but concluded that choline did not significantly suppress the movements. Growdon *et al.*, and Aquilonius and Eckernas both reported a linear increase in serum choline levels with increasing doses of choline over a 3-15 g/day range. Growdon *et al.* also found that choline levels in the cerebrospinal fluid rose significantly during the period of choline ingestion (Figure 1), although — contrary to a previous report (Aquilonius *et al.*, 1972) — the pretreatment choline levels in the cerebrospinal fluid of these patients were not significantly lower than those of normal subjects.

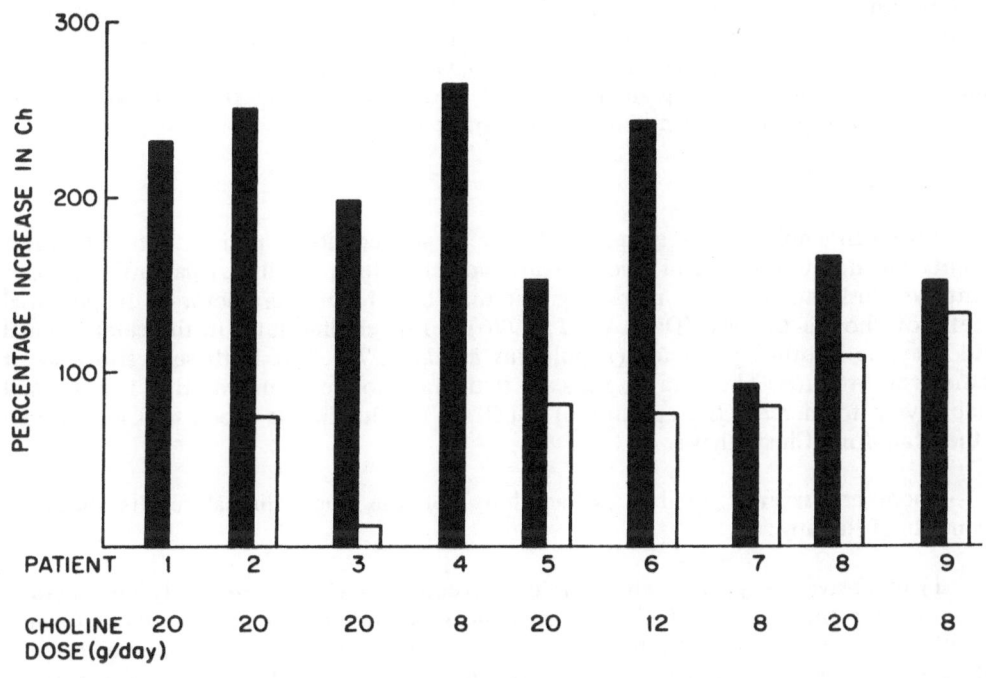

FIGURE 1

Percentage increase in blood and cerebrospinal fluid (CSF) choline (Ch) levels during maximal oral Ch administration in patients with Huntington's disease. (Pretreatment Ch levels were not measured in Patient 10.) Dark bars indicate sera and open bars represent CSF. Samples were collected on separate days 1 hr after a Ch dose. CSF was not collected from Patients 1 and 4. (From Growdon *et al.*, (1977b), reprinted, by permission, from the *Ann. Neurol. 1:*420).

Side Effects

Although acute doses of choline have been used in the past to treat patients with liver disease (De La Huerga and Popper, 1951), these three reports affirm that humans can take large amounts of choline orally for long periods with safety. All patients did develop a "fishy" odor in their urine, sweat, and breath that disappeared when choline ingestion ceased. The odor apparently derived from the action of intestinal bacteria on choline, which produced trimethylamines (Lee *et al.*, 1976). This odor is less likely to develop after lecithin ingestion and, since lecithin also elevates serum choline levels (Hirsch *et al.*, in press; Wurtman *et al.*, 1977), it may provide a more agreeable form of choline therapy.

All investigators noted gastrointestinal symptoms (nausea, abdominal cramps, vomiting, diarrhea) that usually occurred with high doses and ceased when the dosage was lowered or discontinued. Growdon *et al.*, (1977b) did not detect any hematologic, hepatic, or renal signs of toxicity; blood pressure and the electrocardiograms were not significantly altered during choline ingestion. Davis *et al.*, (1976) did report that the P-R interval on the electrocardiogram lengthened during choline ingestion in two patients who did not take peripherally acting antimuscarinic drugs.

Conclusions

Although choline may suppress chorea in an occasional patient with HD, most patients did not improve, and two actually worsened temporarily. A patient's response to intravenously administered physostigmine may be a helpful predictor of the potential benefit of choline therapy (Davis *et al.*, 1976); a low choline level in the cerebrospinal fluid may be another predictor (Aquilonius *et al.*, 1972), but both suggestions await further confirmation. The data do indicate that oral choline administration is a safe and reliable way to increase the amount of substrate choline in the blood that is delivered to the brain for ACh synthesis.

There are several possible explanations for the poor clinical results following this mode of therapy:

1) extensive presynaptic cholinergic destruction — CAT is normally unsaturated, and increasing the amount of choline available to it accelerates ACh synthesis (Cohen and Wurtman, 1976). In HD, however, CAT in the remaining neurons may become fully saturated and thus be unable to increase ACh synthesis further even in the presence of additional amounts of substrate.

2) postsynaptic cholinergic destruction — the number of striatal cholinergic receptor sites may be so reduced (Enna *et al.*, 1976) that any newly synthesized ACh, should it be released, has no target, and thus no effect.

3) faulty theory — it is, of course, possible that choline ingestion does not increase brain ACh content in humans, even though it does in rats. The increase in caudate levels of ACh induced by choline causes increased cholinergic neurotransmission in rats (Ulus and Wurtman, 1976; Ulus *et al.*, 1977), but may not do so in humans. Even if choline does increase ACh levels and release in human subjects, such an effect may not correct the underlying pathophysiology of chorea.

TARDIVE DYSKINESIA

Epidemiology

Tardive dyskinesia is another choreiform disorder. It is characterized by involuntary repetitive movements involving the face (eyelids, tongue, lips, and jaw) and extremities; in severe cases there are muscular spasms of the trunk as well (Crane, 1968). These movements can arise spontaneously, especially in older people ("senile" chorea); occasionally they occur in patients who have taken antihistaminic (Thatch *et al.*, 1975) or anticonvulsant (Chadwick *et al.*, 1976) drugs for long periods. They usually occur, however, after the chronic ingestion of neuroleptic drugs (phenothiazines, haloperidol).

Neuroleptics were introduced into clinical psychiatry in 1952, and the earliest reports of TD appeared 7 years later (Druckman *et al.*, 1962; Sigwald *et al.*, 1959; Uhrbrand and Faurbye, 1960). Evidence that neuroleptics cause TD was overwhelming when the American College of Neuropsychopharmacology task force formally recognized the relationship between these drugs and the disease (Food and Drug Administration, 1973). In contrast to the other neurologic side effects of neuroleptics (idiosyncratic acute dystonic reactions, dose-related Parkinson's syndrome, and akathisia), TD generally occurs after neuroleptics are taken for months or years. TD may occur during drug therapy, but it most often begins when the drug dose is lowered or discontinued.

Dyskinesia means abnormal movement; the term tardive underscores its delayed or late onset. The exact incidence of TD is unknown, and most estimates are based on surveys done in chronic mental hospitals, where the incidence is as high as 40% (Fann *et al.*, 1972). Since TD seems to be most prevalent in the elderly, it is possible that underlying structural brain damage facilitates neuroleptic-induced dyskinesias. Patients with TD have normal CT (computerized tomography) brain scans, however (Gelenberg, 1976), and only minor nonspecific pathologic changes at postmortem examination. Christiansen *et al.*, (1970) did describe an increased incidence of neuronal degeneration and gliosis in the substantia nigra of brains from patients with TD, but this report awaits confirmation.

TD is more often reported in women than in men, but this may merely reflect the sex distribution of the aged populations surveyed in nursing homes and chronic state hospitals. Both the duration of neuroleptic medication and the dose may influence the development of TD, but a careful prospective study has not yet been reported. It is well known, however, that TD can begin in patients who have taken low doses of phenothiazines for less than one year. Another possible variable is the class of neuroleptic. Although all phenothiazines can produce TD, some, such as thioridazine, are considered "safer" than others. The new antipsychotic drug clozapine apparently has few extrapyramidal side effects, and may not cause TD at all (Matz *et al.*, 1974), but its use may be restricted because of its suspected toxicity to bone marrow. Nevertheless, use of this drug does illustrate that it is possible to retain antipsychotic activity and eliminate undesired neurologic side effects.

Symptomatology

TD consists of involuntary choreic movements in the face, limbs, and trunk. There are no laboratory tests for TD; the diagnosis is made on clinical grounds and is most secure when the documented onset of involuntary movements coincides with neuro-leptic therapy. Among the many diseases that may present with choreic movements (Asnis, 1977), patients with psychoses and mental retardation can exhibit mannerisms that are indistinguishable from the movements of patients with TD, and this similarity may cause diagnostic uncertainty. It is also necessary to consider HD and L-DOPA toxicity in patients with Parkinson's disease in the differential diagnosis of TD, since either condition may mimic TD.

TD most often affects the facial musculature. Although the entire face may spas-modically grimace, more often a particular part is involved, and tongue movements are most common. There may be a continuous fine rapid tongue tremor, or slower, large-amplitude rolling tongue movements. The "fly-catcher tongue," in which the tongue protrudes from the mouth and retracts repetitively every second or so, is the most dramatic movement. In some patients, the lips quiver or periodically pucker; there may be a twitch at the corner of the mouth. Jaw movements range from an occasional twitch to a con-tinual tremor; some patients have chewing movements. These motions are usually asymp-tomatic, but an occasional patient may have difficulty speaking and swallowing. Eye blink frequency may increase, and severe blepharoclonus may even cause functional blindness.

The extremities are the next most commonly involved site of chorea in TD. Limb movements generally involve the distal musculature and consist of small-amplitude, irregular finger or foot twitches. In more severe instances, stereotyped finger tapping may occur and, rarely, the arms fling about the body. Limb movements may be seen in con-junction with facial chorea but can occur alone.

Muscle spasms of the neck and trunk are the least common movements in patients with TD but are often the most severe; face and limbs are usually affected as well in these patients. The movements may consist of spasmodic torticollis and retrocollis; opisthotonus also occurs. In severe forms, patients are completely disabled and may even require assistance eating and dressing.

Natural History

Spontaneous buccal-lingual-masticatory movements of the elderly ("senile" chorea) generally do not improve without medication, whereas movements that are secondary to neuroleptics (TD) may subside spontaneously once the drug has been discontinued. Improvement may take a year or more, however, and no chorea should be called "permanent" until this much time has elapsed. In many patients with TD, however, the symptoms do not subside but persist unchanged for years. The best treatment is preven-tion; physicians should use neuroleptics only for treating psychotic illnesses, prescribe the lowest effective dose, give them for the shortest duration possible, and discontinue the drug (if possible) at the first sign of TD. In addition, there is suggestive evidence that concurrent administration of anticholinergic drugs facilitates the development of TD; these thus should not be given unless a parkinsonian syndrome develops (Klawans, 1973).

Evidence for Neurotransmitter Involvement in TD

In contrast to the data available on HD, no postmortem analyses have been published concerning neurotransmitter enzymes in brains of patients who died with TD. Thus, evidence for the involvement of specific neurotransmitters is more indirect and is based on neuropharmacologic testing; nevertheless, it indicates that an imbalance exists in the postulated reciprocal relation between dopaminergic and cholinergic neurotransmission in the basal ganglia (Davis *et al.*, 1975b; Gerlach *et al.*, 1974; Klawans and Rubovits, 1974).

It is widely believed that neuroleptic drugs, by blocking intrasynaptic DA receptors, cause a reflex overactivity of dopaminergic neurons, which may be due to increased DA turnover (Carlsson, 1975), to "denervation" supersensitivity (Tarsy and Baldessarini, 1974), or to increased DA receptor density (Burt *et al.*, 1977). Thus, drugs used to treat TD include those that block catecholamine synthesis (alpha-methyl-p-tyrosine) (Chase, 1972; Gerlach *et al.*, 1974), deplete the brain of monoamines (reserpine, tetrabenazine) (Kazamatsuri *et al.*, 1972a), or antagonize DA actions on synaptic receptors (phenothiazines, haloperidol) (Kazamatsuri *et al.*, 1972b).

In contrast, drugs that stimulate DA receptors (amphetamine, L-DOPA) often exacerbate TD (Gerlach *et al.*, 1974; Klawans and McKendall, 1971), a finding consistent with the dopaminergic-hyperactivity theory. Indeed, it is possible to suppress TD in most patients by giving adequate doses of a potent neuroleptic (DA-receptor antagonist); this is counterproductive, however, inasmuch as these drugs caused the syndrome in the first place.

Evidence that cholinergic neurons are involved in TD is also indirect and based on the theory that dopaminergic neurons from the substantia nigra inhibit cholinergic interneurons in the striatum (McGeer *et al.*, 1974). With the relative increase in dopaminergic tone postulated to occur as a result of chronic neuroleptic medication, cholinergic neurons are suppressed even further with a resultant decrease in ACh release. Clinical neuropharmacologic testing tends to support this hypothesis, since antimuscarinic drugs (e.g., scopolamine) tend to worsen TD (Gerlach *et al.*, 1974; Klawans and Rubovits, 1974). There are exceptions, however, and some patients with TD apparently improve while taking anticholinergics (Granacher *et al.*, 1975; Uhrbrand and Faurbye, 1960). Attempts to increase cholinergic tone in the striatum at the synapse distal to that employing DA have had some limited success in treating TD. For example, the choline precursor deanol apparently has produced some benefit in a few specific cases (Casey and Denny, 1975; De Silva and Huang, 1975; Fann *et al.*, 1975) but not in most others (Crane, 1975; Escobar and Kemp, 1975), including a recent double-blind study (Tarsy and Bralower, 1977). Intravenously administered physostigmine reportedly decreased choreic movements temporarily in some patients with TD (Davis *et al.*, 1976; Fann *et al.*, 1974; Klawans and Rubovits, 1974), but its route of administration precludes its use in chronic therapy.

Clinical Trials

The demonstration that exogenous choline elevates brain choline and ACh levels in rats suggested that choline administration might increase brain ACh levels in humans as well, and thus provide a practical way to restore deficient cholinergic tone (Davis *et al.*, 1975b; Growdon *et al.*, 1977c). Shortly after the initial publication of the animal data, Davis *et al.* (1975a) reported that choline chloride (16 g/day) suppressed choreic movements in a single patient with TD. These same authors subsequently reported that oral doses of choline chloride (16-20 g/day) suppressed TD in four patients, all of whom had responded favorably to acute physostigmine infusions (Davis *et al.*, 1976). These preliminary findings were consistent with the hypotheses that choline ingestion increased brain levels of ACh in humans as well as in rats; that TD does arise, at least in part, from too much dopaminergic tone at the expense of ACh; and that therapeutic strategies designed to enhance cholinergic tone might be successful in treating diseases, like TD, in which cholinergic tone is presumably deficient.

Two subsequent studies confirmed these general conclusions (Table 2). Tamminga *et al.* (1977) gave choline chloride as a single open-label drug to four patients with TD, and two improved. Choline was discontinued in the other two before adequate doses were reached because of intercurrent depression (Tamminga *et al.*, 1976). Growdon *et al.* (1977d) described the largest clinical trial thus far reported on the use of choline in patients with TD. They gave choline chloride to 20 patients with "permanent" TD according to a double-blind cross-over protocol. They counted the number of buccal-lingual-masticatory facial movements that occurred during 30-sec observation periods before, during, and after both choline and placebo ingestion and reviewed movies taken during each medication period. Ten patients received 150 mg/kg/day of choline chloride in three divided doses for the first week of the study and 200 mg/kg/day during the second week; the other 10 received a bitter-tasting placebo administered in an identical manner. These schedules were reversed after a 10-day interval during which neither choline nor placebo was dispensed. The 12 patients taking neuroleptics when the study began continued the medication, but the six patients taking anticholinergics (trihexyphenidyl, benztropine) discontinued them prior to the study (Table 3). Neither the patients, the ward staff, nor the examining physicians knew which compound — choline or placebo — a patient received during the study. Blood samples for choline measurements were collected from every patient before the drug trial began and again during the final weeks of choline and placebo ingestion. All blood samples were collected before breakfast; during the treatment periods they were obtained 1 hr after the medication was given. Serum samples were separated, frozen, and assayed for choline content by a radioenzymatic method (Shea and Aprison, 1973).

TABLE 2

Effects of Choline Administration to Patients With TD: A Summary of Three Series

Study	Number of TD Patients	Number of Patients Who Improved With Choline	Choline Chloride Dose Range g/day
Davis *et al.* (1976)	4	4	16-20
Tamminga *et al.* (1977)	4	2	3-18
Growdon *et al.* (1977d)	20	9	8-20

TABLE 3

Clinical Characteristics of 20 Patients with Tardive Dyskinesia

Case Number	Age	Sex	Primary Diagnosis	Severity of Tardive Dyskinesia	Current Medication	Dosage (mg/day)
1	36	F	Schizophrenia	Moderate	Thiothixene	100
2	55	F	Schizophrenia	Moderate	Chlorpromazine	300
					Trifluoperazine	40
					Trihexypenidyl[a]	
3	38	F	Schizophrenia	Moderate	Haloperidol	15
					Phenytoin	300
					Phenobarbital	100
					Trihexyphenidyl[a]	
4	75	F	Senile dementia	Severe	Thioridazine	75
5	63	M	Schizophrenia	Severe	Phenytoin	300
					Benztropine[a]	
6	85	F	Senile dementia	Severe	Diazepam	8
					Phenytoin	300
7	79	F	Schizophrenia	Moderate	None	
8	66	F	Mental retardation with psychosis	Severe	Phenytoin	300

TABLE 3 (CONTINUED)

Clinical Characteristics of 20 Patients with Tardive Dyskinesia

Case Number	Age	Sex	Primary Diagnosis	Severity of Tardive Dyskinesia	Current Medication	Dosage (mg/day)
9	73	F	Schizophrenia	Severe	None	
10	48	F	Schizophrenia	Severe	Haloperidol Phenobarbital Benztropine[a]	5 120
11	72	F	Schizophrenia	Moderate	Chlorprothizene	150
12	80	F	Schizophrenia	Severe	Thioridazine Diphenhydramine	50 100
13	63	F	Schizophrenia	Mild	Thioridazine Benztropine[a]	300
14	52	F	Schizophrenia	Mild	Chlorpromazine Phenytoin Phenobarbital	100 300 100
15	62	F	Schizophrenia	Moderate	None	
16	37	M	Schizophrenia	Mild	Fluphenazine	25
17	76	M	Senile dementia	Severe	Diphenhydramine	50

TABLE 3 (CONTINUED)

Clinical Characteristics of 20 Patients with Tardive Dyskinesia

Case Number	Age	Sex	Primary Diagnosis	Severity of Tardive Dyskinesia	Current Medication	Dosage (mg/day)
18	32	M	Mental retardation with psychosis	Moderate	Haloperidol Phenytoin Trihexyphenidyl[a]	40 300
19	37	F	Mental retardation with psychosis	Severe	Phenytoin Phenobarbital	300 160
20	66	M	Schizophrenia	Mild	Thioridazine	400

[a]Discontinued before choline protocol began.

From Growdon et al., (1977d), reprinted, by permission, from the N. Engl. J. Med. 297:525.

During the second week of choline ingestion, buccal-lingual-masticatory move-ments decreased greatly in five patients and moderately in four others; the movements were unchanged in ten and worse in one (Table 4). Thus, nine of 20 patients with TD improved during choline ingestion even in the presence of neuroleptics. Four of the five patients who greatly improved took both choline and their usual neuroleptic dose. The number of movements per 30 sec did not change from control values during placebo ingestion in any patient. When choline was discontinued, the number of movements returned to baseline values within 1-2 weeks, both in patients who had improved and in the one who had worsened. One patient who had improved greatly took a second course of choline for 2 weeks, and her number of tongue protrusions decreased from 20 per 30 sec to 6 per 30 sec within 1 week, exactly as they had during the first course.

TABLE 4

Clinical Effect of Choline Administration on the Buccal-Lingual-Masticatory Movements in 20 Patients with Tardive Dyskinesia

Classification	Number of Patients	Mean Number of Movements Per 30 Seconds		Percent Change[a]
		Before Choline	During Choline	Range
Greatly improved	5	12.6	4.2	+74 – +84
Moderately improved	4	21.2	11.7	+41 – +55
Unchanged	10	13.4	13.6	+18 – –21
Worsened	1	4.5	27.5	–511

[a] + Indicates improvement, and – worsening of the chorea.

From Growdon *et al.* (1977d), reprinted, by permission, from the *N. Engl. J. Med. 297:*525.

Mean serum choline levels rose by 170% (P < .001), from 12.4 ± 1.0 (mean ± SEM) to 33.5 ± 2.5 nmole/ml, during choline therapy. Serum choline levels measured during placebo administration and at the end of the 10-day washout period did not differ significantly from control values. These data confirm observations from other studies that oral choline ingestion significantly increases the amount of choline available to the brain (Aquilonius and Eckernas, 1975; Growdon *et al.*, 1977a; Wurtman *et al.*, 1977). The data are also consistent with the expectation that choline would enhance ACh synthesis in humans as well as in rats, and support the theory that increased ACh release might suppress TD.

Not all patients improved, however, and the variety of their responses suggests that the patient sample was heterogeneous at least with respect to cholinergic mechanisms

(Growdon and Wurtman, 1977). No specific features were identified that distinguished patients who improved with choline from those who did not. Baseline serum choline levels of patients who improved did not differ significantly from those of patients who did not improve; both groups had a similar rise in serum choline levels during choline therapy. Other variables — including age, sex, primary diagnosis, concurrent medication, and clinical features of the movements — did not help to predict a favorable response to choline. Intravenous physostigmine was not administered in this study; the results reported by Davis *et al.* (1976), however, suggest that a choreic patient's response to this drug might help to predict his or her potential for benefiting from choline.

Side Effects

Most patients who ingested choline chloride developed a "fishy" odor that disappeared when the treatment was discontinued. Gastronintestinal complaints were common with high doses of choline and consisted of nausea, abdominal cramps, and diarrhea; these symptoms subsided when the dose of choline was lowered. Tamminga *et al.* (1977) reported that two of the four patients in their study became depressed while taking choline and that both attempted suicide. Even though these patients took low doses of choline (3-9 g/day), the investigators thought that choline may have precipitated the depression, and thus discontinued the treatment. Growdon *et al.* (1977d) reported that two of their 20 patients seemed more withdrawn and apathetic during choline therapy; both patients, however, were able to complete the experimental protocol. Choline did not exacerbate underlying psychosis in any of the 20 patients, nor did it diminish the efficacy of the neuroleptics that 13 of them continued to take.

More recently, Growdon and Gelenberg (unpublished observations) detected increased signs of parkinsonism in two of four young patients with TD who were treated with choline while taking neuroleptics. Facial expressions were less lively in one patient, and arm rigidity increased in another; these signs subsided when choline was discontinued. These side effects constitute additional evidence that increased choline consumption accelerates ACh synthesis and release in human subjects as well as in rats.

CONCLUSION

The oral administration of large doses of dietary constituents that are neurotransmitter precursors constitutes a new mode of treatment for neuropsychiatric diseases. Choline is the physiological precursor of the neurotransmitter ACh, and the amount of choline available to the brain determines the amount of ACh that is synthesized. The demonstration that choline administration increased brain ACh levels in rats encouraged physicians to give choline to patients with neuropsychiatric diseases that, like TD and HD, had been associated with deficient cholinergic tone. These studies indicated that most human subjects could ingest large doses of choline safely, and that choline administration significantly increased choline concentrations in the serum and cerebrospinal fluid. Lecithin, the naturally occurring dietary source of choline, also elevated brain levels of ACh in rats; when given to normal human subjects, it increased serum choline levels to a greater extent than did choline chloride alone. These observations underlie current attempts to use choline precursor therapy in patients with TD and HD.

To date, three separate groups of investigators have reported that oral choline administration suppressed choreiform movements in many patients with TD. Patients with HD responded less well, although a few did improve with choline treatment. Although choline was administered in the form of choline chloride in both the TD and HD clinical trials, lecithin may be even more effective and surely will be tested in future studies. These preliminary trials indicate that choline (or compounds that contain choline, such as lecithin) may be prescribed for any disease in which the physician may wish to enhance cholinergic tone.

ACKNOWLEDGEMENTS

These studies were supported in part by grants from ADAMHA (MH-28783), the National Aeronautics and Space Administration (NGR-22-009-627), and the Ford Foundation.

REFERENCES

Ansell, G.B., and Spanner, S., 1967, The metabolism of labeled ethanolamine in the brain of the rat *in vivo*, *J. Neurochem. 14:*873.

Aquilonius, S.M., and Eckernas, S.A., 1975, Plasma concentration of free choline in patients with Huntington's chorea on high doses of choline chloride, *N. Engl. J. Med. 293:*1105.

Aquilonius, S.M., and Eckernas, S.A., 1977, Choline therapy in Huntington's chorea, *Neurology 27:*887.

Aquilonius, S.M., Nystrom, B., Schuberth, J., and Sundwall, A., 1972, Cerebrospinal fluid choline in extrapyramidal disorders, *J. Neurol. Neurosurg. Psychiatry 35:*720.

Arregui, A., Bennett, J.P., Bird, E.D., Yamamura, H.I., Iversen, L.I., and Snyder, S.H., 1977, Huntington's chorea: selective depletion of activity of angiotensin converting enzyme in the corpus striatum, *Ann. Neurol. 2:*294.

Asnis, G.M., 1977, Tardive dyskinesia: is it or is it not? *Dis. Nerv. Syst. 38:*856.

Bird, E.D., and Iversen, L.L., 1974, Huntington's chorea: postmortem measurement of glutamic acid decarboxylase, choline acetyltransferase, and dopamine in basal ganglia, *Brain 97:*457.

Bjornsted, P., and Bremer, J., 1966, *In vivo* studies on pathways for the biosynthesis of lecithin in the rat, *J. Lipid Res. 7:*38.

Bruyn, G.W., 1968, Huntington's chorea, in *"Handbook of Clinical Neurology" Vol. 6, "Diseases of the Basal Ganglia,"* (P.J. Vinken and G.W. Bruyn, eds.), pp. 298-378, John Wiley and Sons, New York.

Burt, D.R., Creese, I., and Snyder, S., 1977, Antischizophrenic drugs: chronic treatment elevates dopamine receptor binding in brain, *Science 196:*326.

Carlsson, A., 1975, Some aspects of dopamine in the basal ganglia, *Res. Publ. Assoc. Res. Nerv. Ment. Dis. 55:*181.

Casey, D.E., and Denny, D., 1975, Deanol in the treatment of tardive dyskinesia, *Am. J. Psychiatry 132:*864.

Chadwick, D., Reynolds, E.H., and Marsden, C.D., 1976, Anticonvulsive-induced dyskinesias: a comparison with dyskinesias induced by neuroleptics, *J. Neurol. Neursurg. Psychiatry 39:*1210.

Chase, T.N., 1972, Drug-induced extrapyramidal disorders, *Res. Publ. Assoc. Res. Nerv. Ment. Dis. 50:*448.

Chase, T.N., 1973, Biochemical and pharmacologic studies of monoamines in Huntington's chorea, in *"Advances in Neurology,"* Vol. 1, *"Huntington's Chorea, 1872-1972,"* (A. Barbeau, T.N. Chase, and G.W. Paulson, eds.), pp. 533-542, Raven Press, New York.

Christiansen, E., Moller, J.E., and Faurbye, A., 1970, Neuropathological investigation of 28 brains from patients with dyskinesia, *Acta Psychiatr. Scand. 46:*14.

Cohen, E.L., and Wurtman, R.J., 1975, Brain acetylcholine: increase after systemic choline administration, *Life Sci. 16:*1095.

Cohen, E.L., and Wurtman, R.J., 1976, Brain acetylcholine: control by dietary choline, *Science 191:*561.

Cotzias, G.C., Papavasiliou, P.S., and Gellene, R., 1969, Modification of Parkinsonism: chronic treatment with L-DOPA, *N. Engl. J. Med. 280:*337.

Crane, G.E., 1968, Tardive dyskinesia in patients treated with major neuroleptics: a review of the literature, *Am. J. Psychiatry 124(8):*Suppl:40.

Crane, G.E., 1975, Deanol for tardive dyskinesia, *N. Engl. J. Med. 292:*926.

Critchley, M., 1973, Great Britain and the early history of Huntington's chorea, *Adv. Neurol. 1:*13.

Davis, K.L., Berger, P.A., and Hollister, L.E., 1975a, Choline for tardive dyskinesia, *N. Engl. J. Med. 293:*152.

Davis, K.L., Hollister, L.E., Berger, P.A., and Barchas, J.D., 1975b, Cholinergic imbalance hypotheses of psychoses and movement disorders: strategies for evaluation, *Psychopharmacol. Commun. 1:*533.

Davis, K.L., Hollister, L.E., Barchas, J.D., and Berger, P.A., 1976, Choline in tardive dyskinesia and Huntington's disease, *Life Sci. 19:*1507.

De La Huerga, J., and Popper, H., 1951, Urinary excretion of choline metabolites following choline administration in normals and patients with hepatobiliary diseases, *J. Clin. Invest. 30:*463.

De Silva, L., and Huang, C.Y., 1975, Deanol in tardive dyskinesia, *Br. Med. J. 3:*466.

Druckman, R., Seelinger, D., and Thulin, B., 1962, Chronic involuntary movements induced by phenothiazines, *J. Nerv. Ment. Dis. 135:*69.

Enna, S.J., Bird, E.D., Bennett, J.P., Byland, D.B., Yamamura, H.I., Iversen, L.L., and Snyder, S.H., 1976, Huntington's chorea: changes in neurotransmitter receptors in the brain, *N. Engl. J. Med. 294:*1305.

Escobar, J.I., and Kemp, K.F., 1975, Dimethylaminoethanol for tardive dyskinesia, *N. Engl. J. Med. 292:*317.

Fahn, S., 1972, Treatment of choreic movements with perphenazine, *Dis. Nerv. Syst. 33:*653.

Fann, W.E., Davis, J.M., and Janowsky, D.S., 1972, The prevalence of tardive dyskinesia in mental hospital patients, *Dis. Nerv. Syst. 33:*182.

Fann, W.E., Lake, C.R., and Gerber, C.J., 1974, Cholinergic suppression of tardive dyskinesia, *Psychopharmacologia 37:*101.

Fann, W.E., Sullivan, J.L. III, Miller, R.D., and McKenzie, G.M., 1975, Deanol in tardive dyskinesia: a preliminary report, *Psychopharmacologia 42:*135.

Food and Drug Administration Task Force, American College of Neuropsychopharmacology, 1973, Neurological syndromes associated with anti-psychotic drug use: a special report, *Arch. Gen. Psychiatry 28:*463.

Freeman, J.J., Choi, R.L., and Jenden, D.J., 1975, Plasma choline: its turnover and exchange with brain choline, *J. Neurochem. 24:*729.

Gelenberg, A.J., 1976, Computerized tomography in patients with tardive dyskinesia, *Am. J. Psychiatry 133:*578.

Gerlach, J., Reisby, N., and Randrup, A., 1974, Dopaminergic hypersensitivity and cholinergic hypofunction in the pathophysiology of tardive dyskinesia, *Psychopharmacologia 34:*21.

Granacher, R.P., Baldessarini, R.J., and Cole, J.O., 1975, Deanol for tardive dyskinesia, *N. Engl. J. Med. 292:*926.

Growdon, J.H., and Wurtman, R.J., 1977, Choline for tardive dyskinesia (letter to the editor), *N. Engl. J. Med. 297:*1236.

Growdon, J.H., Cohen, E.L., and Wurtman, R.J., 1977a, Effects of oral choline administration on serum and CSF choline levels in patients with Huntington's disease, *J. Neurochem. 28:*229.

Growdon, J.H., Cohen, E.L., and Wurtman, R.J., 1977b, Huntington's disease: clinical and chemical effects of choline administration, *Ann. Neurol. 1:*418.

Growdon, J.H., Cohen, E.L., and Wurtman, R.J., 1977c, Treatment of brain diseases with dietary precursors of neurotransmitters, *Ann. Int. Med. 86:*337.

Growdon, J.H., Hirsch, M.J., Wurtman, R.J., and Wiener, W., 1977d, Oral choline administration to patients with tardive dyskinesia, *N. Engl. J. Med. 297:*524.

Hirsch, M.J., Growdon, J.H., and Wurtman, R.J., (in press), Relations between dietary choline or lecithin intake, serum choline levels and various metabolic indices, *Metabolism.*

Hornykiewicz, O., 1973, Dopamine in the basal ganglia, *Br. Med. Bull. 29:*172.

Huntington, G., 1872, On chorea, *The Medical and Surgical Reporter 26:*317.

Kazamatsuri, H., Chien, C., and Cole, J.O., 1972a, Treatment of tardive dyskinesia. I. Clinical efficacy of a dopamine-depleting agent, tetrabenazine, *Arch. Gen. Psychiatry 27:*95.

Kazamatsuri, H., Chien, C., and Cole, J.O., 1972b, Treatment of tardive dyskinesia. II. Short-term efficacy of dopamine-blocking agents, haloperidol and thiopropazate, *Arch. Gen. Psychiatry 27:*100.

Klawans, H., 1972, Use of L-DOPA in the detection of presymptomatic Huntington's chorea, *N. Engl. J. Med. 286:*1332.

Klawans, H.L., 1973, The pharmacology of tardive dyskinesia, *Am. J. Psychiatry 130:* 82.

Klawans, H.L., and McKendall, R.R., 1971, Observations on the effect of levodopa on tardive lingual-facial-buccal dyskinesia, *J. Neurol. Sci. 14:*189.

Klawans, H.L., and Rubovits, R., 1972, Central cholinergic-anticholinergic antagonism in Huntington's chorea, *Neurology 22:*107.

Klawans, H.L., and Rubovits, R., 1974, Effect of cholinergic and anticholinergic agents on tardive dyskinesia, *J. Neurol. Neurosurg. Psychiatry 27:*941.

Lee, C.W.G., Yu, J.S., Turner, B.B., and Murray, K.E., 1976, Trimethylaminuria: fishy odors in children, *N. Engl. J. Med. 295:*937.

Matz, R., Rick, W., Oh, D., Thompson, H., and Gershon, S., 1974, Clozapine — a potential antipsychotic agent without extrapyramidal manifestations, *Curr. Ther. Res. 16:*687.

McGeer, P.L., and McGeer, E.G., 1975, Evidence for glutamic acid decarboxylase-containing interneurons in the neostriatum, *Brain Res. 91:*331.

McGeer, P.L., McGeer, E.G., Fibiger, H.C., and Wickson, V., 1971, Neostriatal choline acetylase and acetylcholinesterase following selective brain lesions, *Brain Res. 35:*308.

McGeer, P.L., McGeer, E.G., and Fibiger, H.C., 1973, Choline acetylase and glutamic acid decarboxylase in Huntington's chorea, *Neurology 23:*912.

McGeer, P.L., Grewaal, D.S., and McGeer, E.G., 1974, Influence of noncholinergic drugs on rat striatal acetylcholine levels, *Brain Res. 80:*211.

McMenemy, W.H., 1958, The dementias and progressive diseases of the basal ganglia, in *"Neuropathology"* (J.C. Greenfield, ed.), pp. 502-507, Edward Arnold, London.

Millington, W.R., McCall, A.L., and Wurtman, R.J., (submitted), Deanol acetamidobenzoate inhibits the blood-brain barrier transport of choline, *Ann. Neurol.*

Muller, P., and Seeman, P., 1977, Brain neurotransmitter receptors after long-term haloperidol: dopamine, acetylcholine, serotonin, a-adrenergic and naloxone receptors, *Life Sci. 21:*1751.

Perry, T.L., Hansen, S., and Kloster, M., 1973, Huntington's chorea: deficiency of γ-aminobutyric acid in brain, *N. Engl. J. Med. 288:*337.

Perry, T.L., MacLeod, P.M., and Hansen, S., 1977, Treatment of Huntington's chorea with isoniazid (letter to the editor), *N. Engl. J. Med. 297:*840.

Schuberth, J., and Jenden, D.J., 1975, Transport of choline from plasma to cerebrospinal fluid in the rabbit with reference to the origin of choline and to acetylcholine metabolism in brain, *Brain Res. 84:*245.

Schuberth, J., Sparf, B., and Sundwall, A., 1969, A technique for the study of acetylcholine turnover in mouse brain *in vivo, J. Neurochem. 16:*695.

Schwarcz, R., Bennett, J.P., and Coyle, J.T., 1977, Inhibitors of GABA metabolism: implications for Huntington's disease, *Ann. Neurol. 2:*299.

Shahani, B.T., and Young, R.R., 1976, Physiological and pharmacological aids in the differential diagnosis of tremor, *J. Neurol. Neurosurg. Psychiatry 39:*772.

Shea, P.A., and Aprison, M.H., 1973, An enzymatic method for measuring picomole quantities of acetylcholine in CNS tissue, *Anal. Biochem. 56:*165.

Shoulson, I., Chase, T.N., Roberts, E., and Van Balgooy, J.N.A., 1975, Huntington's disease: treatment with imidazole-4-acetic acid, *N. Engl. J. Med. 293:*504.

Shoulson, I., Kartzinel, R., and Chase, T.N., 1976, Huntington's disease: treatment with dipropylacetic acid and gamma-aminobutyric acid, *Neurology 26:*61.

Sigwald, J., Bouttier, D., Raymondeaud, Cl., and Piot, Cl. 1959, Quatre cas de dyskinesie facio-bucco-linguo-masticatrice a evolution prolongee secondaire a un traitement par les neuroleptiques, *Rev. Neurol. 100:*751.

Stahl, W.L., and Swanson, P.D., 1974, Biochemical abnormalities in Huntington's chorea brains, *Neurology 24:*813.

Stevens, D.L., 1973, The classification of variants of Huntington's chorea, *Adv. Neurol. 1:*57.

Tamminga, C., Smith, R.C., Chang, S., Haraszti, J.S., and Davis, J.M., 1976, Depression associated with oral choline, *Lancet 2:*905.

Tamminga, C.A., Smith, R.C., Ericksen, S.E., Chang, S., and Davis, J.M., 1977, Cholinergic influences in tardive dyskinesia, *Am. J. Psychiatry 134:*769.

Tarsy, D., and Baldessarini, R.J., 1974, Behavioural supersensitivity to apomorphine following chronic treatment with drugs which interfere with the synaptic function of catecholamines, *Neuropharmacology 13:*927.

Tarsy, D., and Bralower, M., 1977, Deanol acetamidobenzoate treatment in choreiform movement disorders, *Arch. Neurol. 34:*756.

Thatch, B.T., Chase, T.N., and Bosma, J.F., 1975, Oral facial dyskinesia associated with prolonged use of antihistaminic decongestants, *N. Engl. J. Med. 293:*486.

Uhrbrand, L., and Faurbye, A., 1960, Reversible and irreversible dyskinesia after treatment with perphenazine, chlorpromazine, reserpine, and electroconvulsive therapy, *Psychopharmacologia 1:*408.

Ulus, I.H., and Wurtman, R.J., 1976, Choline administration: activation of tyrosine hydroxylase in dopaminergic neurons of rat brain, *Science 194:*1060.

Ulus, I.H., Hirsch, M.J., and Wurtman, R.J., 1977, Trans-synaptic induction of adrenomedullary tyrosine hydroxylase activity by choline: evidence that choline administration can increase cholinergic transmission, *Proc. Natl. Acad. Sci. USA 74:* 798.

Walker, J.E., Hoehn, M., Sears, E., and Lewis, J., 1973, Dimethylaminoethanol in Huntington's chorea (letter to the editor), *Lancet 1:*1512.

Whittier, J.R., and Koreny, C., 1968, Effect of oral fluphenazine on Huntington's chorea, *J. Neuropsychiatry 4:*1.

Wurtman, R.J., Hirsch, M.J., and Growdon, J.H., 1977, Lecithin consumption elevates serum free choline levels, *Lancet 2:*68.

Zahniser, N.R., Chou, D., and Hanin, I., 1977, Is 2-dimethylaminoethanol (deanol) indeed a precursor of brain acetylcholine? A gas chromatographic evaluation, *J. Pharmacol. Exp. Ther. 200:*545.

DEANOL TRIALS IN TARDIVE DYSKINESIA

D. E. Casey

Departments of Medical Research and Psychiatry
Portland VA Hospital

Department of Psychiatry, University of Oregon Health Sciences Center
Portland, Oregon

INTRODUCTION

PHARMACOLOGIC PROFILE OF TARDIVE DYSKINESIA: CHALLENGE DRUGS AND DEANOL

Interest in the identification and treatment of movement disorders has greatly increased in recent years. As the knowledge of the biochemistry of neurotransmitters continues to develop, new approaches to treatment are being suggested. One trend of major interest has been the evaluation of the interaction of dopamine (DA) and acetyl-choline (ACh) in tardive dyskinesia. In the past few years deanol, a putative precursor of ACh (Haubrich et al., 1975; Pfeiffer et al., 1957), has been used to study the role of cholinergic influences in this syndrome. Since the results with deanol have been con-flicting, the purpose of this chapter is two-fold: to demonstrate a method of utilizing short-acting challenge drugs to develop a pharmacologic profile of tardive dyskinesia that may predict the response to deanol, and to summarize the available data in the limited number of clinical trials to determine the efficacy of deanol as a treatment for tardive dyskinesia.

Tardive dyskinesia is a disorder of the motor system which occurs late in the course of treatment with neuroleptics. It is usually characterized by abnormal, involuntary, irregular movements of the mouth, face, and tongue, and may also have associated choreoathetoid dyskinesias of the limbs and trunk. Factors predisposing to tardive dyskinesia have been widely studied, but the results are conflicting. The prevalence rate is highly variable, ranging from 0.5% to 56% (Jus et al., 1976a). Rare cases have been reported after only a few months of neuroleptic treatment (Simpson, 1973), but the syndrome is generally not seen unless patients have been taking neuroleptic drugs for two or more years (Tarsy and Baldessarini, 1976). Some studies demonstrate a correlation between age at the time of diagnosis or age at the onset of neuroleptic treatment and tardive dyskinesia (Jus *et al.*, 1976a; Crane, 1973). Duration of drug treatment or total drug dose has been associated with prevalence rates in some reports (Crane and Smeets, 1974), but not in others (Jus *et al.*, 1976b). The parameters of sex, psychiatric diagnosis, type of neuroleptic drug, previous organic brain disease, lobotomy, and acute neuroleptic-induced dyskinesias reflect an inconsistent relationship to the occurrence of tardive dyskinesia (Tarsy and Baldessarini, 1976). At present we know that some individuals who have been treated with neuroleptics will develop tardive dyskinesia, but we cannot predict in advance of the disorder's onset who those individuals will be.

Tardive dyskinesia was initially hypothesized to result from DA receptor denervation supersensitivity (Klawans and McKendall, 1971). Presumably DA receptors in the striatum gradually become oversensitive following the long-term partial receptor blockade with neuroleptic drugs. Although there is ample evidence to support a dopaminergic role in tardive dyskinesia, the receptor supersensitivity theory has expanded to account for counterbalancing cholinergic influences in the pathophysiology of tardive dyskinesia. This concept evolves from the general notion that normal movement results from a properly functioning balance between counterbalancing dopaminergic and cholinergic influences in the striatum. Specifically, the increased spontaneous involuntary movements of tardive dyskinesia result from the relative predominance of an overactive DA system over cholinergic influences (Gerlach *et al.*, 1974). Much of the data resulting from the pharmacologic manipulations of dopaminergic and cholinergic influences in humans with tardive dyskinesia supports this notion.

DA agonists often aggravate the symptoms (Klawans and McKendall, 1971; Hippius and Logemann, 1970), while DA depletors (Kazamatsuri *et al.*, 1972a; Sato *et al.*, 1971) and DA receptor blockers (Kazamatsuri *et al.*, 1972b) usually lead to improvement. Anticholinergic drugs often worsen the symptoms (Gerlach *et al.*, 1974; Klawans and Rubovits, 1974; Klawans, 1973), while the dyskinesias may be reduced by increasing available ACh through enzyme inhibition (Fann *et al.*, 1974; Gerlach *et al.*, 1974; Klawans and Rubovits, 1974) or by administering the putative precursors of acetylcholine, deanol (Casey and Denney, 1974; Miller, 1974) or choline (Growdon *et al.*, 1977; Davis *et al.*, 1975; Davis *et al.*, 1976).

However, not all reports are consistent with the above findings. Three patients had their tardive dyskinesia symptoms gradually improve while taking the DA agonist L-DOPA (levodopa) (Alpert *et al.*, 1976), and apomorphine, a DA agonist, failed to aggravate dyskinetic symptoms in another group of patients (Smith *et al.*, 1977). Additionally, patients with tardive dyskinesia occasionally may become worse with neuroleptics (Claveria *et al.*, 1975; Lal, 1974; Kazamatsuri *et al.*, 1973; Singer and Cheng, 1971). Anticholinergic drugs also have been helpful (Granacher *et al.*, 1975; Gerlach *et al.*, 1974; Uhrbrand and Faurbye, 1960), and increasing ACh with physostigmine worsened some patients (Tarsy *et al.*, 1974).

To develop a method utilizing short-acting challenge drugs that may produce a pharmacological profile of tardive dyskinesia and predict a response to deanol, the following study was carried out. The aim of this investigation was to study quantitatively the dopaminergic-cholinergic counterbalancing hypothesis in tardive dyskinesia with an objective measuring device. The approach included: (a) short-term challenges of dopaminergic and cholinergic agonists and antagonists; (b) long-term single-blind deanol and placebo administration; and (c) an evaluation of the relationship between drug challenges and response to deanol.

MATERIALS AND METHODS

Subjects

Six patients with a clinical diagnosis of tardive dyskinesia were admitted to the inpatient ward and given physical, neurological, mental status, and routine laboratory exams. Criteria for selection were: (a) no medical contraindication; (b) visible dyskinetic movements following prolonged exposure to neuroleptic drugs; (c) no family history of inheritable neurodegenerative disease; (d) no exposure to other known causes of dyskinesia; and (e) informed consent.

Drug Schedule

Dyskinetic movements were evaluated in patients under the following conditions:

1. Throughout the entire study, each patient was continued on his maintenance neuroleptic and anticholinergic drugs.

2. Phase I began with admission to the study and a 2-week baseline period taking only maintenance medications. During the following week, a different challenge drug was given each morning for 5 days. The order of the administration was rotated to control for sequential effects. They were: (a) DA agonist, L-DOPA 500 mg p.o.; (b) DA antagonist, droperidol 2.5 mg I.V.; (c) cholinergic agonist, physostigmine, 1.0 mg I.V. mixed with methscopolamine 0.75 mg I.V. to block peripheral cholinergic side effects; (d) cholinergic antagonist, benztropine 2.0 mg I.V.; and (e) placebo, two yellow capsules p.o.

3. Phase II began the week after the challenge drug with deanol 800 mg/day in divided q.i.d. doses. If this dose was insufficient to suppress the movements completely, the dose was increased by 400 mg/day every 7 days, up to 2000 mg/day over 4 weeks. If side effects occurred, the dose was held at the level which did not produce side effects and continued for the remainder of the 4 weeks. This was followed by a 2-week single-blind placebo period. At the end of the placebo period, deanol was restarted for 2 weeks at the previous dose and again followed by a 2-week period of placebo.

Evaluation of Dyskinesias

Changes in movement were evaluated by a modification of a previously described system (Denney and Casey, 1975). An air-filled balloon, approximately 1 x 4 cm, was placed in the mouth to record bucco-lingual dyskinesias. Preliminary testing showed the patients could remove and accurately replace the mouth balloon and yield consistent results. If limb dyskinesias were present, another balloon was taped between the fingers or toes with markings on the tape and digits to insure accurate placement each session. The balloons caused a minimal dampening of the dyskinesias as they provided a slight passive resistance. The recording system consisted of a balloon attached to an air-tight pneumatic transducer whose signal was AC coupled, amplified, and integrated. The waveform and its integration were plotted on a polygraph for a visual display, and recorded on magnetic tape. Calibrations done before and after each recording session included pneumatic calibration of the transducer to insure against air leaks and electrical calibration of the amplifiers.

Data Analysis

Dyskinetic movements during the initial baseline, deanol, and placebo periods were evaluated by calculating the average integrations/minute during 15-min recording sessions twice weekly. Percentage changes were determined by comparing deanol and placebo values with the initial baseline values.

Prechallenge baselines for each day were determined for 20 min prior to the challenge. Challenge drug effects were calculated as the average integrations/minute during 10-min blocks. The drug effect was evaluated by continuous recording for 2 hr after its administration. Percentage change for each challenge drug was calculated by comparing the prechallenge baseline score with the 15-min average score in the 45-60 min period following the challenge drug. The L-DOPA score was calculated from the 90-105 min period due to the slower onset of action of this drug.

Recordings during the initial baseline and placebo challenges showed a variation of less than 50% from day to day. Thus, a 50% change from baseline was arbitrarily defined as significant. Although this cut-off point may have reduced the likelihood of detection of subtle drug responses, it was considered imperative to limit definitions of drug effect to unequivocal responses.

RESULTS

Challenge Drugs

Results of the drug challenges are presented in Table 1. Only patients 1 and 3 significantly responded to L-DOPA. Both developed increased movements, but there was an unequal response between mouth and limb movements. None of the patients admitted to any side effects, and there was no evidence of a change in mental status.

Of the four patients who responded to droperidol, two had reduced movements (patients 1 and 2) and two had increased movements (patients 4 and 6). Figure 1 shows the benefit in patient 2, while Figure 2 illustrates the increased movements of patient 6. Only patient 5 reported a side effect, slight fatigue. There were no changes in mental status.

Each patient had a marked response to physostigmine. Three patients (1-3) improved and three showed increased movements (4-6). Figure 1 illustrates the improvement in patient 2, and Figure 2 shows the increase in dyskinesia in patient 6. As with the other challenge drugs, changes in mouth and extremity movements were not necessarily correlated.

TABLE 1

Drug Effects on Tardive Dyskinesia: % Change

No.	Area	Challenge Drugs							Deanol			
		Lev (DA+)	Dro (DA−)	Phy (ACh+)	Benz (ACh−)	Pla	Dnl	1 Pla	(mg)	Dnl	2 Pla	(mg)
Group 1												
1	M	+87*	−71*	+22	−33	+22	−27	+47	800	+7	0	800
	F	0	−75*	−55*	−33	+26	−83*	−72*	800	−83*	−89*	800
2	M	+17	−53*	−63*	−14	+8	−88*	−96*	1600	−92*	−96*	1600
3	M	+139*	−26	−77*	+19	−14	−67*	−10	1600			
	T	+95*	0	−80*	+74*	+20	−92*	−81*	1600			
Group 2												
4	M	+33	+175*	+1000*	−86*	+13	+125*	+50*	2000	+150*	+125*	800
	F	+20	+525*	+1000*	−44	+25	+400*	+675*	2000	+525*	+600*	800
5	M	+20	+33	+38	−10	+22	+24	+147*	1200	+124*	+306*	1200
	T	+23	−15	+55*	−61*	+8	+19	+26	1200	0	+26	1200
6	M	−10	+283*	+266*	−50*	+11	−13	+25	1600			

Abbreviations: M–mouth; F–fingers; T–toes; +–increase movements; −–decrease movements; *–50% or more change; Lev–Levodopa; Dro–droperidol; Phy–physostigmine; Benz–benztropine; Pla–placebo; Dnl–deanol; DA+–dopamine agonist; DA−–dopamine antagonist; ACh+–acetylcholine agonist; ACh−–acetylcholine antagonist.
Reprinted with permission from Casey, D.E., and Denney, D., 1977.

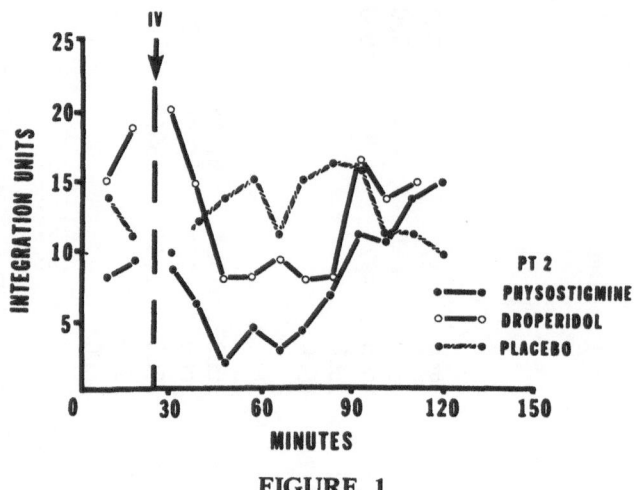

FIGURE 1

Effect of physostigmine, droperidol, and placebo on tardive dyskinesia in patient 2. Reprinted with permission from Casey, D.E., and Denney, D., 1977.

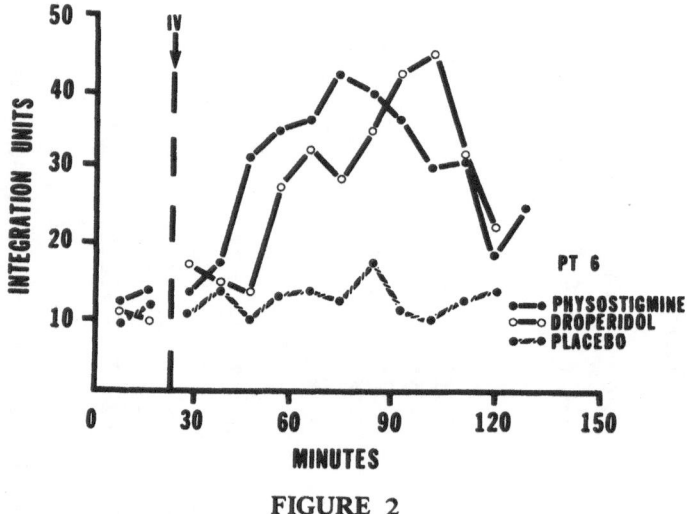

FIGURE 2

Effect of physostigmine, droperidol, and placebo on tardive dyskinesia in patient 6. Reprinted with permission from Casey, D.E., and Denney, D., 1977.

Patient 4 had a striking increase in dyskinesia following physostigmine which lasted about 30 min. Prior to physostigmine, the movement disorder consisted of a random assortment of irregular chewing movements plus finger or toe choreoathetosis. During the period of exacerbation the movements changed in magnitude and frequency and developed a much more rhythmical pattern consisting of chewing, head nodding, rocking back and forth in the chair, stroking the face and hair with both hands, and moving the legs and feet as if walking in place. The patient reported that he "felt restless for awhile." Patient 5 also demonstrated a moderate shift toward more regular and stereotyped movements which appeared similar to akathisia, but had no subjective awareness of feeling restless. Side effects included mild nausea in patient 3 and light-headedness in patient 5.

Of the four patients who responded to benztropine, one had increased movements (patient 3) and three had reduced movements (4-6). There were no side effects.

No patient responded with 50% or greater change in movements to all the challenges. However, all six patients responded 50% or more to two challenge drugs and four patients responded 50% or more to three out of the four challenges. Significantly, the responses that were 50% or more subgrouped into two types. Both of these groups were characterized by the pairing of responses to DA antagonist-ACh agonist (DA^--ACh^+) or DA agonist-ACh antagonist (DA^+-ACh^-). Group 1 patients (1-3) tended to improve with the DA^- or ACh^+ drugs and to worsen with the DA^+ or ACh^- agents. Group 2 patients (4-6) showed the opposite response: improvement with DA^+ or ACh^- and aggravation with DA^- or ACh^+. Although not all patients demonstrated a change of 50% or more to all the challenge drugs, of those who did, there were no exceptions to the pairing of DA and ACh agonists and antagonists. This pairing is also seen in Figure 1 and Figure 2.

Deanol

During the first deanol period three patients improved (Group 1), one became worse (patient 4), and two showed no effects (patients 5 and 6). There was often a quantitative discrepancy between the mouth and limb responses. The patient who became strikingly worse with physostigmine also became worse with deanol. During the first 2-week placebo period the three patients who had improved with deanol generally maintained that improvement. However, patient 3 demonstrated further discrepancy between mouth and limb movements, as seen in Figure 3. During the placebo period his mouth movements returned to the pretreatment level but his limb movements did not. Patient 4, who became worse with deanol, showed improvement in mouth movements with placebo, but his finger movements worsened. Patient 5, who had no significant response to deanol, had increased mouth movements during placebo while movement of his toes remained unaffected.

Four of the six patients completed the second deanol and placebo cycle. The two with significant improvement during the first deanol and placebo period continued to maintain the improvement throughout the second deanol and placebo period. The patients who became worse with the first deanol-placebo period also became worse in the second period. Patient 5 again demonstrated an increase in mouth movements with the placebo as if there were a rebound "off response" after deanol treatment was stopped.

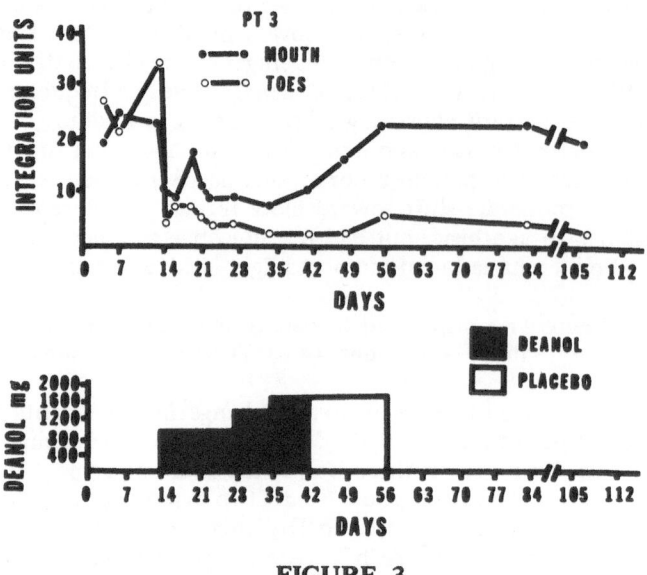

FIGURE 3

Effect of deanol and placebo on tardive dyskinesia in patient 3. Reprinted with permission from Casey, D.E., and Denney, D., 1977.

The subgrouping of patients' responses to deanol resembled that of the challenge drug subgroups. Those patients who improved with the $DA^- - ACh^+$ agents also improved with deanol, and those who worsened with the $DA^- - ACh^+$ became worse or had no response to deanol. The Spearman Rank Order Correlation Coefficient for response between physostigmine and deanol is 0.89, $p < 0.05$. Other drug comparisons were not statistically significant.

The dosage range for deanol was 800-2000 mg/day, with upper limits determined by side effects. It was noted that a deanol response, when present, occurred within the first week and further dosage increases had only small additive effects. This was true both for the initiation of deanol and for the effects observed during placebo. No patient had complete suppression of movements. The major changes in the dyskinesias during the deanol period were readily visible. While there was a relationship between the recordings and the visible changes, the recordings detected the trends earlier.

Side effects, which included mild insomnia, irritability, and mood changes, occurred in the dosage range of 1200-2000 mg/day. Patients 1-4 reported depressive mood changes while patients 5 and 6 reported elevation of mood with an increased activity level. Reducing the drug dosage alleviated the side effects within a week without affecting the dyskinesias.

DISCUSSION

Tardive dyskinesia was initially thought to be the result of dopaminergic receptor denervation supersensitivity (Klawans and McKendall, 1971). This concept has expanded to include the notion that tardive dyskinesia results from a disturbance in the inversely related balance between dopaminergic and acetylcholinergic mechanisms in the striatum (Casey and Denney, 1975; Fann et al., 1974; Gerlach et al., 1974; Klawans, 1973).

All six patients responded to challenges with drugs affecting a cholinergic system and five of six responded to challenges with drugs that alter a dopaminergic system. The data are clearly consistent with the postulated balance hypothesis.

The absence of response of some patients to some challenges has been found by others (Fann et al., 1974; Gerlach et al., 1974; Klawans and Rubovits, 1974; Tarsy et al., 1974). It is possible that the doses of challenge drugs were too low in individual cases. Also, from clinical necessity, the patients were maintained on neuroleptics and sometimes also on antiparkinsonian medication. Since there are no clinical methods for quantitatively comparing the central antidopaminergic and anticholinergic actions of these agents in human subjects, it is likely that the challenge drug effects may vary depending on individual differences and the unknown equilibrium between DA and ACh striatal influences produced by the patient's treatment.

Additionally, it is possible that some patients may have progressed to a point at which brief alterations in neurohumoral turnover in the striatum cannot be produced by any means. This is well known in parkinsonism, in which responsiveness to L-DOPA decreases and finally disappears as clinical severity increases.

The pattern of response to the challenge drugs suggests a division of patients into two groups. Responses in Group 1 imply the underlying pathophysiological state is an absolute or relative dominance of dopaminergic effects associated with cholinergic hypofunction, while responses in Group 2 suggest the opposite: absolute or relative dominance of cholinergic effects and dopaminergic hypofunction. Careful examination of the literature yields occasional patients who do not respond to neuroleptic and anticholinergic drugs in the traditional (Group 1) pattern. In two studies with the phenothiazine thiopropazate, a few patients had their dyskinesias increase (Lal, 1974; Singer and Cheng, 1971). The butyrophenone haloperidol increased tardive dyskinesia in two patients (Kazamatsuri et al., 1973), as has the new investigational neuroleptic pimozide (Claveria et al., 1975). Some patients improved during and following treatment with the DA precursor levodopa (Alpert et al., 1976), and others improved or were unaffected by the DA agonist apomorphine (Carroll et al., 1977; Smith et al., 1977). Investigations with drugs that affect the cholinergic system have also produced conflicting results as Gerlach et al., (1974) and Tarsy et al., (1974) described patients adversely affected by cholinergic augmentation with physostigmine. High doses of choline can also increase tardive dyskinesia (Growdon et al., 1977). Others have experienced unexpected improvement from the anticholinergics benztropine (Granacher et al., 1975; Uhrbrand and Faurbye, 1960) and scopolamine (Gerlach et al., 1974).

Cools and Van Rossum (1976) and Klawans *et al.*, (this volume) have proposed that two distinct dopaminergic neuron pools with excitatory or inhibitory characteristics coexist. These subgroups can be differentiated on the basis of electrophysiological, biochemical, pharmacological, neuroanatomical, and functional data. It may be that subgroups of tardive dyskinesia are the final neurological expression of alterations in separate dopaminergic neuron populations (Casey, 1976).

The stereotyped hyperkinetic response to physostigmine that occurred in two of the Group 2 patients was qualitatively similar to akathisia and possibly related to the "paradoxical" hyperkinetic stereotypies reported in animals (Scheel-Kruger and Randrup, 1968; Schiorring and Randrup, 1968). There may be a symptom complex that appears similar to akathisia and is an integral part of the tardive dyskinesia syndrome. Since akathisia is somewhat responsive to anticholinergic agents, it is possible that cholinergic augmentation would selectively aggravate the akathisia-like symptoms of tardive dyskinesia. Alternatively, this response may be an acutely induced akathisia that becomes dominant over the tardive dyskinetic symptoms during a physostigmine challenge.

The concept of cholinergic receptor hypersensitivity might be raised in tardive dyskinesia. The phenomenon of central nervous system cholinergic denervation supersensitivity has been demonstrated in the septohippocampal pathway of the rat (Bird and Aghajanian, 1975). Prolonged exposure to anticholinergic agents or large doses of neuroleptics intrinsically high in anticholinergic properties, e.g., thioridazine (Snyder *et al.*, 1974), may ultimately alter cholinergic receptors. Perhaps patient 4, who was taking a large dose of thioridazine, demonstrated a clinical manifestation of this phenomenon since he had a dramatic aggravation of symptoms with physostigmine and deanol. An analogous situation in the dopaminergic system is the increase in dyskinesias with DA agonists. This observation, if confirmed, suggests that prior treatment with drugs that affect the cholinergic system may have long-term effects on cholinergic receptors, and that a dyskinetic response to physostigmine would argue against treating patients with this subgroup of dyskinesias with drugs that increase central nervous system ACh turnover.

A different approach of the question of subgroups is to ask if patients in Group 2 actually had tardive dyskinesia. Perhaps there is another movement disorder that closely mimics tardive dyskinesia but is seldom recognized. Hyperkinetic reactions other than akathisia very infrequently have been reported to occur during the early phase of neuroleptic treatment (Denham and Carrick, 1961; Sarwer-Foner, 1960). If this hyperkinetic dyskinesia was similar in temporal relationship to other extrapyramidal syndromes associated with the start of neuroleptic treatment, it might be expected that they all would have a common underlying mechanism. The acute neuroleptic-induced reactions of dystonia, akathisia, and parkinsonism are thought to result from a dopaminergic deficit and an cholinergic excess, and indeed, this is also the pharmacological characterization of Group 2. Thus it is possible that the symptoms which comprise the tardive dyskinesia syndrome actually derive from heterogeneous etiologies. The implication is that at least two separate but clinically similar hyperkinetic dyskinesias that are pharmacologically opposite can occur with neuroleptic therapy. One dyskinesia is pharmacologically similar to the acute neuroleptic-induced extrapyramidal dyskinesias that are characterized by relative dopaminergic hypofunction or cholinergic hyperfunction; the other is related to the traditional pharmacology of tardive dyskinesia characterized by relative dopaminergic hyperfunction or cholinergic hypofunction.

The dyskinetic symptoms changed in five out of six patients with tardive dyskinesia during deanol therapy, in agreement with initial reports (Casey and Denney, 1974; Miller, 1974). Although deanol has been reported to be ineffective in many cases, significant exacerbation of dyskinesias has not been described. The continued improvement in some patients during the 2-week placebo period raises the questions of sustained drug effects and spontaneous remissions. The same issues have also been associated with a prolonged reduction of L-DOPA-induced dyskinesias in some patients treated with deanol (Miller, 1976; Klawans et al., 1975). Although temporary tardive dyskinesias that resolved within a period of weeks to months after neuroleptics were stopped (Quitkin et al., 1977; Moline, 1975; Jacobson et al., 1974) may account for the variably persisting course of the syndrome reflected in the literature, the patients in this study were different because they were maintained on their neuroleptic drugs and their dyskinesias had remained stable.

The similarity of responses to physostigmine and deanol supports the notion that both drugs affect the same system, though not necessarily by the same mechanism. Physostigmine increases available synaptic ACh by inhibition of acetylcholinesterase (AChE), but the mechanism of action of deanol is much less clear and will be discussed in depth below.

Since a positive response to deanol is associated with Group 1 patients who benefited from cholinergic enhancement or dopaminergic blockade, it is possible that deanol may also indirectly affect DA or other neurotransmitters. Cholinergic neurons function as interneurons between ascending dopaminergic neurons and descending feedback gamma-aminobutyric acid (GABA)-mediated neurons. Thus, any effect on the cholinergic interneuron would ultimately be reflected in changes in both DA and GABA turnover.

The mood alterations seen at higher doses of deanol are interesting in light of the cholinergic-adrenergic balance hypothesis of mood disorders (Janowsky et al., 1972). Physostigmine has also been shown to reduce mania and produce transient depression (Janowsky et al., 1973; Davis et al., 1978). Large doses of choline have also produced depression (Tamminga et al., 1976). While deanol-related depression in these cases would be further support for the hypothesis, the elevated mood and activity level are contrary to expectations. The dyskinesia response during the deanol period was independent of the mood alterations because reducing the dosage eliminated the affective changes without influencing the movement disorder.

In the present study some general points merit discussion. The subgrouping of responses to challenge drugs and deanol was not related to degree of dyskinesia, psychiatric diagnosis, or maintenance medications. These aspects do not seem to be good indicators for making decisions in clinical management because they do not reflect the plasticity of the underlying pathophysiology. The repeated observation that a discrepancy existed between drug effects on the mouth and limb movements bears further evaluation. This discrepancy has been noted by others (Gardos et al., 1976; Fann et al., 1974; Gerlach et al., 1974) and is difficult to explain. Gerlach et al., (1974) have proposed that age is an important factor in determining which symptoms are present and what the drug response will be. The worsening or "off response" of the dyskinesia in one patient at the initiation of placebo periods is similar to the response seen when the neuroleptics are suddenly discontinued. It was also observed that the movements were only quantitatively affected. No patients had their symptoms completely suppressed with any drug, nor did anyone have new movements appear as a result of the drugs.

It is technically feasible and worthwhile to investigate tardive dyskinesia by systematic drug challenges and objective measurement of responses. The data from the combined approach have added support to the concept of unbalanced dopaminergic and cholinergic influences in tardive dyskinesia and have raised additional questions.

REVIEW OF PHARMACOLOGICAL STUDIES AND CLINICAL TRIALS

Treating tardive dyskinesia by augmenting central nervous system ACh logically derives from the theory of counterbalancing striatal dopaminergic-cholinergic influences. Investigations with deanol have produced inconsistent findings both in the pharmacologic evaluations of the drug's ability to increase brain ACh and in the clinical trials treating tardive dyskinesia. An overall examination of the data may, perhaps, clarify some of the seemingly disparate findings and suggest directions for further research.

PHARMACOLOGICAL STUDIES

Deanol was originally proposed as an ACh precursor by Pfeiffer et al., (1957). To date there is evidence both for and against this postulation, as summarized in Table 2. Whole brain ACh was significantly increased following the acute (Goldberg and Silbergeld, 1974) and long-term administration of deanol (Danysz et al., 1967), and striatal choline and ACh were significantly raised following the acute administration of deanol (Haubrich et al., 1975). However, other investigations have not found significant increases in whole brain choline or ACh, or only a slight increase in striatal ACh following very high (900 mg/kg in the mouse) acute doses of deanol (Zahniser et al., 1977). In addition, whole brain ACh was unchanged following 45 days of deanol intake (Pepeu et al., 1960). Further evidence against deanol being an immediate direct precursor of brain choline or ACh is the demonstration that only a small proportion of the total deanol administered is incorporated into brain tissue as deanol itself (Zahniser et al., 1977).

Since the brain does not synthesize choline de novo, choline must be derived from peripheral tissues (Freeman and Jenden, 1976). It has been shown that the primary source for choline synthesis is the liver where phosphatidyldeanol is an immediate precursor of phosphatidylcholine (Bremer et al., 1960). Also, exogenous deanol can function as a precursor to phosphoryl and phosphatidylcholine in the liver (Dormard et al., 1975; Bjornstad and Bremer, 1966; Ansell and Spanner, 1962; DuVigneaud et al., 1946). These phosphorylated forms of choline could conceivably cross the blood brain barrier, be hydrolyzed back to choline and contribute to the choline pool available for synthesis to ACh (Zahniser et al., 1977). While there is evidence to support this point of view, both the role of deanol as a potential precursor for phosphatidylcholine and the contribution of phyosphatidylcholine as a source of brain choline remain unknown. Therefore, it is not yet apparent how much deanol must be given to augment the pool of brain choline available for ACh synthesis.

TABLE 2

Comparison of Experimental Conditions and Results of Studies Investigating the Effect of Deanol Administration on Brain Acetylcholine (ACh) and Choline (Ch) Levels

Authors	Sex/Species	Dose[a]	Tissue Assayed	ACh Assay	Results[b]
Pepeu et al., (1960)	M/rat	Deanol,[c] 1 or 500 mg/kg (1 hr) 0.03 M (p.o.) (45 days)	Whole brain	Bioassay	↗ ACh
Danysz et al., (1967)	M/mouse	Deanol, 175 or 350 mg/kg (8, 11, 14, 17, 20, 23 days)	Whole brain	Bioassay	ACh
Goldberg and Silbergeld (1974)	M/mouse	Deanol, 300 mg/kg (30 min)	Whole brain	Enzyme	ACh
Haubrich et al., (1975)	M/rat	Deanol,[c] 214 mg/kg (15 min) Deanol, 550 mg/kg (15 min)	Striatum	Enzyme	ACh; Ch
Zahniser and Hanin (1976)	M/mouse (30 min)	Deanol, 300 mg/kg	Whole brain	GC	→ ACh; → Ch
Zahniser et al., (1977)	M or F/mouse	Deanol, 300 mg/kg (30 min) Deanol, 900 mg/kg (30 min)	Whole brain; striatum Whole brain; striatum	GC	→ ACh; → Ch → ACh → ACh → ACh
	M/rat	Deanol, 550 mg/kg (15 min)	Whole brain; cortex; striatum; hippocampus	GC	↑ ACh → ACh → ACh → ACh

[a] Dosage was administered i.p. as the p-acetamidobenzoate salt unless otherwise noted; time in parentheses.
[b] ↑ indicates a statistically significant increase in the level of ACh or Ch when compared with control; → indicates no statistically significant difference in the level of ACh or Ch when compared with control.
[c] Deanol administered as the free base.
Reprinted with permission from Zahniser, N., et al., 1977.

An important aspect of further understanding the pharmacologic role of deanol in cholinergic function involves the effects of long-term drug administration. Since the time course for a clinical response to deanol in humans is usually a matter of days rather than minutes as seen in animal brain ACh, the effect of deanol on brain choline may well be mediated via lipid pathways instead of functioning as an immediate precursor. However, continued research is needed to clarify the initial conflicting findings in long-term deanol administration, as one study found an increase in brain ACh (Danysz et al., 1967), but another did not (Pepeu et al., 1960). Two additional and incompletely investigated aspects important to interpreting laboratory data and understanding cholinergic function are that changes in the turnover rate of ACh can occur without altering the steady-state levels, and an increase in tissue ACh may be due to a decrease in the turnover rate (Hanin and Costa, 1976). In conclusion, it must be said that there are many unknowns regarding the mechanism of action of deanol, and its role as a cholinergic precursor remains an open question.

The effect of deanol in acutely produced hyperdopaminergic states in animals has also been used as a method to evaluate the ability of this drug to alter central nervous system cholinergic influences. Single doses of deanol (500-1200 mg/kg) failed to modify the dose-response relationship of amphetamine-induced stereotyped behavior in guinea pigs. It was concluded that acutely administered deanol exerts no significant central cholinergic effects (Weiner et al., 1976). However, the model of acute amphetamine-induced stereotypies does not directly approximate the pathophysiology of tardive dyskinesia because the animals are not previously exposed to neuroleptic drugs. Deanol has yet to be studied in the animal models of tardive dyskinesia that utilize neuroleptic-induced DA hypersensitivity (Klawans and Rubovits, 1972) and DA receptor binding parameters (Burt et al., 1977).

Symptoms of peripheral cholinergic excess in humans provide indirect support for the proposal that deanol augments cholinergic function. Side effects of increased sweating, salivation, or bronchial secretions have been reported in four patients, none of whom experienced any improvement in their tardive dyskinesia (Casey, 1977; Mehta et al., 1976; Nesse and Carroll, 1976).

CLINICAL TRIALS

The initial reports by Miller (1974) and Casey and Denney (1974) using deanol for tardive dyskinesia were encouraging, but subsequent reports (see Tables 3 and 4) did not consistently replicate the early findings. Deanol has now been evaluated in 19 reports. Table 3 summarizes the findings of 14 open trials and one single-blind placebo-controlled evaluation in a total of 49 patients. The dosage range was 200-2000 mg/day over a duration range of 5 days to 16 weeks. The overall results show that 25 patients improved during deanol therapy (51%), 23 were unaffected (47%), and one became worse (2%). Four of the 49 patients did not have the dyskinesias return when deanol was stopped (8%).

Table 4 summarizes the findings of four double-blind placebo-controlled trials in 39 patients. The dosage range was 1200-1500 mg/day over a duration range of 3-5 weeks. Three reports noted no significant drug versus placebo effects in 28 patients (72%) when symptoms were globally assessed. One report found significant improvement in the orofacial dyskinesias in 7 of 11 patients, but no change in the limb or truncal dyskinesias.

TABLE 3

Deanol in Tardive Dyskinesia: Open and Single-Blind Trials[a]

Investigator-Year	Patients	Dose mg/day	Duration	Results
Miller (1974)	2	600	1 week	Improved in first week
Casey and Denney (1974)	1	1600	8 weeks	Improved in first week
Escobar and Kemp (1975)	2	1200	2 weeks	No change
Crane (1975)	11	1200-1600	18 days	No change
Curran et al., (1975)	1	500	8 weeks	Improved in first week
Fann et al., (1975)	10	500	5 days	Improved in first week
DeSilva and Huang (1975)	4	800-1000	2 weeks	Improved in first week
Laterre and Fortemps (1975)	1	225-900	14 weeks	Improved with low dose; worsened with high dose
Davis et al., (1975)	4	1600-2000	3-5 weeks	No change
Widroe and Heisler (1976)	2	200-300	3-8 weeks	1 improved; 1 no change
Nesse and Carroll (1976)	1	1500	19 days	No change; cholinergic side effects
Kumar (1976)	1	1200	12 weeks	Improved; dyskinesia did not return when drug was stopped
Mehta et al., (1976)	2	600-800	3-5 weeks	No change; cholinergic side effects in one patient
Casey and Denney (1977)	6	800-2000	4 weeks	3 improved; 2 unchanged; 1 worsened. Response correlated with physostigmine response
McLean and Casey (1978)	1	2700	16 weeks	Improved; dyskinesias did not return when drug was stopped

[a] All reports involve open investigations except Casey and Denney (1977) which was single-blind placebo-controlled. Adapted from Casey, D.E., 1977; reprinted with permission.

TABLE 4

Deanol in Tardive Dyskinesia: Double-Blind Trials

Investigator-Year	Patients	Dose mg/day	Duration	Results
Cole *et al.*, (1976)	12	1500	5 weeks	No significant differences
Bockenheimer and Lucius (1976)	11	1500	5 weeks	7 improved; 4 unchanged; orofacial dyskinesias improved; limb dyskinesias unchanged
Simpson *et al.*, (1977)	10	1200	8 weeks	No significant differences
Tamminga *et al.*, (1977)	6	1500	3 weeks	No significant differences

Adapted from Casey, D.E., (1977) reprinted with permission.

The discrepant results between the open and double-blind trials merit further discussion. The factor of unintentional observer bias in open conditions may favor a trend toward a favorable outcome and must be acknowledged. Another point for consideration is that the double-blind studies tended to report results for the group as a whole. Thus a prominent drug effect in a few patients could be diluted in an analysis of group data. The nature of patient selection for open or double-blind investigations is another factor to be considered in comparing results. Since double-blind trials require a strict adherence to lengthy protocols, patients who are hospitalized for long periods of time, and who may represent a more severely affected subgroup, are more likely to be studied. On the other hand, patients treated under open conditions are more likely to be outpatients and to represent a less severely affected cohort whose symptom resolution could occur independent of, or be enhanced by, drugs. Direct examination of the possibility that different patient populations were being studied cannot be adequately evaluated because most of the double-blind studies and many of the open studies did not report sufficient data regarding age, sex, length of and total dose of neuroleptic treatment, or duration and severity of tardive dyskinesia symptoms. However, indirect support for this notion comes from the observations of temporary tardive dyskinesias. Self-limiting dyskinesias have been associated with withdrawing neuroleptics in patients taking these drugs less than 3 years (Moline, 1975; Jacobson *et al.*, 1974). In addition, dyskinetic symptoms gradually disappeared in the majority of outpatients when their neuroleptic drugs were discontinued at the first signs of tardive dyskinesia (Quitkin *et al.*, 1977). If an all or none position is taken that rigidly defines tardive dyskinesia as a permanent condition, it can be argued that a diagnosis of tardive dyskinesia should not be made if symptoms resolve. However, defining a syndrome by an arbitrarily determined time period imposes a limitation that actually may not exist. A more parsimonious explanation is that tardive dyskinesia occurs along a continuum of permanence. Symptoms that gradually resolve reflect a temporary alteration in function whose return to normal is independent of, or facilitated by drugs, while symptoms that persist reflect a permanent alteration in function that is minimally responsive to drugs.

Although the failure of dyskinesias to return to their previous level in some patients after deanol was stopped can be interpreted as a spontaneous change independent of drug effect, it is important to consider that deanol may also have some long-term effects on involuntary dyskinesias. Such an effect has been noted in treating both tardive dyskinesia (this report; McLean and Casey, 1978; Bockenheimer and Lucius, 1976; Kumar, 1976) and L-DOPA-induced dyskinesias (Miller, 1976; Klawans et al., 1975) with deanol. The finding that L-DOPA-induced dyskinesias remained reduced during a 2-week placebo period following 4 weeks of deanol was interpreted as a fluctuation in the dyskinesias independent of deanol (Klawans et al., 1975). However, the observation that L-DOPA-induced dyskinesias did not return to their previous level for up to 2 months following substantial doses of deanol (up to 1800 mg/day) for 3 months was considered as evidence that deanol may have a long-lasting effect (Miller, 1976). Support for a persisting effect from deanol treatment comes from the report that choline reduced tardive dyskinesia symptoms which did not return to their pretreatment level for many weeks into the placebo period, even though the choline blood level returned to normal within 48 hr of discontinuing choline (Davis et al., 1976). Speculative but interesting avenues of further inquiry include the possibilities that deanol, like choline, may affect tyrosine hydroxylase (Ulus and Wurtman, 1976; Lewander et al., 1975) and thus affect amine turnover, or that these drugs might affect myelinization processes. Since deanol and choline are so similar structurally, discovering the mechanisms of action in one may clarify our understanding of the other.

Failures of deanol treatment are somewhat difficult to interpret. Although most patients who responded did so within the first few weeks of treatment at a dose level below 1000 mg/day, it is possible that the dosage for a particular patient may have been too low or given for too short a period to be effective. This could result from disorders of absorption or increased states of drug metabolism. Conversely, patients may have received a potentially adequate dose, but were incapable of responding because the underlying pathophysiologic process had progressed to an unalterable or unresponsive stage. It has been observed that one patient's tardive dyskinesia was unresponsive to 6000 mg/day of deanol, though he developed peripheral cholinergic symptoms of excessive sweating and salivation at this dose (Casey, 1977). Perhaps monitoring deanol or metabolite blood levels would be helpful in determining the amount of deanol required for each patient to produce a clinical response.

Until adequate methodology can be developed to assist in managing the deanol dosage with blood level determinations, it might be worthwhile to investigate physostigmine as a predictive test for deanol. This investigation demonstrated that the response to physostigmine significantly correlated with the deanol response. Improvement with physostigmine was also associated with improvement in two patients with Huntington's disease taking deanol (Walker et al., 1973). Additionally, symptom reduction with physostigmine in four patients with tardive dyskinesia and two patients with Huntington's disease correlated with improvement during choline therapy (Davis et al., 1976). Although the mechanism of action of physostigmine, an acetylcholinesterase inhibitor, is clearly different from the putative cholinergic precursors, it may be that a response to a challenge dose of physostigmine is a reflection of the integrity and plasticity of the nigro-striato-nigral feedback system. Thus, physostigmine could be a predictive test to measure the capacity of the striatum to respond to cholinergic augmentation.

SUMMARY

Incontrovertible conclusions cannot be drawn about the roles of deanol as a cholinergic precursor or as a therapeutic agent for tardive dyskinesia. Some investigations demonstrate that brain choline and ACh are elevated following acute and chronic doses of deanol; other studies do not corroborate these findings. In the clinical setting, approximately one-half of the patients treated under open or single-blind conditions improved while taking deanol. The results of double-blind studies in 39 patients are less encouraging with 18% significantly benefiting. To date, we are unable to predict which patients will benefit from deanol and which ones will not.

Future research should be directed at both the basic science and clinical levels. Further biochemical and pharmacological inquiries should attempt to clarify the discrepancies regarding the acute and long-term effects of deanol on brain choline and ACh. A particular inquiry should investigate the role of deanol in the phosphatidylcholinergic metabolic pathways. Additionally, the effect of deanol on indolamine, catecholamine and GABA influences deserves attention. The animal models of tardive dyskinesia using stereotypies and receptor binding parameters may also elucidate the effect of deanol. At the human level of investigation, studies need to correlate clinical effects, or the lack thereof, with deanol and metabolite blood levels. Inquiries into the effect of deanol on cerebral spinal fluid amine and cholinergic metabolites may also be worthwhile. Patient characteristics of age, sex, duration and type of neuroleptic and anticholinergic treatment, and duration and type of tardive dyskinesia symptoms need to be reported as thoroughly as possible to develop a profile of factors that identify patients who are likely to benefit from drug therapy. In addition, further evaluation of physostigmine as a predictive test for responsiveness to deanol in particular, and cholinergic augmentation in general, is warranted. To date, deanol as a putative cholinergic precursor has been a useful research tool for advancing our understanding of tardive dyskinesia. However, we have clearly not found the ideal drug to treat this perplexing syndrome.

ACKNOWLEDGEMENTS

The author wishes to acknowledge the contributions that made this work possible. Duane Denney, M.D. greatly assisted with data analysis and Marian Karr provided expert technical assistance with the manuscript. Riker Laboratories generously provided the deanol and placebo drugs. This work was supported in part by funds from the Portland Veterans Administration Hospital Research Committee, Portland, Oregon, MRIS #1314-01 and in part by funds from The Grass Foundation. Parts of Section 1 have been previously published and are reprinted with permission from Springer-Verlag Co.

REFERENCES

Alpert, M., Diamond, F., and Friedhoff, A.J., 1976, Tremographic studies in tardive dyskinesia, *Psychopharmacol. Bull. 12:*5.

Ansell, G.B., and Spanner, S., 1962, The effect of 2-dimethylaminoethanol on brain phospholipid metabolism, *J. Neurochem. 9:*253.

Bird, D., and Aghajanian, G., 1975, Denervation supersensitivity in the cholinergic septohippocampal pathway: a microiontophoretic study, *Brain Res. 100:*355.

Bjornstad, P., and Bremer, J., 1966, *In vivo* studies on pathways for the biosynthesis of lecithin in the rat, *J. Lipid Res. 7:*38.

Bockenheimer, S., and Lucius, G., 1976, Zur Therapie mit Dimethylaminoethanol (Deanol) bei neuroleptikainduzierten extrapyramidalen Hyperkinesen, *Arch. Psychiatr. Nervenkr. 222:*69.

Bremer, J., Figard, P.H., and Greenberg, D.M., 1960, The biosynthesis of choline and its relation to phospholipid metabolism, *Biochim. Biophys. Acta 43:*477.

Burt, D.R., Creese, I., and Snyder, S.H., 1977, Antischizophrenic drugs: chronic treatment elevates dopamine receptor binding in brain, *Science 196:*326.

Carroll, B.J., Curtis, G.C., and Kokmen, E., 1977, Paradoxical response to dopamine agonists in tardive dyskinesia, *Am. J. Psychiatry 134:*785.

Casey, D.E., 1976, Tardive dyskinesia: are there subtypes? *N. Engl. J. Med. 259:*1078.

Casey, D.E., 1977, Deanol in the management of involuntary movement disorders: a review, *Dis. Nerv. Syst. 38(2):*7.

Casey, D.E., and Denney, D., 1974, Dimethylaminoethanol in tardive dyskinesia, 1974, *N. Engl. J. Med. 291:*797.

Casey, D.E., and Denney, D., 1975, Deanol in the treatment of tardive dyskinesia, *Am. J. Psychiatry 132:*864.

Casey, D.E., and Denney, D., 1977, Pharmacological characterization of tardive dyskinesia, *Psychopharmacology 54:*1.

Claveria, L.E., Teychenne, P.F., Calne, D.B., Haskayne, L., Petrie, A., Pallis, C.A., and Lodge-Patch, I.C., 1975, Tardive dyskinesia treated with pimozide, *J. Neurol. Sci. 24:*393.

Cole, J.O., Gardos, G., and Granacher, R., 1976, Drug evaluations in tardive dyskinesia: papaverine and deanol, presented at the 129th annual meeting of the American Psychiatric Association, Miami Beach, Florida.

Cools, A.R., and VanRossum, J.M., 1976, Excitation-mediating and inhibition-mediating dopamine-receptors: a new concept towards a better understanding of the electrophysiological, biochemical, pharmacological, functional, and clinical data, *Psychopharmacologia 45:*243.

Crane, G.E., 1973, Persistent dyskinesia, *Br. J. Psychiatry 122:*395.

Crane, G.E., 1975, Deanol for tardive dyskinesia, *N. Engl. J. Med. 292:*926.

Crane, G.E., and Smeets, R.A., 1974, Tardive dyskinesia and drug therapy in geriatric patients, *Arch. Gen. Psychiatry 30:*341.

Curran, D.J., Nagaswami, S., and Mohan, K.J., 1975, Treatment of phenothiazine-induced bulbar persistent dyskinesia with deanol acetamidobenzoate, *Dis. Nerv. Syst. 36:*71.

Danysz, A., Kocmierska-Grodzka, D., Kostro, B., Polocki, B., and Kruszewska, J., 1967, Pharmacological properties of 2-dimethylaminoethanol (bimanol-DMAE), *Diss. Pharm. Pharmacol. 19:*469.

Davis, K.L., Berger, P.A., and Hollister, L.E., 1975, Choline for tardive dyskinesia, *N. Engl. J. Med. 293:*152.

Davis, K.L., Hollister, L.E., Barchas, J.D., and Berger, P.A., 1976, Choline in tardive dyskinesia and Huntington's disease, *Life Sci. 19:*1507.

Davis, K.L., Berger, P.A., Hollister, L.E., and De Fraites, 1978, Physostigmine in mania, *Arch. Gen. Psychiatry 35:*119.

Denham, J., and Carrick, D.J., 1961, Therapeutic value of thioproperazine and the importance of the associated neurological disturbances, *J. Ment. Sci. 107:*326.

Denney, D., and Casey, D.E., 1975, An objective method for measuring dyskinetic movements in tardive dyskinesia, *Electroencephalogr. Clin. Neurophysiol. 38:*645.

DeSilva, L., and Huang, C.Y., 1975, Deanol in tardive dyskinesia, *Br. Med. J. 3:*466.

Dormard, Y., Levron, J.C., and LeFur, J.M., 1975, Pharmacokinetic study of maleate acid of 2-(N,N-dimethylaminoethanol-14C$_1$)-cyclohexylpropionate (cyprodenate) and of N,N-dimethylaminoethanol-14C$_1$ in animals. II. Study and identification of the metabolites of 14C-cyprodenate and 14C-dimethylaminoethanol in animals, *Arzneim. Forsch. 25:*201.

DuVigneaud, V., Chandler, S.P., Simmonds, S., Moyer, A.W., and Cohn, M., 1946, The role of dimethyl- and monomethylaminoethanol in transmethylation reactions *in vivo, J. Biol. Chem. 164:*603.

Escobar, J.I., and Kemp, K.F., 1975, Dimethylaminoethanol for tardive dyskinesia, *N. Engl. J. Med. 292:*317.

Fann, W.E., Lake, C.R., Gerber, C.J., and McKenzie, G.M., 1974, Cholinergic suppression of tardive dyskinesia, *Psychopharmacologia 37:*101.

Fann, W.E., Sullivan, J.L., Miller, R.D., and McKenzie, G.M., 1975, Deanol in tardive dyskinesia: a preliminary report, *Psychopharmacologia 42:*135.

Freeman, J.J., and Jenden, D.J., 1976, The source of choline for acetylcholine synthesis in brain, *Life Sci. 19:*949.

Gardos, G., Cole, J.O., and Sniffen, C., 1976, An evaluation of papaverine in tardive dyskinesia, *J. Clin. Pharmacol. 16:*304.

Gerlach, J., Reisby, N., and Randrup, A., 1974, Dopaminergic hypersensitivity and cholinergic hypofunction in the pathophysiology of tardive dyskinesia, *Psychopharmacologia 34:*21.

Goldberg, A.M., and Silbergeld, E.K., 1974, Neurochemical aspects of lead-induced hyperactivity, *Trans. Amer. Soc. Neurochem. 5:*185.

Granacher, R.P., Baldessarini, R.J., and Cole, J.O., 1975, Deanol for tardive dyskinesia, *N. Engl. J. Med. 292:*926.

Growdon, J.H., Hirsch, M.J., Wurtman, R.J., and Wiener, W., 1977, Oral choline administration to patients with tardive dyskinesia, *N. Engl. J. Med. 297:*524.

Hanin, I., and Costa, E., 1976, Approaches used to estimate brain acetylcholine turnover rate *in vivo;* effects of drugs on brain acetylcholine turnover rate, in *"Biology of Cholinergic Function"* (A. Goldberg and I. Hanin, eds.), pp. 355-377, Raven Press, New York.

Haubrich, D.R., Wang, P.F.L., Clody, D.E., and Wedeking, P.W., 1975, Increase in rat brain acetylcholine induced by choline or deanol, *Life Sci. 17:*975.

Hippius, H., and Logemann, G., 1970, Zur Wirkung von Dioxyphenylalanin (L-DOPA) auf extrapyramidalmotorische Hyperkineses nach langfristiger neuroleptische Therapie, *Arzneim. Forsch. 20:*894.

Jacobson, G., Baldessarini, R.J., and Manschreck, T., 1974, Tardive dyskinesia associated with haloperidol, *Am. J. Psychiatry 131:*910.

Janowsky, D.S., Davis, J.M., El-Yousef, M.K., and Sekerke, H.J., 1972, A cholinergic-adrenergic hypothesis of mania and depression, *Lancet 2 (7778):*632.

Janowsky, D.S., El-Yousef, M.K., Davis, J.M., and Sekerke, H.J., 1973, Parasympathetic suppression of manic symptoms by physostigmine, *Arch. Gen. Psychiatry 28:*542.

Jus, A., Pineau, R., Lachance, R., Pelchat, G., Jus, K., Pires, P., and Villeneuve, R., 1976a, Epidemiology of tardive dyskinesia: Part I, *Dis. Nerv. Syst. 37:*210.

Jus, A., Pineau, R., Lachance, R., Pelchat, G., Jus, K., Pires, P., and Villeneuve, R., 1976b, Epidemiology of tardive dyskinesia: Part II, *Dis. Nerv. Syst. 37:*257.

Kazamatsuri, H., Chien, C., and Cole, J.O., 1972a, The treatment of tardive dyskinesia. I. Clinical efficacy of a dopamine-depleting agent, tetrabenazine, *Arch. Gen. Psychiatry 27:*95.

Kazamatsuri, H., Chien, C., and Cole, J.O., 1972b, The treatment of tardive dyskinesia. II. Short-term efficacy of dopamine-blocking agents haloperidol and thiopropazate, *Arch. Gen. Psychiatry 27:*100.

Kazamatsuri, H., Chien, C.P., and Cole, J.O., 1973, Long-term treatment of tardive dyskinesia with haloperidol and tetrabenazine, *Am. J. Psychiatry 130:*479.

Klawans, H.L., 1973, The pharmacology of tardive dyskinesia, *Am. J. Psychiatry 130:*82.

Klawans, H.L., and McKendall, R., 1971, Observations on the effect of L-DOPA on tardive lingual-facial-buccal dyskinesia, *J. Neurol. Sci. 14:*189.

Klawans, H.L., and Rubovits, R., 1972, An experimental model of tardive dyskinesia, *J. Neural Transm. 33:*235.

Klawans, H.L., and Rubovits, R., 1974, Effect of cholinergic and anticholinergic agents on tardive dyskinesia, *J. Neurol. Neurosurg. Psychiatry 27:*941.

Klawans, H.L., Topel, J.L., and Bergen, D., 1975, Deanol in the treatment of L-DOPA-induced dyskinesias, *Neurology 25:*290.

Kumar, B.B., 1976, Treatment of tardive dyskinesia with deanol, *Am. J. Psychiatry 133:*978.

Lal, S., 1974, Comparison of thiopropazate and trifluoperazine on oral dyskinesia — a double-blind study, *Curr. Ther. Res. 16:*990.

Laterre, E.C., and Fortemps, E., 1975, Deanol in spontaneous and induced dyskinesias, *Lancet 1 (7919):*1301.

Lewander, T., Joh, T.H., and Reis, D.J., 1975, Prolonged activation of tyrosine hydroxylase in noradrenergic neurons of rat brain by cholinergic stimulation, *Nature 258:*440.

McLean, P., and Casey, D.E., 1978, Tardive dyskinesia in an adolescent, *Am. J. Psychiatry 135:*969.

Mehta, D., Mehta, S., and Mathew, P., 1976, Failure of deanol in treating tardive dyskinesia, *Am. J. Psychiatry 133:*1467.

Miller, E., 1974, Deanol: a solution for tardive dyskinesia? *N. Engl. J. Med. 291:*796.

Miller, E., 1976, Effectiveness of deanol on L-DOPA-induced dyskinesias: a placebo-controlled double-blind crossover study, in *"Advances in Parkinsonism"* (W. Birkmayer, and O. Hornykiewics, eds.), pp. 582-590, Hoffmann-LaRoche, Basle, Switzerland.

Moline, R., 1975, Atypical dyskinesia, *Am. J. Psychiatry 132:*534.

Nesse, R., and Carroll, B.J., 1976, Cholinergic side-effects associated with deanol, *Lancet 2(7975):*50.

Pepeu, G., Freedman, D.X., and Giarman, N.J., 1960, Biochemical and pharmacological studies of dimethylaminoethanol (deanol), *J. Pharmacol. Exp. Ther. 129:*291.

Pfeiffer, C.C., Jenney, E.H., Gallacher, W., Smith, R.P., Bevan, J., Killam, E.K., Killam, K.F., and Blackmore, W., 1957, Stimulant effect of 2-dimethylaminoethanol — possible precursor of brain acetylcholine, *Science 126:*610.

Quitkin, F., Rifkin, A., Gochfeld, L., and Klein, D.F., 1977, Tardive dyskinesia: are first signs reversible? *Am. J. Psychiatry 134:*84.

Sarwer-Foner, G.J., 1960, Recognition and management of drug-induced extrapyramidal reactions and "paradoxical" behavioral reactions in psychiatry, *Can. Med. Assoc. J. 83:*312.

Sato, S., Daly, R., and Peters, H., 1971, Reserpine therapy of phenothiazine-induced dyskinesia, *Dis. Nerv. Syst. 32:*680.

Scheel-Kruger, J., and Randrup, A., 1968, Pharmacological evidence for a cholinergic mechanism in brain involved in a special stereotyped behavior of reserpined rats, *Br. J. Pharmacol. 34:*217.

Schiorring, E., and Randrup, A., 1968, Paradoxical stereotyped activity of reserpined rats, *Int. J. Neuropharmacol. 7:*71.

Simpson, G.M., 1973, Tardive dyskinesia, *Br. J. Psychiatry 122:*618.

Simpson, G.M., Voitashevsky, A., Young, M.A., and Lee, H.J., 1977, Deanol in the treatment of tardive dyskinesia, *Psychopharmacology 52:*257.

Singer, K., and Cheng, M.N., 1971, Thiopropazate HCL in persistent dyskinesia, *Br. Med. J. 4:*22.

Smith, R.C., Tamminga, C., Haraszti, J., Pandey, G.N., and Davis, J.M., 1977, Effects of dopamine agonists in tardive dyskinesia, *Am. J. Psychiatry 134:*763.

Snyder, S., Greenberg, D., and Yamamura, H., 1974, Antischizophrenic drugs and brain cholinergic receptors, *Arch. Gen. Psychiatry 31:*58.

Tamminga, C., Smith, R.C., Chang, S., Haraszti, J.S., and Davis, J.M., 1976, Depression associated with oral choline, *Lancet 2(7991):*905.

Tamminga, C., Smith, R.C., Ericksen, S.E., Chang, S., and Davis, J.M., 1977, Cholinergic influences in tardive dyskinesia, *Am. J. Psychiatry 134:*769.

Tarsy, D., and Baldessarini, R.J., 1976, The tardive dyskinesia syndrome, in *"Clinical Neuropharmacology"* (H.L. Klawans, ed.), Vol. 1, pp. 29-61, Raven Press, New York.

Tarsy, D., Leopold, N., and Sax, D.S., 1974, Physostigmine in choreiform movement disorders, *Neurology 24:*28.

Uhrbrand, L., and Faurbye, A., 1960, Reversible and irreversible dyskinesia after treatment with perphenazine, chlorpromazine, reserpine and electroconvulsive therapy, *Psychopharmacologia 1:*408.

Ulus, I.H., and Wurtman, R.J., 1976, Choline administration: activation of tyrosine hydroxylase in dopaminergic neurons of rat brain, *Science 194:*1060.

Walker, J.E., Hoehn, M., Sears, E., and Lewis, J., 1973, Dimethylaminoethanol in Huntington's chorea, *Lancet 1(7818):*1512.

Weiner, W.J., Kanapa, D.J., and Klawans, H.L., 1976, The effect of dimethylaminoethanol (deanol) on amphetamine-induced stereotyped behavior, *Life Sci. 19:*1371.

Widroe, H.J., and Heisler, S., 1976, Treatment of tardive dyskinesia, *Dis. Nerv. Syst. 37:*162.

Zahniser, N.R., and Hanin, I., 1976, Deanol and the cholinergic system: a gas chromatographic evaluation, *Fed. Proc. 35:*801.

Zahniser, N.R., Chou, D., and Hanin, I., 1977, Is 2-dimethylaminoethanol (deanol) indeed a precursor of brain acetylcholine? A gas chromatographic evaluation, *J. Pharmacol. Exp. Ther. 200:*545.

ORAL PHYSOSTIGMINE AND INHERITED ATAXIAS

R. A. P. Kark[1], M. Rodriguez-Budelli[1], J. P. Blass[2,3] and M. A. Spence[2,4]

Departments of [1]Neurology, [2]Psychiatry, [3]Biochemistry and [4]Biomathematics [1]Reed Neurological Research Center and [1,2]Mental Retardation Center, UCLA School of Medicine, Los Angeles, California 90024

BACKGROUND

The study of ataxias with physostigmine was originally based entirely on theoretical considerations. A great deal of evidence relates abnormalities of pyruvate metabolism to ataxia (for reviews see Blass et al., 1976a; Blass et al., 1975; Kark et al., (in press). Certain inherited ataxias are associated with defects of the pyruvate dehydrogenase multi-enzyme complex and especially its pyruvate decarboxylase and lipoamide dehydrogenase components (Blass et al., 1970; Blass et al., 1971; Blass et al., 1976b; Rodriguez-Budelli et al., in press; Blass et al., in press; and Kark et al., in press). Experiments on brain slices and whole animals have shown that the synthesis of acetylcholine (ACh) is decreased by each of a number of conditions that impair the oxidation of pyruvate or glucose. ACh synthesis is reduced before there is any change in energy-charge or levels of ATP or creatine phosphate (Gibson and Blass, 1976a, 1976b). The conditions that decrease ACh synthesis include mild hypoxia, hypoglycemia, and various poisons that inhibit the pyruvate dehydrogenase complex (Gibson and Blass, 1976a, 1976b; Gibson et al., 1975). It was tempting to speculate that there might be insufficient ACh in some central nervous pathway in inherited ataxias associated with defects of pyruvate oxidation, and perhaps in other ataxias as well. If so, physostigmine might lessen the severity of one or more aspects of the ataxia.

Others had analyzed diseases of the central nervous system with physostigmine (Duvoisin, 1967; Duvoisin and Katz, 1968; McDowell and Markham, 1971), especially Klawans and Rubovits (1972) in their study of Huntington's chorea. These studies had shown that systemic use of physostigmine could modulate the signs of progressive degenerative diseases of the central nervous system in doses that produced few side effects. The results implied that central cholinergic pathways might be involved in the pathophysiology of the diseases.

As described below, physostigmine appears to ameliorate the signs of the ataxia in several of the inherited ataxias whether there is evidence of decreased pyruvate oxidation or not.

METHODS

Preparations of Drugs

Physostigmine

Physostigmine was prepared for intravenous use and for oral use. The intravenous preparation was a sterile solution of 1 mg physostigmine salicylate in 10 ml of normal saline. The oral preparations were tablets made from inert bases and binders, starch granules, microcrystalline Plasdone C, and magnesium stearate, plus 1 mg physostigmine salicylate (Kark et al., 1977).

Other Drugs

Methylscopolamine was given intravenously as a sterile solution of 1 mg drug in 10 ml normal saline. Placebo for the intravenous drug studies were normal saline. Placebo tablets for the other drug studies were made of the inert bases and binders without the drug and were identical in appearance and taste to the physostigmine tablets.

Diagnosis of Ataxias

The clinical and radiological criteria for the clinical diagnosis of Friedreich's ataxia have been presented elsewhere (Kark et al., in press). Clinical diagnoses of other inherited ataxias were based on the combination of an appropriate clinical picture (Greenfield, 1954; Victor et al., 1959; Brain and Walton, 1969; Konigsmark and Weiner, 1970; Kark et al., 1974) plus evidence of appropriate anatomical changes. Evidence for the latter came from neuropathological changes found at autopsy in affected relatives, from changes seen at pneumoencephalography with linear, biplanar tomography of the posterior fossa with a Mimer tomogram, or from both sources.

Evaluation of Ataxia

Examinations of various body movements (Table 1) were recorded on videotape before and after giving drugs or placebo. One to two years later, 60 tests of speed, dysrhythmia or dysmetria were scored from each tape on a semi-quantitative scale. This was done independently by three physicians who did not know the drug codes and who viewed the tapes in random sequence. Separate scores were averaged for the three physicians who did not know the drug codes and who viewed the tapes in random sequence. Separate scores were averaged for the three physicians and statistical analyses were performed before drug codes were broken. The scale was designed where 0 equals normal, and 5 equals such severe ataxia that a movement could not be completed. Movements that were atypical for some reason other than ataxia, like weakness, were not scored. The scale is non-linear in that a change from two to three arbitrary units, for example, represents approximately a two-fold increase in the severity of ataxia rather than a 50% increase.

TABLE 1

Tests Used for Ataxia Scores

Speech

Conversation
"Commonwealth of
  Massachusetts"
"Schenectady, New York"
"Santiago, Chile"
"Around the rugged rock
  the ragged rascal ran"

Eyes

Nystagmus
Dysmetria

Tongue Movements

Speed
Precision

**Diaphragmatic and
Laryngeal Ataxia**

Truncal Ataxia

Upper Extremities

Undressing (speed,
  precision, rhythm)
Use of gesture
Finger-to-nose
  (eyes closed, eyes open)
Finger-to-thumb crease
Alternate patting
  (speed, rhythm, fineness
  of movement)
Handwriting
  (speed, effect)
Spirals (rhythm, effect)

Lower Extremities

Toe-to-finger
Heel-knee-shin
Tap rhythm
Stance
Gait
Tandem gait
  (and with aid)

SINGLE BLIND TRIAL

Intravenous Physostigmine

Three patients were given physostigmine intravenously, alternating with placebo, in a single-blind design. After baseline examinations and with monitoring by electro-cardiograms, 1 mg methylscopolamine was given intravenously over two min followed in ten min by 1 mg physostigmine or 10 ml normal saline (placebo). The examination was recorded again 20, 40 and 90 min later. This was done in the morning of one day, and repeated in the afternoon with the other test solution, placebo or physostigmine. The tests were repeated in full the next day with physostigmine and placebo given in the opposite order.

The responses for the three patients were similar and one is illustrated in Figure 1. Maximal effects of physostigmine on the overall score were seen at 40 min. These were always greater than the placebo effect. The order of test solutions did not influence the results. However, the side effects of methylscopolamine, especially dry mouth, blurred vision and abdominal discomfort, troubled the patients for two to four hr and the methylscopolamine did not always block the peripheral effects of physostigmine (Kark *et al.*, 1977). We therefore tested oral physostigmine in a single-blind design.

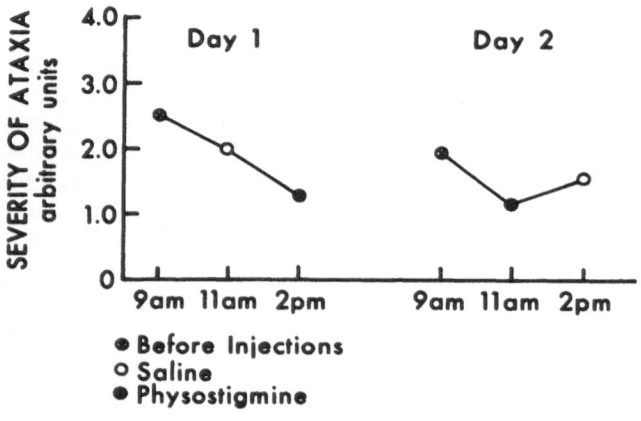

FIGURE 1

Response of Ataxia Scores to Intravenous Physostigmine and Saline in a Patient. The arbitrary scale of severity and doses of drugs are described in the test. Examinations were recorded before injections (x), and 40 min after test injections of methylscopolamine plus physostigmine (filled circles) or methylscopolamine plus saline placebo (open circles). Test injections were given 6 hr apart. Note that the same test injections were given again 24 hr later, but in the opposite order.

Oral Physostigmine

Ten patients were examined, given a tablet of physostigmine, and were reexamined 15 to 90 min later. They did not know whether the tablet was placebo or physostigmine and we hinted it was the former. Maximal effects were seen by 40 min and none were demonstrable after two hr. There were no peripheral side effects.

Every patient's score improved with a single dose of physostigmine (Figure 2). The average scores for the 13 patients in the single-blind, short term studies changed from 2.67 ± 0.01 before the drug to 1.69 ± 0.00 afterwards ($p < .0005$). The diagnoses of these patients were: Friedreich's ataxia, 5; olivopontocerebellar atrophy, 5; cerebellar cortical atrophy, 1; cerebellar and cerebral atrophy, 1; and the Ramsay-Hunt syndrome, 1. These observations suggested that there might be deficient activity of some cholinergic mechanism in the ataxic patient. The results with methylscopolamine suggested the mechanism was central. However, a placebo effect could not be entirely excluded.

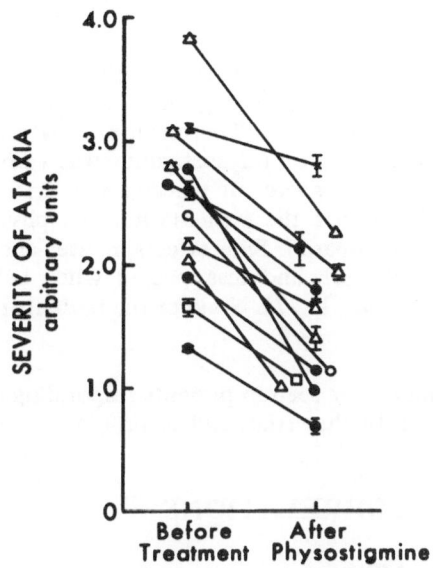

- Friedreich's Ataxia × Ramsey-Hunt Syndrome
- △ Olivopontocerebellar Atrophy
- ○ Cerebellar Cortical Atrophy
- □ Cerebellar and Cerebral Cortical Atrophy

FIGURE 2

Ataxia Scores Before and After Single Doses of Physostigmine. Each symbol represents the mean score for one patient on one occasion. Bars represent S.E.M. (not shown if smaller than the symbol). Diagnoses are as indicated in the Figure. The patients represented in the left hand column by the first full circle, the open circle and the fourth triangle from the top received physostigmine intravenously. The other patients received it orally. Data in the right-hand column represent scores 40 min after the drug.

DOUBLE BLIND, RANDOMIZED TRIAL

Eleven patients received tablets of physostigmine or placebo for four periods, each of three months' duration. The nature of the tablets was assigned at the start of each period and videotape recordings of examinations were made before and after each period. Doses of tablets were increased progressively over the first month of each period from one tablet three times daily, to one tablet eight times daily (every two hr while awake). The latter dosage was maintained for the last two months. Data on the first five patients have been reported (Kark *et al.*, 1977).

Ataxia in nine of the patients responded better to physostigmine than to placebo by the semi-quantitative scores. In two patients, there was no response to the drug. Diagnoses are given in the legend to Figure 3. The mean pretreatment score for the 11 patients was 2.14 ± 0.19; the mean score on physostigmine was 1.56 ± 0.11 ($p < .00005$ vs. pretreatment scores); and the mean score on placebo was 2.16 ± 0.26 ($p < .01$ vs. physostigmine scores, Figure 3). Neither the patients nor the physicians could detect changes until the videotapes were compared. Side effects, nausea and vomiting, occurred only in one patient, a nine-year-old girl, and disappeared when half-tablet doses were substituted for whole doses (Kark *et al.*, 1977). None of the patients had fasciculations or changes in strength.

The pattern of changes that can be seen in patients responding to the drug is shown in Figure 4. These data are from a further trial, still in progress, conducted in a double-crossover, double-blind pattern.

CORRELATIONS

Between Observers and Over Time

There were three observers. For scores over all patients, observer A correlated with B with a correlation coefficient, $r = 0.9$ ($p < .001$ vs. no correlation). Observer A correlated with C with $r = 0.8$ ($p < .001$); and observer B correlates with C with $r = 0.9$ ($p < .001$). Scores for observer A have been correlated over the four years of the study and $r = 0.85$ ($p < .001$) over time.

Over Tests for Ataxia

To investigate redundancy among the ataxia tests of Table 1, subscores for each test were compared in each patient each time he went from one drug to the other (e.g. physostigmine to placebo). Subscores for every test improved and worsened appropriately in one patient or more. Conversely, there was no single test that changed appropriately and significantly in every patient. In this sense, all 60 tests are of value and none has proved redundant.

The scores for the 12 tests of Table 2 correlated with switches on and off physostigmine over all the patients with $p < .05$. These are mainly tests of distal, fine movements. Most patients are disabled by ataxia of gross, proximal movements. The discrepancy may account for the paradoxical improvement of scores in patients who could not discern improvement.

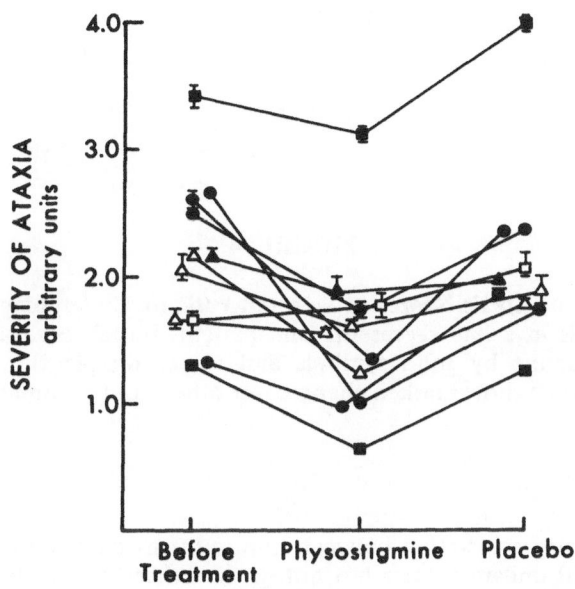

FIGURE 3

Ataxia Scores Before and After Long-Term Double-Blind Use of Physostigmine and Placebo. Symbols and Diagnoses are as in Figure 2. Solid squares represent biopsy-proven ragged-red neuromuscular disease with ataxia (ragged-red ataxia). Data in the first column represent the results of a single examination of each patient. Data in the second and third columns are the means of the examinations scored after one to three trial periods (each of 3 months' length).

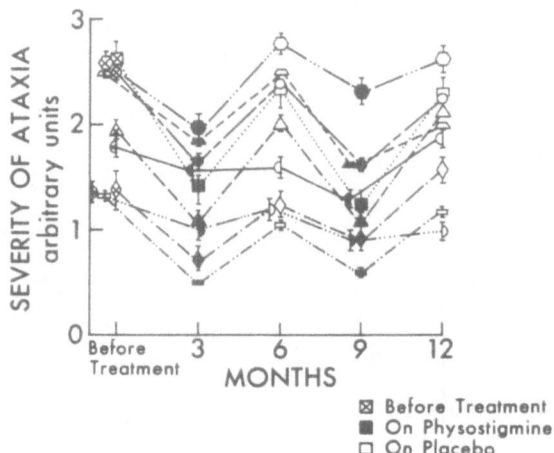

FIGURE 4

Pattern of Changes in Ataxia Scores in Selected Patients Undergoing a Cross-over Trial.
Each set of symbols in a line represents one patient. Initial scores are indicated by X, scores on physostigmine by solid symbols and scores on placebo by open symbols. Note that some patients show marked changes but others, only minimal ones.

There is a strong association between improvement on one side and improvement on the other in eight unilateral tests but not in the other three tests. (Table 3). Two of the latter are dependent in part on handedness and all our patients appear to have strong dominance.

SUSTAINED USE OF PHYSOSTIGMINE

Thirty patients are currently taking physostigmine, 1 to 2 mg eight times a day and have done so for six to 36 months. Several have reported improvement in function after six to 18 months. Speech, handwriting or gait are said to be better and occasionally all three improve anecdotally. Two patients have reported worsening when the drug was stopped for a month and have regained a function after resuming the drug. Unfortunately, distance prevented videotape examinations of the anecdotal changes.

TABLE 2

Correlation of Subtests with Overall Scores

1) Every subtest correlated across treatments in *some* of the patients.
2) The following correlated over *all* patients with $p < .05$:

       "Santiago, Chile"
       Nystagmus
       Tongue movements
       Undressing
       Use of gesture
       Truncal ataxia (seated)
       Finger-to-nose test, eyes closed (right arm)
       Speed of finger-to-nose test with eyes open
       Finger-to-thumb test
       Alternating patting of hands
       Speed of toe-to-finger test
       Rhythm of foot tap (right side)

TABLE 3

Scores of Severity of Ataxia:
Correlations Between Right-sided and Left-sided Tests

A. **Strong Correlation**

    1) nystagmus
    2) ocular dysmetria
    3) finger-to-nose test with eyes open
    4) finger-to-thumb test
    5) alternate patting
    6) toe-to-finger test
    7) heel-knee-shin test
    8) tap rhythm with foot

B. **No Correlation**

    1) finger-to-nose test with eyes closed
    2) speed and quality of handwriting
    3) speed and quality of drawing spirals

It has been possible to score examinations on ten patients from videotape before and after a six months' sustained use of physostigmine (Table 4). All had semi-quantitative improvement and the mean scores improved by 30% ± 5% (p < .005). Patients with a mean improvement of more than 0.5 arbitrary units have reported subjective improvement; the others have not.

TABLE 4

Effects of Sustained Physostigmine

Patients	Before Treatment	Six Months Prolonged Treatment	Δ
1.	2.4 ± .26	1.4 ± .06	1.0
2.	1.5 ± .10	0.8 ± .15	0.7
3.	1.7 ± .15	1.0 ± .03	0.7
4.	2.1 ± .10	1.4 ± .10	0.7
5.	2.1 ± .01	1.5 ± .08	0.6
6.	2.5 ± .12	1.9 ± .14	0.6
7.	2.0 ± .13	1.5 ± .18	0.5
8.	2.1 ± .29	1.6 ± .06	0.5
9.	2.2 ± .15	1.7 ± .05	0.5
10.	1.5 ± .12	1.1 ± .10	0.4
MEAN ± S.E.M.	2.0 ± .11	1.4 ± .11	0.6 ± .05
% of Pretreatment		70% ± 5%	

Legend: Patients 1 through 6 reported subjective improvement. Diagnoses were: Friedreich's ataxia, patients 3, 6, 7 and 9; Friedreich's variant, patients 1 and 5; Olivopontocerebellar atrophy, patients 2, 4 and 10; and ragged-red ataxia, patient 8.

CONCLUSIONS

Physostigmine improves the symptoms of ataxia by semi-quantitative measurements within one hr of a single dose over a three months' span in randomized, cross-over trials, and over a six months' span with sustained use of the drug but without controls. The changes take place whether or not the patients are aware of improvement, and the effects of physostigmine are significantly greater than placebo effects. Methylscopolamine does not block the effects of single doses, and no neuromuscular changes were seen with the long-term use of physostigmine. Hence physostigmine appears to act on ataxia through some central cholinergic mechanism. Too little is known of the anatomy of cholinergic pathways within the cerebellum, or of cholinergic influences on the connections from the cerebellum to other parts of the nervous systems to speculate on likely sites of action of the drug in ataxic patients. While most of the patients we have studied have had defects of enzymes related to pyruvate metabolism, some patients who have responded to physostigmine do not. Studies with other cholinergic agents, agonists and antagonists, are needed to characterize the mechanism of action of physostigmine. To determine the clinical efficacy of physostigmine in the inherited ataxias, there must be large scale, formal, controlled trials.

REFERENCES

Blass, J.P., Avigan, J., and Uhlendorf, B.W., 1970, A defect in pyruvate decarboxylase in a child with an intermittent movement disorder, *J. Clin. Invest. 49:*423.

Blass, J.P., Kark, R.A.P., and Engel, W.K., 1971, Clinical studies of a patient with pyruvate decarboxylase deficiency, *Arch. Neurol. 25:*449.

Blass, J.P., Cederbaum, S.D., and Gibson, G.E., 1975, Clinical and metabolic abnormalities accompanying deficiencies in pyruvate oxidation, in *"Normal and Pathological Development of Energy Metabolism"* (F.A. Hommes and C.J. Van den Berg, eds.), pp. 193-210, Academic Press, New York.

Blass, J.P., Gibson, G.E., and Kark, R.A.P., 1976a, Pyruvate decarboxylase deficiency, in *"Thiamine"* (C.J. Grubler, M. Fujiwara and P.M. Dreyfus, eds.), pp. 321-334, John Wiley and Sons, New York.

Blass, J.P., Kark, R.A.P., and Menon, N.K., 1976b, Low activities of the pyruvate and oxoflutarate dehydrogenase complexes in five patients with Friedreich's ataxia, *N. Engl. J. Med. 295:*62.

Blass, J.P., Kark, R.A.P., and Rodriguez-Budelli, M., in press, Pyruvate dehydrogenase deficiency in six of 14 patients with spino-cerebellar degeneration, *Neurology (Minneap).*

Brain, the late Lord, and Walton, J.N., 1969, *"Brain's Diseases of the Nervous System,"* 7th edition, Oxford University Press, New York.

Duvoisin, R.C., 1967, Cholinergic-anticholinergic antagonism in Parkinsonism, *Arch. Neurol. 17:*124.

Duvoisin, R.C., and Katz, R., 1968, Reversal of central anticholinergic syndrome in man by physostigmine, *JAMA 206:*1963.

Gibson, G.E., and Blass, J.P., 1976a, Impaired synthesis of acetylcholine in brain accompanying mild hypoxia and hypoglycemia, *J. Neurochem. 27:*37.

Gibson, G.E., and Blass, J.P., 1976b, A relation between $[NAD^+]/[NADH]$ potentials and glucose utilization in rat brain slices, *J. Biol. Chem. 251:*4127.

Gibson, G.E., Jope, R., and Blass, J.P., 1975, Decreased synthesis of acetylcholine accompanying impaired oxidation of pyruvic acid in rat brain minces, *Biochem. J. 148:*17.

Greenfield, J.G., 1954, *"The Spino-cerebellar Degenerations,"* Blackwell, Oxford.

Kark, R.A.P., Blass, J.P., and Engel, W.K., 1974, Pyruvate oxidation in neuromuscular diseases: evidence of a genetic defect in two families with the clinical syndrome of Friedreich's ataxia, *Neurology (Minneap) 24:*964.

Kark, R.A.P., Blass, J.P., and Spence, M.A., 1977, Physostigmine in familial ataxias, *Neurology (Minneap) 27:*70.

Kark, R.A.P., Rodriguez-Budelli, M., and Blass, J.P., in press, A primary defect of lipoamide dehydrogenase in Friedreich's ataxia, in *"The Inherited Ataxias: Biochemical, Viral and Pathological Studies"* (R.A.P. Kark, R.N. Rosenberg and L.J. Schut, eds.), Raven Press, New York.

Klawans, H.L., and Rubovits, R., 1972, Central cholinergic-anticholinergic antagonism in Huntington's chorea, *Neurology (Minneap) 22:*107.

Konigsmark, B.W., and Weiner, L.P., 1970, The olivopontocerebellar atrophies: a review, *Medicine (Baltimore) 49:*227.

McDowell, F.H., and Markham, C.H., 1971, *"Recent Advances in Parkinson's Disease,"* Contemporary Neurology Series, F.A. Davis Company, Philadelphia.

Rodriguez-Budelli, M., Kark, R.A.P., and Blass, J.P., in press, "Kinetic evidence for a structural abnormality of lipoamide dehydrogenase in two patients with Friedreich's ataxia," *Neurology (Minneap)*.

Victor, M., Adams, R.D., and Mancall, E.L., 1959, A restricted form of cerebellar cortical degeneration occurring in alcoholic patients, *Arch. Neurol. 1:*579.

ALTERATIONS IN MUSCARINIC CHOLINERGIC RECEPTOR BINDING IN HUNTINGTON'S DISEASE

H. I. Yamamura, G. J. Wastek and R. E. Hruska

Department of Pharmacology, College of Medicine,
The University of Arizona Health Sciences Center,
Tucson, Arizona 85724

INTRODUCTION

Dramatic advances have been made in recent years in the identification and isolations of hormonal receptors (Sica *et al.*, 1976) and of the nicotinic cholinergic receptors of invertebrates (Changeux, 1975). Patrick and Lindstrom (1973) have administered a solubilized and purified form of the nicotinic cholinergic receptor from the electric organ of the eel or fish into animals and have produced a flaccid paralysis which electromyographically and pharmacologically exhibits similar symptoms to myasthenia gravis. Tremendous gains have been made towards understanding the autoimmune aspects of this debilitating disease (Elias and Appel, 1976, Lindstrom *et al.*, 1976).

Few studies have been performed demonstrating and identifing the neurotransmitter receptors within the mammalian central nervous system (CNS). This is probably due to the lack of a highly stable and specific neurotransmitter receptor ligand. Recently however, it has been possible to demonstrate the presence of neurotransmitter receptors within the CNS by biochemical means. One of these procedures involves studying the responses of the cyclic AMP and cyclic GMP systems in neuronal tissue to applications of various agonists and antagonists (Iversen, 1975; Kuo *et al.*, 1973; Lee *et al.*, 1973). A second method takes into consideration the specificity of a given ligand for the neurotransmitter receptor binding site. Using the latter procedure, it has been possible to demonstrate specific receptor binding sites within the brain (Snyder and Bennett, 1976).

GENERAL PRINCIPLES IN RECEPTOR LABELING

Recent success in the biochemical identification of brain neurotransmitter receptors comes from the solution of several methodological problems. First, it is important to determine whether the binding of a radiolabeled ligand to brain tissue represents specific binding to a neurotransmitter receptor. It has been reported that some radioactive materials bind to membranes in a non-specific manner (Cautrecasas and Hollenberg, 1976; Snyder,

1975). We have attempted to overcome nonspecific binding in studies of the muscarinic cholinergic receptor by using a high-affinity ligand, 3-quinuclidinyl benzilate (QNB), that is radiolabeled to a high specific activity (Yamamura and Snyder, 1974a; Yamamura and Snyder, 1974b). When ^{3}H-QNB is used at relatively low concentrations, we find that there is little or no non-specific binding either to filters or tissue. Non-specific binding can also be eliminated if the tissue is washed several times after incubation. However, if the dissociation rate of the specifically bound ligand is rapid, then all of the bound ligand, whether it is specific or non-specific, may be washed away leaving little ligand binding to the neurotransmitter receptor binding site. For example, Young and Snyder (1973) reported the half-life for the rate of dissociation of the glycine receptor in the mammalian spinal cord to be in the order of about 45 sec at 4°C. Glycine-displacable ^{3}H-strychnine binding must, therefore, be measured under conditions in which the membrane receptors are only surface-washed. For ligands such as ^{3}H-QNB, which have slower dissociation rates, the membranes can be extensively washed without fear of dissociating the ligand from the receptor binding site.

Second, it is important that the binding affinity and biological response be measured in the same tissue under identical *in vitro* conditions. Of course, this is not always feasible. In the case of brain dopamine receptors, the affinity of dopamine analogs can be examined using the dopamine-sensitive adenylate cyclase (Burt *et al.*, 1976). For the muscarinic cholinergic receptor, several laboratories (Richelson, 1977; Strange *et al.*, 1977; Bartfai, personal communication) have examined the ability of the muscarinic cholinergic antagonists to alter agonist-induced cyclic GMP formation in the intact neuroblastoma cell and in slices of rat brain. In their systems, they find a positive correlation in the ability of the muscarinic antagonists to inhibit the formation of cyclic GMP and in inhibiting the binding of ^{3}H-QNB. We have utilized the longitudinal muscle of the guinea pig ileum to measure the ability of a drug to inhibit acetylcholine-induced responses of the guinea pig ileum (Yamamura and Snyder, 1974a). Using the same tissue, we have measured the ability of the drug to inhibit ^{3}H-QNB binding. In this system, we find that the muscarinic cholinergic antagonists have similar dissociation constants (K_D) as in the ^{3}H-QNB displacement assay (Yamamura and Snyder, 1974b).

Third, before it can be stated that one is looking at a physiologically relevant neurotransmitter receptor, several criteria must be satisfied. Specific ligand binding should exhibit saturability with increasing concentrations of the radiolabeled ligand, indicating that there are a limited number of high-affinity neurotransmitter receptor binding sites, while non-specific binding should increase linearly with increasing concentrations of ligand. Specific binding should also be localized to neuronal tissue and should have an uneven distribution which may be similar to that of the neurotransmitter. Lastly, if one is labeling the physiologically-relevant receptors, then drugs which differ in potency, *in vivo*, should exhibit parallel differences in potency in competing for the radiolabeled ligand binding sites. Therefore, we shall consider a neurotransmitter receptor to be specifically labeled only after the above criteria have been met.

DEMONSTRATION AND CHARACTERIZATION OF MUSCARINIC CHOLINERGIC RECEPTORS IN HUMAN BRAIN

Because most of the acetylcholine receptors within the mammalian CNS appear to be muscarinic (Phillis, 1970; Ferrendelli *et al.*, 1970; Kuo *et al.*, 1972), we decided to demonstrate and characterize these cholinergic receptors by direct binding techniques. We utilized the potent and reversible muscarinic antagonist, 3-quinuclidinyl benzilate (QNB), radiolabeled to a high specific activity. We reported previously that ^{3}H-QNB binds specifically to a pharmacologically relevant muscarinic cholinergic receptor in the rat brain (Yamamura and Snyder, 1974a) and in the longitudinal muscle of the guinea pig ileum (Yamamura and Snyder, 1974b).

Before examining neurotransmitter receptor alterations in diseased human brains, we characterized the muscarinic receptors in control human brains. For these studies, several brains were obtained from patients who had been hospitalized at the time of their death. Brains of individuals having any type of a CNS disorder were not used as controls. In all cases, less than 24 hr had elasped between death and autopsy. In most cases, the brain was dissected immediately after autopsy and the various regions were frozen at -80°C until needed for analysis.

Initial ^{3}H-QNB binding studies were done to insure that binding was linear with tissue protein. Figure 1 depicts the time course of specific ^{3}H-QNB binding in three areas of human brain. Binding in the putamen, frontal cortex and hippocampus reached equilibrium after approximately 30 min. All of our studies, however, were done for at least 60 min. to insure that equilibrium had been reached. Figure 2 illustrates the time course of dissociation of ^{3}H-QNB after the addition of either oxotremorine or unlabeled QNB, in the same three brain areas. After the addition of either 100 μM oxotremorine or 0.01 μM unlabeled QNB at 60 min. (0 min. in Figure 2), the $t_{1/2}$ of ^{3}H-QNB-receptor dissociation was calculated to be about 120 min. Determining the dissociation constant (K_D) from the association rate constant divided by the dissociation rate constant, one finds that the K_D is approximately 20-50 pM.

A second method was also used to determine K_D. Figure 3 shows the saturability of specific ^{3}H-QNB binding in the putamen, frontal cortex and hippocampus. It can readily be seen that saturation occurs within the three brain areas, with increasing concentrations of ^{3}H-QNB. When a Scatchard analysis (Figure 4) is done of the saturation data, a K_D of approximately 20-50 pM is obtained. Scatchard analysis shows that the total density of specific binding sites for the hippocampus, frontal cortex and putamen are 300, 500 and 600 fmoles/mg protein, respectively. A Hill plot of the saturation data (data not shown) gave a Hill coefficient of 1.0, indicating no positive or negative cooperativity of ^{3}H-QNB binding. QNB binding is inhibited by non-radioactive QNB with half-maximal inhibition occuring at approximately 0.1 nM (Figure 5). This value is approximately the half-maximal value obtained from saturation curves and also from equilibrium data. Other pharmacologically active muscarinic antagonists inhibited ^{3}H-QNB binding. Figure 5 illustrates that scopolamine as well as atropine inhibit QNB binding at nM concentration. By contrast, the muscarinic agonists, oxotremorine, pilocarpine and acetylcholine are less effective in displacing ^{3}H-QNB from the receptor. The IC_{50} values are approximately 1 μM for oxotremorine, and 10 μM for pilocarpine and acetylcholine.

The regional variation in ^{3}H-QNB binding to the muscarinic cholinergic receptor in post-mortem human brain samples is illustrated in Table 1. Muscarinic cholinergic receptor binding of ^{3}H-QNB is highest in the caudate nucleus and putamen. Binding in these two areas is approximately 20 times greater than that in the substantia nigra. QNB binding in the hippocampus and frontal cortex is about 34% and 58% of the value in the caudate nucleus. The lowest ^{3}H-QNB binding occurs in the cerebellum and lower brain stem areas

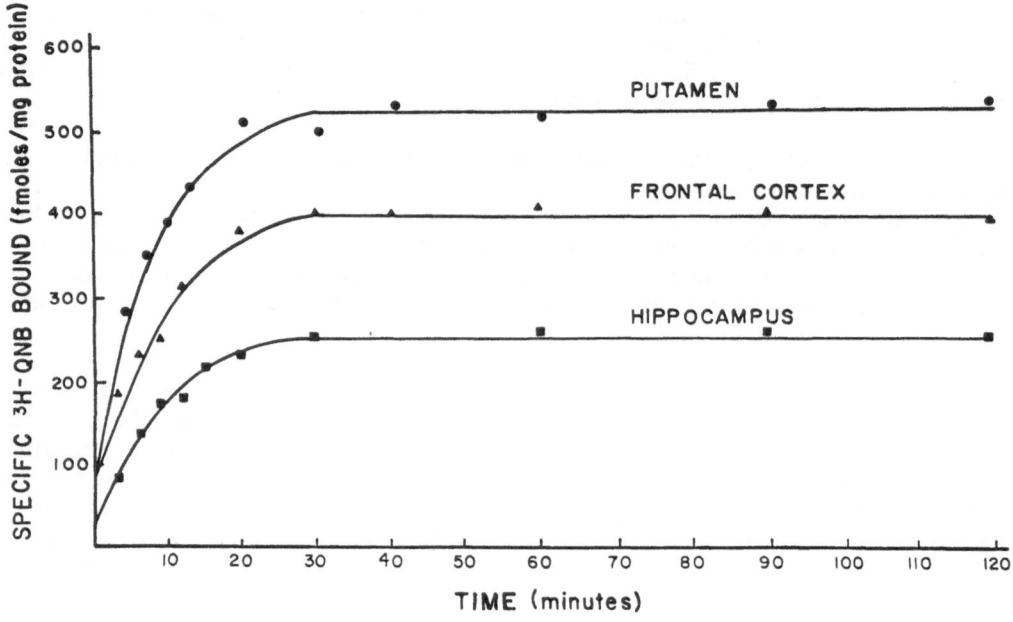

FIGURE 1

Rate of association of ^{3}H-QNB with three human brain regions. The incubation was performed at 37°C for the specified lengths of time using 0.2 nM ^{3}H-QNB with 0.01 μ M unlabeled QNB as the specific displacer. A tissue concentration of approximately 0.1 mg protein/assay was used for each of the specified regions.

where only negligible binding is detected. This pattern of QNB binding is similar to that previously reported for the monkey (Yamamura *et al.*, 1974).

Table 2 shows the choline acetyltransferase (ChAc) activity in post-mortem human brain. Choline acetyltransferase activity is highest in the extrapyramidal regions, closely resembling previous observations in the monkey and rat brain (Yamamura *et al.*, 1975; Yamamura and Snyder, 1974a). In other brain regions, ChAc activity is uniform and substantially lower than in the putamen and caudate nucleus, with no values greater than 20% of the levels in the putamen as reported by others (Aquilonius *et al.*, 1975).

Being satisfied that we had characterized the muscarinic cholinergic receptor binding site in control human brain, we performed muscarinic binding assays in post-mortem brain samples of patients who died of Huntington's disease.

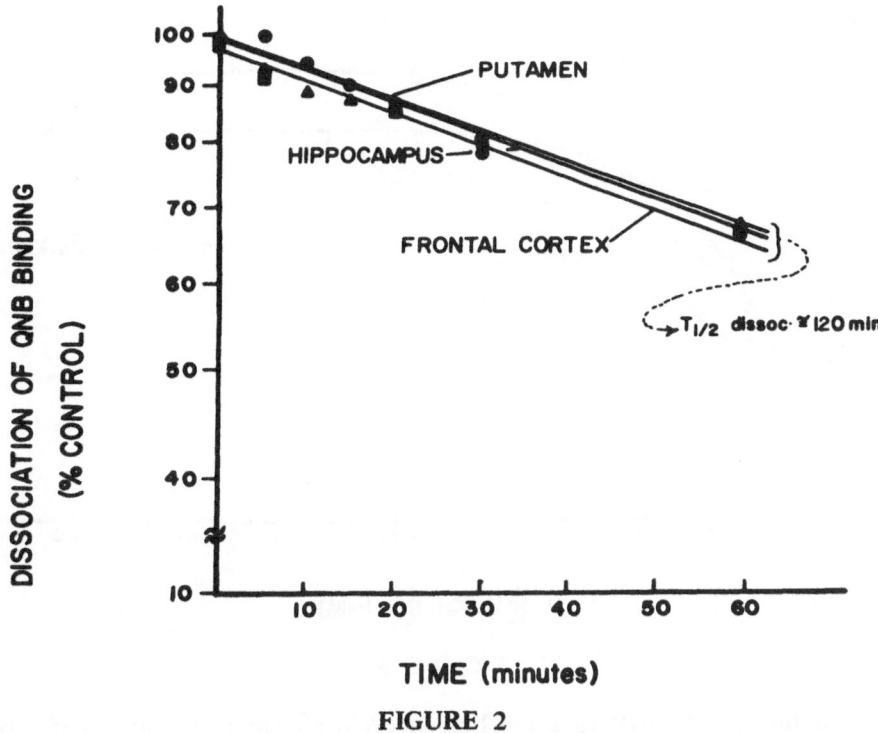

TIME (minutes)

FIGURE 2

Rate of dissociation of ^{3}H-QNB from the receptor in three human brain regions. 0.15 nM ^{3}H-QNB was allowed to equilibrate with 0.3 mg protein/assay of each region for 60 min. at 37°C. At 60 min. 0.1 μM atropine was added to the incubation media to specifically displace ^{3}H-QNB binding. The appropriate samples were then filtered over a vacuum at the specified time periods in order to determine the rate of dissociation of specifically bound ^{3}H-QNB.

MUSCARINIC RECEPTOR ALTERATIONS IN HUNTINGTON'S DISEASE

Huntington's disease (H.D.) is an autosomal dominantly-inherited progressive neurological disorder characterized by involuntary choreiform movements and dementia. It appears to occur at a frequency of approximately 10 in 10,000, and manifests itself in two forms (Shoulson and Chase, 1975). The more frequently occuring form is the adult-onset which becomes symptomatic in the fourth or fifth decade of life. The early-onset form, or Westphal variant, which occurs in less than 5% of those individuals with H.D., has a rapid course. Rigid hypokinetic movements accompanied by seizures and severe mental retardation, frequently characterize this form.

The brain of an adult patient with Huntington's disease shows marked pathological

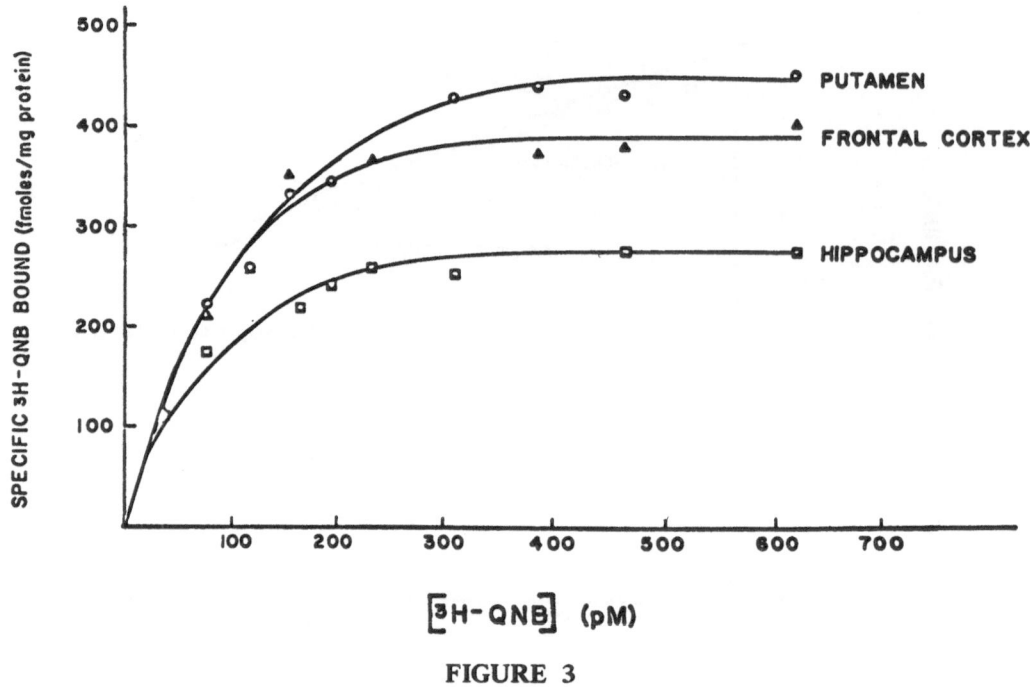

FIGURE 3

Specific binding of ^{3}H-QNB to three human brain regions as a function of ^{3}H-QNB concentration. Varying concentrations of ^{3}H-QNB were incubated with 0.15 mg protein/ assay of each region, with 0.01 μM unlabeled QNB as the specific displacer, for 60 min. at 37°C. The percent of total free ligand bound ranges from 20%, at the lowest free ligand concentration, to 9% at the highest ligand concentration.

changes in the basal ganglia, with some neuronal loss occurring in the cerebral cortex. A significant amount of information has been accumulated regarding the neurochemical abnormalities of the adult-onset form of the disease (Enna *et al.*, 1977; Urquhart *et al.*, 1975; Bird and Iverson, 1974; Bird and Iverson, 1976; Barbeau, 1973). As a result of these studies, it seems probable that the most profound neuronal alterations are due to a severe degeneration of neurons, within the basal ganglia, which utilize acetylcholine and gamma-aminobutyric acid (GABA) as their neurotransmitters.

Dramatic improvements have been obtained in individuals suffering from Parkinson's disease by treating these patients with L-DOPA. For this therapy to be effective, however, it is necessary that the receptor binding site for dopamine be unaltered by this disease. Because of the profound neuronal loss in the basal ganglia in Huntington's disease, the synaptic neurotransmitter receptor binding sites for acetylcholine are also decreased (Hiley and Bird, 1974; Enna *et al.*, 1976; Wastek *et al.*, 1976).

We have further characterized the alterations in ^{3}H-QNB binding in H.D. brains. The caudate nucleus and putamen of choreic brains show marked reductions of specific ^{3}H-QNB binding, while no significant alterations were seen in other brain regions (Table I).

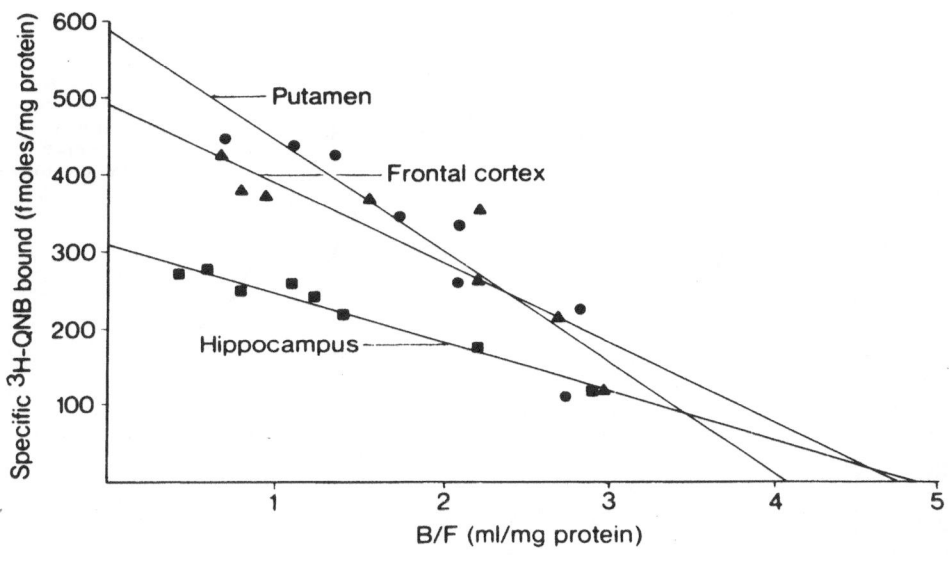

FIGURE 4

Scatchard plot of ^{3}H-QNB binding to three human brain regions.

Significant decreases in choline acetyltransferase activity were found in the caudate nucleus, putamen and globus pallidus of choreic brains (Table II). No significant alterations in choline acetyltransferase activity were observed in other brain regions.

One might ask if the decreases in specific QNB binding and choline acetyltransferase activity reflect non-specific post-mortem changes. The post-mortem stability of choline acetyltransferase has been well documented (McGeer and McGeer, 1976). We have also shown that there is no significant decrease in muscarinic cholinergic receptor binding for up to three months in frozen intact tissue from rat and monkey brain (Enna et al., 1976). However, biochemical alterations of these parameters might occur prior to freezing of the tissue. To examine this, we have sacrificed rats and left them at room temperature for up to 6 hr prior to removal and freezing of the brain (Enna et al., 1976). We found no significant differences in the density of the muscarinic cholinergic receptor binding sites in these rat brains.

Reduction in specific ^{3}H-QNB binding could also result from a decreased receptor affinity rather than from a decrease in the density of receptors. We tested this hypothesis by varying the concentration of ^{3}H-QNB (data not shown). Using the dissociation constant derived from Scatchard analysis, we obtained a K_D of approximately 0.07 nM for the choreic brains which is not significantly different from the K_D obtained in control human brains. This indicates that the decreased binding of ^{3}H-QNB appears to be due to a decrease in the number of receptor binding sites.

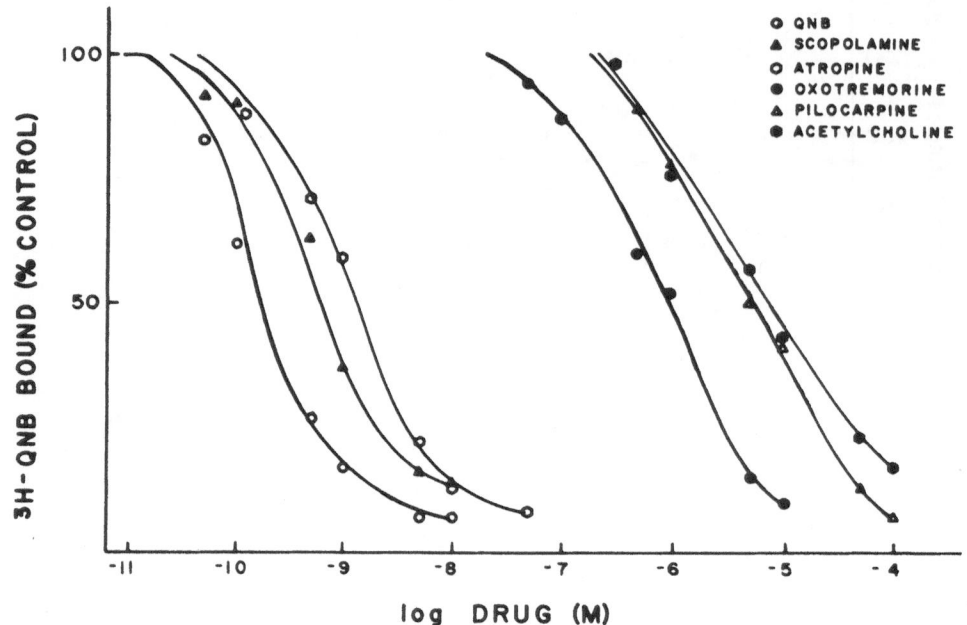

FIGURE 5

Inhibition of specific ^{3}H-QNB binding by various muscarinic agonists and antagonists in human frontal cortex. 39 pM ^{3}H-QNB was incubated with 0.1 mg protein/assay of frontal cortex and varying concentrations of unlabeled drugs for 60 min. at 37°C. The total amount of ^{3}H-QNB bound at each unlabeled drug concentration was calculated as the percent of ^{3}H-QNB bound when no displacer was present.

We have also studied receptor alterations by looking at the ability of dexetimide, the active isomer of benzetimide, to inhibit ^{3}H-QNB in control and H.D. brains. These data are illustrated in Figure 6. There appears to be no alterations in the ability of dexetimide to inhibit ^{3}H-QNB binding, however, there is a significant (50%) reduction in the density of binding sites in H.D. brains. These data provide ample proof that the reduction in ^{3}H-QNB binding in choreic brains is due to a decrease in the number of binding sites rather than to a change in receptor affinity.

Further evidence supporting the idea that the decreases in QNB binding and ChAc activity in the extrapyramidal sites is selective, and not due to the result of non-specific post-mortem changes, is our finding that these affected areas are the only ones showing significant decreases in QNB binding and ChAc activity while all other areas showed no changes (Table I and II). Since atrophy of the basal ganglia is a prominent feature of H.D.,

TABLE I

Regional Variations of Specific ^{3}H-QNB Binding in Control and Huntington's Diseased Brains

Region	Control				H.D.[d]			
Caudate Nucleus	(6)[a]	949.67	±	44.03[c]	(5)	314.00	±	68.76[b]
Putamen	(9)	706.78	±	95.83	(6)	250.83	±	19.98[b]
Parietal Cortex	(3)	559.67	±	103.57	(4)	532.25	±	90.36
Occipital (Calcarine) Cortex	(8)	540.25	±	85.51	(5)	540.80	±	112.56
Frontal Cortex	(9)	520.55	±	89.19	(5)	624.60	±	81.21
Amygdala	(7)	471.00	±	105.15	(6)	479.83	±	60.03
Precentral Gyrus	(4)	389.75	±	73.97	(4)	388.50	±	101.83
Postcentral Gyrus	(4)	386.00	±	84.12	(4)	400.00	±	101.31
Hippocampus	(9)	319.89	±	59.43	(6)	305.17	±	50.11
Pulvinar of Thalamus	(2)	219.00	±	60.00	(2)	197.50	±	40.5
Tectum of Midbrain	(3)	141.67	±	21.17	(3)	229.67	±	152.32
Hypothalamus	(3)	129.00	±	35.51	(3)	61.67	±	28.90
Globus Pallidus	(9)	124.89	±	47.63	(5)	69.20	±	13.91
Basis Pons	(7)	85.43	±	33.57	(6)	114.17	±	36.23
Tegmentum of Medulla	(6)	68.50	±	25.54	(3)	31.33	±	18.80
Mammillary Body	(6)	60.33	±	13.87	(3)	37.00	±	17.06
Substantia Nigra	(9)	46.33	±	16.43	(4)	43.75	±	16.45
Red Nucleus	(6)	38.33	±	12.98	(3)	16.33	±	16.33
Inferior Olivary Nucleus	(9)	20.55	±	8.14	(5)	36.00	±	30.30
Basis Medulla	(3)	20.33	±	13.17	(2)	20.50	±	20.50
Interpeduncular Area	(7)	20.14	±	13.96	(3)	42.00	±	15.14
Corpus Callosum	(7)	15.86	±	8.11	(4)	36.75	±	10.82
Cerebellar Hemisphere	(7)	14.71	±	9.50	(4)	22.75	±	13.70
Posterior Cerebellar Vermis	(8)	13.00	±	6.71	(5)	30.40	±	13.16
Dentate Nucleus	(6)	12.17	±	7.78	(6)	20.83	±	10.73
Anterior Cerebellar Vermis	(8)	9.50	±	5.44	(6)	18.50	±	9.40

[a]Number in parenthesis, n = number of samples analyzed

[b]Significant to a level of $P < 0.01$ from the corresponding control value as measured by Student's "t" test.

[c]Values are mean ± S.E.M.

[d]H.D. = Huntington's Disease.

TABLE II

Regional Distribution of Choline Acetyltransferase Activity in Control and Huntington's Diseased Brains (fmoles/mg protein)

Region	Control				H.D.[e]		
Putamen	(5)[a]	42.33	±	6.38[d]	(6)	16.34	±	11.09[c]
Caudate Nucleus	(5)	38.99	±	7.34	(5)	12.26	±	4.36[b]
Globus Pallidus	(5)	13.43	±	3.14	(5)	4.52	±	1.18[c]
Dentate Nucleus	(3)	8.23	±	5.02	(6)	2.57	±	0.67
Amygdala	(4)	7.29	±	2.11	(6)	8.96	±	4.29
Hypothalamus	(5)	5.18	±	2.01	(4)	3.52	±	0.83
Posterior Cerebellar Vermis	(5)	5.10	±	2.08	(5)	2.40	±	0.55
Tegmentum of Pons	(5)	4.84	±	0.79	(4)	6.41	±	1.82
Anterior Cerebellar Vermis	(6)	4.70	±	1.46	(6)	2.89	±	0.71
Hippocampus	(5)	3.99	±	1.12	(6)	3.04	±	1.04
Thalamus	(5)	3.93	±	0.90	(4)	2.61	±	0.42
Basis of Pons	(5)	3.18	±	0.89	(6)	2.86	±	0.79
Red Nucleus	(4)	2.81	±	0.53	(3)	3.06	±	1.20
Inferior Olivary Nucleus	(6)	2.79	±	0.38	(3)	3.76	±	1.86
Substantia Nigra	(5)	2.57	±	0.52	(5)	3.22	±	1.38
Frontal Cortex	(5)	2.23	±	0.55	(4)	3.24	±	0.75
Cerebellar Hemisphere	(5)	1.78	±	0.32	(4)	1.50	±	0.40

[a]Number in parenthesis, n = number of samples analyzed

[b]Significant to a level of $P < 0.01$ from the corresponding control value as measured by Student's "t" test.

[c]$P < 0.05$

[d]Values are mean ± S.E.M.

[e]H.D. = Huntington's Disease.

alterations in QNB binding might simply reflect the fact that there is less tissue in these areas, resulting in fewer receptor binding sites with which QNB can interact. However, we have demonstrated previously that ^{3}H-GABA and ^{3}H-dihydroalprenolol binding is unchanged in the neostriatum of H.D. brains (Enna *et al.*, 1976). Therefore, our results support the theory that H.D. involves the degeneration of cholinergic interneurons within the neostriatum.

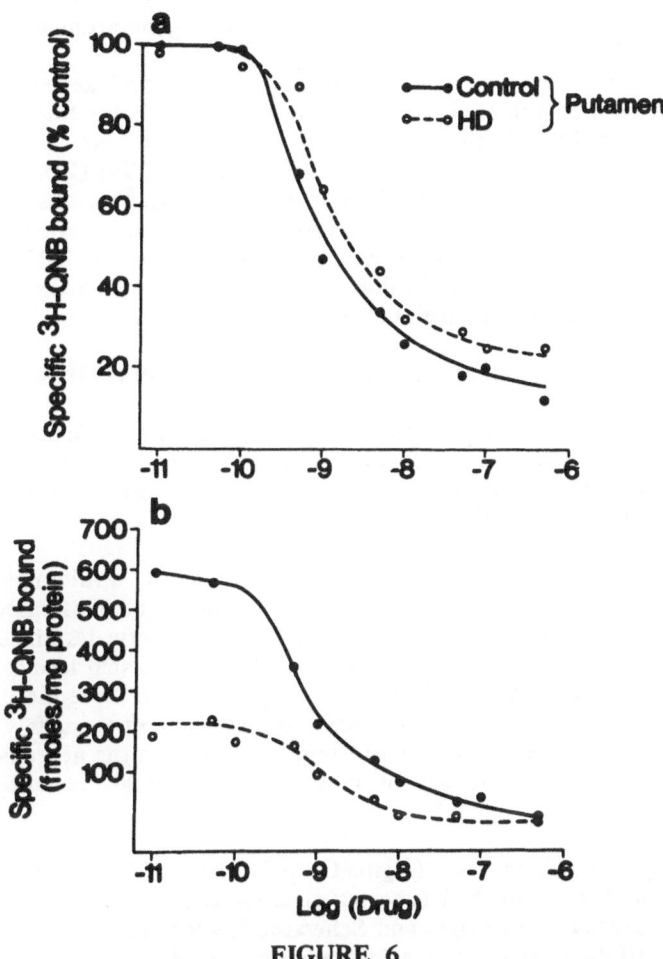

FIGURE 6

Inhibition of specific ^{3}H-QNB binding by dexetimide in control and H.D. putamen (fmoles/mg protein). 0.02 nM ^{3}H-QNB was incubated with 0.3 mg protein/assay of both normal and H.D. putamen plus varying concentrations of dexetimide for 60 min. at 37°C. The amount of ^{3}H-QNB bound at each dexetimide concentration was calculated as both specific ^{3}H-QNB bound and as percent control.

In previous studies, changes in neurotransmitter receptor binding were also examined in the frontal cortex of post-mortem choreic brain (Enna *et al.*, 1976). We found no alterations in the density of β-adrenergic, GABAergic, muscarinic cholinergic or serotonergic receptors in the frontal cortex of choreic brain. However, we have recently examined the frontal cortex for the existence of dopamine receptors, using ^{3}H-spiroperidol. We found a 65% decrease in ^{3}H-spiroperidol binding and no alterations in choline acetyltransferase activity (Reisine *et al.*, in press). We suggest that the decrease in ^{3}H-spiroperidol binding which presumably reflects a change in a dopaminergic receptor in the frontal cortex of choreic brains, may be associated with the neuronal degeneration found in that area.

Finally, our results suggest that cholinomimetic drugs such as oxotremorine, deanol or choline might be useful in some cases for the symptomatic treatment of Huntington's disease. These drugs have been administered in H.D. patients with varying success (Aquilonius and Eckernas, 1977; Laterre and Fortemps, 1975; Growdon et al., 1977; Davis et al., 1975; Davis et al., 1976, Walker et al., 1973). Previous clinical trials with the reversible cholinesterase inhibitor, physostigmine, have been equivocal (Aquilonius and Sjostrom, 1971; Klawans and Rubovits, 1972; Tarsy et al., 1974). Our data explains why this may be the case. Physostigmine non-responders could represent patients who had marked alterations in the density of striatal muscarinic receptors.

AN ANIMAL MODEL OF HUNTINGTON'S DISEASE

There are only a few animal models for H.D. (Dill et al., 1976; Coyle and Schwarcz, 1976). The degeneration of neurons in the rat caudate nucleus after kainic acid injection appears to resemble that in the neostriata of post-mortem brain samples from patients with Huntington's disease (Coyle et al., 1977).

Recently, Coyle and his associates (1977) reported that a microinjection of kainic acid, a rigid analogue of glutamic acid, into the rat caudate nucleus causes degeneration of 85% of the neuronal cell bodies while leaving axons and nerve terminals intact. Neurochemical examination of the rat caudate nucleus after kainic acid lesions shows that the activity of both glutamic acid decarboxylase (GAD) and ChAc are reduced approximately 70% while the activity of tyrosine hydroxylase is elevated approximately 50%. Since the striatal injections of kainic acid produce profound decreases in the neurochemical markers of the caudate nucleus, we looked for muscarinic cholinergic receptor alterations in lesioned caudate nucleus.

Two micrograms of kainic acid (Sigma Corp.) in 1 μl of sodium phosphate buffered saline, were microinjected into the left corpus striatum (coordinates = 7.9 A; 2.6 L; 4.8 V) according to the procedure of Coyle and Schwarcz (1976). The animals were allowed to recover for 5 or 10 days after kainic acid injections, at which time they were sacrificed by decapitation and their brains rapidly removed and dissected in a cold room. The muscarinic cholinergic receptor was measured in washed striatal homogenates using ^{3}H-QNB as the ligand. As can be seen from Table 3, the specific binding of ^{3}H-QNB to membrane preparations of kainic acid injected caudate nuclei is reduced approximately 40% below values of the contralateral non-lesioned caudate nuclei. The decline in ^{3}H-QNB binding, induced by kainic acid lesions, appears to parallel the reduction in binding of ^{3}H-QNB in the H.D. caudate nucleus.

We also examined the effects of kainic acid lesions on the apparent K_D as well as on the total number of binding sites (Bmax). The K_D's were 11 and 13 pM for the lesioned

TABLE III

Muscarinic Cholinergic Receptor Binding in Caudate Nuclei from Kainic Acid Lesioned Rats and Huntington's Disease Patients

Kainic Acid Lesions[d] Specific ^{3}H-QNB Bound (fmol/mg tissue)			H.D.[c]
Lesioned	Non-Lesioned	Δ%	Δ%
43 ± 5.1	77.0 ± 11.6	-43**	-52; -64*[a,b]

[d]Rats received a unilateral injections of 2 μg in 1 μl of kainic acid and were sacrificed after 5 days. Data are the mean ± S.E.M. from 14 Scat analyses.

[c]For Huntington's Disease (H.D.) caudate nuclei, the values are taken from [a]Wastek *et al.*, (1976) and [b]Enna *et al.*, (1976).

* P < 0.01

**P < 0.025 by Student's "t" test.

and non-lesioned rat caudate nuclei, respectively, as determined from the rate constant of association (7 X 10^8 M^{-1} min^{-1} for both the lesioned and non-lesioned caudate nuclei) and from the rate constant of dissociation (8 X 10^{-3} min^{-1} for the lesioned and 9 X 10^{-3} min^{-1} for the non-lesioned caudate nucleus). The apparent K_D was also determined from saturation isotherms as shown in Figure 7. Scatchard analyses of the saturation isotherms revealed a K_D of approximately 60 pM for both lesioned and non-lesioned caudate nuclei (Figure 8), and about a 40% reduction in ^{3}H-QNB binding. Therefore, the kainic acid lesions had no significant effect on the apparent K_D. This is similar to our previous findings in post-mortem H.D. brain samples (Wastek *et al.*, 1976). However, kainic acid lesions do appear to markedly decrease the density of specific ^{3}H-QNB binding sites.

Since the alterations in muscarinic cholinergic receptor binding caused by kainic acid lesions of the rat caudate nucleus parallel those found in H.D. caudate nucleus, kainic acid lesions appear to be a useful animal model of H.D.

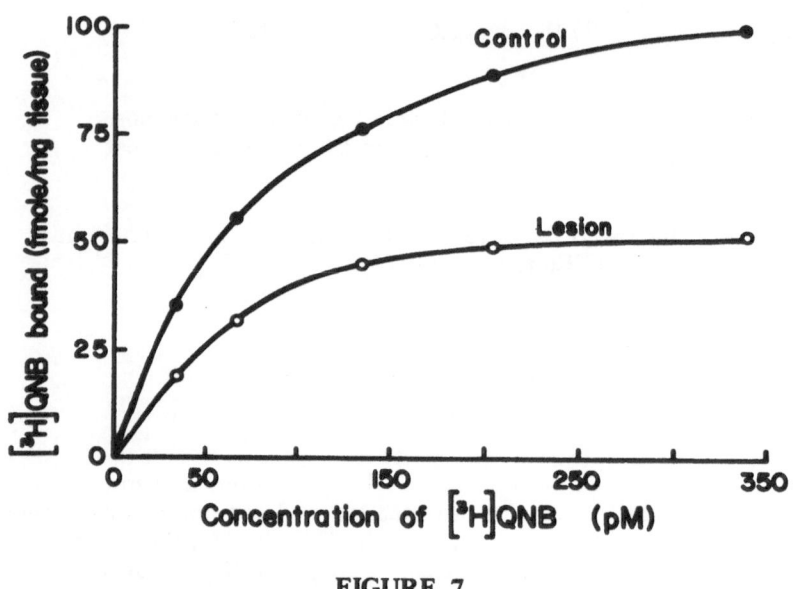

FIGURE 7

Specific binding of ^{3}H-QNB to control and kainic acid lesion caudate nuclei of rat brain as a function of ^{3}H-QNB concentration.

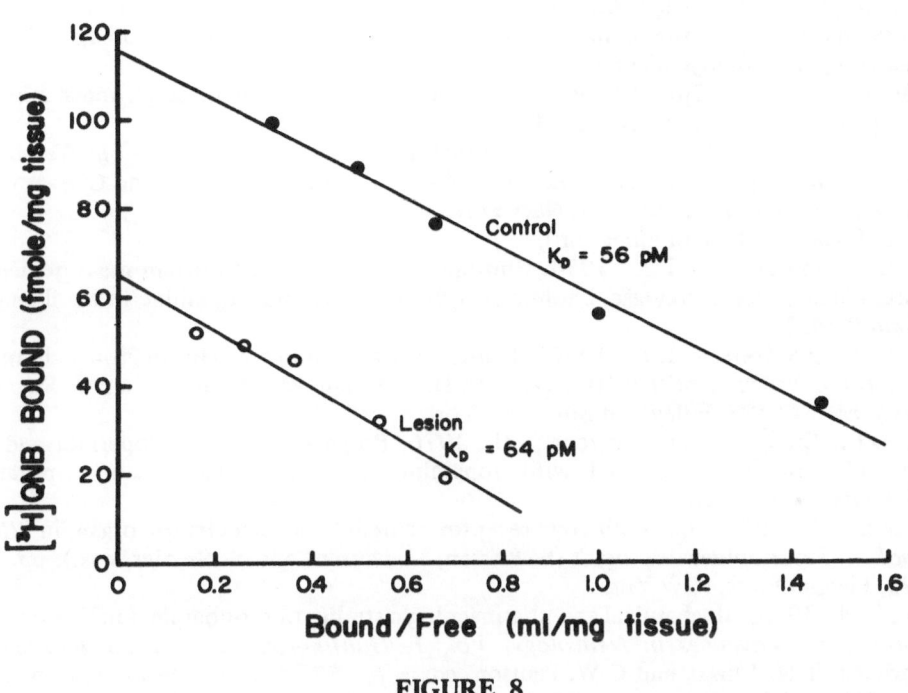

FIGURE 8

Scatchard plot of ^{3}H-QNB binding to control and kainic acid lesioned rat caudate nuclei.

ACKNOWLEDGEMENTS

Portions of the research were supported by USPHS grants and the Committee to Combat Huntington's Disease. Henry I. Yamamura is the recipient of a Research Career Development Award (RSDA) from the NIMH. Gregory J. Wastek and Robert E. Hruska are supported by Pre-doctoral and Post-doctoral Fellowships, respectively from the NIH.

REFERENCES

Aquilonius, S.M., and Eckernas, S.A., 1977, Choline therapy in Huntington's chorea, *Neurology 27:*887.

Aquilonius, S.M., Eckernas, S.A., and Sundwall, A., 1975, Regional distribution of choline acetyltransferase in the human brain: changes in Huntington's chorea, *J. Neurol. Neurosurg. Psychiatry 38:*669.

Aquilonius, S.M., and Sjostrom, R., 1971, Cholinergic and dopaminergic mechanisms in Huntington's chorea, *Life Sci. 10:*405.

Barbeau, A., 1973, Biochemistry of Huntington's chorea, in *"Advances in Neurology, Vol. 1, Huntington's chorea 1872-1972"* (A. Barbeau, T.N. Chase, and G.W. Paulson, eds.), pp. 473-516, Raven Press, New York.

Bartfai, T. (personal communication).

Bird, E.D., and Iversen, L.L., 1974, Huntington's chorea: postmortem measurement of glutamic acid decarboxylase, choline acetyltransferase and dopamine in basal ganglia, *Brain 97:*457.

Bird, E.D., and Iversen, L.L., 1976, Neurochemical findings in Huntington's chorea, in *"Essays in Neurochemistry"* (M. Youdim, D. Sharman, W. Lovenberg, and J. Ragnodo, eds.), pp. 177-195, Wiley and Son, New York.

Burt, D.B., Creese, I., and Snyder, S.H., 1976, Properties of ^{3}H-haloperidol and ^{3}H-dopamine binding associated with dopamine receptors in calf brain membrances, *Mol. Pharmacol. 12:*631.

Changeux, J.P., 1975, The cholinergic receptor protein from fish electric organ, in *"Handbook of Psychopharmacology"* (S. Iversen, L. Iversen, and S. Snyder, eds.), pp. 235-293, Plenum Press, New York.

Chase, T.N., 1973, Biochemical and pharmacologic studies of monoamines in Huntington's chorea, in *"Advances in Neurology, Vol. 1, Huntington's Chorea 1872-1972"* (A. Barbeau, T.N. Chase, and G.W. Paulson, eds.), pp. 533-542, Raven Press, New York.

Coyle, J.T., and Schwarcz, R., 1976, Lesion of striatal neurones with kainic acid provides a model for Huntington's chorea, *Nature 263:*244.

Coyle, J.T., Schwarcz, R., Bennett, J.P., and Campochiaro, P., 1977, Clinical, neuropathologic and pharmacologic aspects of Huntington's disease: correlates with a new animal model, *Neuropsychopharmacology 1:*1.

Cuatrecasas, P., and Hollenberg, M., 1976, Membrane receptors and hormone action, *Adv. Protein Chem. 30:*251.

Davis, K.L., Hollister, L.E., Berger, P.A., and Barchas, J.D., 1975, Cholinergic imbalance hypotheses of psychoses and movement disorders: strategies for evaluation, *Psychopharmacol. Comm. 1(5):*533.

Davis, K.L., Hollister, L.E., Barchas, J.D., and Berger, P.A., 1976, Choline in tardive dyskinesia and Huntington's chorea, *Life Sci. 19:*1507.

Dill, R.E., Dorris, R.L., and Phillips-Thonnard, I., 1976, A pharmacologic model of Huntington's chorea, *J. Pharm. Pharmacol. 28:*646.

Elias, S.B., and Appel, S.H., 1976, Recent advances in myasthenia gravis, *Life Sci. 18:* 1031.

Enna, S.J., Bennett, J.P., Bylund, D.B., Snyder, S.H., Bird, E.D., and Iversen, L.L., 1976, Alterations of brain neurotransmitter receptor binding in Huntington's chorea, *Brain Res. 116:*531.

Enna, S.J., Bird, E.D., Bennett, J.P., Bylund, D.B., Yamamura, H.I., Iversen, L.L., and Snyder, S.H., 1976, Huntington's chorea: changes in neurotransmitter receptors in the brain, *N. Engl. J. Med. 294:*1305.

Enna, S.J., Stern, L.Z., Wastek, G.J., and Yamamura, H.I., 1977, Neurobiology and pharmacology of Huntington's disease, *Life Sci. 20:*205.

Ferrendelli, J.A., Steiner, A.L., McDough, D.B., and Kipnis, D.M., 1970, The effect of oxotremorine and atropine on cGMP and cAMP levels in mouse cerebral cortex and cerebellum, *Biochem. Biophys. Res. Commun. 41:*1061.

Growdon, J.H., Cohen, E.L., and Wurtman, R.J., 1977, Huntington's disease: clinical and chemical effects of choline administration, *Ann. Neurol. 1:*418.

Hiley, C.R., 1976, The muscarinic receptor for acetylcholine in Huntington's chorea, in *"Biochemistry and Neurology"* (H. Bradford, and C. Marsden, eds.), pp. 103-109, Academic Press, New York.

Hiley, C.R., and Bird, E.D., 1974, Decreased muscarinic receptor concentration in post-mortem brain in Huntington's chorea, *Brain Res. 80:*355.

Iversen, L.L., 1975, Dopamine receptors in the brain, *Science 188:*1084.

Klawans, H.L., and Rubovits, R., 1973, Central cholinergic-anticholinergic antagonism in Huntington's chorea, *Neurology 22:*107.

Kuo, J.F., Lee, T.P., Reyes, P.L., Walton, K.G., Donnalley, T.E., and Greengard, P., 1972, Cyclic nucleotide-dependent protein kinases X. An assay method for the measurement of guanosine 3, 5-monophosphate in various biological materials and a study of agents regulating its level in heart and brain, *J. Biol. Chem. 247:*16.

Laterre, E.C., and Fortemps, E., 1975, Deanol in spontaneous and induced dyskinesias, *Lancet 1(7919):*1301.

Lee, T.P., Kuo, J.F., and Greengard, P., 1972, Role of muscarinic cholinergic receptors in regulation of guanosine 3, 5-cyclic monophosphate content in mammalian brain, heart muscle, and intestinal smooth muscle, *Proc. Natl. Acad. Sci. USA 69:*3287.

Lindstrom, J.M., Seybold, M.E., Lennon, V.A., Whittingham, S., and Duane, D.P., 1976, Antibody to acetylcholine receptor in myasthenia gravis, *Neurology 26:*1054.

McGeer, P.L., and McGeer, E.G., 1976, Enzymes associated with the metabolism of catecholamines, acetylcholine and GABA in human controls and patients with Parkinson's disease and Huntington's chorea, *J. Neurochem. 26:*65.

Patrick, J., and Lindstrom, J., 1973, Autoimmune response to acetylcholine receptor, *Science 18:*871.

Phillis, J.W., 1970, Pharmacological studies on neurons in the brain and spinal cord. – Part 1: Cholinergic mechanisms, in *"The Pharmacology of Synapses"* (G.A. Kerkut, ed.), pp. 149-185, Oxford Pergamon Press, New York.

Reisine, T.D., Fields, J.Z., Stern, L.Z., Johnson, P.C., Bird, E.D., and Yamamura, H.I., in press, Alterations in dopaminergic receptors in Huntington's disease, *Life Sci.*

Richelson, E., 1977, Antipsychotics block muscarinic acetylcholine receptor-mediated cyclic GMP formation in cultured mouse neuroblastoma cells, *Nature 266:*371.

Shoulson, I., and Chase, T.N., 1975, Huntington's disease, *Ann. Rev. Med. 26:*419.

Sica, V., Cuatrecasas, P., Nola, E., Parikh, I., and Puca, G.A., 1976, Purification of estrogen receptor by affinity chromatography, in *"Receptors and Mechanisms of Action of Steroid Hormones"* (J. Pasqualini, ed.), pp. 85-107, M. Dekker, New York.

Snyder, S.H., and Bennett, J.P., 1976, Neurotransmitter receptors in the brain: biochemical identification, *Ann. Rev. Physiol. 38:*153.

Strange, P.G., Birdsall, N.J.M., and Burgen, A.S.V., 1977, Occupancy of muscarinic acetylcholine receptors stimulates a guanytale cyclase in neuroblastoma cells, *Biochem. Soc. Trans. 5:*189.

Tarsy, D., Leopold, N., and Sax, D.S., 1974, Physostigmine in choreiform movement disorders, *Neurology 24:*28.

Urquhart, N., Perry, T.L., Hansen, S., and Kennedy, J., 1975, GABA content and glutamic acid decarboxylase activity in brain of Huntington's chorea patients and control subjects, *J. Neurochem. 24:*1071.

Walker, J.E., Hoehn, M., Sears, E., and Lewis, J., 1973, Dimethylaminoethanol in Huntington's chorea, *Lancet 1(7818):*1512.

Wastek, G.J., Stern, L.Z., Johnson, P.C., and Yamamura, H.I., 1976, Huntington's disease: regional alterations in muscarinic cholinergic receptor binding in human brain, *Life Sci. 19:*1033.

Yamamura, H.I., Kuhar, M.J., Greenberg, D., and Snyder, S.H., 1974, Muscarinic cholinergic binding: regional distribution in monkey brain, *Brain Res. 66:*541.

Yamamura, H.I., and Snyder, S.H., 1974a, Muscarinic cholinergic binding in rat brain, *Proc. Natl. Acad. Sci. USA 71:*1725.

Yamamura, H.I., and Snyder, S.H., 1974b, Muscarinic cholinergic receptor binding in the longitudinal muscle of the guinea pig ileum with ^{3}H-quinuclidinyl benzilate, *Mol. Pharmacol. 10:*861.

Young, A.B., and Snyder, S.H., 1973, Strychnine binding associated with glycine receptors of the central nervous system, *Proc. Natl. Acad. Sci. USA 70:*2832.

BRAIN ACETYLCHOLINE AND COGNITIVE FUNCTION

CHOLINERGIC EXCITABILITY AND MEMORY: ANIMAL STUDIES AND THEIR CLINICAL IMPLICATIONS

J. A. Deutsch and J. B. Rogers

Department of Psychology, University of California, San Diego
La Jolla, California 92093

INTRODUCTION

When an organism learns, we presume that there must be a change within its nervous system. Such a change will then produce an alteration in the behavior of the organism on future occasions. When we search for the change that underlies learning, it would seem plausible to look for some change in the pattern of connectivity between the components of the nervous system. The synapse interconnects components of the nervous system. The plasticity of such interconnections could be mediated by the growth of new synapses, alteration in electrophysiological properties at the synapse, or systematic change in pharmacological synaptic sensitivity. Its lability makes the synapse a plausible target for investigations into the substrates of memory.

The most direct test of the idea that memory change is due to synaptic change would be electrophysiological observation of a synapse during the process of learning, subsequent memory storage and retrieval. However, there are two major difficulties of a technical nature that render such observation difficult. First, one would have to find a synapse that was modified during a particular instance of learning in order to correlate the synaptic change with the behavioral modification. Second, having found such a synapse one should ideally be able to observe it over a time span which corresponds with the time span of the behavioral change. While it has been possible to find neural units whose activity changes as learning proceeds, these experiments have been limited to simple behaviors in simple preparations — for example, habituation in Aplysia (Kandel, 1976). The implications of this research for understanding such complex phenomena as associative learning and memory in man are, as yet, remote. In studies with higher animals, it has not been possible to show that the changes in activity observed in particular units during or subsequent to learning actually stem from changes in the units themselves. They might simply mirror activity relayed to the units under observation from any number of other regions in the brain.

The experimental strategy of pharmacological intervention provides a useful alter-

175

native or adjunct to electrophysiological methods. The basis for this belief follows primarily from indications that changes in the substrate of memory are somewhat gradual. Ribot's law, implying the existence of such gradual changes, is based on clinical observation, but its correctness has been strikingly confirmed in an ingenious experimental paradigm by Squire (1975). More recent events (measured on a time scale of years or months) are more likely to be forgotten following traumatic injury to the central nervous system. Since it would be difficult to see how memories of different age could be differentially affected if the change underlying memory were all-or-none, it is reasonable to believe that the substrate of memory keeps changing over a long time span. It also seems that, on the whole, the greater the severity of injury, the longer the retrograde amnesia. Taking these facts together we might hypothesize that if the changes underlying memory are synaptic and take place gradually over time, then memories of different age should be differentially sensitive to the same dose of synaptically active pharmacological agent, just as they are differentially sensitive to a given level of trauma.

Assuming the above hypothesis, which of the ever-growing number of confirmed or putative neurotransmitters and transmitter systems should one begin examining for synaptic changes associated with memory? There are several reasons why work in our laboratory has focused on the cholinergic system. To begin with, cholinergic neurotransmission is perhaps the longest studied and best understood. Indeed, the very concept of a chemical neurotransmitter in part owes to work with acetylcholine (ACh), Loewi's "Vagusstoff" (Loewi, 1921). Since the pioneering work of Dale, Koelle, Nachmansohn, and others, increasingly fine detail of the mechanisms controlling ACh synthesis, storage, release, receptor interactions, and enzymatic inactivation has been provided. Secondly, a very large number of animal studies have suggested that cholinergic agents may systematically influence recall. As this book itself attests, the work has come from many different laboratories. Converging lines of evidence have been provided by the use of a variety of cholinergic drugs including scopolamine, methscopolamine, physostigmine, neostigmine, diisopropylfluorophosphate (DFP), a-neurotoxin, atropine, 3-isopropylphenyl N-methyl carbamate (Compound 10854), carbaryl, carbachol, mecamylamine, and hemicholinium-3. In addition, several of the protein synthesis inhibitors reported to disrupt memory have recently been shown to have moderate to highly potent anticholinesterase properties (Moss *et al.*, 1974a, 1974b; Moss and Fahrney, 1976).

TRANSIENT VERSUS PERMANENT EFFECTS OF PSYCHOPHARMACOLOGICAL AGENTS

In order to evaluate properly the mnemonic effects of various cholinergic drugs, it is critical to differentiate permanent aftereffects of a drug with transient agonist/antagonist interactions during the drug's metabolic life in the nervous system. Administration of 6-hydroxydopamine, for example, produces a permanent aftereffect: degeneration of catecholamine containing nerve terminals. On the other hand, the cholinergic agents discussed in the present paper are viewed in terms of their agonist/antagonist properties which are likely to persist only for so long as the drugs' presence in the nervous system can be demonstrated. Radioactive labeling of the anticholinesterase (acetylcholinesterase inhibitor) physostigmine, for instance, demonstrates that it is metabolized and excreted from the body within hours of its administration. In order to make use of physostigmine's anticholinesterase properties, we therefore inject it 10-30 min before recall test (or training).

Failure to differentiate permanent aftereffect and current metabolic interaction of cholinergic agents may lead to serious interpretive and experimental error. For example, in one series of experiments Signorelli (1976) administers physostigmine 24-72 hr before recall test. His failure to obtain any subsequent effect on memory is, therefore, hardly surprising. This is particularly true given that we had published the very same result some 10 years earlier (Deutsch, 1966). To avoid such misunderstanding, we have divided the present discussion of our work into four broad areas based on time of administration of the cholinergically active drug. These are: injection immediately before recall test, injection one or more days before recall test, injection immediately before training, and injection immediately before both training and recall test.

ADMINISTRATION OF CHOLINERGIC AGENTS IMMEDIATELY BEFORE RECALL TEST

The first set of experiments we report here show that there is a variation in the sensitivity of habits to cholinergic agents according to the age of such habits. These experiments are simple. Rats are trained on a particular behavioral task, then retested on that task at some later time. All animals are intraperitoneally-injected with drug 10-30 min before retest*, and each rat is retested only on one occasion. Thus, there are two experimental variables: time between training and retest (age of habit) and drug condition at retest.

Such experiments have now been repeated a number of times (Deutsch et al., 1966; Hamburg, 1967; Wiener and Deutsch, 1968; Squire, 1970; Biederman, 1970, 1974; Stanes et al., 1976; Puerto et al., 1976). Basically, the results show that habits are differentially affected by the same dose of anticholinesterase depending simply on their age (Figure 1). Animals given anticholinesterase and retested three days after training evidence no impairment of memory; but other animals given anticholinesterase and retested 7-14 days after training perform significantly worse than vehicle-injected controls. This relationship between age of habit and vulnerability to drug reverses if an anticholinergic (ACh receptor blocker) is given before retest instead of an anticholinesterase (Figure 2). With anticholinergics, three-day old habits are disrupted whereas seven-day old habits are unaffected. In addition, 28 days after training, when control animals appear to have forgotten the task, anticholinesterase-injected subjects evince quite good recall.

Similar facilitation of memory when tested in a delayed-response situation has been shown by Alpern and Marriott (1973). Physostigmine produced increasing facilitation of memory the poorer memory became in control animals. The effects were observed within a 25-min delay interval, suggesting cholinergic storage even at very short times after learning.

Several anticholinesterases, anticholinergics, subject species, and behavioral tasks have been employed in these studies where drug is injected immediately before retest. In general, the pattern of results has been the same although temporal parameters may vary somewhat depending on task and level of training. This can be seen on comparison of Figure 1 and 3. The former presents data obtained using a Y-maze brightness discrimination task; the latter, data from step-through passive avoidance (Rogers and Deutsch,

*In the case of the long-lasting, irreversible cholinesterase inhibitor DFP, intracerebral injections may be as much as 24 hours before retest.

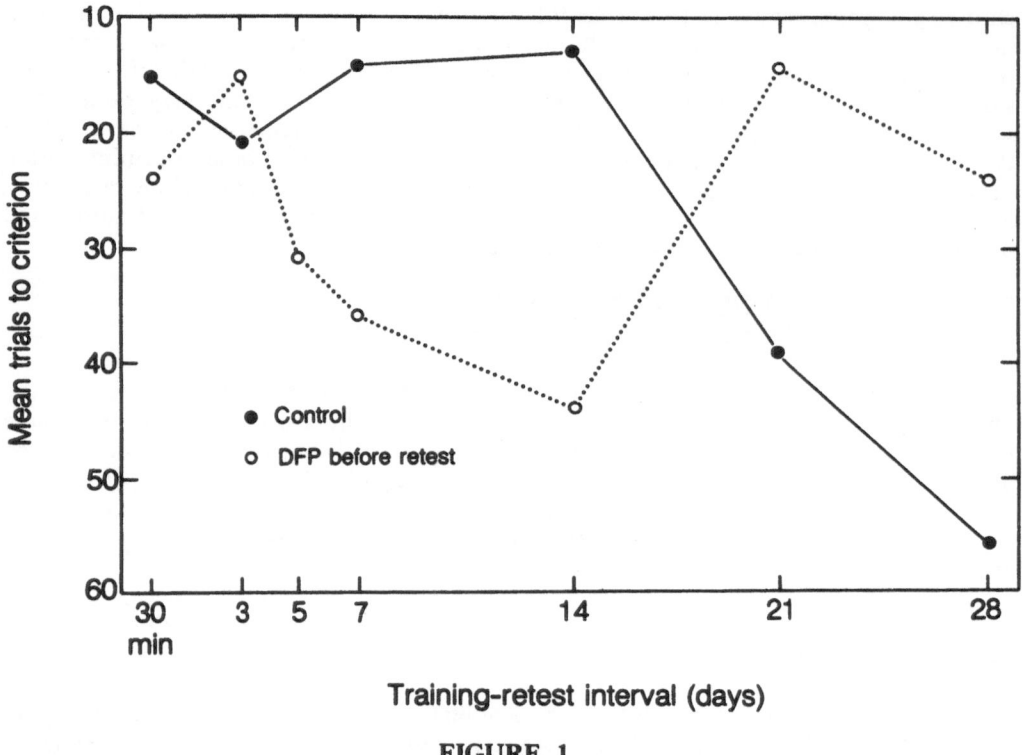

FIGURE 1

Effect on memories of different age when the anticholinesterase DFP is intracranially-injected before retest. Control animals receive intracranial injections of the peanut oil vehicle only. Rats are trained and retested until they research a criterion of 10 out of 10 consecutive errorless trials on a Y-maze brightness discrimination task. The measure of recall (Y axis) is mean trials to the 10/10 criterion at retest.

in preparation). Note that regardless of task, the better the performance of control animals, the worse the performance of anticholinesterase-injected animals and vice-versa.

Not only do there seem to be differences in susceptibility to cholinergic agents as functions of time and behavioral task, but also it has been shown that there are such variations depending on the speed of initial learning. Stanes *et al.,* (1976) have reported that fast learners and slow learners differ in the time it takes to produce a maximum of amnesia with physostigmine. Using an appetitive Y-maze light discrimination task, it has been found that rats which learned quickly were maximally susceptible to the amnesia effects of physostigmine approximately four days after initial learning whereas slow learners reached the same point approximately seven days after initial learning. Further, it seems that slow learners do not reach the same high level of synaptic transmission attained by fast learners as judged by their susceptibility to memory block by the same dose of physostigmine. However, such a conclusion may be due to the small number of

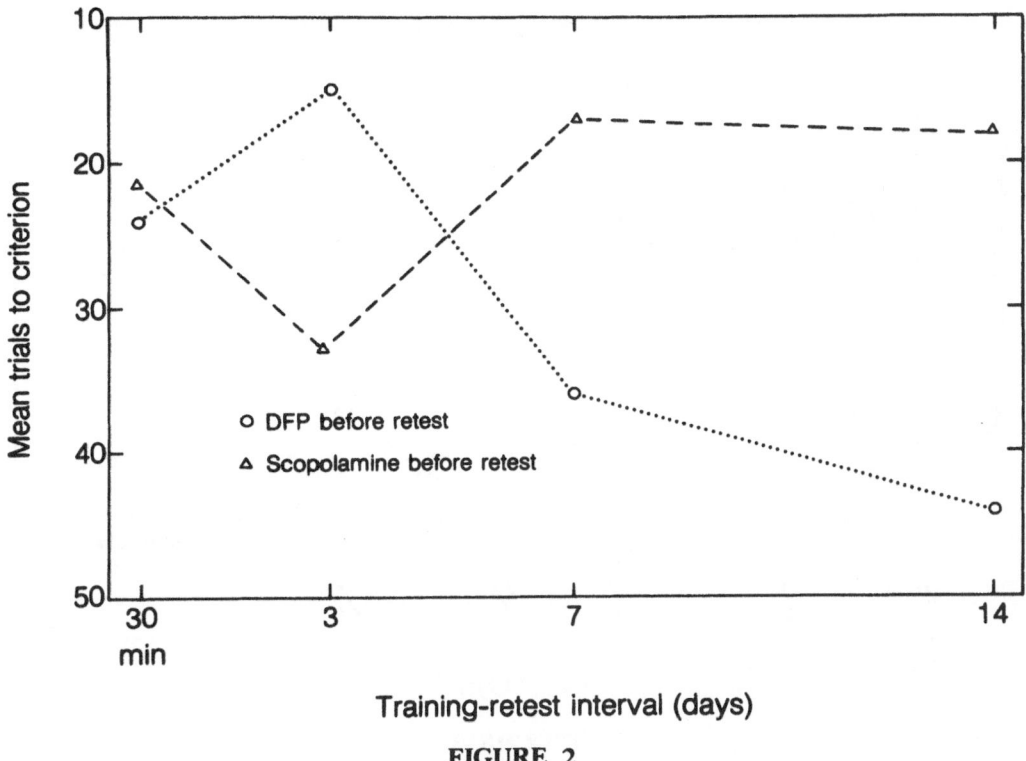

FIGURE 2

Effect on memories of different age when the anticholinesterase DFP or the anticholinergic scopolamine is intracranially-injected before retest. Same task and criterion as Figure 1.

time intervals sampled (4, 7 and 35 days) in the study.

Interpretation of these results follows directly from the known physiological and pharmacological effects of anticholinesterases and anticholinergics on peripheral synapses. Anticholinesterases reduce the rate of destruction of acetylcholine (ACh). In poorly conducting synapses this can be advantageous: more transmitter survives thereby helping assure adequate pre- and postsynaptic communication. Such an action is used to good effect in clinical treatment of myasthenia gravis, a condition characterized by reduced postsynaptic sensitivity to ACh. On the other hand, in synapses with normal cholinergic sensitivity, ACh accumulation may become excessive after anticholinesterase treatment. The postsynaptic membrane may not be able to repolarize and synaptic blockade may ensue. Thus, an anticholinesterase dose which is therapeutic for a myasthenic patient might be lethal to a normal subject. The anticholinergics, of course, have quite different actions on the synapse. These agents compete with ACh for cholinergic receptor sites and thereby reduce cholinergic synaptic excitability. Cholinergic agonists and antagonists, particularly the anticholinesterases, can therefore be used as a means for testing cholinergic synaptic sensitivity.

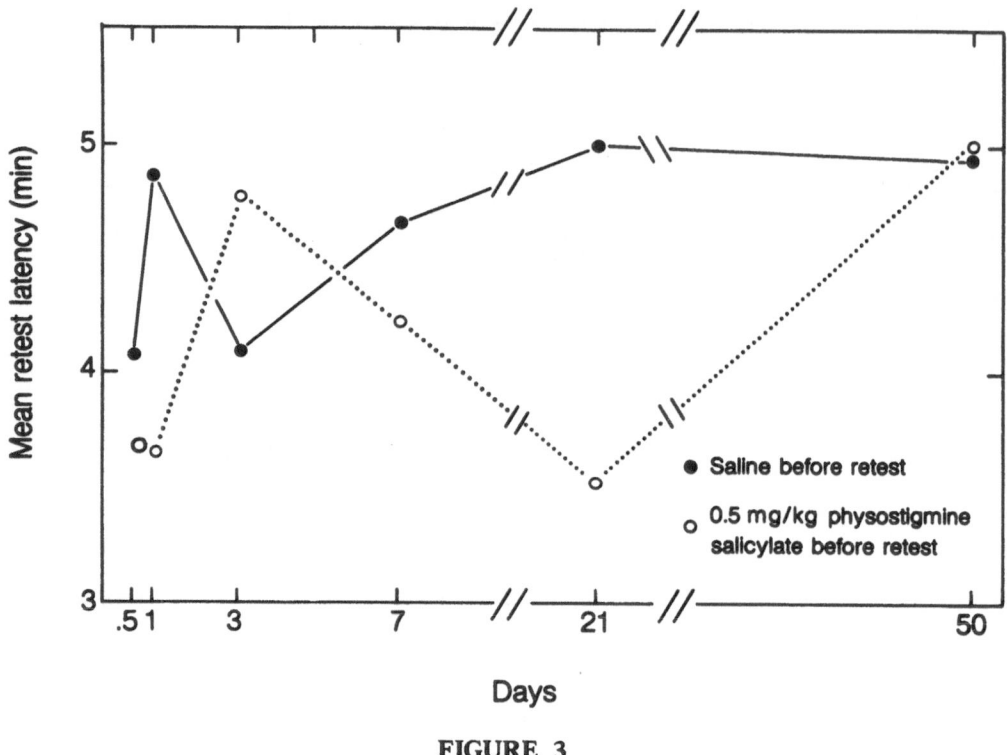

FIGURE 3

Effect on memories of different age when the anticholinesterase physostigmine is intra-peritoneally-injected before retest. The task is one-trial step-through passive avoidance.

Our behavioral data indicate 1) that cholinergic synapses represent an essential component or link in mnemonic substrates and 2) that variations in memory strength over time are positively associated with variations in cholinergic sensitivity (Figure 4). The better the recall, the greater the cholinergic sensitivity of the mnemonic substrate. The greater the cholinergic sensitivity, the greater the probability of disruption, presumably by synaptic blockade, on administration of anticholinesterase. Similarly, we infer that such states as forgetting must be characterized by reduced cholinergic excitability since, here, anticholinesterases facilitate the expression of memory. Anticholinergics reduce cholinergic sensitivity and, therefore, we would predict that they should also decrease memory strength for as long as they are active in the nervous system. This, too, is borne out by our behavioral data. Three days after training, when strength of recall has not yet reached optimum, rats given scopolamine appear to forget. At intervals where strength of recall is near optimum, the same dose of scopolamine has no significant effect on recall, presumably because of ceiling effects. Much higher doses of anticholinergic, even at intervals of optimum recall, should produce some memory impairment, and informal studies in our laboratory suggest that this is so.

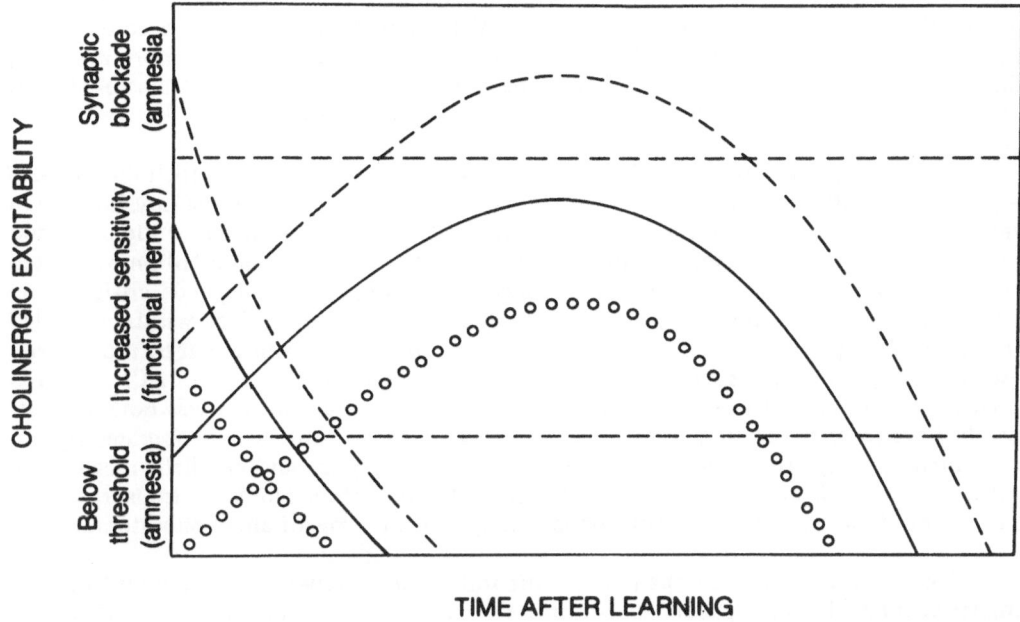

TIME AFTER LEARNING

FIGURE 4

Hypothesized changes in strength of memory as a function of changes in cholinergic excitability and age of the memory.

Several other experimental strategies have been used to confirm and extend the above conclusions. With regard to facilitation of memory, for example, there is another way to manipulate strength of recall without waiting for the memory to decay. This is to train rats to differing degrees. If the modification of memory synapses is graded rather than all-or-none, then low degrees of learning should produce synapses that conduct relatively poorly, whereas increased amounts of training should produce synapses that conduct well. Consequently, a poorly learned habit should be facilitated by the same dose of physostigmine that blocks the same habit when it has been learned well. That this is the case has been shown in two separate experiments (Deutsch and Lutzky, 1967; S.F. Leibowitz, doctoral thesis).

Another means of testing the synaptic blockade hypothesis of anticholinesterase impairment of recall is by the use of massed and spaced trials in the memory task. Electrophysiological studies by Bacq and Brown (1937) have shown that moderate anticholinesterase doses produce blockade of peripheral cholinergic synapses only when the intervals between test pulses are short. No blockade occurs when such pulses are widely spaced. As previously described, this follows directly from the mode of action of anticholinesterases: they slow the rate of hydrolysis of ACh. Acetylcholinesterase (AChE) is, however, one of the most powerful enzymes known. Even under very high levels of inhibition, given sufficient time, that portion of AChE activity remaining may be adequate to clear the synapse of accumulated ACh. When stimuli follow each other at short intervals, however, only part of the excess ACh may be cleared. Thus, as trials and trains of stimuli progress, excess ACh accumulates, soon producing synaptic blockade.

We can apply the same principle to the recall situation. If we retest anticholinesterase-injected rats with short intervals between trials we should expect a memory block. On the other hand, if we space the trials out sufficiently in time, no memory block should be apparent. Of course we initially did not know what the precise amount of time between trials should be for memory block and successful retrieval. This depends critically on ACh hydrolysis rates under various anticholinesterase concentrations within the CNS (as opposed to peripheral neurotransmission where such parameters might be more easily ascertained). Our previous work had shown, however, that accumulation of ACh occurred even with trials spaced as far apart as 30 sec. Thus, the only question was how long we would have to wait between trials to get no block. It turned out that we obtained significant memory impairment if we massed retest trials at 25 sec and excellent recall if we spaced retest trials at 50 sec (Figure 5A). Except for the interval between trials, rats were run under identical conditions both behaviorally and in terms of anticholinesterase dose.

That memory may be impaired by anticholinesterase depending simply on length of intertrial interval (ITI) appears to confirm the synaptic blockade hypothesis. However, there is another more trivial explanation of our results in terms of performance variables. It could be that massed trials under anticholinesterase are very taxing, the short intervals between trials not allowing the rat to recover from stress. This could produce a difference in performance between massed and spaced retest animals. Alternatively, it might also be argued that both 25- and 50-sec ITI subjects were amnesic; but with 50 sec between trials the rats were able to relearn the task so quickly that they appeared to have good initial recall. The Y-maze task employed in the experiment is, after all, shock-escape motivated. Increased ITI's might, therefore, represent increased reward. To eliminate these alternatives, we employed a variation in our experimental paradigm.

When an animal is trained to discriminate between two stimuli, it can then be trained to reverse the discrimination between them. For example, we might initially train a rat to avoid shock by avoiding the unlighted arms of a Y-maze and escaping into a lighted arm. To reverse the animal, we simply reverse the lighting/shock contingencies: an unlighted arm becomes safe, whereas shock is received in the two lighted arms. When animals are first taught such a reversal, an interesting property emerges. The number of trials required to learn the reversal is approximately double that required to learn the original discrimination. The reason for such an increase in trials during reversal is that the animal remembers the original discrimination and this memory hampers it in the acquisition of the reversal.

In our situation, therefore, if the results in the massed condition reflect a genuine amnesia then reversal acquisition should be faster for a drugged group under massed trial conditions compared to either an undrugged group under massed trial or a drugged group under spaced trials. This is because for the massed, drugged group there should be no memory of the original discrimination to interfere with the acquisition of the reversal habit. Note that the reversal paradigm provides effective control for the performance variables described above. As an example, let us assume the hypothesis that massed trials are simply more taxing for drugged subjects. In massed, drugged, reversal training, therefore, acquisition would be hampered not only by the memory of the original habit but also by the interaction of the drugged state with the short period of recovery between trials. In spaced, drugged, reversal training, memory of the original habit should also slow acquisition; but the longer period between trials would facilitate performance. Thus, this alternative explanation in terms of performance variables would predict that the massed, drugged group would be inferior on reversal to the spaced, drugged group. Our hypothesis of synaptic blockade predicts just the opposite result.

Figure 5B presents data for Y-maze reversal acquisition under drugged and undrugged, spaced and massed trial conditions. With 50-sec ITI's, both anticholinesterase and saline groups took almost twice as long to reverse as they took to learn the original habit. This indicates good recall for the original discrimination. With 25-sec ITI's anticholinesterase-injected rats learned the reversal as quickly as they had the original habit. The results of the reversal experiment, therefore, are not consistent with an hypothesis invoking performance variables, but are consistent with the known peripheral pharmacological effects of anticholinesterase — in this case, synaptic blockade — and the notion that such blockade of certain central synapses produces amnesia.

Our conclusion from the above set of experiments is that at the time of learning some as yet unknown mechanism stimulates a particular group of synapses to alter their state and, without further practice, to begin to increase their cholinergic conductivity. However, after a certain lapse of time this original stimulus to increase conductivity loses its effectiveness and the synapses gradually return to their original less sensitive state. If such an hypothesis is correct we may ask why it has not been noted that in the undrugged state habits are better remembered one week rather than three days after learning. This should be the case if one-week old habits are more susceptible to anticholinesterase block than three-day old habits. One reason for a lack of such evidence is that animal training has, in general, stretched over many days so that the age of a habit was rather indeterminate. Further, it is difficult to find studies where the age of the habit has been used as an independent variable in studies of retention. In our own control groups where such a variable has been studied, an effect of increasing recall has sometimes been difficult to observe for the methodological reason that our animals were trained initially to a very high level of performance, ten out of ten correct trials. As retention was already almost perfect at three days, there was little or no room for the control rats to show improvement at seven days.

To overcome this methodological limitation we have employed two strategies. In the first (Rogers and Deutsch, in preparation), rats were trained and tested on a passive avoidance paradigm. The test for memory in this task involves the time taken to make a response; the stronger the memory, the longer the time taken. We could therefore observe an improvement in memory with less interference from ceiling effects (Figure 3). Although, as might be expected, the temporal parameters for recall of the one trial passive avoidance habit differ somewhat from discrimination tasks employing many training trials, the pattern of results is the same. Mean recall three days after training is far less than optimum, but improves steadily to reach good performance by 21 days. Anticholinesterase-injected rats' mean performance is, of course, the mirror image of control performance, decreasing steadily to reach significant impairment by 21 days.

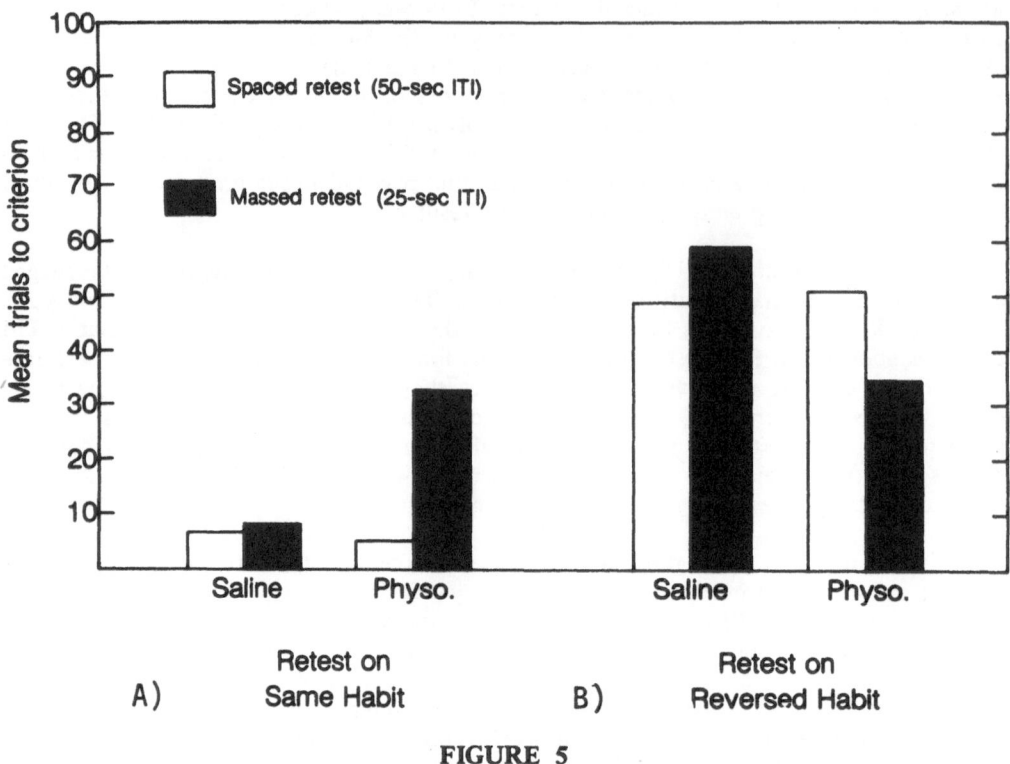

FIGURE 5

Left (A) – Effect of the anticholinesterase physostigmine on recall of a Y-maze bright-ness discrimination task when the time between trials is either 25 or 50 sec. Right (B) – Same as A, except that subjects are retested on the reverse habit (i.e., if training were to a lighted alley, then retest would be to a darkened alley and vice-versa).

A second method has been initially to undertrain subjects on a Y-maze brightness discrimination task. Escape from shock was used as motivation. During initial training the rats were given 15 acquisition trials. They were then divided into a number of groups, and each group was made to wait a different number of days before being placed back in the Y-maze. When they were returned to the Y-maze we counted the number of trials that such groups took to reach the ten out of ten trials correct criterion we had employed in previous studies. In this case, no drugs were used. We found that the rats took only about half the number of trials to reach criterion when they waited seven to ten days as when they waited three days (Figure 6). It appears that memory of the initial training improves simply as a function of the passage of time since that training. Similar results have been obtained on mice by Crabbe and Alpern (1975) and Fox and Crabbe (1976).

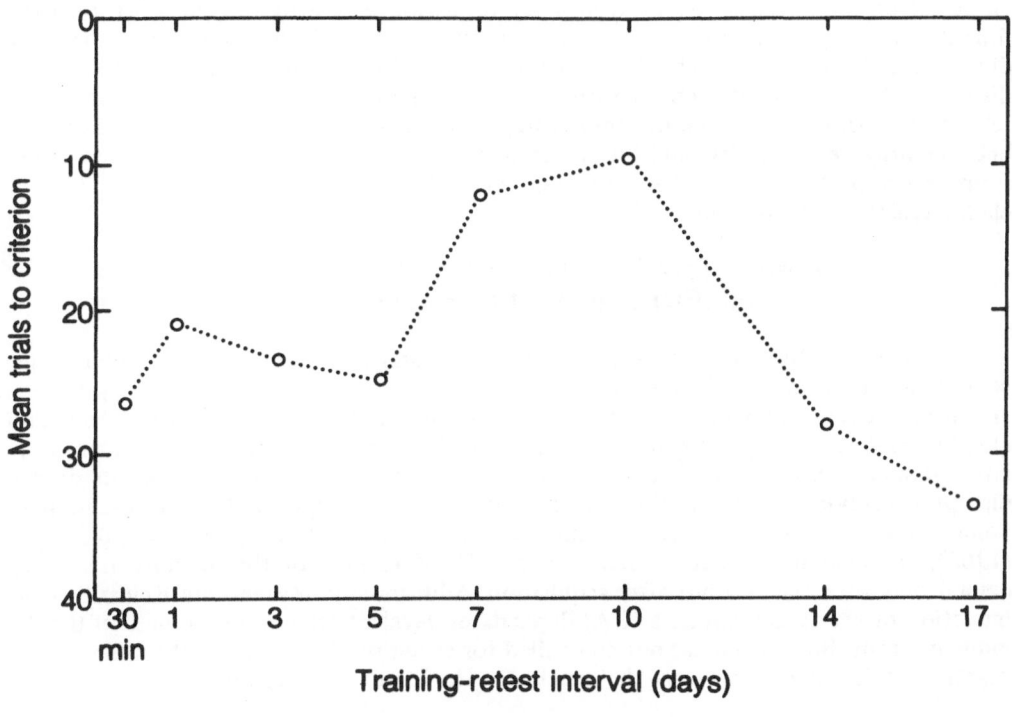

FIGURE 6

Strength of memory as a function of time since learning. The task is Y-maze brightness discrimination as in previously-discussed experiments. In order to minimize ceiling effects, however, rats were initially undertrained by giving only 15 acquisition trials. Note that no drugs were employed.

ADMINISTRATION OF CHOLINERGIC AGENTS
ONE OR MORE DAYS BEFORE RECALL TEST

Do the effects of anticholinergics and anticholinesterases on recall outlive their presence in the nervous system? That is, do transient cholinergic agonist or antagonist actions permanently disrupt the memory trace? To answer this question, we have adminis-tered the anticholinesterase physostigmine to rats several days after training but one or more days before recall test. As previously mentioned, radioactively labeled physostigmine is metabolized and excreted from the body within hours of its administration. To date, results from our laboratory (Deutsch, 1966) and from other investigators (Signorelli, 1976) suggest that anticholinesterases affect memory only transiently. Even with the relatively long lasting, irreversible cholinesterase inhibitor DFP, we find that memory returns after the drug has worn off.

Based on these results it will be asked if we are dealing with an effect on recall or an effect on memory. Clearly, if a memory returns after a drug has worn off, then the drug did not disrupt the memory but only recall. However, in the present case the drugs did not simply disrupt a mechanism which retrieves information from memory: the drugs disrupted the retrieval of memories differentially depending on their age. This fact then tells us something about the memory storage process itself. The interaction we observe between drug, retrievability, and the age of memories is precisely what would be predicted from the hypothesis that memory storage critically involves changes in the ability of cholinergic synapses to conduct.

ADMINISTRATION OF CHOLINERGIC AGENTS
IMMEDIATELY BEFORE TRAINING

If, as shown by effects on retrieval, memory storage employs an essential cholinergic component, it becomes of interest to determine whether or not cholinergic agents can also influence acquisition or consolidation of memories. As previously mentioned, Signorelli (1976) administers physostigmine one or more days before recall test but many days after training. Observing no recall deficit, he concludes that cholinergic agents do not disrupt consolidation. But is this a reasonable test? McGaugh (1966) and others have pointed out that the length of consolidation may be quite short. Chorover and Schiller (1965), for example, conclude that the period of lability of the memory trace may extend only for a few seconds after acquisition. Additionally, it seems quite clear that the induction of retrograde amnesia (RA) depends on level of trauma or strength of the RA inducing agent. Because he has not controlled for either of these two variables, Signorelli's negative results may not warrant the conclusions he has drawn from them.

The testing of effects of cholinergic agents on consolidation presents something of a methodological difficulty since there is a considerable lag between the end of training and the time it takes to administer a drug and have it penetrate the nervous system. In our laboratory, administration of cholinergic agents immediately before training was initially undertaken primarily as a further measure for demonstrating control over performance variables; doses of anticholinesterase which impair recall do not impair the rate or manner in which rats acquire a brightness discrimination habit (Figure 7). Nonetheless, these same rats which have been injected before training demonstrate marked impairment of recall when subsequently retested. This holds true for both passive avoidance (Figure 8) and Y-maze (Table 1, 2, and 3) tasks (Rogers and Deutsch, in preparation). Whether these data have anything to do with effects on consolidation cannot as yet be stated. It is true, however, that administration of anticholinesterase just before training is one means for assuring the drug's presence in the nervous system immediately after training when the vulnerability of the memory consolidation process is at a maximum.

It can be seen that rats injected with anticholinesterase before training do not remember their training as well as rats injected only with saline. In fact, at all points in time after initial training, recall performance of drug-trained rats is worse than controls by an almost constant amount. It is most unlikely that this impaired recall is due to anticholinesterase synaptic blockade since at the time of recall test there would be no anticholinesterase left in the nervous system to produce blockade. Further, synaptic blockade predicts inverse or mirror image variation of recall when drugged animals are compared with controls. Rats injected before training, however, do not show such a

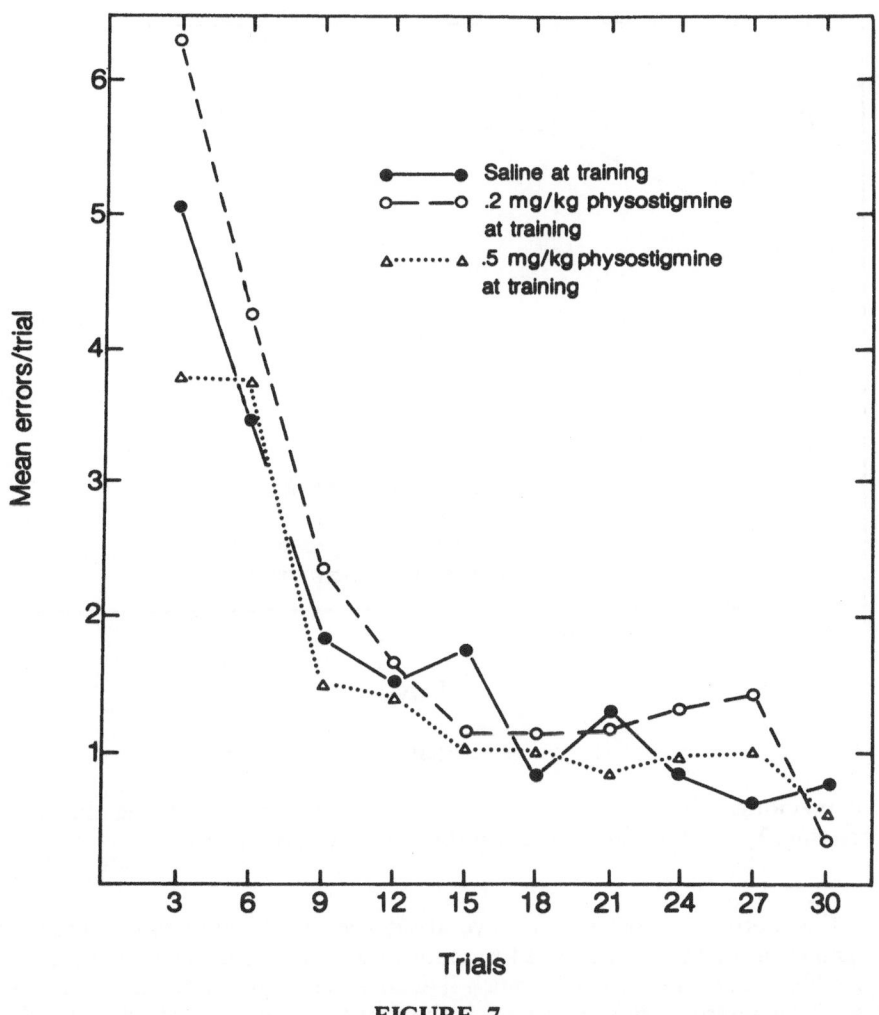

FIGURE 7

Acquisition performance under two levels of anticholinesterase or under saline. The Y-axis represents mean errors per subject summed over sets of three trials.

mirror image pattern in strength of recall; rather, their mean performance over time is always parallel to and lower than controls'. This parallel and lower curve suggests that anticholinesterase injected before training produces a weakened memory trace which subsequently undergoes temporal variations in strength similar to those for normal memory traces.

A weakened memory trace might arise from direct neurophysiological effects on memory such as interference with consolidation, or from non-associative drug side effects such as analgesic properties of physostigmine. Since escape from the pain of

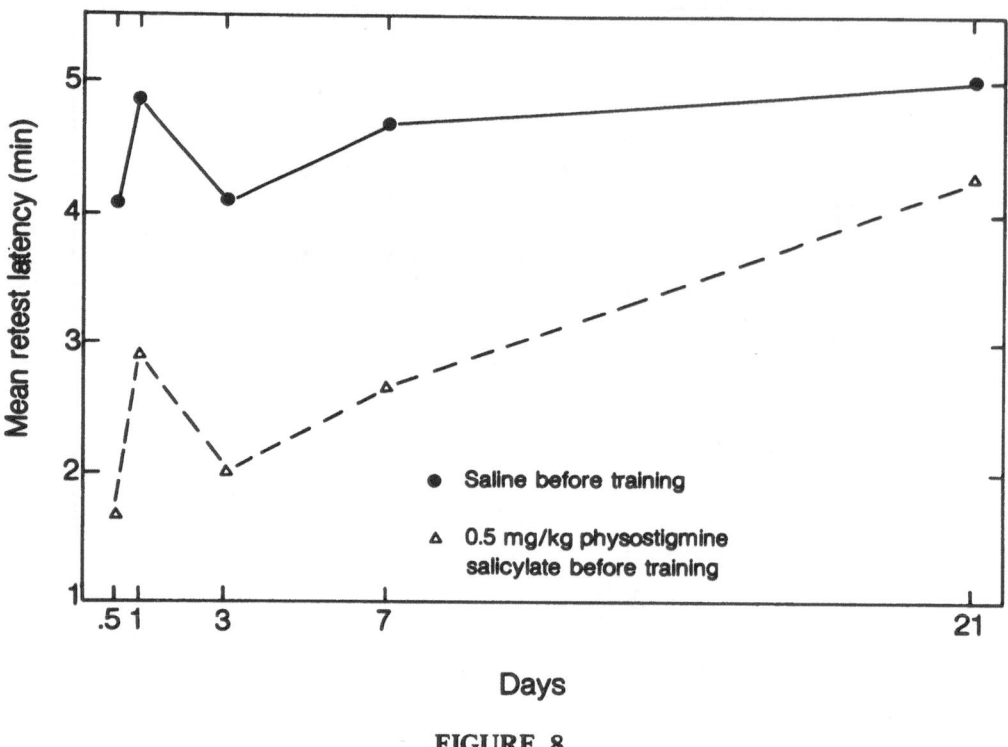

FIGURE 8

Effect on memories of different age when the anticholinesterase physostigmine is injected before training. The task is one-trial step-through passive avoidance.

shock is the motivation for both passive avoidance and Y-maze tasks, animals under physostigmine might be less motivated because of analgesic drug side effects and, therefore, resemble undertrained subjects much like those given fewer training trials. Arguing against such an interpretation, however, is the fact that animals trained under the drug acquire the task at the same rate and in the same manner as control animals (Figure 7). If physostigmine animals were less motivated, then we would expect them to take more trials to reach the training criterion.

There are at least as many difficulties in arguing for a direct effect on memory of anticholinesterase injected before training. For example, it will be remembered that when injected before retest, the anticholinergics, having a pharmacological effect opposite to the anticholinesterases, also have an opposite set of effects on recall (Figure 2). This predictability of behavioral effect from known pharmacological action provides a converging line of evidence that cholinergic drugs may interact directly with memory. However, when given before training, both anticholinergics and anticholinesterases appear to produce similar, debilitating effects on subsequent ability to recall the task. Thus, a converging line of evidence for the direct effects on memory of cholinergic drugs given before training cannot, at least on the present data alone, be established. Alternatively, if mnemonic processes involve an essential cholinergic component, then it is not unreasonable to suspect that pretraining administration of cholinergic agents should affect subsequent recall. One of the earliest observations of mnemonic cholinergic properties, in fact, was that women given scopolamine before childbirth had hazy recollections of the event. Further, it is worth noting that the opposite effects of anticholinesterases and anticholinergics given before retest only emerged when age of habit was employed as a variable. With regard to injection of anticholinergic before training, we know of only one study (Dennis, 1974) in which age of habit has been considered. For this reason we turned to the set of experiments described in the next section.

ADMINISTRATION OF CHOLINERGIC AGENTS IMMEDIATELY BEFORE TRAINING AND/OR RECALL TEST

We knew from studies with undertrained habits and forgotten habits that anticholinesterase administration before retest could result in good recall of memories unavailable without the drug; put more simply, anticholinesterases may facilitate weakened memories. Therefore, if anticholinesterase before training produces a weakened memory trace by somehow interfering with the normal mechanism for increasing cholinergic synaptic excitability as a result of learning, then a second injection of the drug immediately before retest should result in good recall. Our initial experiments using both passive avoidance and Y-maze tasks suggested that this was so (Tables 1 and 2). Further, as will be seen, administration of cholinergic agents before both training and retest provides a means by which the effects on memory of anticholinesterases and anticholinergics may be better discriminated, and by which drug state dependence may be further ruled out as an explanation of our results.

TABLE 1

Retest Passive Avoidance Latency
(5 Minute Maximum Latency) One Day After Training

Physostigmine Dose (mg/kg) (0 = Saline)		N	Mean Retest Latency
Training	Retest		
0	0	44	4.86
0	.5	18	3.64
.5	0	16	2.87
.5	.5	16	4.40
0	.2	8	5.00
.2	0	8	2.93
.2	.2	8	4.91

TABLE 2

Training and Retest Trials To A 9/10 Criterion On A
Y-Maze, Brightness Discrimination Task

Physostigmine (mg/kg) (0 = Saline)		N	Training Trials To Criterion	Retest Trials To Criterion
Train	Test			
0	0	8	31.0	13.8
0	.5	8	29.1	23.0
.5	0	8	26.8	25.1
.5	.5	8	26.4	14.5
0	.2	8	30.6	14.4
.2	0	8	29.5	13.9
.2	.2	8	28.8	14.9

The homeostatic properties of the nervous system are well-documented. For example, the addictive opiates produce transient changes in neural function while they are metabolically active. After such opiate injection, however, a long period may follow during which those systems acted upon by opiate manifest compensatory changes in function. Decreased sensitivity to opiate, the requirement for ever-increasing doses to achieve the same behavioral effect, and the other phenomena of drug tolerance result. Our present hypothesis concerning mnemonic effects of cholinergic agents administered before training follows from the concepts of neuropharmacological homeostasis and varying synaptic sensitivity. We believe it possible that the effects of cholinergic agents given before training result from a combination of two factors, both of which alter cholinergic synaptic sensitivity. The first is simply a tolerance response: the agonist action of physostigmine is followed by a longer-term compensatory desensitization. The second is an alteration in sensitivity with time of particular sets of cholinergic synapses as a result of learning. In other words, habits acquired under anticholinesterase, like habits acquired without drug, undergo changes in strength associated with changes in cholinergic sensitivity. Superimposed on this, however, there is an additional cholinergic component: a compensatory cholinergic desensitization, a homeostatic rebound from the agonist effects of the drug at training. The summation of changing cholinergic sensitivity as a result of learning with changing cholinergic sensitivity as a result of tolerance explains 1) why anticholinesterase injected before training always results in recall impairment, 2) why anticholinesterase injected before training results, when viewed over time, in habit strength variations which parallel the normal, and 3) why anticholinesterase injected before training results, at all intervals so far examined, in weakened memory traces which are fully retrievable by a second dose of anticholinesterase before retest.

Can the above hypothesis be supported by converging pharmacological evidence? Our most recent studies suggest it can. In the first (Rogers, in preparation), we have administered scopolamine, saline, or physostigmine at training and then scopolamine, saline or physostigmine at retest. The experimental design is factorial such that nine different drug conditions are represented. In all, three groups received scopolamine at training, one getting a second scopolamine dose before retest, another getting saline before retest, and the last receiving physostigmine before retest. In similar fashion, three saline-trained groups are divided into one administered scopolamine, one administered saline, and one administered physostigmine before retest. Three physostigmine-trained groups are also divided in this way. Mean retest trials to criterion for the various groups are presented in Table 3.

TABLE 3

Retest Trials To A 9/10 Criterion On A
Y-Maze Brightness Discrimination Task
(N = 126)

Training Drug	Scopolamine	Retest Drug Saline	Physostigmine
Scopolamine	16.1	30.6	36.9
Saline	21.8	14.9	23.6
Physostigmine	20.7	25.4	15.2

We may begin analysis of the data by noting that the results from several of the experimental conditions replicate our previously published work. Anticholinesterase immediately before retest causes significant impairment of one day old habits. Anticholinergic before retest at best only marginally impairs one day old. Anticholinesterase before training results in significant recall deficits one day after training; anticholinesterase before training and before retest produces good recall. Replicating previous work of others, anticholinergics before training disrupt subsequent recall, but do not do so if doses are also administered before retest.

The mixed-drug conditions are those which hold the greatest theoretical interest. As previously mentioned, it is highly desirable to demonstrate opposite mnemonic effects of drugs with opposite actions on the nervous system. Our hypothesis posits a rebound cholinergic desensitization in response to doses of cholinergic agonist administered before training. Administration of agonist before retest should then transiently restore synaptic transmission to normal and good recall should result. We should also predict an opposite effect of antagonist administration before training when followed by agonist injection before retest. Here, the compensatory response to the anticholinergic should be to increase cholinergic sensitivity. Since this would sum with the increased sensitivity due to learning, we might predict that physostigmine before retest would result in massive synaptic blockage and total amnesia if training had taken place under scopolamine. In fact, synaptic blockade should be more evident under this antagonist-agonist condition than under any other condition. Examination of the data reveals that antagonist-agonist rats were significantly recall-impaired compared not only to control animals but also to saline-agonist subjects (and that the latter were, themselves, significantly worse than non-drug controls). Indeed, scopolamine-physostigmine subjects' retest scores were nearly identical to their training scores. It may also be worth noting that these results are not likely to be due to drug state dependence (discussed further in the next section): among several reasons, one in particular is that drug state dependence predicts equality between scopolamine-physostigmine and physostigmine-scopolamine groups. The opposite is true.

While sensitization and tolerance effects have been reported for many neuropharmacological agents, they have not been for cholinergic drugs. One possible exception is clinical reports of "cholinergic rebound" — here meaning behavioral depression — following anticholinesterase treatment of psychotics. Rebound follows an initial heightening of mood during the period of the drug's presence in the nervous system (Shopsin et al., 1975).

As an explanation of this phenomenon it is suggested that behavioral systems which increase their activity under cholinergic agonist subsequently decrease activity below normal levels once agonist actions have subsided. This is essentially the same mechanism suggested by our memory studies with rats.

In addition to our behavioral evidence and the human clinical observations, we felt that nonbehavioral physiological assays should be undertaken to establish that compensatory responses to cholinergic agonists and antagonists occur. To accomplish this we (Rogers and Moss, in preparation) first obtained an estimate of the LD_{50} (lethal drug dose to 50% of subjects) for intraperitoneal physostigmine injection. Published tables of LD_{50} for various drugs provide surprisingly little data for cholinergic agents in rats. In our rats the physostigmine LD_{50} fell within such a narrow range that we ended up testing two drug doses, an LD_{81} and an LD_{31}. These doses were, respectively, 2.41 and 2.10 mg/kg.

One day before injection with LD_{81} or LD_{31} physostigmine, subjects were given either saline, 0.5 mg/kg physostigmine, or 2.0 mg/kg scopolamine. These were the drug doses used in our previous memory experiments and which we postulated had produced sensitization or tolerance effects. Twenty-four hours later, LD_{81} or LD_{31} physostigmine was injected and the animals observed for 30 min. During this time subjects were rated once per minute for discernable physostigmine effects. Rating was on a scale encompassing progressively more severe symptoms of anticholinesterase toxicity, from no effect through twitching of ears only, body tremors, convulsions, unconsciousness, and death. The study was conducted blind; that is, the experimenters did not know which drug (saline, physostigmine, or scopolamine) a given animal had previously been exposed to. Overall, 72% of scopolamine, 57% of saline, and 48% of physostigmine pretreated rats died. Results are presented in Figure 9. These appear to support the hypothesis that administration of cholinergic agonist (physostigmine) and antagonist (scopolamine) results, respectively, in relatively long-term decrease or increase in cholinergic sensitivity. We note that this must be a long-term compensatory response since when they are administered together scopolamine is normally antidotal for physostigmine and vice-versa. Here, where the toxic anticholinesterase dose follows long after excretion of previous physostigmine or scopolamine, we find that animals previously exposed to agonist are less likely to die and suffer less severe symptoms of toxicity than controls. The opposite is true if prior exposure is to antagonist.

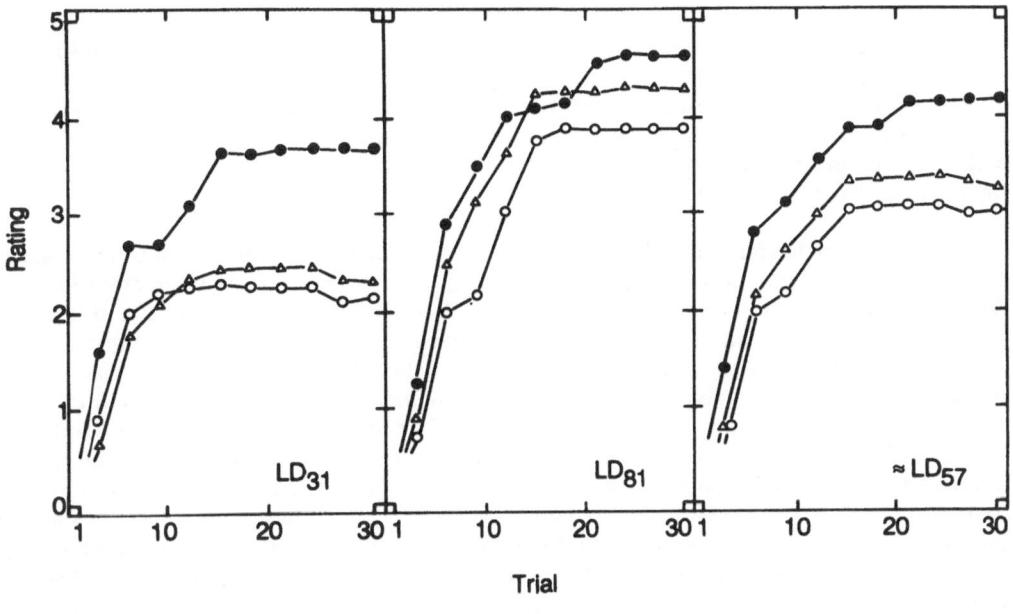

FIGURE 9

Left (A) — Mean toxicity response to a 2.1 mg/kg physostigmine injection one day after injections with 2.0 mg/kg scopolamine (filled circles), 0.5 mg/kg physostigmine (open circles), or saline (open triangles). Center (B) — Mean toxicity response to a 2.4 mg/kg physostigmine injection one day after injections with 2.0 mg/kg scopolamine (filled circles), 0.5 mg/kg physostigmine (open circles), or saline (open triangles). Right (C) — The experiment shows a significant effective of pretreatment drug on severity, but not rate of onset of toxic responses (same Figure legends as A and B).

PERFORMANCE OR MEMORY?

Are the effects of cholinergic agents on retest due to changes in memory or just alterations in the ability to perform? When an animal scores more poorly after the administration of a pharmacological agent this might be due to decreased motivation, malaise, poorer attention, motor incoordination or perceptual disturbance. Any changes in the score are not necessarily due to an alteration of memory or recall.

There are seven main reasons which persuade us that we are observing changes in memory or recall in our series of experiments.

1. The time between initial training and retest is varied between conditions in most of our experiments. In others degree of learning is varied. The time between drug injection and retest is always kept fixed. Since we observe differences in performance after drug as we vary the time between training and retest (or as we vary amount of training) we must conclude that the differences we observe are due to an interaction of

the drug with the recency (or amount) of training.

2. Our most striking effects are obtained from one week to a month after initial training both with escape and appetitive habits. It is difficult to imagine non-associative effects of training that would persist for so long, interacting with the drug to affect performance. In addition, control procedures examining possible interactions of drug with training and retest stress from footshock have shown the latter not to be significant factors (Puerto et al., 1976).

3. Our behavioral data is supported by a converging line of pharmacological evidence. That is, cholinergic drugs with similar modes of action (e.g., physostigmine and DFP) produce similar effects on memory; cholinergic drugs with opposite modes of action (e.g., physostigmine and scopolamine) have opposite effects on memory. Were such non-associative drug effects as drug state dependence significant factors in our results, then we should expect similar effects on memory of cholinergic agonists and antagonists. The opposite is true. Agonists given before retest facilitate poorly-remembered habits, disrupt well-remembered habits, and have no observable effect on memories of intermediate strength; antagonists given before retest depress poorly-remembered habits, have no observable effect on well-remembered habits, and depress memories of intermediate strength. Further, drug state dependence predicts equivalent effects of a drug on memory regardless of the strength or age of that memory. Again, the opposite is true.

4. Several behavioral tasks — for example, fixed-ratio responding, Y-maze escape, passive avoidance, and delayed response situations — have been employed. Some of these would appear to be oppositely biased for non-associative drug side effects; yet all of them produce essentially similar results.

5. A further argument to support the notion that we are dealing with a mnemonic function derives from our results with reversal training under physostigmine. An animal is trained with one cue as positive and the other as negative. After the animal has reached a certain criterion showing that it has learned the discrimination, the values of the two cues are reversed. When this is done it generally takes the animal twice as many trials to reach the criterion after reversal than it took the animal to reach such a criterion during original training. Original learning is faster because then the animal has nothing to unlearn. During reversal learning the animal has first to unlearn what it learned during original training before it can acquire the reverse habit. If we could erase the memory or prevent the recall of the original habit during reversal training, then reversal training should take no longer than original training. This is actually what happens when reversal training is done under physostigmine. If physostigmine impaired performance without affecting memory, then reversal training under physostigmine should take longer than reversal training without drug. It should take more than twice as long. This prediction is completely contrary to the obtained result.

6. The dose of anticholinesterase which produces amnesia or facilitation of memory is a dose which produces no effect on the rate of initial acquisition of the habit when injected prior to original training. If the drug had an effect on performance through motivational, attentional, perceptual, or motor mechanisms, similar effects should be evident during original training. In fact, original training should be much more susceptible

to disruption by such variables than an already established habit.

7.   Even if the above arguments are completely disregarded and we wish to maintain that some factor has affected performance and produced the effects we observe, there is another consideration that must be borne in mind. Any factor which could produce such results must be a factor that cannot only diminish retest scores but also greatly boost them. The effects we have observed with the same dose of drug, administered at the same time before retest, have demonstrated extreme improvement of scores over control levels as well as extreme deterioration of performance compared to control levels. Whether facilitation or deterioration is obtained has depended only on the recency (or amount) of initial training. It is difficult to see how a factor affecting performance alone could produce two quite contradictory effects, depending simply on the strength and age of the habit being tested.

We therefore conclude that some memory process is being manipulated by cholinergic administration. Since the change in memory disappears when the pharmacological agent has worn off we conclude that memory storage was not affected. The effect we observe is one on recall. However as the recall of a habit varies with the age and strength of the memory, such an effect provides information about the nature of memory storage itself. The observed effect supports the hypothesis that an essential component of information storage in the nervous system consists of the increase in sensitivity of specific cholinergic synapses.

NEUROPHYSIOLOGICAL BASES FOR CHOLINERGIC SYNAPTIC CHANGE

We believe our research strongly suggests that as a result of learning there is some systematic change in cholinergic synaptic excitability, and that this change represents an essential component in mnemonic processes. But what of the neurophysiological mechanism which might underlie such a change? We suspect that it is probably not nicotinic since the potent, irreversible nicotinic blocker a-neurotoxin (Moss and Rogers, 1975) does not have a reliable effect on recall. Specific to our research, however, little else has so far been established. Nonetheless, during the period of our behavioral work, neurophysiological and neurochemical studies have demonstrated a great capacity for plastic change possessed by cholinergic systems, and these we think worth briefly reviewing here. For purposes of this chapter, only four broad areas and a few specific examples within each will be covered. The areas are ACh release, AChE control, cholinergic receptor (AChR) changes, and heterosynaptic cholinergic/catacholaminergic interactions.

ACh Release

Kosower (1972) has provided an elaborate mechanism for synaptic change which would result in increased release of transmitter through structural modification of vesicle-release sites. He suggests that short term memory might result from the conversion of dithiol sites in the presynaptic membrane to disulfides, thus activating vesicle-release mechanisms. Based upon the rate constants for thiol-disulfide interchange and the concentration of the reactants, Kosower computes the half life of the activated release to be between 10 sec and 30 hr. Long-term memory was also suggested to result from expansion of the region of presynaptic transmitter release by insertion of a "synaptomeric protein" into the presynaptic membrane. An increase in release would increase synaptic effectiveness, and represent a stable information store.

There is abundant evidence for increased ACh release for a short period following natural, electrical, or pharmacological stimulation (Pepeu, 1973). Post-stimulus durations range from milliseconds (synaptic facilitation) to several hours (Pepeu and Bartolini, 1968; Beani et al., 1968). The basis for this increase might involve Ca^{2+} flux, feedback onto presynaptic receptors, and/or long-loop feedback (Pepeu, 1973). The permanence of such effects, however, is at best unclear.

AChE Regulation

AChE is an enzyme of approximately 260,000 molecular weight with multiple subunits (Kremzner and Wilson, 1964; Mooser et al., 1972). More important, it is an enzyme subject to allosteric control, regulation by means other than direct (steric) interactions at the catalytic site (Changeux, 1966; Kitz et al., 1970). A substance mediating allosteric modulation is thought to bind at some site distinct from the catalytic site, and to induce a conformational change in the enzyme. The latter would then modify the efficiency with which the enzyme could convert substrate to product. Large molecular weight enzymes with multiple subunits and allosteric control properties are usually found where physiological function requires elaborate control.

The possibility that cholinergic synaptic function might be controlled, at least in part, by the inhibition of AChE is not a new idea, having been proposed by Cohen and Hagan (1964) with regard to substrate inhibition of the enzyme, and by Aprison (1961) with regard to allosteric AChE inhibition by serotonin. The latter possibility is supported by recent experiments of Fahrney and Moss (personal communication) demonstrating that the concentration of serotonin required to reduce AChE activity to 50% of uninhibited control values varies from 0.5 mM to 4.2 mM with a 100 fold range in substrate concentration. Further, experiments with the sulfonyl fluorides — active site specific, irreversible inhibitors — strongly suggest that serotonin is bound only at some allosteric site on rat brain AChE. However, in view of a recent failure to obtain any change in endogenous ACh concentration after various treatments affecting serotonin concentration (Pepeu et al., 1974), the hypothesis that serotonin modulates concentrations of ACh by inhibiting AChE may be suspect — at least with regard to in vivo functional significance.

Cohen and Hagen (1964) have attempted to assign physiological significance to the fact that AChE is substrate inhibited (i.e., in the presence of high ACh concentrations, AChE activity is greatly reduced, further prolonging the effects of ACh). Inhibition of AChE by substrate represents a mechanism through which a synaptic response could be exaggerated once previous synaptic activity had resulted in accumulation of ACh. However, because of the great speed with which AChE hydrolyzes ACh, substrate inhibition does not seem a likely mechanism for long-term cholinergic sensitivity changes.

Finally, it is of interest to note that many "specific", purportedly noncholinergic agents used by neuroscientists to affect memory, in fact have potent anticholinesterase properties. This is particularly true of the protein synthesis inhibitors (Moss et al., 1974a; 1974b; Moss and Fahrney, 1976).

AChR Changes

DeRobertis (1971) has suggested that ACh acts by way of phospholipid hydrolase to hydrolyze phosphoinositides. It can therefore change the microenvironment of receptor proteolipids in synaptic pathways which are repeatedly activated. DeRobertis notes that the effect of ACh on phosphoinositides might subserve memory by causing relatively permanent changes in receptors. Over one-third of the brain's phospholipids are phosphoinositides. Additionally, studies with isotopically labeled precursors indicate a high rate of synthesis in brain of inositol-containing phospholipids and gangliosides. The presence of these complex lipids in close association with proteins, and their high metabolic turnover suggests they might play a role in some brain membrane structures, with their rapid metabolism reflecting membrane activity during function (Hawthorne and Kemp, 1964; White *et al.*, 1968).

In addition to a proposed mechanism for increased ACh release after learning (discussed earlier), Kosower (1972) has also proposed postsynaptic mechanisms further augmenting AChR response to increased ACh. An increase in average quantity of transmitter arriving at the postsynaptic membrane over an extended period of time could lead to an increase in the number of receptor sites and an expansion of the postsynaptic receptor region through conversion of receptor monomers into receptor polymers. Indeed, expansion of synapses in response to activity has been reported (Cragg, 1967; Illis, 1969; Schapiro and Vulkovich, 1970).

The possibility that a change in synaptic sensitivity is mediated by a change in aggregation of cholinergic receptors in postsynaptic membranes is supported by ample physiological and biochemical precedent. As thoroughly reviewed by Michelson and Zeimal (1973), the pattern of arrangement of individual acetylcholine receptors in cholinoceptive membranes changes with phylogenetic status of the source animal, its development level, and the functional status of the synapses sampled. In these several experiments, arrangement of ACh receptors has been studied by using cholinomimetics and cholinolytics which have either one or two cationic centers. This strategy follows from the fact that there is one anionic center in each receptor site of each AChR. If cholinoreceptors have a specific and regular arrangement in the membrane, then a compound with two cationic centers a certain distance apart becomes a very powerful agonist or antagonist as compared to compounds having only one cationic site. Were there no specific arrangement, and thus no regular occurrence of AChR anionic centers a certain distance apart, then sensitivity to bis-quaternary compounds should only be slightly greater than that to mono-quaternary compounds. This experimental technique, when applied to cholinoreceptors of various muscles, has demonstrated three primary AChR arrangements: 1) no detectable arrangement, 2) an arrangement wherein anionic centers of cholinoreceptors are approximately 20 Å or 16 carbon atoms apart (C-16 structure), 3) a double arrangement wherein the anionic center of one cholinoreceptor is 20 Å from one neighboring cholinoreceptors, 16 Å from others (C-10 structure), with C-10 predominating (Michelson and Zeimal, 1973). There is also evidence for a C-6 structure in rat and mouse brain (Paton and Zeimis, 1949).

In immaturely born mammals, C-10 structure is not fully formed. The process of C-10 structure formation extends for several days or even weeks after parturition in rats and dogs (Fedorov, 1968; Michelson and Zeimal, 1973). Within mammals there is also evidence that increasingly sophisticated receptor aggregation is associated with increased functional significance, the most obvious example being provided by denervation. After denervation cholinoreceptors in the vicinity of the endplate appear to lose their C-10 structure. The new cholinoreceptors which appear over the entire muscle membrane and which cause denervation sensitivity lack the C-10 structure of a functional endplate (Khromov-Borisov and Michelson, 1966). Denervation reduces the rate of rise of the action potential, reduces its rate of depolarization, and prolongs its duration (Thesleff, 1973). When denervated muscle is reinnervated, cholinoreceptors in the area of the new endplate form C-10 aggregates and other cholinoreceptors on the muscle membrane disappear (Fex *et al.*, 1966; Fex and Thesleff, 1967). Cholinoreceptors in C-10 arrangements respond faster than cholinoreceptors in C-16 or no arrangements (Feltz and Mallart, 1971a, 1971b). The work of Katz and Thesleff (1957) suggests that cholinoreceptors may interact cooperatively; that is, receptors may interact such that binding of an agonist to one receptor makes it more likely that another receptor will become occupied. Such cooperative effects might make an aggregate system of receptors much more responsive than a simple collection of individual receptors. In sum, denervation effects suggest that changes in AChR aggregation subserve relatively permanent changes in cholinergic sensitivity; developmental studies suggest that changes in AChR aggregation may have important functional significance. For a more complete and authoritative review of the literature on AChR aggregation — much of which has previously been available only in Russian — the reader is referred to Michelson and Zeimal's *Acetylcholine: An Approach to its Molecular Mechanism of Action* (1973).

Myasthenia gravis, a disease characterized by extreme muscular weakness, has recently been shown to be due to an autoimmune response toward the body's own nicotinic cholinergic receptors (Lennon, 1977). This condition in some ways serves as a model system for the central effects our behavioral work has posited since it establishes 1) that cholinergic systems can undergo long-term changes in sensitivity, 2) that such changes can be due to changes in postsynaptic sensitivity, and 3) that cholinergic agonists in doses that would produce synaptic blockade in normal subjects prove to have facilitory, therapeutic effects when applied to the deteriorating cholinergic sensitivity of the myasthenic patient.

Heterosynaptic Cholinergic/Catacholaminergic Interactions

Interactions of various neurotransmitters have begun to be explored as possible mechanisms for long-term changes in neural response. Three of the most recent examples involve possible or known interactions of ACh and one or more of the catecholamines.

Long-lasting potentiation of response to cholinergic afferents at frog 10th sympathetic ganglion (Schulman and Weight, 1976) and rabbit superior cervical ganglion (Libet *et al.*, 1975) is induced by prior stimulation of additional, probably noncholinergic afferents converging on the principal ganglion cell. In the work of Libet *et al.*, (1975), such potentiation lasts for the life of the preparation (several hours) and is most likely mediated by a dopamine interneuron. Input to the dopamine interneuron is by way of muscarinic cholinergic innervation. Further, application of cyclic GMP (cGMP) disrupts the phenomenon in a time dependent manner: cGMP administration within minutes of the conditioning stimulation (i.e., output of the dopamine interneuron onto the principal neuron) disrupts subsequent potentiation of the principal neuron response to cholinergic afferents, but later administration of cGMP has no effect. Cyclic GMP is believed to act as a secondary messenger in ganglionic muscarinic cholinergic neurotransmission (Greengard, 1975). Libet et al., (1975) view their ganglion preparation as exhibiting properties necessary to a neural memory substrate including "read-in", "storage", and "read-out" functions. Since both read-in and read-out require cholinergic input (the former by way of a dopamine interneuron), both should show susceptibility to influence by applications of cholinergic agents, whereas storage should not. This is analogous to our behavioral findings wherein applications of cholinergic agents at time of acquisition or recall influence recall performance, but the same agents do not seem to affect memory storage.

Oesch et al., (1975) have presented evidence that nicotinic cholinergic stimulation may regulate dopamine synthesis in certain brain pathways. This induction of new dopamine is long-term, becoming maximal at around 48 hr after nicotinic stimulation (Mueller et al., 1969). The effect is mediated by intranuclear synthesis of new tyrosine hydroxylase, the rate limiting enzyme in dopamine production. Several days may be taken for axonal transport of this new enzyme to presynaptic sites of dopamine synthesis (Oesch et al., 1975). Whether this process would result in long-term increased responsiveness to stimulation or simply represents a means by which adequate supplies of transmitter are maintained over periods of maximum stimulation is an open question.

HUMAN AND ANIMAL AMNESIA

Cholinergic drugs affect the recall of memories as a function of the age of those memories. In the case of memories in the passive avoidance situation such memories last for a considerable portion of the lifespan of the rat. The substrate of such memories also changes as evinced by the changes in latency of response as the memory becomes older and by its changing susceptibility to anticholinesterases. Thus, a number of experiments on the rat support the hypothesis that specialized cholinergic synapses whose conductance increases with time after learning represent an essential component in the memory process.

It is tempting to generalize such ideas to human memory storage. If humans store their memories in a similar manner this would lead to a specific theory of human retrograde amnesia. As we have seen in the rat, anticholinesterases block older memories. On the other hand, such older memories are spared by anticholinergics but more recent ones are blocked. In human retrograde amnesia it is the older memories that are spared. This would lead us to infer that human retrograde amnesia is due to a state of cholinergic insufficiency. If that is the case, treatment with cholinergic agonists should produce a temporary reversal (at least partially) of clinical retrograde amnesia. However, the view that retrograde amnesia is due to cholinergic insufficiency is not without its difficulties.

Squire and Chase (1975) and Squire et al., (1975, 1976) have shown that ECS treatment in patients leads to retrograde amnesia. Further, animal research strongly suggests that electroconvulsive shock (ECS) has its amnesic effect via a change in the cholinergic system. For instance it has been shown that the release of bound acetylcholine as a result of ECS increases the activity of cholinergic neurons (Richter and Crossland, 1969). As a result of the release of such acetylcholine, there may be an induction of the enzyme acetylcholinesterase (Adams et al., 1969). These workers found an elevation in acetylcholinesterase levels after a series of four ECS treatments. Such an elevation did not subside to normal levels unitl 96 hr after treatment. In another experiment using a behavioral assay for memory, they trained rats for 20 trials to avoid footshock when a light appeared. After training, three ECS treatments were administered and the rats were retested four hours later. Half an hour before retest the rats were injected with either physostigmine, scopolamine or saline. While ECS amnesia was not affected by saline, physostigmine enhanced and scopolamine reduced such amnesia.

While the result showing that ECS treatment elevates acetylcholinesterase levels is consistent with the hypothesis that retrograde amnesia is produced by cholinergic insufficiency, the fact that physostigmine enhances ECS amnesia speaks against such an interpretation as does a subsequent study. In this study, Davis et al., (1971) explored the interaction of physostigmine or scopolamine and ECS on the acquisition of a one trial passive avoidance task and its retention, four hours later. When no ECS was given after learning, scopolamine administered before the learning trial produced amnesia. But administered before the retention trial, scopolamine had no amnesic effect. The administration of physostigmine when no ECS was given had an almost opposite effect — almost no amnesia was observed when the drug was given before the training trial but some amnesic effect was found when it was administered before the retention trial. On the other hand, when ECS was administered after the training trial then scopolamine administered before training had little effect in reducing amnesia during retention. But when scopolamine was administered prior to the retention trial amnesia was materially reduced. By way of contrast, physostigmine in the ECS condition administered before the training trial materially reduced amnesia when administered before the learning trial. But physostigmine injected before the retention trial had no seeming effect on recall. While the results of this study are in the main consistent with the belief that cholinergic excitability must be within a certain optimum range for a memory to be retrievable, it would seem that ECS amnesia is due to an excess rather than an insufficiency of acetylcholine. In addition, Wiener (1970) found ECS treatment given before retest analogous to anticholinesterase injection in its effects on recall of memories of different age.

While the literature on ECS in rats gives no clear guide as to what to expect in human retrograde amnesia, there are indications that the cholinergic system is somehow involved in the effects of ECS, and this alone may make it worthwhile to look for a connection in clinical amnesias. Indeed the evidence from experiments on human volunteers is consistent with the notion that the cholinergic system is somehow implicated when material is to be remembered for short intervals of time. For instance, Safer and Allen (1971) and Drachman and Leavitt (1974) found no impairment of a memory span for digits under scopolamine but delayed recall of digits and words was impaired. Ostfeld and Araguete (1962) showed an impairment of performance on several subtests of the Wechsler Memory Scale after scopolamine administration. Ghoneim and Mewaldt (1975, 1977) also report learning deficits after scopolamine injection, which were almost completely antagonized by a further injection of physostigmine. Drachman and Leavitt found that 1 mg of physostigmine injected subcutaneously had no effect on memory. However, Sianska et al., (1972) found physostigmine to improve story recall. Davis et al., (1976) showed a significant decrease in memory span for digits after an intravenous dose of 3 mg.

Based on our findings in animals, several research strategies suggest themselves. First of all, if human clinical amnesias are due to disorders of cholinergic synaptic functioning, then drugs that alter the level of transmission across such synapses should alter the amnesic state. For instance, the suggestion was made above that human amnesia was due to a state of cholinergic insufficiency. Moderate doses of centrally acting anticholinesterases should then produce restoration of some or all of the memory lost to retrieval.

Second, in investigations of cholinergic agents on the memory of human volunteers, the main effects to look for would be on materials learned at various times before the session in which the drug was actually administered, or on materials learned to various degrees of mastery a long time before retest under drug. For instance, a group of subjects could be taught a different list of words or shown different pictures every two weeks for two months before the drug session, with perhaps four sessions during the last two weeks. Tests during the drug session would then be made of the memory for the word lists or pictures. The memory for the material would then be compared to that of controls to see if there were differences based on the age of the memory during retest. Different groups of subjects should be given differing amounts of training. Unfortunately, it is improbable that the intervals found to be useful in the rat studies will be similar to those that can be anticipated in human memory: it would seem likely from human retrograde amnesia observed clinically that rather long time intervals will be involved.

In memory tests with physostigmine it was shown in animal experiments that recall of the same item at closely spaced intervals produced amnesia whereas recall at more widely spaced intervals produced no interference with memory. A similar strategy could be adopted with human volunteers by observing the effects of repetitious recognition of the same items in close succession as compared with such recognition spaced apart in time. The advantage of this research strategy is that learning is allowed to occur in the undrugged state. If learning and retest take place in the drugged state, as in most of the human studies hitherto, the performance of the subject during recall may be due either to a disorder of initial registration or some general performance deficit during recall. If learning occurs in the undrugged state then altered recall cannot be due to a disorder of initial registration. Further, if the results show that the drug blocks or facilitates the recall of the learned material depending on the amount or time of initial learning then a trivializing explanation in terms of some general performance deficit at the time of recall cannot be invoked.

REFERENCES

Adams, H.E., Hobbit, P.R., and Sutker, P.B., 1969, Electroconvulsive shock, brain acetylcholinesterase activity and memory, *Physiol. Behav. 4:*113.

Alpern, M.P., and Marriott, J.G., 1973, Short-term memory: facilitation and disruption with cholinergic agents, *Physiol. Behav. 11:*571.

Aprison, M.H., 1961, On a proposed theory for the mechanism of action of serotonin in brain, *Recent Adv. Biol. Psychiat. 4:*133.

Bacq, S.M., and Brown, G.C., 1937, Pharmacological experiments on mammalian voluntary muscle in relation to the theory of chemical transmission, *J. Physio. 89:*45.

Beani, L., Bianchi, C., Santinoceto, L., and Marchetti, P., 1968, The cerebral acetylcholine release in conscious rabbits with semipermanently unplanted epidural cups, *Int. J. Neuropharmac. 7:*469.

Biederman, G.B., 1970, Forgetting of an operant response: physostigmine-produced increases in escape latency in rats as a function of time of injection, *Q. J. Exp. Psychol. 22:*384.

Biederman, G.B., 1974, The search for the chemistry of memory: recent trends and the logic of investigation in the role of cholinergic and adrenergic transmitters, *Prog. Neurobiol. 2*:289.

Changeux, J.P., 1966, Responses of acetylcholinesterase from Torpedo marmorata to salts and curarizing drugs, *Mol. Pharmacol. 2*:369.

Chorover, S.L., and Schiller, P.H., 1965, Short-term retrograde amnesia in rats, *J. Comp. Physiol. Psychol. 59*:73.

Cohen, L.H., and Hagen, P.B., 1964, A physiological role for the presynaptic localization of acetylcholinesterase and for its inhibition by excess substrate, *Can. J. Physiol. Pharmacol. 42*:593.

Crabbe, J.C., and Alpern, H.P., 1975, Improvement over days after partial training on an appetitive task in mice. Annual Meeting of the Western Psychological Association, Sacramento, California (April, 1975).

Cragg, B.G., 1967, Changes in visual cortex on first exposure of rats to light, *Nature 215*:251.

Davis, J.W., Thomas, R.K., Jr., and Adams, H.E., 1971, Interactions of scopolamine and physostigmine with ECS and one trial learning, *Physiol. Behav. 6*:219.

Davis, K.L., Hollister, L.E., Overall, J., Johnson, A., and Train, K., 1976, Physostigmine: effects on cognition and affect in normal subjects, *Psychopharmacology 51*:23.

Dennis, S.G., 1974, Temporal aspects of scopolamine-induced one-way memory dissociation in mice, *J. Comp. Physiol. Psychol. 86*:1052.

DeRobertis, E., 1971, Molecular biology of synaptic receptors, *Science 171*:963.

Deutsch, J.A., 1966, Substrates of learning and memory, *Dis. Nerv. Syst. 27*:20.

Deutsch, J.A., Hamburg, M.D., and Dahl, H., 1966, Anticholinesterase-induced amnesia and its temporal aspects, *Science 151*:221.

Deutsch, J.A., and Lutzky, H., 1967, Memory enhancement by anticholinesterase as a function of initial learning, *Nature 213*:742.

Drachman, D.A., and Leavitt, J., 1974, Human memory and the cholinergic system, *Arch. Neurol. 30*:113.

Fedorov, V.S., 1968, The potency of mono- and bis-quaternary compounds blocking neuro-muscular transmission in newborn and adult rats and mice, *J. Evol. Biochem. Physiol. 4*:236.

Feltz, A., and Mallart, A., 1971a, An analysis of acetylcholine responses of junctional and extrajunctional receptors of frog muscle fibres, *J. Physiol. 218*:85.

Feltz, A., and Mallart, A., 1971b, Ionic permeability changes induced by some cholinergic agonists on normal and denervated frog muscles, *J. Physiol. 218*:101.

Fex, J., and Thesleff, S., 1967, The time required for innervation of denervated muscles by nerve implants, *Life Sci. 6*:635.

Fex, J., Sonesson, B., Thesleff, S., and Zelena, J., 1966, Nerve implants in botulinum poisoned mammalian muscle, *J. Physiol. 184*:872.

Fox, R.A., and Crabbe, J.C., 1976, Curvilinear retention function for partial escape-avoidance training in hybrid mice at test-retest delay intervals up to 30 days. Annual Meeting of the Western Psychological Association, Los Angeles, California (April, 1976).

Ghoneim, M.M., and Mewaldt, S.P., 1975, Effects of diazepam and scopolamine on storage retrieval, and organizational processes in memory, *Psychopharmacologia 44*:257.

Ghoneim, M.M., and Mewaldt, S.P., 1977, Studies on human memory: the interactions of diazepam, scopolamine and physostigmine, *Psychopharmacology 52*:1.

Greengard, P., 1975, Cyclic nucleotides, protein phosphorylation, and neuronal function, in *"Advances in Cyclic Nucleotide Research"* (G.A. Robison, ed.), pp. 585-602, Raven Press, New York.

Hamburg, M.D., 1967, Retrograde amnesia produced by intraperitoneal injection of physostigmine, *Science 156:*973.

Hawthorne, J.N., and Kemp, P., 1964, The brain phosphoinositides, *Adv. Lipid Res. 2:* 127.

Illis, L.S., 1969, Enlargement of spinal cord synapses after repetitive stimulation of a single posterior root, *Nature 223:*76.

Kandel, E.R., 1976, *"Cellular Basis of Behavior: An Introduction to Behavioral Neurobiology,"* Freeman, San Francisco.

Katz, B., and Thesleff, S., 1957, A study of the "desensitisation" produced by acetylcholine at the motor end plate, *J. Physiol. 138:*63.

Khromov-Borisov, N.V., and Michelson, M.J., 1966, The mutual disposition of cholinoreceptors of locomotor muscles, and the changes in their disposition in the course of evolution, *Pharmacol. Rev. 18:*105.

Kitz, R.J., Braswell, L.M., and Ginsburg, S., 1970, On the question: is acetylcholinesterase an allosteric protein?, *Mol. Pharmacol. 6:*108.

Kosower, E.M., 1972, A molecular basis for learning and memory, *Proc. Natl. Acad. Sci. USA 69:*3292.

Kremzner, L.T., and Wilson, I.B., 1964, A partial characterization of acetylcholinesterase, *Biochemistry 3:*1902.

Leibowitz, S.F., 1967, Doctoral Thesis, New York University.

Lennon, V.A., 1977, Myasthenia gravis: A prototype immunopharmacological disease, International Symposium on Organ-Specific Autoimmunity, Cremona, Italy (June, 1977).

Libet, B., Kobayashi, H., and Tanaka, T., 1975, Synaptic coupling into the production and storage of a neuronal memory trace, *Nature 258:*155.

Loewi, O., 1921, Über humorale Ubertragbarkeit der Herznervenwirkung, *Pfluegers Arch. 189:*239.

McGaugh, J.L., 1966, Time-dependent processes in memory storage, *Science 153:*1351.

Michelson, M.J., and Zeimal, E.V., 1973, *"Acetylcholine: An Approach to the Molecular Mechanism of Action,"* Pergamon Press, New York.

Mooser, G., Schulman, H., and Sigman, D.S., 1972, Fluorescent probes of acetylcholinesterase, *Biochemistry 11:*1595.

Moss, D.E., and Fahrney, D., 1976, Anisomycin, acetoxycycloheximide, cycloheximide, and puromycin as inhibitors of rat brain acetylcholinesterase *in vitro, J. Neurochem. 26:*1155.

Moss, D.E., and Rogers, J.B., 1975, Effect of cobra neurotoxin on retention of a brightness discrimination in rats, *Pharmacol. Biochem. Behav. 3:*1147.

Moss, D.E., Moss, D.R., and Fahrney, D., 1974a, Puromycin as an inhibitor of rat brain acetylcholinesterase, *Pharmacol. Biochem. Behav. 2:*271.

Moss, D.R., Moss, D.E., and Fahrney, D., 1974b, Puromycin as an inhibitor of acetylcholinesterase, *Biochem. Biophys. Acta 350:*95.

Mueller, R.A., Thoenen, H., and Axelrod, J., 1969, Increase in tyrosine hydroxylase after reserpine administration, *J. Pharmacol. Exp. Ther. 169:*74.

Oesch, F., Otten, U., Mueller, R.A., Goodman, R., and Thoenen, H., 1975, In *"Golgi Centennial Symposium Proceedings"* (M. Santini, ed.), Raven Press, New York.

Ostfeld, A.M., and Araguete, A., 1962, Central and peripheral effects of muscarinic cholinergic agents in man, *Anesthesiology 28:*568.

Paton, W.D.M., and Zeimis, E.J., 1949, The pharmacological action of polymethylenebistrimetylammonium salts, *Br. J. Pharmacol. 4:*381.

Pepeu, G., 1973, The release of acetylcholine from the brain: an approach to the study of the central cholinergic mechanisms, *Prog. Neurobiol. 2:*259.

Pepeu, G., and Bartolini, A., 1968, Effect of psychoactive drugs on the output of acetylcholine from the cerebral cortex of the cat, *Eur. J. Pharmacol. 4:*254.

Pepeu, G., Garau, L., and Mulas, M.L., 1974, Does 5-hydroxytryptamine influence cholinergic mechanisms in the central nervous system? *Adv. Biochem. Psychopharmacol. 10:*247.

Puerto, A., Molina, F., Rogers, J.B., and Moss, D.E., 1976, Physostigmine induced amnesia for an escape response 12 to 72 hours after training, *Behav. Biol. 16:*85.

Richter, D., and Crossland, J., 1969, Variation in acetylcholine content of the brain physiological state, *Am. J. Physiol. 159:*247.

Rozanova, V.D., 1968, Maturation of function of the neuro-muscular synapse in ontogenesis, *J. Physiol. USSR 54:*313.

Safer, D.J., and Allen, R.P., 1971, The central effects of scopolamine in man, *Biol. Psychiatry 3:*347.

Schapiro, S., and Vulkovich, K.R., 1970, Early experience effects upon cortical dendrites: a proposed model for development, *Science 167:*292.

Schulman, J., and Weight, F.F., 1976, Synaptic transmission: long-lasting potentiation by a postsynaptic mechanism, *Science 194:*1437.

Shopsin, B., Janowsky, D., and Davis, J., 1975, Rebound phenomena in manic patients following physostigmine: preliminary observations, *Neuropsychobiology 1:*180.

Sianska, J., Vojtechovsky, M., and Votova, Z., 1972, The influence of physostigmine on individual phases of learning in man, *Activ. Nerv. 14:*110.

Signorelli, A., 1976, Influence of physostigmine upon consolidation of memory in mice, *J. Comp. Physiol. Psychol. 99:*658.

Squire, L.R., 1970, Physostigmine: effects on retention at different times after brief training, *Psychonomic Sci. 19:*49.

Squire, L.R., and Chase, P.M., 1975, Memory functions six to nine months after electroconvulsive therapy, *Arch. Gen. Psychiatry 32:*1557.

Squire, L.R., and Miller, P.L., 1974, Diminution in anterograde amnesia following electroconvulsive therapy, *Br. J. Psychiatry 125:*490.

Squire, L.R., Slater, P.C., and Chase, P.M., 1975, Retrograde amnesia: temporal gradient in very long-term memory following electroconvulsive therapy, *Science 187:*77.

Squire, L.R., Slater, P.C., and Chase, P.M., 1976, Anterograde amnesia following electroconvulsive therapy: no evidence for state dependent learning, *Behav. Biol. 17:*31.

Stanes, M.D., Brown, C.P., and Singer, G., 1976, Effect of physostigmine on Y-maze discrimination retention in the rat, *Psychopharmacologia 46:*269.

Thesleff, S., 1973, Functional properties of receptors in striated muscle, in *"Drug Receptors"* (H.P. Rang, ed.), pp. 121-133, University Park Press, Baltimore.

White, A., Handler, P., and Smith, E.L., 1968, *"Principles of Biochemistry, Fourth Edition"*, McGraw-Hill, New York.

Wiener, N.I., 1970, Electroconvulsive shock induced impairment and enhancement of a learned escape response, *Physiol. Behav. 5:*971.

Wiener, N.I., and Deutsch, J.A., 1968, Temporal aspects of anticholinergic and anticholinesterase induced amnesia for an appetitive habit, *J. Comp. Physiol. Psychol. 66:*613.

BRAIN ACETYLCHOLINE AND DISORDERS OF MEMORY

K. L. Davis[1,2] and J. A. Yesavage[1,2]

[1] Veterans Administration Hospital, 3801 Miranda Avenue,
Palo Alto, California 94304

[2] Department of Psychiatry and Behavioral Sciences, Stanford University
School of Medicine, Stanford, California 94305

INTRODUCTION

There is neurochemical and pharmacological evidence linking changes in brain cholinergic function with aging and changes in memory function. This data has clear implications for the treatment of senile dementia and age related cognitive deficits. This paper reviews this data and discusses its implications.

NEUROCHEMICAL STUDIES

Human Studies

There are several reports of age related changes in central cholinergic enzymes. Choline acetyltransferase (CAT) and acetylcholinesterase (AChE) activities have been measured in several different brain areas from patients dying of non-neurological causes or sudden death (McGeer and McGeer, 1976). A reduction of up to 66% was found in CAT activity as subjects' age approached 50 years (MGeer and McGeer, 1976). The largest changes in CAT activity were found in the amygdala and septal areas. Although the extrapyramidal system has an extensive cholinergic innervation, CAT activity in this area was little affected. CAT activity in subjects between age 63 and 98 has also been measured (Bowen et al., 1976). Interestingly CAT activity does not appear to decrease over these years. This is in marked contrast to the younger subjects (McGeer and McGeer, 1976).

AChE activity has been determined in subjects between 20 and 50 years of age. With increasing age there is a trend toward diminishing AChE activity. However, this decrement is not as consistent as that reported for CAT. Furthermore, the physiological significance of a decrement in AChE activity is less certain than it is for CAT. CAT has been regarded as a marker for cholinergic neurons (Kuhar, 1976). AChE can be found in noncholinergic neurons. Furthermore, AChE exists in both a membrane bound and soluble form (Hickey *et al.*, 1976). The two states may have different roles. Therefore, although CAT depletion indicates a loss of cholinergic neurons, no similar conclusion can be drawn regarding AChE.

Patients with Alzheimer's disease have changes in CAT activity that may be an exaggeration of the age related alterations found in normal elderly people. Four separate studies by independent groups of investigators have found a significant reduction in CAT activity in brains of patients with Alzheimer's disease compared to age matched controls dying of non-neurological causes (Davies and Maloney, 1976; Perry *et al.*, 1977; White *et al.*, 1977; Reisine *et al.*, in press). The areas of greatest depletion are the caudate, putamen, frontal cortex and hippocampus. Behavioral correlates of cortical and hippocampal lesions make the cholinergic losses in these areas particularly relevant to the cognitive abnormalities of patients with Alzheimer's disease. The possibility that these neuronal changes are specific to cholinergic neurotransmission is suggested by the absence of any change in glutamic acid decarboxylase, tyrosine hydroxylase, monoamine oxidase, L-aromatic acid decarboxylase and dopamine β-hydroxylase (Davies and Maloney, 1976; Reisine *et al.*, in press).

Recent advances in neurochemical techniques have made possible the measurement of the post synaptic muscarinic receptor (Yamamura and Snyder, 1974). Determination of the status of this receptor has obvious implications for rational treatment of both age related deficits in cognition and Alzheimer's disease. In a population without neurological or psychiatric disease, no decrease in muscarinic receptor binding was found with increasing age from 65 to 95 (White *et al.*, 1977). Three investigations of muscarinic receptor binding in patients with senile dementia or Alzheimer's disease have been conducted (Perry *et al.*, 1977; White *et al.*, 1977; Reisine *et al.*, in press). The results of these studies differ. Muscarinic receptor binding in the caudate, parietal cortex and frontal cortex were not found to significantly differ from normal age matched controls in two studies (Perry *et al.*, 1977; White *et al.*, 1977). It is not clear whether these studies directly assessed muscarinic receptor binding in the hippocampus. In the one study that unambiguously measured hippocampal muscarinic receptor binding, a significant reduction in receptor binding was found for this brain area in patients with Alzheimer's disease (Reisine *et al.*, in press). A reduction in muscarinic receptor binding in the caudate, putamen and frontal cortex was also seen, although this did not reach statistically significant levels. These discrepant results may reflect differences in assay technique. However, another possibility is that the degree of decreased muscarinic receptor binding varies extensively from patient to patient. If there is diminished muscarinic receptor binding in patients with senile dementia and Alzheimer's disease this would be analogous to the neurochemical condition of patients with Huntington's disease in which there is both diminished CAT and muscarinic receptor binding in the corpus striatum (Enna *et al.*, 1976).

Animal Studies

A number of studies report that with increasing age there is a loss in CAT activity in both rats and chickens (Hollander and Barrows, 1968; Vernadakis, 1973; Meek *et al.*, 1977). As is true in humans, the areas of greatest loss are the caudate and cortex. No consistent relationship between AChE and age has been found (Hollander and Barrows, 1968; Vernadakis, 1973). A simultaneous increase in AChE and decrease in CAT might account for the report that despite these enzyme changes, brain acetylcholine (ACh) concentration was unchanged (Meek *et al.*, 1977). Rat brain monoamine oxidase activity is reported to increase with age. Thus, in the rat, as in man changes in CAT activity do not reflect a non-specific phenomena.

PHARMACOLOGICAL STUDIES

Human Studies

Evidence is growing that drugs which decrease central cholinergic activity worsen the ability of normal subjects to store information in long-term memory (LTM), and cholinomimetics improve this aspect of LTM functioning (Ostfeld and Araguete, 1962; Soukapova *et al.*, 1970; Crow and Grove-White, 1971; Hrbek *et al.*, 1971; Dundee and Pandit, 1972; Hrbek *et al.*, 1974; Davis *et al.*, 1978; Sitaram *et al.*, 1978). The effects of cholinergic agents on memory function are extremely sensitive to dose. Thus, although a low dose of physostigmine improves LTM functioning, a high dose significantly impairs both LTM and short-term memory (STM) (Davis *et al.*, 1976; Davis *et al.*, 1978). Similarly a low dose of atropine or scopolamine selectively impairs LTM, but a larger dose also causes an impairment of STM (Safer and Allen, 1971; Drachman and Leavitt, 1974).

The deficit that a dose of 1 mg of scopolamine, given subcutaneously, produced in normal young subjects was compared to the memory loss seen in elderly individuals (Drachman and Leavitt, 1974). The supraspan digit test, a procedure that assesses the ability of a subject to store new information into LTM, was most affected by scopolamine. Scopolamine produced a deficit in LTM in young normal subjects that was almost identical to the performance on the supraspan digit test by elderly control subjects. The scopolamine-induced memory loss was found to be a specific cholinergic deficit. It was reversible by physostigmine, but unaffected by amphetamine (Drachman, 1977). On the basis of these results, and the large cholinergic contribution to the hippocampus, it was suggested that an abnormality in cholinergic activity underlies the age related memory loss observed in the elderly. Therefore, elderly subjects were given 0.8 mg of physostigmine intravenously in the hope of improving their LTM. A trend toward increased ability to store information in LTM was found, but this effect was not statistically significant (Drachman, 1976). The lack of significance could be attributable to the small number of patients studied, and a large standard deviation in their scores. However, it may also reflect the variable extent that post-synaptic cholinergic receptor degeneration might be present in the elderly population. Clearly the absence of the cholinergic receptor would negate the action of physostigmine, which increases acetylcholine levels.

Consequently the most likely group of subjects to demonstrate a cholinomimetic facilitation of LTM function would be young people. Both low doses of arecoline, a muscarinic agonist, and physostigmine have been demonstrated to improve a subject's ability to transfer information from STM to LTM (Davis *et al.*, 1978; Sitaram *et al.*, 1978). Since arecoline and physostigmine increase cholinergic activity by different mechanisms, the concordance of these two findings is strong support that increasing cholinergic activity can positively affect LTM.

The possibility that cholinomimetics might be used therapeutically in some memory disorders is supported by a case report of a young patient with a post-encephalitic memory loss. A double blind study was conducted in which the patient received either 0.8 mg of physostigmine subcutaneously or a saline control (Peters and Levin, 1977). On all three trials when this dose of physostigmine was administered, there was a marked improvement of all aspects of LTM. In contrast, placebo or other doses of physostigmine were ineffective.

Animal Studies

A large and confusing animal literature describes the effects of altered cholinergic activity on memory. The data from a few studies on the effects of AChE inhibition is presented in Table 1. Although this data is open to many interpretations, some important points have been made. Pretreatment with agents that block muscarinic cholinergic activity impairs passive avoidance learning (Buresova *et al.*, 1964; Meyers *et al.*, 1964; Meyers, 1965; Bohdanecky and Jarvick, 1967; Ilyutchenok, 1968). It has been asserted that normal cholinergic transmission is a prerequisite for passive avoidance conditioning (Carlton, 1963; Carlton, 1968; Carlton, 1969; Carlton and Markiewicz, 1973). Small doses of cholinesterase inhibitors appear to facilitate acquisition of maze learning, while larger doses may decrease the speed at which animals learn to traverse the maze (Deutsch, 1973; Cox and Tye, 1974). There are no effects of either large or small dosages of cholinesterase inhibitors on maze learning immediately after training (Deutsch, 1973; Cox and Tye, 1974). However, physostigmine in large doses (0.4 mg/kg) inhibited maze learned behavior 2 or 5 days after the learning trial (Deutsch, 1973; Signorelli, 1976). In one study inhibition was still found 14 days after training, but another study found facilitation 11 days after training (Deutsch, 1973; Signorelli, 1976). Part of these contradictory results may be due to different learning paradigms, or to the possibility that physostigmine may have more effect on rats which are "slow" rather than "fast" learners (Cox and Tye, 1974). Further complications arise from the use of different dosages of different cholinomimetics and different learning paradigms across groups: the results are not exactly the same for diisopropylfluorophosphate (DFP) and physostigmine nor are they exactly the same in approach versus avoidance paradigms.

Anticholinergic agents generally inhibit maze learning in rats (Hingten and Aprison, 1976). These results have also been confirmed in a paradigm dependent upon appetite or nociception (Van der Poel, 1972). These findings are consistent with the human studies that have found anticholinergic agents to impair LTM. Numerous methodological problems limit the usefulness of these studies. Cholinergic manipulation affects appetitive behavior, nociception and even locomotor activity (Karczmar, 1976). Thus, results attributing a change in memory to an alteration in cholinergic activity may be reporting an artifact of the effect of cholinergic activity on another aspect of behavior. For this reason with the exception that cholinergic agents can profoundly affect the outcome of T-maze studies, operant behavior paradigms or avoidance tasks, little else can be concluded.

DISCUSSION

Behavioral studies leave a clear impression that the storage or acquisition of new information into LTM can be altered by drugs that either increase or decrease cholinergic

TABLE 1

Diisopropylfluorophosphate (DFP) and Physostigmine Effects on T Maze

					Time After Training						
	-30 min.	1	3	4	5	7	12	14	21	28	35
Avoidance											
Signorelli (1975)			− (.4)				+ (.4)				
Deutsch (1973)			+ 0 (.4)(.4) +' 0 DFP DFP		− (.4) 0 DFP	− (.4) − DFP		− (.4) − DFP		+ DFP	
Deutsch (1973)			+ + DFP DFP		− DFP		+ DFP		+ DFP		
Approach											
Cox & Tye (1973) Slow & fast learners		0 (.1) 0 (.2)		− (.1) 0 (.2)		− (.1) 0 (.2)		0 (.1) 0 (.2)		0 (.1) 0 (.2)	
Slow learner		0 (.1)		+ (.05-.1) 0 (.2)		0 (.05) 0 (.2)					+ (.05) 0 (.2)

Continued

TABLE 1 (CONTINUED)

Diisopropylfluorophosphate (DFP) and Physostigmine Effects on T Maze

Approach		Time After Training									
		-30 min. 1	3	4	5	7	12	14	21	28	35
	Fast learner	0 (.1)		(.05-.1) 0 (.2)		0 (.05) - (.2)					0 (.05) + (.2)
Stanes & Brown (1976)	Effect acquisition	+ (.02-.06) (.1)	0 (.02-.06) 0 (.1)								

Dose Physostigmine in Mg/kg

0 no effect of drug
+ improvement with drug
- decrement with drug

activity. When these results are coupled with neurochemical data that there are age related changes in CAT activity, a hypothesis relating hippocampal cholinergic alteration and memory dysfunction in the elderly becomes apparent. However, as in all such hypotheses, it is no doubt oversimplified. A number of considerations add complexity to the relationship between memory and cholinergic activity.

There is only a limited dose range in which an increasing or decreasing cholinergic activity improves or worsens the storage process of LTM. Furthermore, animal studies indicate that the time between learning and the administration of a cholinergic agent is also crucial to the effect of manipulating cholinergic activity on memory. Pharmacological studies in humans indicating a cholinergic link to LTM are based on young normal subjects. The extent to which these findings are applicable to the geriatric population is unclear. Specifically, if patients with Alzheimer's disease have a loss of post synaptic cholinergic receptors, treatment with cholinomimetics will not yield the same effect on LTM as it does in normal subjects.

Thus, a number of studies are needed to clarify these issues. Correlating the extent of LTM impairment around the time of death with the degree of CAT activity and muscarinic receptor binding would be extremely valuable. Determination of the incidence of muscarinic receptor loss in both Alzheimer's disease and age related cognitive changes is also indicated. Obviously, the behavioral effects in the geriatric population of a wide spectrum of possible cholinomimetics including physostigmine, arecoline, choline chloride and possibly oxotremorine should be investigated. Finally, consideration should be given to the possibility that only subgroups of patients with a loss in memory function will respond to cholinomimetics. Consequently statistical techniques seeking significant differences between all control and all experimental subjects can be misleading.

In summary, studies from divergent disciplines have led to a consensus that there is a relationship between central cholinergic activity and LTM. Future research may lead to the therapeutic exploitation of this relationship.

ACKNOWLEDGEMENTS

This research was supported in part by the Medical Research Service of the Veterans Administration, the National Institute of Mental Health Specialized Research Center grant MH-30854, and the Kate Pande Memorial Research Fund.

REFERENCES

Bohdanechy, Z., and Jarvick, M.E., 1967, Impairment of one trial passive avoidance learning in mice by scopolamine, scopolamine methylbromide and physostigmine, *Int. J. Neuropharmacol.* 6:217.

Bowen, D.M., Smith, C.B., White, P., and Davison, A.N., 1976, Neurotransmitter-related enzymes and indices of hypoxia in senile dementia and other abiotrophies, *Brain 99:* 459.

Buresova, O., Bures, J., Bohdanechy, Z., and Weiss, T., 1964, The effect of atropine on learning extinction, retention and retrieval in rats, *Psychopharmacologia 5:*255.

Carlton, P.L., 1963, Cholinergic mechanisms in the control of behavior by the brain, *Psychol. Rev. 70:*19.

Carlton, P.L., 1968, Brain acetylcholine and habituation, *Prog. Brain Res. 28:*48.

Carlton, P.L., 1969, Brain acetylcholine and inhibition, in *"Reinforcement and Behavior"* (J.T. Tapp, ed.), pp. 286-327, Academic Press, New York.

Carlton, P.L., and Markiewicz, B., 1973, Behavioral effects of atropine and scopolamine, in *"Pharmacological and Biophysical Agents and Behavior"* (E. Furchtgott, ed.), pp. 345-373, Academic Press, New York.

Cox, T., and Tye, N., 1974, Effects of physostigmine on the maintenance of discriminator behavior in rats, *Neuropharmacology 13:*205.

Crow, T.J., and Grove-White, I.G., 1971, Differential effect of atropine and hyoscine on human learning capacity, *Br. J. Pharm. 43:*464.

Davies, P., and Maloney, A.J.F., 1976, Selective loss of central cholinergic neurons in Alzheimer's disease (a letter), *Lancet 2:*1403.

Davis, K.L., Hollister, L.E., Overall, J., Johnson, A., and Train, E., 1976, Physostigmine: Effects on cognition and affect in normal subjects, *Psychopharmacology 51:*23.

Davis, K.L., Mohs, R., Tinklenberg, J.R., Pfefferbaum, A., Hollister, L.E., and Kopell, B.S., 1978, Physostigmine: Improvement of long-term memory processes in normal humans, *Science 201:*272.

Deutsch, J.A., 1973, The cholinergic synapse and the site of memory, in *"The Physiological Basis of Memory"* (J.S. Deutsch, ed.), pp. 59-78, Academic Press, New York.

Drachman, D., 1976, Memory and cholinergic function, in *"Neurotransmitter Function"* (W.S. Fields ed.), pp. 353-372, Stratton Intercontinental Medical Book Corporation, New York.

Drachman, D.A., 1977, Memory and cognitive function in man: Does the cholinergic system have a specific role? *Neurology 27:*783.

Drachman, D.A., and Leavitt, J., 1974, Human memory and the cholinergic system, *Arch. Neurol. 30:*113.

Dundee, J.W., and Pandit, S.K., 1972, Anterograde amnesic effects of pethidine hyoscine and diazepam in adults, *Br. J. Pharmacol. 44:*140.

Enna, S.J., Bird, E.D., Bennett, J.P., Bylund, D.B., Yamamura, H.I., and Iversen, L.L., 1976, Huntington's chorea: Changes in neurotransmitter receptors in the brain, *N. Engl. J. Med. 294:*24:1305.

Hickey, S.W., Ansell, G.B., Mitchell, K., and Pearce, G.W., 1976, Subcellular fractions of normal human substantia nigra and caudate nucleus: A study of their morphology and some enzymes including glutamate decarboxylase and choline acetyltransferase, *J. Neurochem. 27:*957.

Hingten, J.N., and Aprison, M.H., 1976, Behavioral and environmental aspects of the cholinergic system, in *"Biology of Cholinergic Function"* (A.M. Goldberg and I. Hanin, eds.), pp. 515, Raven Press, New York.

Hollander, J., and Barrows, C.H., 1968, Enzymatic studies in senscent rodent brains, *J. Gerontol 23:*174.

Hrbek, J., Komenda, S., and Macakova, J., 1974, The effect of scopolamine (0.6 mg) and physostigmine (1.0 mg) on higher nervous activity in man followed up during five hours after application, *Activ. Nerv. Sup. (Praha) 16:*213.

Hrbek, J., Komenda, S., and Siroka, A., 1971, On the interaction of scopolamine and physostigmine in man, *Activ. Nerv. Sup. (Praha) 13:*200.

Ilyutchenok, R.Y., 1968, Cholinergic brain mechanisms and behavior, in *"Progress in Brain Research. Vol 28: Anticholinergic Drugs and Brain Function in Animals and Man"* (P.B. Bradley and M. Fink, eds.), pp. 134, Elsevier, Amsterdam.

Karczmar, A., 1976, Central actions of acetylcholine cholinomimetics and related drugs, in *"Biology of Cholinergic Function"* (A.M. Goldberg and I. Hanin, eds.), pp. 395, Raven Press, New York.

Kuhar, M.J., 1976, The anatomy of cholinergic neurons, in *"Biology of Cholinergic Function"* (A.M. Goldberg and I. Hanin, eds.), pp. 3027, Raven Press, New York.

McGeer, E., and McGeer, P.L., 1976, Age changes in the human for some enzymes associated with metabolism of catecholamines, GABA, and acetylcholine, in *"Neurobiology of Aging"* (J.M. Ordee and R.R. Brizee, eds.), pp. 389, Raven Press, New York.

Meek, J.L., Bertilsson, L., Cheney, D.L., Zsilla, G., and Costa, E., 1977, Aging-induced changes in acetylcholine and serotonin content of discreet brain nuclei, *J. Gerontol. 32:*129.

Meyers, B., 1965, Some effects of scopolamine on passive avoidance response in rats, *Psychopharmacologia 8:*111.

Meyers, B., Roberts, K.R., Riciputi, R.H., and Domino, E.F., 1964, Some effects of muscarinic cholinergic blocking drugs on behavior and the electrocorticogram. *Psychopharmacologia 5:*289.

Ostfeld, A.M., and Araguete, A., 1962, Central nervous system effects of hyoscine in man, *J. Pharmacol. Exp. Ther. 137:*133.

Perry, E.K., Perry, R.H., Blessed, G., and Tomlinson, B.E., 1977, Necropsy evidence of central cholinergic deficits in senile dementia, *Lancet 1:*189.

Peters, B.H., and Levin, H.S., 1977, Memory enhancement after physostigmine treatment in the amnesic syndrome, *Arch. Neurol. 34(4):*215.

Reisine, T.D., Yamamura, H.I., Bird, E.D., Spokes, E., and Enna, S.J., (in press), Pre- and post synaptic neurochemical alterations in Alzheimer's disease, *Brain Res.*

Safer, D.J., and Allen, R.P., 1971, The central effects of scopolamine in man, *Biol. Psychiatry 3:*347.

Signorelli, A., 1976, Influence of physostigmine upon consolidation of memory in mice, *J. Comp. Physiol. Psychol. 90:*658.

Sitaram, N., Weingartner, H., and Gillin, J.C., 1978, Human serial learning: Enhancement with arecoline and impairment with scopolamine correlated with performance on placebo, *Science 201:*274.

Soukupova, B., Vojtechovsky, M., and Safratova, V., 1970, Drugs influencing the cholinergic system and the process of learning and memory in man, *Activ. Nerv. Sup. (Praha) 12:*91.

Van der Poel, A.M., 1972, Centrally acting cholinolytics and the choice behavior of the rat, *Prog. Brain Res. 36:*127.

Vernadakis, A., 1973, Comparative studies of neurotransmitter substances in the maturing and aging central nervous system of the chicken. *Prog. Brain Res. 40:*231.

White, P., Hiley, C.R., Goodhardt, M.J., Carrasco, L.H., Keet, J.P., Williams, I.E.I., Bowen, D.M., 1977, Neocortical cholinergic neurons in elderly people, *Lancet 1:*668.

Yamamura, H.I., Snyder, S.U., 1974, Muscarinic cholinergic binding in rat brain, *Proc. Natl. Acad. Sci. USA 71:*1725.

CARBOHYDRATES AND ACETYLCHOLINE SYNTHESIS: IMPLICATIONS FOR COGNITIVE DISORDERS

J. P. Blass and G. E. Gibson

Department of Neurology, Division of Chronic and Degenerative Disease, Cornell University Medical College and Dementia Research Center, Burke Rehabilitation Center, White Plains, New York 10605

INTRODUCTION

The hypothesis put forward in this chapter is based on correlations of an experimental finding with a set of clinical, a set of pharmacological, and a set of chemical pathological observations. The experimental finding is that even minimal impairment of glucose oxidation by the brain leads to a proportional impairment of the synthesis of the neurotransmitter acetylcholine (ACh). The clinical observations are that even mild impairment of cerebral carbohydrate oxidation impairs mentation and specifically cognitive function. The pharmacological observations are that even low doses of drugs which impair cholinergic function (such as atropine and scopolamine) impair mental function, leading to impairments of cognitive abilities very similar to those seen in early senility. The chemical pathological finding is recent evidence of a specific loss of cholinergic cells in senile dementia. Put together, these sets of observations suggest that impairment of cholinergic function in the brain has an important role in the cognitive dysfunction which characteristically accompanies impairment of cerebral carbohydrate oxidation. These observations also suggest that chronic low-grade hypoxia or vascular insufficiency can selectively damage cholinergic cells in the brain and contribute in some elderly people to the development of so called "senile dementia." These hypotheses are of great potential importance clinically, since conditions in which the supply of oxygen and/or glucose to the brain are impaired are among the major causes of neuropsychiatric disability in the U.S. today (Adams and Victor, 1977). On the other hand, there is no direct evidence linking these sets of data to each other. In the following discussion, each set of observations is described in turn, and then the hypothesis linking them and its experimental and clinical implications are discussed.

LINKAGE OF ACETYLCHOLINE SYNTHESIS TO CARBOHYDRATE OXIDATION

In the 1940's, Ochoa and Nachmansohn and their coworkers demonstrated that the neurotransmitter ACh was made from the condensation of acetyl-coenzyme A with choline (Nachmansohn, 1959), and it was recognized that the normal source of this acetyl-coenzyme A was from the oxidation of pyruvate derived from glucose by glycolysis (Quastel *et al.*, 1936; Harpur and Quastel, 1949). Subsequent work by Cheng, Tucek, Nakamura and their coworkers indicated that pyruvate or compounds which gave rise to pyruvate such as lactate or glucose were far and away the most efficient precursors of the acetyl moiety of ACh, *in vivo* (Tucek and Cheng, 1974) and *in vitro* (Nakamura *et al.*, 1970). The ketone bodies acetoacetate and β-hydroxybutyrate also proved to be efficient precursors of ACh in the brains of very young but not adult animals (Itoh and Quastel, 1970). Normally less than 1% of the glucose or ketone body which was oxidized was incorporated into the acetyl moiety of ACh. While it was generally accepted that some oxidative metabolism was necessary to sustain the synthesis of ACh, it seemed unlikely that anything less than very severe impairment of carbohydrate catabolism would alter the rate of ACh synthesis.

However, during the course of studies of the effects on the brain of inborn errors of pyruvate oxidation, we discovered that even mild impairment of carbohydrate oxidation in the brain led to a proportional fall in the synthesis of ACh, despite a 100 to 200 fold difference in the fluxes to CO_2 and to ACh (Gibson *et al.*, 1975; Blass and Gibson, 1978).

In Vitro Studies

This relationship was first demonstrated in brain slices from adult rats (Figure 1). It was evident with all methods of inhibiting pyruvate oxidation (Gibson *et al.*, 1975): with 3-bromopyruvate, a noncompetitive inhibitor of pyruvate dehydrogenase, the enzyme which produces acetyl-coenzyme A and CoA from pyruvate (Maldonado *et al.*, 1972); with 2-ketobutyrate, a competitive inhibitor of pyruvate dehydrogenase (Blass and Lewis, 1973); with other 2-keto-acids, which probably inhibit pyruvate oxidation indirectly by their effects on the further oxidation of acetyl-coenzyme A (Gibson and Blass, 1976a); and with barbiturates, which appear to inhibit pyruvate oxidation secondary to their effects on the electron transport chain (Gibson *et al.*, 1975).

The close linkage between carbohydrate oxidation and ACh synthesis also held when brain slices were incubated with glucose as substrate instead of pyruvate (Gibson and Blass, 1976b). It was seen with all inhibitors of glucose oxidation tested, including lowering the concentrations of oxygen or glucose in the incubation flask, or adding cyanide (which inhibits cytochrome oxidase), as well as with the inhibitors of pyruvate oxidation listed above. With either glucose or pyruvate as substrates, the close relationship between carbohydrate oxidation and ACh synthesis was evident whether one followed the synthesis of ACh by measuring the incorporation of radioactive precursors or by measuring the mass of ACh by gas-liquid-chromatography-mass-spectrometry (Gibson *et al.*, 1975; Gibson and Blass, 1976b).

The linkage between oxidative metabolism and ACh synthesis was also seen when the substrate was a ketone body, 3-hydroxybutyric acid (Gibson and Blass, in press). In these experiments, slices from both weanling and adult animals were studied, since it is well established that the brains of young animals utilize ketone bodies more effectively than do the brains of adults (Itoh and Quastel, 1970). These experiments were complicated

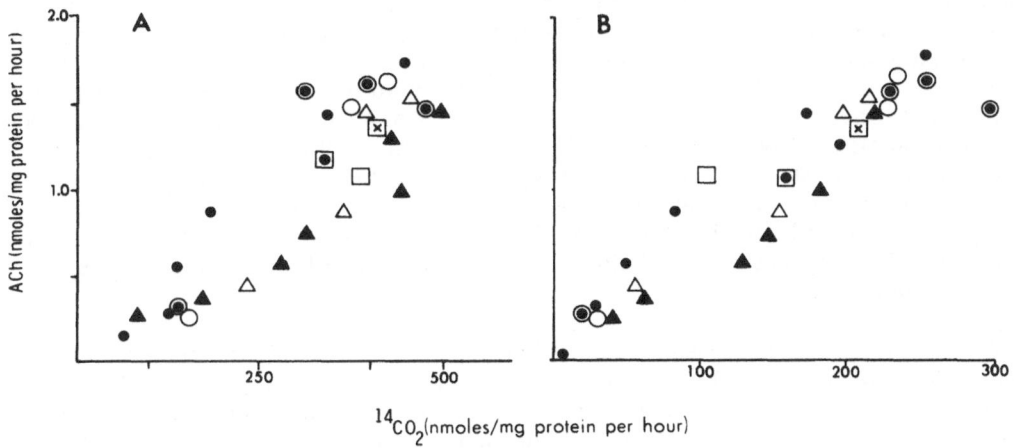

FIGURE 1

Proportional Inhibition of Pyruvate Oxidation and Acetylcholine Synthesis.

Rat brain slices were incubated with $[1\text{-}^{14}C]$ pyruvate (A) or $[2\text{-}^{14}C]$ pyruvate (B) and the production of $^{14}CO_2$ and of ACh determined, as described in detail by Gibson *et al.* (1975). Each value is the mean of at least two experiments done in triplicate. Inhibitors were: 5 mM-leucine (⊠); 5 mM-2-oxo-3-methylpentanoic acid (□); 5 mM-2-oxo-3-methyl-butanoate (◙); 0.05, 0.2, and 1.0 mM-pentobarbital (○) 1, 5, and 20 mM-2-oxo-4-methylpentanoate (△); 0.1, 0.2, 0.3, 0.4, 0.5, and 1.0 mM-3-bromo-pyruvate (●); 1.0, 5.0, and 20.0 mM-2-oxo-butyrate (▲); and 0.05, 0.2, and 1.0 mM-amobarbital (◉). Reprinted by permission of the editors of the *Biochemical Journal.*

by the fact that maximal utilization of ketone bodies by brain slices requires the presence of glucose as cosubstrate. These studies demonstrated that reducing the oxidation of glucose by adding 3-hydroxybutyrate led to a proportional fall in the synthesis of ACh from glucose. Inhibiting the oxidation of 3-hydroxybutyrate (with methylmalonic acid, an inhibitor of 3-hydroxybutyrate dehydrogenase) led to a proportional fall in the synthesis of ACh from this ketone body. These effects occurred although the total oxidation of either glucose or 3-hydroxybutyrate was one to two orders of magnitude greater than the incorporation of either precursor into ACh. These effects were seen at physiological concentrations of these normal substrates, and therefore are not seen only with artificial inhibitors.

In Vivo Studies

The close linkage between carbohydrate oxidation and ACh synthesis also exists *in vivo* (Gibson and Blass, 1976c). In these studies carbohydrate oxidation was impaired in the brains of rats or mice *in vivo* in any of several ways. The concentration of glucose was reduced by making the animals hypoglycemic with large doses of insulin (Ferrendelli and Chang, 1973). Oxygen utilization was impaired by treating animals with potassium cyanide ("histotoxic hypoxia"). The oxygen-carrying capacity of the blood was reduced by injecting animals with sodium nitrite, which oxidizes hemoglobin to methemoglobin and induces a reversible "anemic hypoxia." In these studies, animals were sacrificed by microwave irradiation to the head, and the synthesis of ACh was followed by measuring the incorporation of deuterated choline into ACh using gas-liquid-chromatography-mass-spectrometry. In all three conditions (hypoglycemia, histotoxic hypoxia, and anemic hypoxia) there was a dose-related fall in the synthesis of ACh. The effects of reducing oxygen tension could not be studied in this system, since the geometry of the microwave apparatus did not allow manipulation of the composition of the air which the experimental animals breathed.

Recent studies have demonstrated that impaired ACh synthesis accompanies even very mild hypoxia, so mild that it does not alter the levels of compounds such as lactic acid or AMP whose concentrations are sensitive indicators of hypoxia (Gibson et al., in press b). In these experiments, a double-label technique was used to measure the synthesis of ACh in the brains of adult mice. The mildest conditions of (anemic) hypoxia studied led to a drop in the incorporation of [U-^{14}C] glucose (but not of [^{2}H$_4$] choline) into ACh (Table 1). There was an associated doubling of the concentration of cyclic GMP [probably due in part to stimulation of guanylate cyclase by the NO$_2$- ion (Kimura et al., 1975)], but the concentration of cyclic AMP did not change. More severe hypoxia led to a decrease in the incorporation of both [U-^{14}C] glucose and [^{2}H$_4$] choline into ACh and ultimately to a drop in the level of ACh.

Physiological Significance

The decrease in ACh synthesis which accompanies impaired carbohydrate oxidation appears to be functionally significant. When mice were pretreated with physostigmine (eserine — a cholinesterase inhibitor and cholinergic agonist) before the induction of hypoglycemia with insulin (Gibson and Blass, 1976c), the physostigmine treatment reduced the number of mice dying (from 14 of 40 to 3 of 40, $P < .005$ by χ^2 test). The effect was not on absorption of insulin, since the levels of blood glucose were identical in the insulin-physostigmine and insulin-alone groups. Physostigmine also delayed the onset of seizures and death in animals with histotoxic or anemic hypoxia. Again, the effect did not appear to be on absorption of sodium nitrite or of the potassium cyanide (Gibson and Blass, 1976c). These effects of physostigmine are particularly notable because a fall in the total amount of ACh in the brain was only detected with very severe impairments of carbohydrate catabolism. Taken together, these observations suggest that the decrease in ACh synthesis which accompanies impaired carbohydrate oxidation reflects a decrease in a small, rapidly turning-over, but functionally very significant pool of cerebral ACh. The existence of such pools is supported by work by many others. A large body of evidence supports the existence of "bound" and "free" forms of ACh in nervous tissues (Barker, 1976). Jenden et al., (1974) found kinetic evidence during turnover studies for fast and slowly turning-over pools of cerebral ACh. Molenaar and Polak (1976) reported that the specific activity of ACh released into the media bathing tissue slices was higher than the specific activity of ACh remaining in the slices when radioactive glucose was the substrate, but not with radioactive pyruvate, which agrees with our inference that glucose labels a physiologically important pool of ACh more effectively than does pyruvate.

TABLE 1

Effect of Minimal Hypoxia on Cerebral Acetylcholine, Cyclic Nucleotides, and Other Metabolites

Metabolite	Control	Hypoxic	
		(75 mg NaNO2/kg)	(150 mg NaNO2/kg)
$[14_C]$-Acetylcholine (dpm/nanomol)	180 ± 17	103 ± 25**	57 ± 8**
$[^2H_4]$-Acetylcholine (picomol/mg protein)	6.3 ± 0.4	7.1 ± 0.5	3.0 ± 0.2**
Total Acetylcholine (picomol/mg protein)	196 ± 7	211 ± 9	179 ± 15
Cyclic GMP (picomol/mg protein)	0.68 ± 0.005	1.23 ± 0.20*	1.17 ± 0.12*
Cyclic AMP (picomol/mg protein)	10.6 ± 0.6	8.5 ± 1.6	8.8 ± 1.3
ATP (nanomol/mg protein)	24.8 ± 0.5	25.1 ± 0.3	23.9 ± 0.4
AMP (nanomol/mg protein)	0.53 ± 0.06	0.62 ± 0.07	0.74 ± 0.07
Lactate (nanomol/mg protein)	11.7 ± 0.7	11.6 ± 0.5	16.3 ± 4.4

Values are the mean $\pm$ SEM for at least 6 mice in each group. Cyclic nucleotides were measured by radioimmunoassay; ATP, AMP, and lactate enzymatically; and ACh and its labelled derivatives by a combination of gas-liquid-chromatographic-mass spectrometric, radiochemical, and enzymatic methods. Animals were sacrificed by focused microwave irradiation to the head, except for the measurement of ATP and AMP, which was done on animals immersed in liquid N_2. Details of the procedures and values at other levels of hypoxia and for other metabolites are in Gibson and Blass (1976c) and Gibson et al. (1978b). *, $P < 0.01$ vs. controls; **, $P < 0.001$ vs. controls.

The close relationship between carbohydrate oxidation and ACh metabolism has been confirmed in synaptosomes by Jope and Jenden (1977) and by Barker *et al.* (1978).

Mechanisms

Direct studies of the mechanisms linking ACh synthesis to carbohydrate oxidation (despite the gross disparity of fluxes) has demonstrated compartmentation of glucose metabolism with respect to ACh synthesis and thus supports the existence of metabolic pools related to ACh (Gibson *et al.*, in press a). The pathway from glucose to ACh is known to be (in outline):

$$\text{glucose} \longrightarrow \text{pyruvate} \longrightarrow \text{acetyl-coenzyme A} \longrightarrow \text{ACh}$$

Mice were injected with [U-^{14}C] glucose, sacrificed at appropriate intervals, the whole brains extracted, and the specific activity determined for cerebral glucose, pyruvate and the acetyl moiety of ACh (Figure 2). (Specific activities were calculated in DPM/ nanoatom, to allow for the decreasing number of carbon atoms in each of these compounds.) The specific activity of glucose fell exponentially, as expected. The specific activity of ACh rose until it equalled that of cerebral glucose and then fell along with that of glucose, in a typical precursor-product relationship. By contrast, the specific activity of pyruvate never rose as high as that of either glucose or acetylcholine. This observation (higher specific activity in a product than in its known precursor) fulfills the classical criteria for demonstration of compartmentation of metabolism (Berl *et al.*, 1975). Apparently there are at least two compartments of pyruvate in the brain (Figure 3). The smaller compartment or pool is associated with cholinergic structures and is earmarked for ACh synthesis. The larger pool is not associated with cholinergic structures. The two pools mix relatively slowly, if at all, but both are effectively labelled by exogenous glucose. The inhibitors we studied happen to affect pyruvate oxidation equally in both pools, leading to a proportionality between the impairment of CO_2 production (derived largely from the second, large pool) and acetylcholine synthesis (derived from the first, small pool). Compartmentation of glucose metabolism with respect to ACh synthesis provides a simple and attractive explanation for the close linkage of ACh synthesis and carbohydrate oxidation (Blass and Gibson, 1978).

The intimate molecular mechanism linking oxidation and ACh synthesis has been studied (Gibson and Blass, 1976b). ACh synthesis was inhibited *in vivo* and *in vitro* by reducing the supply or utilization of oxygen or the supply of glucose. A variety of potential regulatory parameters were measured. There was no relation between the concentrations of [ATP], [ADP], [AMP], or the adenylate energy charge potential and the synthesis of ACh. Indeed, these parameters did not change at all under most of the experimental conditions examined. The cytoplasmic and mitochondrial [NADH] / [NAD$^+$] ratios were also determined, from the concentrations of the components of the [lactate] / [pyruvate] couple and of the [NH$_3$] [2-ketoglutarate] / [glutamate] couple, using the methods and assumptions of Krebs and coworkers (Miller *et al.*, 1973; Wilson *et al.*, 1974). There was a good correlation between the cytoplasmic [NADH] /[NAD$^+$] ratio and the rate of ACh synthesis *in vivo* but not *in vitro* (Gibson and Blass, 1976b; 1976c). The only parameter which correlated well with the rate of ACh synthesis *in vitro* as well as *in vivo* was the transmitochondrial [NADH] / [NAD$^+$] potential in volts. It was calculated from the [NADH] / [NAD$^+$] ratios using the Nernst equation (Gibson

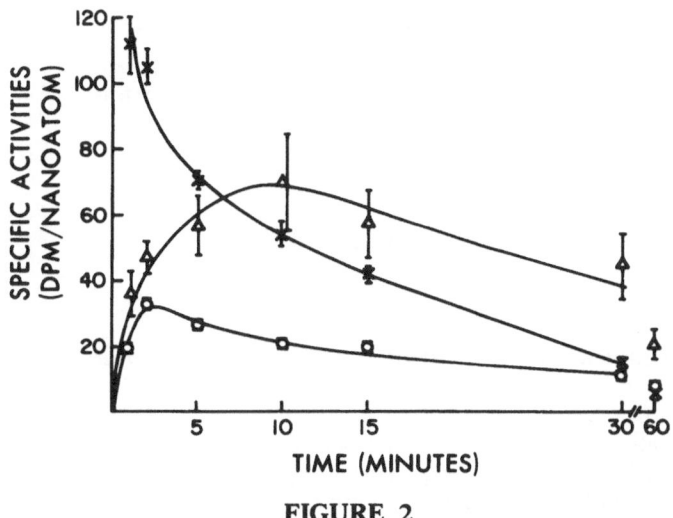

FIGURE 2

Relations Among Specific Activities of Glucose, Pyruvate, and Acetylcholine in Mouse Brains *In Vivo.*

Adult mice were injected intravenously with $[U\text{-}^{14}C]$ glucose, and the specific activities (in dpm/nanoatom) of glucose, of pyruvate, and of the acetyl moiety of ACh were determined by a combination of enzymatic and radiochemical techniques. Details of the methods are described in Gibson *et al.* (1978a). Each point represents the mean for at least 10 animals except the value at 60 min which is for 4 animals. Error bars represent S.E.M.

and Blass, 1976b; 1976c). This value for the transmitochondrial [NADH] / [NAD$^+$] potential is roughly equal to the value for the transmitochondrial [H$^+$] potential, as it should be, since H$^+$ ion participates in the NAD$^+$-NADH equilibrium (Mitchell, 1968). It is now widely accepted that transmitochondrial potentials have an important role in critical biological processes such as oxidative phosphorylation and transport of intermediates between the mitochondria and the cytoplasm. It is tempting to speculate that transmitochondrial potentials might prove to be important regulatory parameters in intermediary metabolism.

Indirect support for the role of [H$^+$] potentials in mediating the effects of hypoxia on cerebral acetylcholine is provided by experiments in which mice were treated with the buffer ion THAM (Figure 4). Pretreatment of mice with alkaline THAM (pH 10.3) significantly delayed the loss of sighting reflex in animals with anemic hypoxia (from 21 ± 1 to 27 ± 2 min, p < .01) and markedly reduced the proportion of animals who lost their sighting reflex from histotoxic hypoxia (from 10 of 12 to 2 of 12, p < .01). Pretreatment with alkaline THAM also ameliorated the changes in cerebral ACh and cyclic GMP (Figure 4). Pretreatment with THAM at an acidic pH (pH 4.5) was without effect. THAM is a well known buffer ion, called in biochemistry tris (or formally tris (hydroxymethyl)aminomethane). It is known to enter cells. Since it was effective at

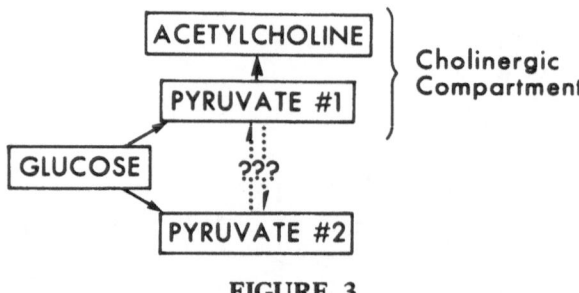

FIGURE 3

Scheme of Compartmentation of Glucose and Pyruvate with Respect to Acetylcholine Synthesis.

The scheme indicates that there are at least two metabolic pools of pyruvate in the brain. Glucose is the precursor of both pools. The first pyruvate pool, in cholinergic structures, is involved in ACh synthesis, while the second pool, in non-cholinergic structures, is not. The pools mix slowly if at all, so what happens to the second and presumably larger pool has little direct effect on ACh synthesis. The inhibitors listed in the legend to Figure 1 appear to affect the oxidation of pyruvate in both pools. The experiments of Nakamura *et al.* (1970) and Tucek and Cheng (1974) suggest that exogenous acetate mixes readily with the acetyl-Co A produced from pyruvate oxidation in the second pool but not the first.

alkaline but not at acid pH, its effects appear to be mediated by changes in intracellular H^+ ion concentrations. These observations also suggest that treatment with THAM or with an analogous compound might prove to benefit patients suffering from chronic mild cerebral hypoxia (Gibson *et al.*, 1977), which may be a major cause of dementia in aging (see Anticholinergic Agents section, below).

Relevance

The importance of this linkage for the control of ACh synthesis in normal and pathological states has been the subject of some discussion. Several lines of evidence support the proposal that the rate of acetylcholine synthesis is normally determined by the principles of mass action (Browning, 1976). The synthetic enzyme, CAT, is present in excess, and the components of the synthetic reaction appear to be present in the cholinergic nerve terminal at or very near equilibrium. There is an important, high-affinity system for the uptake of choline into cholinergic nerve endings where ACh synthesis takes place (Barker, 1976). The rate of ACh synthesis may normally be determined by changes in the ratio of choline to ACh in the cholinergic nerve endings (Browning, 1976; Barker, 1976; Jope and Jenden, 1977). On the other hand, under pathological conditions, impairments of carbohydrate oxidation can apparently reduce acetylcholine synthesis by reducing the supply of acetyl-coenzyme A.

These observations raise the question of whether the clinical and pathological effects of impaired cerebral carbohydrate catabolism can be correlated with the known

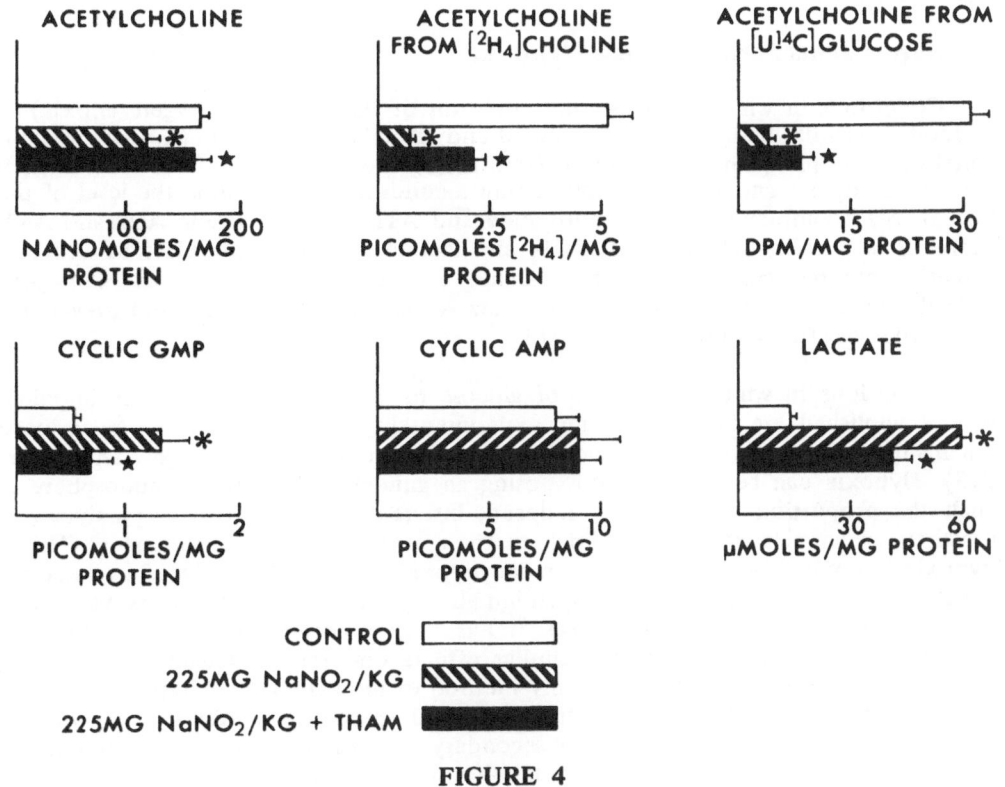

FIGURE 4

Effect of Alkaline THAM on Brain Metabolism in Anemic Hypoxia.

Adult mice were sacrificed by microwave irradiation 20 min after the injection of $NaNO_2$ and 1 min after the injection of a mixture of $[U-^{14}C]$ glucose and $[^2H_4]$ choline. THAM or an equivalent volume of isotonic saline was injected 30 min before the induction of hypoxia. Error bars represent SEM. *, $P < 0.01$ vs. controls; ★, $P < 0.01$ vs. animals treated with $NaNO_2$ without prior treatment with THAM.

effects of pharmacological or pathological states of cholinergic deficiency. The rest of this discussion deals with such states and the possible correlations among them.

HYPOXIA, HYPOGLYCEMIA, AND RELATED CONDITIONS

The effects of even mild hypoxia on acetylcholine synthesis are of particular interest because of the sensitivity of the nervous system to even mild hypoxia. The extreme dependence of the central nervous system on a continuing supply of oxygen and glucose has been recognized for decades (McIlwain and Bachelard, 1971). However, it is only within the last fifteen years that a profound difference has been recognized to exist between conditions in which carbohydrate oxidation is completely abolished and conditions in which it is only midly to moderately reduced.

Experimental Studies

Complete Versus Partial Graded Hypoxia

Conditions in which there is total abolition of the supply of oxygen (*an*oxia) or of blood (*oli*gemia) have been much studied and are relatively easy to approach experimentally, ie, by plunging an animal into 100% nitrogen or by cutting off its head. Experimentally, complete anoxia or oligemia within seconds leads to a fall in the level of the "high-energy" compounds creatine-phosphate and ATP and to a rise in ADP and AMP (Duffy *et al.*, 1972; Cohen, 1973). NH_3 and lactate rise promptly, pH falls and biosynthetic activities cease. Irreversible damage ensues, with cell death and autolysis. Clinically, unconsciousness follows even a few seconds of total anoxia, and irreversible damage follows after 4-6 min (Cohen, 1973).

Conditions in which the supply of glucose or oxygen to the brain are impaired but not abolished are harder to study experimentally. Hypoglycemia can be induced with insulin or so called "hypoglycins" such as 5-pentenoic acid (Glasgow and Chase, 1975). Hypoxia can be induced by exposing an animal to an artificial atmosphere in which the proportion of oxygen is reduced, but requires ventilation of paralyzed or anaesthetized animals or placing animals in the appropriately gassed containers. This is "hypoxic hypoxia." As noted above, graded hypoxia can also be induced by injecting animals with agents such as cyanide which impair oxygen utilization (histotoxic hypoxia) or oxygen transport (anemic hypoxia). It has been reported that chemical hypoxia induced with carbon monoxide has similar effects on brain metabolism to hypoxic hypoxia (MacMillan, 1977). However, any method of inducing graded hypoxia or hypoglycemia is relatively difficult to control compared to complete anoxia or oligemia, in part because in the steady state there are secondary changes in pCO_2 and in body temperature which themselves affect cerebral metabolism (Siesjo and Plum, 1971).

Biochemical Affects of Graded Hypoxia

Nevertheless, it has been well established that mild to moderate hypoxia or hypoglycemia can profoundly impair brain function without any change at all in the concentration of [ATP] or in the adenylate energy charge potential in the brain (Siesjo and Plum, 1971). This point has been demonstrated in at least eight laboratories (Gurdjian *et al.*, 1944; Albaum *et al.*, 1953; Schmahl *et al.*, 1966; Duffy *et al.*, 1972; Ferrendelli and Chang, 1973; Norberg and Siesjo, 1975; Yatsu *et al.*, 1975; Gibson and Blass, 1976c) including ours (Gibson and Blass, 1976c) and documented in great detail by Siesjo and his collaborators in Lund (MacMillan *et al.*, 1974; Siesjo *et al.*, 1974; Norberg and Siesjo, 1975). They have demonstrated that in lightly anaesthetized, artificially ventilated animals, lowering the tension of inspired oxygen to levels which severely alter the EEG does not alter the concentration of [ATP] or the energy charge (Siesjo *et al.*, 1974). Siesjo claims that the measurements are so accurate that if there is a small pool of cerebral ATP which is reduced, it could not reflect more than 1 - 2% of the total in the brain. This degree of hypoxia is associated with a rise in brain lactate, a fall in pH, and a 20% drop in phosphocreatine. The fall in phosphocreatine has been attributed to the fall in pH, since the equilibrium reaction:

$$ATP + creatine \rightleftharpoons ADP + phosphocreatine$$

is pH dependent. Hypoxia of this degree does, however, impair the synthesis of a physiologically important pool of ACh, as noted above.

Physiological Effects of Graded Hypoxia

Physiological studies have also demonstrated the sensitivity of cholinergic transmission to hypoxia or hypoglycemia. In extensive studies of the superior cervical ganglion, Dolivo (1974) has demonstrated that removing oxygen or glucose from the bathing medium severely impairs the response to transsynaptic transmission across the cholinergic synapse while the response of axonal conduction to direct stimulation remains intact. The loss of transmission is a presynaptic rather than a postsynaptic effect, since addition of exogenous ACh restores the response. The loss of transmission is associated with a loss of presynaptic vescicles which contain ACh. Similar results were obtained by Perri *et al.* (1970) who used thiamine deficiency to impair carbohydrate catabolism. They studied rats at the early stage of deficiency, after the onset of weight loss but before the appearance of neurological abnormalities. The only abnormality they detected in the deficient ganglia was a defective response to rapid repetitive but not slow stimulation. They interpreted this deficiency as secondary to an impairment of the capacity for rapid resynthesis of ACh, secondary to the impairment of pyruvate oxidation induced by thiamine deficiency. Studies in the central nervous system are less precise, but it is an electrophysiologist's cliche that polysynaptic transmission is more sensitive to minimal hypoxia than is direct conduction (Cohen, 1973).

Clinical Studies of Impaired Carbohydrate Oxidation

Clinical Effects of Graded Hypoxia

Graded hypoxia was studied in great detail particularly in the 1930s and 1940s when it became apparent that a major limitation on the performance of warplanes in World War II would be the potential effects of hypoxia on the pilots and crews. As hypoxia increases, the first physiological alteration which has been described is delayed dark adaptation, which occurs when the percentage of oxygen in the air is reduced from 20% to 18% at sea level (Siesjo *et al.*, 1974). (The drop in oxygen tension is equivalent to ascending to about 4000 ft.) At these or slightly lower oxygen tensions there is a loss of judgment which is hard to quantify but which has, for instance, taken the form of a pilot indulging in inappropriate aerial acrobatics which endangered him and others in his formation (McFarland, 1932; Collier, 1947). When oxygen is reduced to 15% of inspired air (equivalent to about 8000 ft.) there is a well documented reduction in ability to carry out a complex task (Cohen, 1973; Siesjo *et al.*, 1974). At 13% oxygen, short-term memory is impaired. Below 10% there is severe loss of judgment, and below 8% unconsciousness ensues. It is important to note the analogies between changes in mental function with hypoxia and those which occur in impaired ACh function and aging, as discussed below.

Clinical Effects of Hypoglycemia

Hypoglycemia can also lead to impairments of memory and judgment, although personality changes and other psychiatric abnormalities are generally more prominent (Himwich, 1951; Sourkes, 1962). The neuropsychiatric abnormalities which have been associated with hypoglycemia are immensely varied. They range from irritability, lack of concentration, and poor judgement to frank coma. These reactions are typically episodic and transient when the hypoglycemia is episodic and transient, as with an insulin-secreting tumor. Criteria for the diagnosis of hypoglycemia have been put forward by a joint committee of the Diabetes Association, the Endocrine Society, and the American Medical Association (Ad hoc committee on hypoglycemia, 1973). Unfortunately, these criteria are ignored among certain groups for whom hypoglycemia has become an "in" diagnosis, often based on what may be normal variations in the 5 or 6 hr glucose tolerance test, and subsequently attached to a wide variety of anxiety states and other neurasthenic syndromes. However, the fad for this diagnosis should not obscure the real occurrence of clinically significant hypoglycemia.

Inhibitors of Cerebral Carbohydrate Oxidation

Inhibitors of cerebral carbohydrate oxidation have also been studied clinically in some detail. Some of them act directly and others indirectly. Carbon monoxide displaces oxygen from red cell hemoglobin and leads in effect to anemic hypoxia. Severe poisoning can cause stupor, coma, and death. Somewhat milder poisoning characteristically causes severe and permanent brain damage. Any of an immense variety of neurological sequelae can occur. Mild carbon monoxide poisoning leads to a loss of judgment and control similar to that in dementia. For instance, the chief inspector of mines for Great Britain became poisoned by carbon monoxide while inspecting a mine disaster, and although he knew he was in danger sat down in the area contaminated with carbon monoxide to write farewell notes in which he misspelled the word "good-bye" (Slater and Roth, 1969).

Cyanide, which inhibits the enzyme cytochrome oxidase and impairs oxygen utilization on a cellular level, can lead to rapid loss of consciousness and death (Slater and Roth, 1969). Chronic low-level cyanide poisoning has been reported to be the cause of a spinocerebellar degeneration in Nigeria. Several of the patients with this syndrome studied by Osuntokun (1969) had "slow cerebration" and impaired memory, and one patient had a paranoid psychosis. The neuropsychiatric characteristics of these patients were not studied in great detail, in part because tests of intelligence and personality have not been well standardized for the rural African population involved.

A number of other neurotoxins, such as heavy metals (Slater and Roth, 1969) and a number of nutritional deficiencies, notably thiamine deficiency (Williams et al., 1943), impair mental function and also have as one of their metabolic effects impairment of cerebral carbohydrate metabolism. They also have a number of other effects on cerebral metabolism, and the relation between their effects on behavior and their effects on carbohydrate catabolism is a subject for research.

Inborn Errors of Carbohydrate Catabolism

Inborn errors of carbohydrate catabolism have been described during the last ten years, by us and others (Blass et al., 1976, in press). These have typically been associated with severe mental deficiency, generally presenting in early childhood. Recently milder deficiencies of the same enzymes have been reported in about a third of the patients who present with the syndrome of Friedreich's ataxia or other spinocerebellar disorders (Blass et al., 1976). It is of interest that Sjogren (1943) reported that 2/3 of his large series of Swedish patients with spinocerebellar ataxias developed progressive clinically significant dementia. He concluded that there was a similar high incidence of dementia in patients described in the literature, who had their disorder for more than 20 years. Davies (1949a) reported that low intelligence occurred in 20% or more of a series of English patients with Friedreich's ataxia, and a somewhat smaller proportion had an affective or thought disorder (Davies, 1949b). More recently Barbeau *et al.* (1976) have reported a verbal I.Q. of 82 in four patients with Friedreich's ataxia and deficient pyruvate oxidation, and a verbal I.Q. of 114 in four patients with the same syndrome but normal pyruvate oxidation.

Summary

In summary, hypoxic hypoxia, hypoglycemia, poisons which impair cerebral carbohydrate oxidation, and inherited disorders of carbohydrate catabolism, all impair cerebral function. In their milder forms, they lead to a clinical pattern of dementia with loss of judgment and memory and deterioration of personality.

ANTICHOLINERGIC AGENTS

The idea that impairment of cholinergic systems by mild hypoxia may relate to the impairment of cognitive functions which accompanies mild hypoxia is in accord with the known effects of centrally-active anticholinergic agents. The effects of anticholinergic agents have been well documented. They are described in standard textbooks of pharmacology and medicine (Innes and Nickerson, 1965; Koch-Weser, 1974). Low doses of anticholinergic agents which cross the blood-brain barrier impair memory and judgment. This effect is exploited in standard preoperative medication, which typically includes scopolamine to impair memory of the operation, as well as for the peripheral effects of this drug on reducing secretions. Larger doses of centrally active anticholinergic agents can induce toxic delerium or psychosis, which often has paranoid features and has prompted hospitalization for "schizophrenia" (Koch-Weser, 1974). The combination of peripheral and central anticholinergic actions typically leads to the "cherry-red psychosis" characteristic of poisoning with the belladonna alkaloids atropine or scopolamine.

Drachman and Leavitt (1974) have reported that the effects of a low dose of scopolamine (1 mg) are particularly great on memory storage and resemble the effects of normal aging. They studied 23 students aged 18 to 26. Scopolamine caused a marked impairment of memory storage, as revealed by significant falls in both the digit storage index (from 100 to 73, $p < .05$) and the free recall word storage index (from 100 to 49, $p < .001$). Methylscopolamine, an anticholinergic agent which does not cross the blood-brain barrier, did not alter either the digit storage index (98) or the word storage index (93). There was also an effect on retrieval and on general intelligence, with mean full-scale WAIS I.Q. falling from 118.8 to 106.5 ($p < .001$). With methylscopolamine, which does not cross into the brain, the value was 122.1. Scopolamine had no effect on immediate memory; single trial digit span test scores were 7.2 for control subjects and 6.8 for scopolamine-treated subjects. The pattern of defects in young people treated with scopolamine was strikingly similar to that in aged subjects. The effects of scopolamine were antagonized by the cholinesterase inhibitor physostigmine but not by amphetamine, which acts on adrenergic systems and increases alertness (Drachman and Leavitt, 1975; Drachman, 1977). Drachman (1977) has reviewed the literature on the role of cholinergic transmission in memory functions in humans and animals. He has put forward the view that cholinergic systems have a relatively specific role in memory, due both to the role of acetylcholine in the hippocampus and to the plasticity of cholinergic synapses.

The neuropsychiatric effects of cholinergic agonists and antagonists are reviewed in detail elsewhere in this volume. However, it is important for the purposes of this chapter to note that pharmacologic evidence supports a critical role of cholinergic systems in cognitive function. Even mild impairment of cholinergic function leads to mental changes similar to those seen in "dementias."

HYPOXIA AND CHOLINERGIC FUNCTION IN DEMENTIA

Impairment of mentation is a characteristic result of impaired oxidative metabolism by the brain at any age (Richardson et al., 1959). Hypoxia and related conditions in neonates are a major cause of mental retardation (Adams and Victor, 1977). Dementia often follows hypoxia in young adults, sometimes after an interval of apparently normal function (Plum et al., 1962). The relationship of senile dementia to chronic, low grade impairment of cerebral oxidative metabolism is controversial but is of particular importance for the purposes of this discussion, because of the recent work of Davison and his coworkers implicating a selective failure of cholinergic systems in some patients with this condition (Bowen et al., 1976).

Carbohydrate Oxidation in Senile Dementia

The relationship of impaired carbohydrate catabolism to aging in the brain and specifically to senile dementia and Alzheimer's disease has been a subject of discussion for decades (Freyhan et al., 1951; Arab, 1954; Lassen et al., 1957; Sokoloff, 1966). Two points in this debate are now generally accepted. First, although many elderly people suffer from both atherosclerosis of the large cerebral vessels and from neurofibrillary cerebral degeneration of the Alzheimer type, these appear to be independent processes (Arab, 1954). Clinically, the stepwise degenerative course of multi-infarct dementia associated with atherosclerosis can be distinguished from the relentless progress of Alzheimer's disease (Brizzee, 1975). The incidence of either of these conditions at autopsy is not influenced by the occurrence of the other (Arab, 1954). Secondly, the cerebral metabolic rate (CMR_{O_2}) is abnormally low in patients with senile dementia (or arteriosclerotic dementia). The fall is related to disease rather than simply to age. Sokoloff (1966) reported that CMR_{O_2} (ml O_2/100 gm brain per min) was 3.5 ± 0.2 for elderly subjects with no symptomatic atherosclerosis, and 2.7 ± 0.2 for patients with chronic brain syndrome. In patients with presenile dementia CMR_{O_2} was 2.4 (Butler, 1966). Lassen et al. (1957) found a good correlation between mental function in demented patients and CMR_{O_2} in the left (dominant) hemisphere but not the right. For instance, the correlation between performance on the picture arrangement test was +0.77 with the left hemisphere CMR_{O_2} and -0.13 with right hemisphere CMR_{O_2}. Ingvar and Gustafson (1970) found some evidence for a correlation between dementia and a regional decrease in cerebral blood flow and presumably in oxidative metabolism in temporal areas which may be associated with memory. It should be stressed that CMR_{O_2} is a measure of oxygen utilization per unit brain, so that decreases in it cannot be attributed simply to reductions in the size of the brain due to nonselective atrophy. There is a definite reduction in cerebral oxygen utilization accompanying senile dementia.

The mechanisms leading to the fall in oxygen utilization and the significance of that decrease are less clear. Lassen *et al.* (1960) proposed that the fall reflects a selective loss of neurones, which have a higher rate of oxidative metabolism than do the glia which replace them. By contrast, Freyhan, Woodford and Kety (1951) proposed that "senile psychoses are . . . probably the result of a significant reduction in cerebral oxygen utilization," and suggested that the reduction in oxygen utilization is secondary to an increase in cerebral vascular resistance. Angiopathy of the microvasculature is a very frequent although not constant finding in patients with Alzheimer's disease, occurring in upwards of 75% of carefully studied cases (Klassen *et al.*, 1968; Miyakawa *et al.*, 1974; Brizzee, 1975; Mandybur, 1975; Lang and Carlo, 1975). It has been proposed that the degenerative changes and perhaps even senile plaques (Hassler, 1965; Miyakawa *et al.*, 1974; Brizzee, 1975; Ordy and Kaack, 1975; Brizzee *et al.*, 1975) may be due to such "angiopathic dysphorique" (Arab, 1954). Histochemical and electronmicroscopic studies have shown high levels of mitochondria and mitochondrial enzymes in senile plaques (Friede and Magee, 1962; Friede, 1965; Brizzee, 1975), and Friede and Magee (1962) suggested that "degeneration of plaques probably results from a disproportion between metabolism . . . [and blood] supply." Gottfries *et al.* (1974) found elevated levels of lactate and elevated lactate/pyruvate ratios in the CSF of 6 of 15 demented patients, indicating hypoxia of cerebral tissue in these patients. The degree of dementia was proportional to the increase in lactate and therefore to the degree of hypoxia. Suzuki *et al.* (1965) reported that brain slices from a biopsy of a patient with Alzheimer's disease had a Q_{O_2} of 8.9 *versus* 11.1 for slices from a 30 year old control studied under identical conditions. Comparison with literature values were difficult, since in most other studies of slices of human brain the incubation media did not contain the high concentrations of potassium ion which Suzuki *et al.* (1965) used to stimulate respiration. Unfortunately, none of these experiments can determine to what extent the decrease in oxidative metabolism which accompanies senile dementia is a cause rather than a consequence of the condition.

Loss of Cholinergic Neurones in Senile Dementia

Recent studies have implicated a selective loss of cholinergic neurones in senile dementia. In an exhaustive study of 56 brains removed at autopsy, Bowen *et al.* (1976) found that the degree of morphological senile change correlated with reductions in the activity of CAT, which is localized to, and therefore an excellent marker of, cholinergic cells (McGeer and McGeer, 1975). They found no decrease in the high affinity binding of cholinergic agonists indicating that postsynaptic structures were not affected (White *et al.*, 1977). The decrease in CAT activity was marked: from 67 ± 9 pmol/min per mg protein for controls (mean ± SEM), to 28 ± 6 in patients with senile dementia. Others have found similar results (Davies and Maloney, 1976; Perry *et al.*, 1977). The activity of CAT seemed relatively unaffected by agonal changes, but it does decrease in cortex with aging (McGeer and McGeer, 1975). The decreases in CAT in senile dementia have led to the suggestion that senile dementia is an abiotrophy of cholinergic systems (Bowen *et al.*, 1976) and to the suggestion that treatment with cholinergic agonists might be of benefit (Perry *et al.*, 1977; Ferris *et al.*, 1977; White *et al.*, 1977). Preliminary trials with cholinergic agonists have been inconclusive (Boyd *et al.*, 1977; Ferris *et al.*, 1977). Spillane *et al.* (1977) have put forward the view that even histologically-proven senile dementia is a heterogeneous condition, and that it is important to develop techniques to detect those patients who are deficient in cholinergic structures during life.

Summary

It has been suggested that the loss of cholinergic cells in senile dementia represents "brain failure" secondary to circulatory failure (Anonymous editorial, 1977). This suggestion fits with the sensitivity of acetylcholine synthesis to conditions which impair carbohydrate oxidation. Whether or not chronic, low grade hypoxia leads to permanent loss of cholinergic neurones has not yet been tested by direct experimentation. Such studies are clearly in order.

CONCLUSION

Relationships Between Impairments of Oxidation, Acetylcholine Synthesis and Cognitive Function

Several lines of data indicate that there is an interrelationship among impaired cerebral carbohydrate catabolism, impaired cholinergic function, and cognitive deficiencies. Experimentally, acetylcholine synthesis in animals has been shown to be exquisitely sensitive to conditions which impair carbohydrate oxidation. Cognitive deficiencies, particularly of judgment and memory, accompany even mild deficiencies of cerebral carbohydrate oxidation or treatment with even low doses of anticholinergics in man. The deficiencies in judgment and memory are similar in detail to those which occur in aging and particularly in the earlier stages of senile dementia. There is direct evidence for impaired carbohydrate oxidation and for impaired cholinergic function in the brains of patients with senile dementia. It is tempting to speculate that damage to cholinergic systems due to chronic, low-grade hypoxia is a common mechanism in many common disorders including senile dementia.

Other Neurotransmitters

Although this discussion has focused on acetylcholine, there is evidence that the metabolism of other neurotransmitters is also sensitive to even mild impairment of oxidative metabolism. The hydroxylases which synthesize catecholamines have a Km for oxygen close to the physiological pO_2 in the brain. Davis and Carlson (1973) have reported that the rate of synthesis of catecholamines is reduced by even mild reductions in the supply of oxygen to the brain. However, the increased turnover of catecholamines which accompanies stress is not inhibited by mild hypoxia (Davis, 1976). Impairing cerebral carbohydrate oxidation also alters the metabolism of the amino acids which interact with the Krebs tricarboxylic acid cycle and which may be neurotransmitters (Clarke et al., 1970; Cheng et al., 1972; Lust et al., 1975). Hypoxia may have particularly important effects on GABA metabolism (Bowen et al., 1976). Glutamate decarboxylase, the enzyme that forms GABA from glutamate, appears to be particularly susceptible to agonal pneumonia, suggesting that GABA-minergic neurones may be particularly susceptible to certain kinds of hypoxia (Bowen et al., 1976). We have recently found that minimal hypoxia doubles the level of cyclic GMP in mouse brain without any effect on cyclic AMP (Gibson et al., in press b). Since the cyclic nucleotides are second messengers for a number of neurotransmitters, this finding also suggests that impaired carbohydrate oxidation may affect the metabolism of other neurotransmitters as well as ACh. Synaptic endings are known to have high rates of oxidative metabolism compared to the rest of the nervous system (Sharp, 1976), and McNamara and Appel (1977) have postulated that synaptic damage or deficiency is a common mechanism in many dementias. It is again tempting to speculate that synaptic damage secondary to chronic, low-grade impairment of carbohydrate oxidation may be an important part of the pathophysiology in many disorders which impair cognitive function.

Clinical Significance

A more detailed understanding of the mechanisms of brain damage in hypoxia is likely to have widespread and important clinical implications, since some degree of hypoxia accompanies many common conditions which can impair cerebral function. Hypoxia typically accompanies fetal distress and hyaline membrane disease and is one of the most important causes of organic mental retardation (Schwartz, 1961; Hilliard and Kirman, 1965; Vanucci and Plum, 1975). Impaired cerebral perfusion typically accompanies shock, heart failure, many cardiac arrhythmias, pulmonary failure, cerebral edema secondary to shock or tumor, and cerebrovascular disease including arteriovenous malformations (Olivecrona and Riives, 1948; Richardson *et al.*, 1959; Anonymous editorial, 1977). As noted above, chronic low-grade hypoxia, perhaps secondary to microangiopathy, may play an important role in the development of senile dementia. Nutritional and toxic states including alcohol abuse may also impair cerebral carbohydrate oxidation (Sourkes, 1962; Slater and Roth, 1969). One conclusion is certain. Both theoretical and practical considerations indicate the need for extensive further study of the interrelations between cerebral carbohydrate catabolism and the metabolism of neurotransmitters including specifically ACh.

REFERENCES

Ad hoc committee on hypoglycemia, 1973, Statement on hypoglycemia, *Arch. Int. Med. 131:*591.

Adams, R.D., and Victor, M., 1977, *"Principles of Neurology,"* McGraw-Hill, New York, p. 732.

Albaum, H.G., Noell, W.K., and Chin, H.I., 1953, Chemical changes in rabbit brain during anoxia, *Amer. J. Physiol. 174:*408.

Anonymous editorial, 1977, Cholinergic involvement in senile dementia, *Lancet 1:*408.

Arab, A., 1954, Senile plaques and cerebral arteriosclerosis, *Rev. Neurol. 91:*22.

Barbeau, A., Butterworth, R.F., Ngo, T., Breton, G., Melancon, S., Shapcott, D., Geofrrey, G., and Lemieux, B., 1976, Pyruvate metabolism in Friedriech's Ataxia, *Canad. J. Neurol. Sci. 3:*379.

Barker, L.A., 1976, Subcellular aspects of acetylcholine metabolism, in *"Biology of Cholinergic Function"* (A.M. Goldberg, and I. Hanin, eds.), pp. 203-238, Raven Press, New York.

Barker, L.A., Mittag, T.W., and Krespan, B., 1978, Studies on substrates, inhibitors and modifiers on the high affinity choline transportacetylalion system present in rat brain synaptosomes, in *"Cholinergic Mechanisms and Psychopharmacology"* (D.J. Jenden, ed.), pp. 465-480, Plenum Press, New York.

Berl, S., Clarke, D.D., and Schneider, D., 1975, *"Metabolic Compartmentation and Neurotransmission,"* Raven Press, New York.

Blass, J.P., and Gibson, G.E., 1978, Cholinergic systems and disorders of carbohydrate catabolism, in *"Cholinergic Mechanisms and Psychopharmacology"* (D.J. Jenden, ed.), pp. 791-803, Plenum Press, New York.

Blass, J.P., and Lewis, C.A., 1973, Kinetic properties of the partially purified pyruvate dehydrogenase complex of ox brain, *Biochem. J. 130:*31.

Blass, J.P., Kark, R.A.P., Menon, N., and Harris, S.H., 1976, Low activities of the pyruvate and ketoglutarate dehydrogenase complexes in fibroblasts from five patients with Friedreich's ataxia, *N. Engl. J. Med. 295:*62.

Blass, J.P., Cederbaum, S.D., Kark, R.A.P., and Rodriguez-Budelli, M., in press, Pyruvate dehydrogenase deficiency in 35 patients, *Monogr. Hum. Genet.*

Bowen, D.M., Smith, C.B., White, P., and Davison, A.N., 1976, Neurotransmitter-related enzymes and indices of hypoxia in senile dementia and other abiotrophies, *Brain 99:* 459.

Boyd, W.D., Graham-White, J., Blackwood, G., Glen, I., and McQueen, J., 1977, Clinical effects of choline in Alzheimer senile dementia, *Lancet 2:*711.

Brizzee, K.R., 1975, Aging changes in relation to diseases of the nervous system, in *"Neurobiology of Aging"* (J.M. Ordy, and K.R. Brizzee, eds.), pp. 545-573, Plenum Press, New York.

Brizzee, K.R., Klava, P., and Johnson, J.E., 1975, Changes in microanatomy, neurocytology, and fine structure with aging, in *"Neurobiology of Aging"* (J.M. Ordy, and K.R. Brizzee, eds.), pp. 425-461, Plenum Press, New York.

Browning, E.T., 1976, Acetylcholine Synthesis: Substrate availability and the synthetic reaction, in *"Biology of Cholinergic Function"* (A.M. Goldberg, and I. Hanin, eds.), pp. 187-201, Raven Press, New York.

Butler, R.N., 1966, Psychiatric aspects of cerebrovascular disease in the aged, *Proc. Assn. Res. Nerv. Ment. Dis. 41:*255.

Cheng, S.C., Kumar, S., and Casella, G.A., 1972, Effects of fluoroacetate and fluorocitrate on the metabolic compartmentation of the tricarboxylic acid cycle in rat brain slices, *Brain Res. 42:*117.

Clarke, D.D., Nicklas, W.J., and Berl, S., 1970, Tricarboxylic acid-cycle metabolism in brain: Effect of fluoroacetate and fluorocitrate on the labelling of glutamate, aspartate, glutamine, and γ-aminobutyrate, *Biochem. J. 120:*345.

Cohen, M.M., 1973, *"Biochemistry, Ultrastructure and Physiology of Cerebral Anoxia, Hypoxia and Ischemia,"* Karger, New York.

Collier, J., 1947, Anoxaemia, in *"Price's Textbook of the Practice of Medicine, 7th ed."* p. 439, Oxford University Press, London.

Davies, D.L., 1949a, The intelligence of patients with Friedreich's Ataxia, *J. Neurol. Neurosurg. Psychiatry 34:*34.

Davies, D.L., 1949b, Psychiatric changes associated with Friedreich's Ataxia, *J. Neurol. Neurosurg. Psych. 12:*246.

Davies, P., and Maloney, A.J.F., 1976, Selective loss of central cholinergic neurones in Alzheimer's Disease, *Lancet 2:*1403.

Davis, J.M., 1976, Brain tyrosine hydroxylation: Alteration of oxygen affinity *in vivo* by immobilization or electroshock in the rat, *J. Neurochem. 27:*211.

Davis, J.M., and Carlsson, A., 1973, Effect of hypoxia on monoamine synthesis, levels, and metabolism in rat brain, *J. Neurochem. 21:*783.

Dolivo, M., 1974, Metabolism of mammalian sympathetic ganglia, *Fed. Proc. 33:*1043.

Drachman, D.A., 1977, Memory and the cholinergic system, in *"Neurotransmitter Function"* (W.S. Fields, ed.), pp. 112-136, Symposia Specialists, Miami, Florida.

Drachman, D.A., and Leavitt, J., 1974, Human memory and the cholinergic system — a relationship to aging, *Arch. Neurol. 30:*113.

Drachman, D.A., and Leavitt, J.L., 1975, Are neurotransmitter systems specific for cognitive functions? *Neurology 25:*349.

Duffy, T.E., Nelson, S.R., and Lowry, O.H., 1972, Cerebral carbohydrate metabolism during acute hypoxia and recovery, *J. Neurochem. 19:*959.

Ferrendelli, J.A., and Chang, M.M., 1973, Brain metabolism during hypoglycemia, *Arch. Neurol. Psychiatry 28:*173.

Ferris, S.H., Sattiananthan, G., Gershon, S., and Clark, C., 1977, Senile dementia: Treatment with deanol, *J. Am. Geriatr. Soc. 25:*241.

Freyhan, F.A., Woodford, R.B., and Kety, S.S., 1951, Cerebral blood flow and metabolism in psychoses of senility, *J. Nerve. Ment. Dis. 113:*449.

Friede, R.L., 1965, Enzyme histochemical studies of senile plaques, *J. Neuropathol. Exp. Neurol. 24:*477.

Friede, R.L., and Magee, K.R., 1962, Alzheimer's disease, Presentation of a case with pathological and enzymatic histochemical observations, *Neurology 12:*213.

Gibson, G.E., and Blass, J.P., 1976a, Inhibition of acetylcholine synthesis and of carbohydrate utilization by metabolites from maple-syrup-urine disease, *J. Neurochem. 26:* 1073.

Gibson, G.E., and Blass, J.P., 1976b, A relation between [NAD$^+$]/[NADH] potentials and glucose utilization in rat brain slices, *J. Biol. Chem. 251:*4127.

Gibson, G.E., and Blass, J.P., 1976c, Impaired synthesis of acetylcholine in brain accompanying hypoglycemia and mild hypoxia, *J. Neurochem. 27:*37.

Gibson, G.E., and Blass, J.P., in press, Proportional inhibition of acetylcholine synthesis accompanying impairment of 3-hydroxybutyrate oxidation in rat brain slices, *Biochem. Pharm.*

Gibson, G.E., Jope, R., and Blass, J.P., 1975, Reduced synthesis of acetylcholine accompanying impaired oxidation of pyruvic acid in rat brain slices, *Biochem. J. 148:*17.

Gibson, G.E., Shimada, M., and Blass, J.P., 1977, Partial reversal by THAM of the effects of hypoxia on neurotransmitter metabolism, *Neurosci. Abstracts 3:*314.

Gibson, G.E., Blass, J.P., and Jenden, D.J., in press a, Measurement of acetylcholine turnover using glucose as precursor: Evidence for compartmentation of glucose metabolism in brain, *J. Neurochem.*

Gibson, G.E., Shimada, M., and Blass, J.P., in press b, Alterations in acetylcholine synthesis and cyclic nucleotides in mild cerebral hypoxia, *J. Neurochem.*

Glasgow, A.M., and Chase, H.P., 1975, Production of the features of Reye's syndrome in rats with 4-pentenoic acid, *Pediatr. Res. 9:*133.

Gottfries, C.G., Kjallquist, A., Poulen, U., Roos, B.E., and Sundbarg, G., 1974, Cerebrospinal fluid pH and monoamine and glycolytic metabolites in Alzheimer's disease, *Br. J. Psychiatry 124:*280.

Gurdjian, E.S., Stone, W.E., and Webster, J.P., 1944, Cerebral metabolism in hypoxia, *Arch. Neurol. Psychiatry 51:*472.

Harpur, R.P., and Quastel, J.H., 1949, Relation between acetylcholine synthesis and the metabolism of carbohydrates and d-glucosamine in the central nervous system, *Nature 164:*779.

Hassler, O., 1965, Vascular changes in senile brains, *Acta Neuropathol. 5:*40.

Hilliard, L.T., and Kirman, B.H., 1965, *"Mental Deficiency,"* Little-Brown, Boston.

Himwich, H.E., 1951, *"Brain Metabolism and Cerebral Disorders,"* Williams and Wilkins, Baltimore, pp. 257-266.

Ingvar, D.H., and Gustafson, L., 1970, Regional cerebral blood flow in organic dementia with early onset, *Acta Neurol. Scand. Suppl. 43:*42.

Innes, I.R., and Nickerson, M., 1965, Drugs inhibiting the action of acetylcholine on structures innervated by post ganglionic parasympathetic nerves (antimuscarinic or atropinic drugs), in *"The Pharmacological Basis of Therapeutics"* (L.S. Goodman, and A. Gilman, eds.), pp. 521-545, Macmillan, New York.

Itoh, T., and Quastel, J.H., 1970, Acetoacetate metabolism in infant and adult rat brain *in vitro, Biochem. J. 116:*641.

Jenden, D.J., Choi, L., Silverman, R.W., Steinborn, J.A., Roche, M., and Booth, R.A., 1974, Acetylcholine turnover estimation in brain by gas chromatography/mass spectrometry, *Life Sci. 14:*55.

Jope, R.S., and Jenden, D.J., 1977, Synaptosomal transport and acetylation of choline, *Life Sci. 20:*1389.

Kimura, H., Mittal, C., and Murad, F., 1975, Activation of guanylate cyclase from rat liver and other tissues by sodium azide, *J. Biol. Chem. 250:*8016.

Klassen, A.C., Sung, J.H., and Stadian, E.M., 1968, Histological changes in cerebral arteries with increasing age, *J. Neuropathol. Exp. Neurol. 27:*607.

Koch-Weser, J., 1974, Common poisons, in *"Harrison's Principles of Internal Medicine"* (M.M. Wintrobe, G.W. Thorn, R.D. Adams, E. Braunwald, K.J. Isselbacher, and R.G. Petersdorf, eds.), p. 655, McGraw-Hill, New York.

Lang, R.W., and Carlo, D.J., 1975, Autoimmunity and again, in *"Neurobiology of Aging"* (J.M. Ordy, and K.R. Brizzee, eds.), pp. 233-251, Plenum Press, New York.

Lassen, N.A., Munch, O., and Tolley, E.R., 1957, Mental function and cerebral oxygen consumption in organic dementia, *Arch. Neurol. Psychiatry 77:*126.

Lassen, N.A., Feinberg, I., and Lane, M.H., 1960, Bilateral studies of cerebral oxygen uptake in young and aged normal subjects and in patients with organic dementia, *J. Clin. Invest. 39:*491.

Lust, W.D., Mrsulja, B.B., Mrsulja, B.J., Passonneau, J.V., and Klatzo, L., 1975, Putative neurotransmitters and cyclic nucleotides in prolonged ischemia of the cerebral cortex, *Brain Res. 98:*394.

MacMillan, V., 1977, Cerebral carbohydrate metabolism during acute carbon monoxide intoxication, *Brain Res. 121:*271.

MacMillan, V., Salford, L.G., and Siesjo, B.K., 1974, Metabolic state and blood flow in rat cerebral cortex, cerebellum, and brainstem in hypoxic hypoxia, *Acta Physiol. Scand. 92:*103.

Maldonado, M.E., Oh, K.J., and Frey, P.A., 1972, Studies on eschirichia coli pyruvate dehydrogenase complex, *J. Biol. Chem. 247:*2711.

Mandybur, T.I., 1975, The incidence of cerebral amyloid angiopathy in Alzheimer's disease, *Neurology 25:*120.

McFarland, R.A., 1932, The psychological effects of oxygen deprivation (anoxaemia) on human behavior, *Arch. Psychol. 145:*440.

McGeer, E.G., and McGeer, P.L., 1975, Age changes in the human for some enzymes associated with metabolism of catecholamines, GABA, and acetylcholine, in *"Neurobiology of Aging"* (J.M. Ordy, and K.R. Brizzee, eds.), pp. 287-306, Plenum Press, New York.

McIlwain, H., and Bachelard, H.S., 1971, *"Biochemistry and the Central Nervous System, 4th ed. ",* Williams and Wilkins, Baltimore.

McNamara, J.O., and Appel, S.H., 1977, Biochemical approaches to dementia, in *"Dementia"* (G.E. Wells, ed.), pp. 155-168, Davis, Philadelphia.

Miller, A.L., Hawkins, R.A., and Veech, R.L., 1973, The mitochondrial redox state of rat brain, *J. Neurochem. 20:*1393.

Mitchell, P., 1968, *"Chemiosmatic Coupling and Energy Transduction,"* Glynn Research, Bodmin, England.

Miyakawa, T., Sumiyoshi, S., Murayama, E., and Deshimoru, M., 1974, Ultrastructure of capillary plaque-like degeneration in senile dementia-Mechanism of amyloid production, *Acta Neuropath. 29:*229.

Molenaar, P.C., and Polak, R.L., 1976, Analysis of the preferential release of newly synthesized acetylcholine by cortical slices from rat brain with the aid of two different labelled precursors, *J. Neurochem. 26:*95.

Nachmansohn, D., 1959, *"Chemical and Molecular Basis of Nerve Activity,"* Academic Press, New York.

Nakamura, R., Cheng, S.C., and Naruse, H., 1970, A study on the precursor of the acetyl moiety of acetylcholine in brain slices. Observations on the compartmentalization of the acetyl-CoA pool, *Biochem. J. 118:*443.

Norberg, K., and Siesjo, B.K., 1975, Cerebral metabolism in hypoxic hypoxia. I. Pattern of activation of glycolysis. Reevaluation, *Brain Res. 86:*31.

Olivecrona, H., and Riives, J., 1948, Arteriovenous aneurysms of the brain, their diagnosis and treatment, *Arch. Neurol. Psychiatry 59:*567.

Ordy, J.M., and Kaack, B., 1975, Neurochemical changes with age, in *"Neurobiology of Aging,"* (J.M. Ordy, and K.R. Brizzee, eds.), pp. 253-285, Plenum Press, New York.

Osuntokun, B.O., 1969, An ataxic neuropathy in Nigeria-a clinical, biochemical, and electrophysiological study, *Brain 91:*215.

Perri, V., Sacchi, O., and Casella, C., 1970, Nervous transmission in the superior cervical ganglion of the thiamine-deficient rat, *J. Exp. Physiol. 55:*25.

Perry, E.K., Perry, P.H., Blessed, G., and Tomlinson, B.E., 1977, Necropsy evidence of central cholinergic deficits in senile dementia, *Lancet 2:*189.

Plum, F., Posner, J.B., and Hain, R.F., 1962, Delayed neurological deterioration after anoxia, *Arch. Intern. Med. 110:*18.

Quastel, J.H., Tennenbaum, M., and Wheatley, A.H.M., 1936, Choline ester formation in, and cholinesterase activities of, tissues *in vitro, Biochem. J. 30:*1668.

Richardson, J.D., Chambers, R.A., and Heywood, D.M., 1959, Encephalopathies of anoxia and hypoglycemia, *Arch. Neurol. 1:*178.

Schmahl, F.W., Betz, E., Dettinger, E., and Hohorst, H.J., 1966, Energy metabolism of the cerebral cortex and the electroencephalogram in acidosis, *Pfluegers Arch. 292:*46.

Schwarz, P., 1961, *"Birth Injuries of the Newborn-Morphology, Pathogenesis, Clinical Pathology, and Prevention,"* Karger, Basel.

Sharp, F.M., 1976, Relative cerebral glucose uptake of neuronal perikarya and neuropil determined with 2-deoxyglucose in resting and swimming rat, *Brain Res. 110:*127.

Sjogren, T., 1943, Clinical and genetic investigations of the heredoataxias, *Acta Psychiatr. Neurol. [Suppl.] 27:*1.

Siesjo, B.K., and Plum, F., 1971, Cerebral energy metabolism in normoxia and in hypoxia, *Acta Anaesthesiol. Scand. Suppl. 45:*81.

Siesjo, B.K., Johannsson, H., Ljunggren, B., and Norberg, K., 1974, Brain dysfunction in cerebral hypoxia and ischemia, in *"Brain Dysfunction in Metabolic Disorders"* (F. Plum, ed.), pp. 75-112, Raven Press, New York.

Spillane, J.A., Goodhart, J.A., White, P., Bowen, D.M., and Davison, A.N., 1977, Choline in Alzheimer's disease, *Lancet 2:*826.

Slater, E., and Roth, M., 1969, *"Clinical Psychiatry,"* Williams and Wilkins, Baltimore, pp. 441-444.

Sokoloff, L., 1966, Cerebral circulatory and metabolic changes associated with aging, *Res. Publ. Assoc. Res. Nerv. Ment. Dis. 41:*237.

Sourkes, T.L., 1962, *"Biochemistry of Mental Disease,"* Hober-Harper, New York, pp. 131-155.

Suzuki, K., Katzman, R., and Korey, S.R., 1965, Chemical studies on Alzheimer's disease, *J. Neuropathol. Exp. Neurol. 24:*211.

Tucek, S., and Cheng, S.C., 1974, Provenance of the acetyl group of acetylcholine and compartmentation of acetyl CoA and Krebs cycle intermediates in the brain *in vivo, J. Neurochem. 22:*893.

Vannucci, R.C., and Plum, F., 1975, Physiology of perinatal-hypoxic brain damage, in *"Biology of Brain Dysfunction, Vol. 3"* (G. Gaull, ed.), pp. 1-46, Plenum Press, New York.

White, P., Goodhardt, M.J., Keet, J.P., Hiley, C.R., Carrasco, L.H., Williams, I.E.I., and Bowen, D.M., 1977, Neocortical cholinergic neurons in elderly people, *Lancet 1:*668.

Williams, R.D., Mason, H.L., Power, M.H., and Wilder, R.M., 1943, Induced thiamine (Vitamin B_1) deficiency in man, *Arch. Int. Med. 71:*38.

Wilson, D.F., Stubs, M., Veech, R.L., Erecinska, M., and Krebs, H.A., 1974, Equilibrium relations between the oxidation-reduction reactions and the adenosine triphosphate synthesis in suspensions of isolated liver cells, *Biochem. J. 140:*57.

Yatsu, F.M., Lee, L.W., and Liao, C.L., 1975, Energy metabolism during brain ischemia. Stability during reversible and irreversible damage, *Stroke 6:*678.

COGNITIVE EFFECTS OF PHYSOSTIGMINE AND CHOLINE CHLORIDE IN NORMAL SUBJECTS

R. C. Mohs[1,2], K. L. Davis[1,2], J. R. Tinklenberg[1,2], A. Pfefferbaum[1,2], L. E. Hollister[1,2] and B. S. Kopell[1,2]

[1] Veterans Administration Hospital, 3801 Miranda Avenue, Palo Alto, California 94304

[2] Department of Psychiatry and Behavioral Sciences, Stanford University School of Medicine, Stanford, California 94305

INTRODUCTION

This chapter presents the results of two studies investigating the effects of cholino-mimetic drugs on cognitive functioning in humans. Experiment I investigated the effects of physostigmine, a drug which inhibits cholinesterase and thereby slows the destruction of acetylcholine (Koelle, 1975). Experiment II investigated the effects of precursor loading with choline chloride; this procedure may increase brain acetylcholine and central cholinergic activity (Cohen and Wurtman, 1976; Haubrich *et al.*, 1975). These studies were undertaken because previous work both with animals and with humans indicates that cholinergic mechanisms play an important role in cognitive activities such as learning and memory. One hypothesis of particular interest to us was that some aspects of human cognitive functioning may be improved by giving drugs that increase the level of central cholinergic activity.

At this point it is appropriate to metion briefly the main lines of research implicating cholinergic mechanisms in cognitive functioning. Only studies designed to measure behavioral changes produced by anticholinergic and cholinomimetic drugs will be mentioned since they are directly related to our experiments with physostigmine and choline chloride.

A large number of studies with animals have shown that anticholinergics and cholinomimetics can have substantial effects on learning and memory performance (see e.g., Deutsch, 1971; Hamburg, 1967; Karczmar, 1975; Matthies *et al.*, 1975; McGaugh, 1973; Wiener and Deutsch, 1968). Results from these animal studies are difficult to summarize concisely and, in most instances, generalizations of these results to human behavior are not straightforward. For present purposes it is sufficient to note that drug-induced changes in central cholinergic activity often affect learning and retrieval from memory in animals.

   Relatively few studies have investigated cholinergic mechanisms in human learning and memory, although some well controlled experiments have appeared recently. Anticholinergic drugs such as scopolamine have been shown to impair memory performance but the degree of impairment varies with the memory requirements of the task. Memory for items within the span of short-term memory is usually unimpaired while learning that requires storage in long-term memory is seriously impaired (Drachman, 1977a, 1977b; Drachman and Leavitt, 1974; Ghoneim and Mewaldt, 1975; 1977; Peterson, 1977; Safer and Allen, 1971). Retrieval from long-term memory is only slightly impaired (Drachman and Leavitt, 1974; Ghoneim and Mewaldt, 1975; 1977; Peterson, 1977). For some time it has been known that physostigmine can relieve the mental confusion produced by scopolamine (Granacher and Baldessarini, 1975; Ketchum *et al.*, 1973; Koelle, 1975; Safer and Allen, 1971), and recent controlled studies (Drachman, 1977a; Ghoneim and Mewaldt, 1977) have shown that it reverses anticholinergic amnesia as well. This suggests that a cholinomimetic alone might improve some aspects of cognitive functioning. Previous studies indicate, however, that the cognitive effects of cholinomimetics are complicated and probably vary both with drug dose and with the kind of task used to assess cognitive performance. Drachman (1977a, 1977b; Drachman and Leavitt, 1974) administered physostigmine (up to 2 mg) subcutaneously to both young and old subjects and found small, non-significant improvements on measures of storage in long-term memory. Other cognitive measures were essentially unchanged. These results are suggestive but inconclusive since a small number of subjects was used in a between groups design; in addition, cognitive tests were administered for up to three and one half hours after drug administration so the effective dose of physostigmine was probably very low (Koelle, 1975).

   A later study indicated that the dose-response function for physostigmine may be biphasic (Davis *et al.*, 1976). These investigators found that either 2 or 3 mg of intravenous physostigmine impaired all aspects of memory performance in normal subjects. A biphasic dose-response function is also suggested in a recent case report by Peters and Levin (1977). They administered physostigmine to a patient who had severe amnesia following an attack of herpes simplex encephalitis. A dose of 0.8 mg intravenous physostigmine significantly improved both storage and retrieval in this patient but doses either higher or lower had no significant effect.

   For both practical and theoretical reasons it is important to specify as precisely as possible the conditions under which cholinomimetics can improve cognitive functioning. The problem is complex, however, since drug effects on performance undoubtedly depend upon several pharmacological, subject selection and behavioral variables. The two studies presented here represent only initial attempts to enhance cognition with physostigmine and choline chloride. The drug doses and methods of administration used in these studies were determined both by practical considerations and by our desire to pick a combination of variables likely to yield a positive result. Several performance measures were obtained in both studies so that differential drug effects on various cognitive activities could be detected. In both studies some tests were used to assess drug effects on short-term memory (STM) while others were used to assess drug effects on long-term memory (LTM). We assume here, along with most current theories of human memory (see e.g., Anderson and Bower, 1973; Atkinson and Shiffrin, 1968; 1971; Baddeley and Hitch, 1974; Milner, 1970; Warrington and Weiskrantz, 1973) that

STM is a memory store of limited capacity used to hold small amounts of information for short periods of time while LTM is a memory store of essentially unlimited capacity where information is held for periods of minutes to years. An attempt was also made to separate drug effects on processes that store information in memory from drug effects on processes involved in retrieving (i.e. using) information already in memory (Postman, 1976).

EXPERIMENT I: PHYSOSTIGMINE IN NORMALS

The purpose of this study was to determine whether a low dose of physostigmine could improve any aspect of cognitive functioning. The study was undertaken to follow up some informal observations made during a previous study (Davis *et al.*, 1976) in which 2 or 3 mg intravenous physostigmine impaired all aspects of memory performance. In most subjects the physostigmine caused nausea and vomiting as well as amnesia. Occasionally, however, subjects reported that the drug produced pleasant subjective effects including a feeling of alertness. When reported, the pleasant effects occurred before the onset of nausea, vomiting and amnesia. These observations suggested that a slow infusion of 1 mg of physostigmine might improve memory performance and sustain the pleasant subjective effects. An important aspect of the procedure for the present study was the method of subject selection. To insure the possibility of finding a statistically significant improvement, only subjects whose baseline memory performance indicated that they could improve on the drug were included in the study.

Method

Nineteen healthy males between 18 and 35 years of age were tested while receiving an infusion of normal saline and while receiving 1 mg of physostigmine dissolved in saline. Subjects were screened for the study with a 20-word verbal learning test identical to one of the tests used to evaluate drug effects. About 20 potential subjects who could recall more than 15 words after a single presentation of the 20 words were excluded since there was little opportunity for them to demonstrate improvement on the drug. Nine subjects received physostigmine on the first test day and saline two days later; the ten remaining subjects received saline on the first day and physostigmine two days later. The drug administration and cognitive testing schedule for a single session are presented in Table 1.

Physostigmine and saline placebo were administered by constant infusion over 60 min. Approximately 20 min prior to the start of the infusion subjects were given 0.5 mg of methscopolamine bromide subcutaneously to minimize the peripheral effects of physostigmine. When the subject's pulse rate reached 100 beats per min the infusion was begun.

Two of the tests, digit span and memory scanning, were used to assess physostigmine's effect on short-term memory. The capacity of short-term memory was measured with a digit span task given 9 min after the start of the infusion. On the first trial three digits were read aloud and the subject was asked to repeat them in correct serial order. The number of digits presented was increased by one on each subsequent trial until the subject could not recall them in correct order. The maximum number recalled correctly was the subject's digit span.

TABLE 1

Schedule of Procedures for a Single Session in Experiment I

Total Dose of Physostigmine Received (mg)	Time (min)	
		Pre-infusion
	–30	Two learning trials on list of 15 concrete nouns
	–16	Methscopolamine (0.5 mg sc)
	0	Infusion
.15	+ 9	Digit span
.30	+18	Two recall trials on list of 15 concrete nouns presented at –30 min
.50	+30	Six learning trials on list of 20 categorized nouns
.70	+42	Short-term memory scanning task
1.00	+60	End infusion
1.00	+80	Two recall trials on list of 15 concrete nouns presented at –30 min

The memory scanning task originally developed by Sternberg (1966; 1969) was used to determine whether physostigmine affected the speed of processing in short-term memory. The procedures used for this task were almost identical to the varied set procedures described by Sternberg (1969). The subject was given a series of 128 trials. At the start of each trial a new memory set of 1-4 digits was presented visually. A 1 sec delay followed the memory set and then a test digit was presented. The subject's task was to press one of two buttons to indicate whether the test digit was a member of the memory set for that trial. If the digit was a member of the memory set the subject made a positive response by pressing one of the buttons; if the digit was not in the memory set, the subject made a negative response by pressing the other button. As in Sternberg's original experiments, subjects nearly always decided correctly (error rate was < 1%). The primary dependent measure was response time (RT) which was calculated separately for trials with each of the four memory set sizes (1-4 digits) and for trials on which positive and negative responses were made.

To assess long-term memory functioning two verbal learning tasks were used. These tasks are assumed to involve long-term memory because the number of words to be learned exceeds the capacity of short-term memory. To determine whether physostigmine affects retrieval from LTM subjects were given a verbal memory test in which learning trials occurred prior to the infusion while recall was tested twice during the infusion. Thirty minutes prior to the infusion and before the administration of methscopolamine subjects were given two learning trials on a list of 15 concrete nouns. On the first learning trial the entire list was presented orally at a one word per 2 sec rate. Then the subject tried to recall the 15 words. On the second learning trial the subject was first reminded of all words not recalled on the first trial and then attempted to recall all 15 words. At 18 min after the start of the infusion and again at 80 min after the start of the infusion subjects were given two recall trials. On each of the four recall trials subjects tried to recall all 15 words without any reminders of missed words. Since no reminders were given, subjects had no opportunity to store more information about the list after the start of the infusion.

The hypothesis that physostigmine enhances storage in long-term memory was tested with a verbal learning task given at 30 min into the infusion. The procedures for this task were originally developed by Buschke (1973; Buschke and Fuld, 1974). Subjects were given six learning trials on a list of 20 words from a single semantic category such as four-footed animals or articles of clothing (Battig and Montague, 1969). On the first trial the list was read to the subject at a one word per 2 sec rate. The subject then tried to recall all 20 words. On the five subsequent trials the subject was first reminded of all words not recalled on the previous trial and then attempted to recall all 20 words.

Results

Performance on the two tests of short-term memory was not affected by physostigmine. On the digit span test, subjects recalled an average maximum of 6.8 digits at 9 min into the infusion on physostigmine days (0.15 mg of physostigmine) and 6.9 digits at 9 min into the infusion on saline days. This indicates that a low dose of physostigmine had no measurable effect on the capacity of STM. The results from the memory scanning task were similar to those obtained in Sternberg's original experiments. As Figure 1 indicates, response time (RT) was a linear increasing function of memory set size and was greater when the test digit was not in memory than when it was a member of the memory set. Specifically, mean RT was well fit by equations of the form

$$RT = a_r + bm$$

[where:

m = the number of digits in the memory set
b = a constant
a_r = a constant that depends on the response r

The slope of the function (b) measures the time necessary to process each additional digit in memory, while the intercepts (a_r) measure the total time necessary to complete processes such as stimulus identification, response selection and response execution which do not depend on memory set size. Neither drug nor response type had a significant effect on the slope of the RT function. Physostigmine had no effect on the intercept of the RT function although intercepts were greater on negative trials than on positive trials ($p < .003$ by analysis of variance). Thus, physostigmine had no quantifiable effect on either the capacity or the speed of processing in short-term memory.

Results from the two tests of LTM are presented in Figure 2. The left hand panel presents the number of words recalled in the test of retrieval on saline and physostigmine days. Scores on the pre-infusion learning trials were nearly identical on the two days indicating that subjects stored approximately the same amount of information in LTM

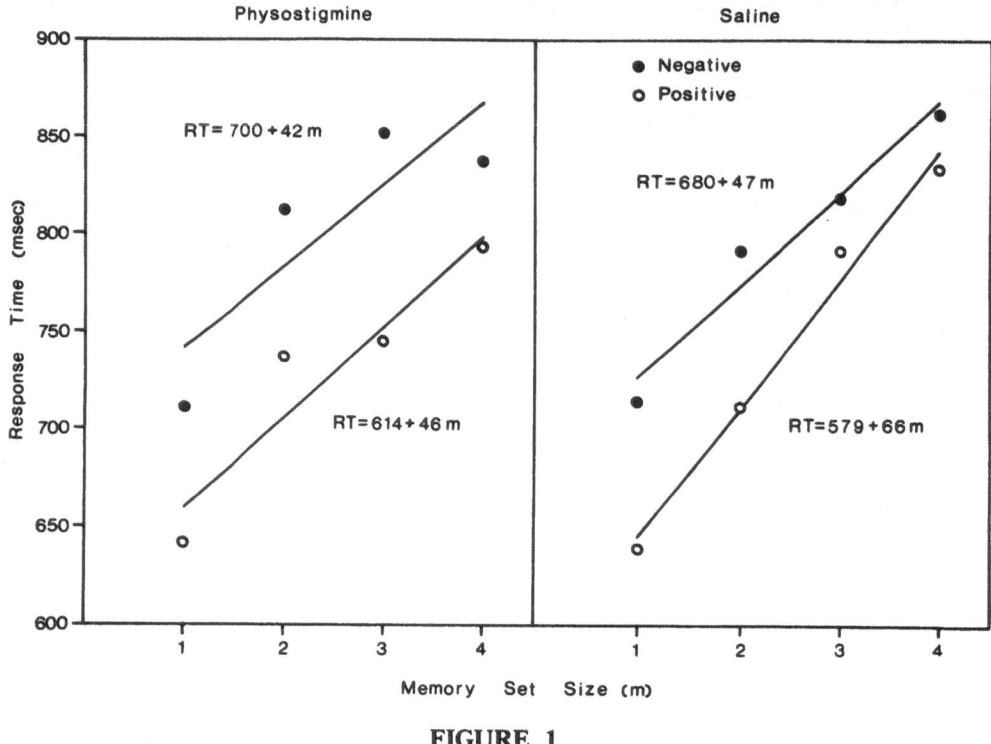

FIGURE 1

Mean response times (RT) for the memory scanning task given in Experiment I.

prior to both infusions. At +18 min and at +80 min subjects were able to recall more words on physostigmine days than on saline days. The differences were small, however, and reached conventional significance levels (p < .03 by analysis of variance) only at +80 min. The right-hand panel of Figure 2 presents the results from the test of storage into LTM which was given at +30 min into the infusion. The figure shows the total number of words recalled on the six learning trials on physostigmine and saline days. The number of words recalled increased significantly over trials (p < .001) as subjects learned the lists and was also greater on physostigmine days than on saline days (p < .006 by analysis of variance).

Post-hoc examination of the data showed considerable variability in the amount of improvement with physostigmine. This is at least partly a result of measurement errors but may also reflect true differences in drug response. The latter hypothesis is supported by the fact that subjective responses to the drug also varied widely; in most cases subjects who reported strong subjective changes in a post-experimental interview also showed larger changes on the verbal learning tests.

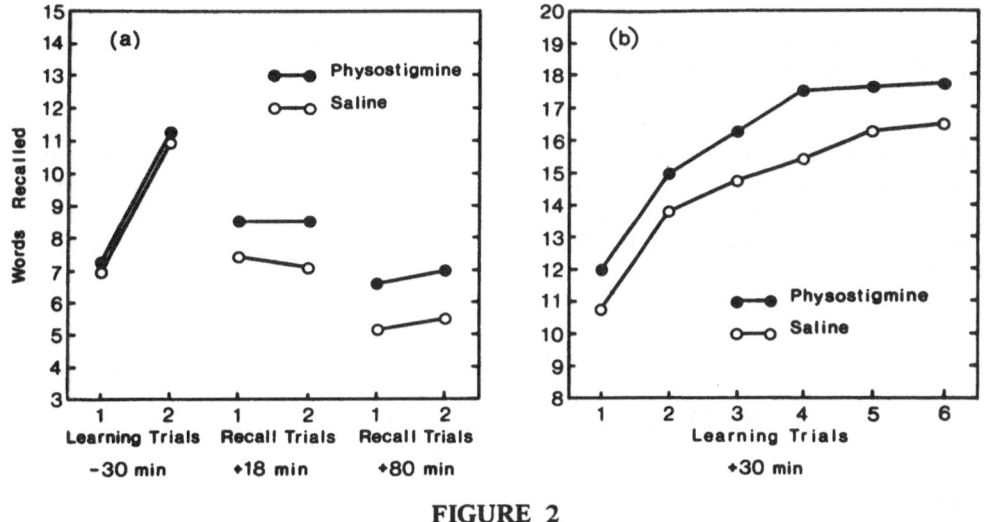

FIGURE 2

Average number of words recalled during the tests of retrieval (a) and storage (b) in Experiment I.

EXPERIMENT II: CHOLINE CHLORIDE IN NORMALS

The experiment with physostigmine demonstrated that a low dose of a cholinomimetic can, at least for some people, enhance storage and retrieval of information in LTM. However, the procedures used to administer physostigmine make it of little practical use in treating patients with memory loss. With this in mind a second experiment was designed to determine whether memory improvement could be obtained with orally administered choline chloride.

As with physostigmine it is likely that any effects of choline chloride on performance will depend on several pharmacological, subject selection and behavioral variables. The present study was designed to duplicate whenever possible the conditions of Experiment I which produced a favorable result. The primary differences were in drug dosage and method of administration which were impossible to equate with those used in Experiment I.

Method

Fifteen of the nineteen subjects who participated in Experiment I returned to participate in this study. The remaining four subjects were unavailable or refused to participate. Subjects were tested three times in a placebo-drug-placebo repeated measures design. Each subject started the study on a Friday and took placebo four times a day for four days. On the fourth placebo day (Monday) cognitive tests were given. For the next three days the subject took 4 g of choline chloride four times a day for a total of 16 g per day. On the third drug day (Thursday) cognitive tests were again administered. Placebos were taken four times a day for the next four days and cognitive tests were given on the last placebo day (Monday). All test sessions for a single subject were scheduled for the same time of day. All testing was double blind.

Three of the memory tests used in Experiment I, digit span and the two tests of LTM, were repeated in this experiment. Alternate forms were constructed for each test so that no subject was tested with the same materials more than once across the two experiments. The memory scanning test, which did not show a drug effect in Experiment I, was not given in Experiment II. The testing schedule for a single session is presented in Table 2.

TABLE 2

Schedule of Procedures for a Single Session in Experiment II

Time (min)	
0	Two learning trials on list of 15 concrete nouns
+15	Digit span
+25	Two recall trials on list of 15 concrete nouns presented at time 0
+30	Ten learning trials on list of 20 categorized nouns
+60	Two recall trials on list of 15 concrete nouns presented at time 0

Results

Average scores on the three memory tests were unaffected by choline chloride. On the digit span test subjects were able to recall 7.0 digits in the pre-drug placebo session, 6.9 digits while on choline and 7.3 digits in the post-drug placebo session. These scores are not significantly different indicating that choline had no measureable effect on the capacity of STM. Since choline was administered over three days the test of retrieval from LTM could not be given with learning prior to drug administration as was done in the physostigmine study. Rather, as Table 2 shows, learning and recall trials both occurred in the same drug state but were separated by intervals during which the subject performed other tasks. As in Experiment I all 15 words were presented on the first trial and all words not recalled on the first trial were presented again on the second trial; no reminders of missed words were given on the four recall trials. The rationale for this procedure was that retrieval could be assessed by measuring the difference between scores on learning and recall trials. Improved retrieval would appear as a reduction in the difference (i.e. forgetting) between learning and recall trials. As the left-hand panel in Figure 3 indicates, however, choline did not affect the number of words recalled on either learning or recall trials. Thus, choline had no measureable effect on the amount of information stored in LTM during learning or on the ability to retrieve information during recall.

These conclusions are supported by the results from the 20-word learning test presented in the right-hand panel of Figure 3. The procedures for this test were the same as those used in Experiment I except that subjects were given 10 learning trials with selective reminding (Buschke, 1973; Buschke and Fuld, 1974) rather than six. The figure shows that average performance on choline was nearly the same as on the two placebo test days.

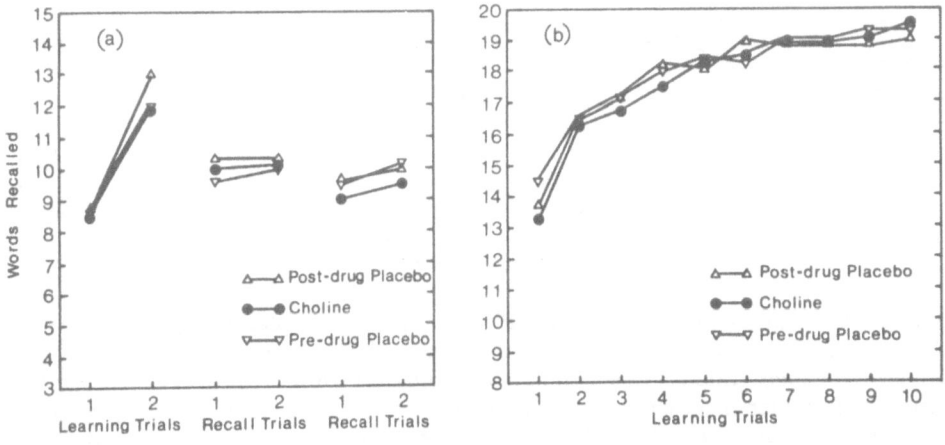

FIGURE 3

Average number of words recalled during the tests of retrieval (a) and storage (b) in Experiment II.

Even though group averages showed no drug effect it is, of course, possible that choline affected performance of individual subjects. As an example, individual drug effects could occur without changes in average performance if some subjects remembered less on choline while others remembered more. Such a possibility must be considered seriously since the studies with physostigmine indicate that cholinomimetics have a biphasic effect on cognitive functioning and that dose-response functions vary among subjects. Figure 4 presents two idealized patterns of individual response data which could both produce average performance that was nearly equal across the three test sessions. Panel (a) depicts a situation in which subjects are divided between those whose performance improves steadily across sessions (e.g. due to practice) and those whose performance deteriorates steadily across sessions (e.g. due to boredom). Panel (b) depicts a situation in which a subject's performance either improves from pre-drug to drug and then returns to normal or deteriorates from pre-drug to drug and then returns to normal during post-drug testing.

Although both patterns seem plausible, only (b) is consistent with the hypothesis that choline had effects on performance that were inconsistent across subjects. That is, the situation in panel (a) indicates that performance changes across time were unrelated to drug intervention. To determine which of these two response patterns characterized the subjects in Experiment II differences between the drug session and the two placebo sessions were examined. Two difference scores were calculated for each subject using the average number of words recalled per trial on the 20-word learning test: d_1 is the average

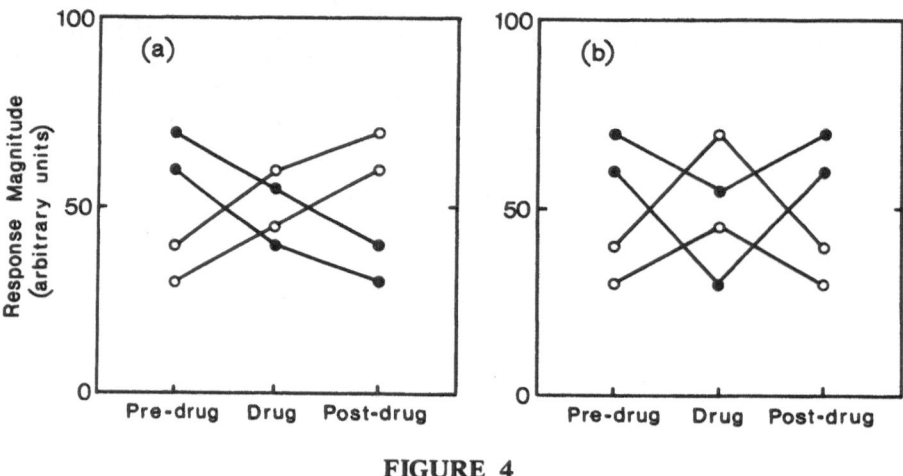

FIGURE 4

Hypothetical response patterns of individual subjects in a placebo-drug-placebo design. Pattern (a) shows a situation in which a subject's performance either improves (open circles) or declines (filled circles) monotonically over three sessions. Pattern (b) shows a situation in which a subject's performance either improves from pre-drug to drug and then returns to normal (open circles) or declines from pre-drug to drug and then returns to normal (filled circles).

recall score on choline minus the average recall score in the pre-drug placebo session, and d_2 is the average score on choline minus the average recall score in the post-drug placebo session. Note that d_1 represents a difference between day 7 performance and day 4 performance while d_2 represents a difference in the opposite direction temporally, between day 7 and day 11. If panel (a) were an adequate representation of individual subjects data, then d_1 and d_2 should be negatively correlated. If, however, panel (b) is the better representation, then the correlation should be positive. The computed correlation was +0.62 ($p < .02$). That is, subjects who got worse from pre-choline placebo to choline got better when they returned to placebo and subjects who scored higher on choline than pre-choline got worse when returned to placebo. It should be noted here that a significant positive correlation between d_1 and d_2 is sufficient to reject response pattern (a), but it is clearly possible for response pattern (b) to be produced even without a drug effect. As an example, pattern (b) could be produced if subjects' performances were accurately represented by a set of stationary time series measured at three time points (see e.g. Box and Jenkins, 1970).

It is also possible to correlate performance changes on choline with performance changes on physostigmine. To do this the average number of words recalled per trial on the 20-word learning test used in Experiment I were calculated for each subject. The difference d_3 is the average score on physostigmine minus the average score on saline. The correlation between d_1 and d_3 was negative ($r = -0.64$) and statistically significant ($p < .02$) while that between d_2 and d_3 was negative ($r = -0.24$) but not statistically significant ($p > .10$). A scatter plot for the larger correlation is presented in Figure 5.

The mean difference scores (based on 15 subjects) were +1.45 and -0.22 words for the physostigmine (d_3) and choline (d_1) studies, respectively. Subjects who improve most with physostigmine (high d_3) tended to show a decrement on choline (negative d_1); subjects with little change on physostigmine (d_3 near 0) showed little change or slight improvement with choline.

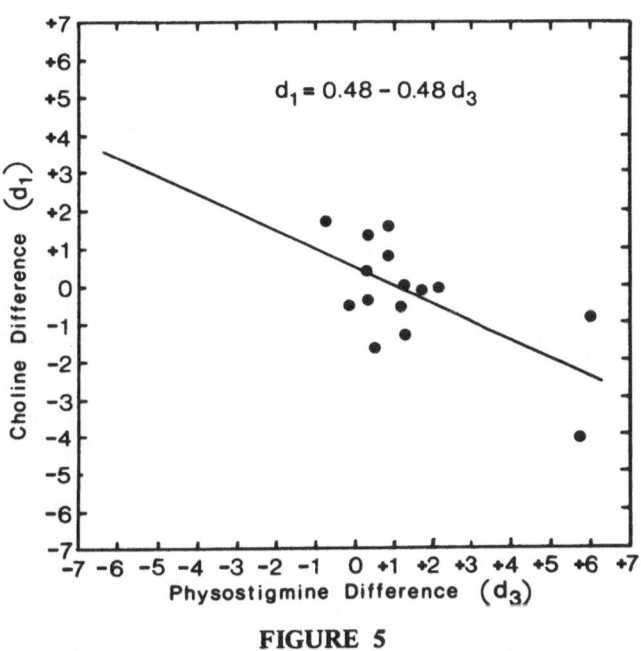

$$d_1 = 0.48 - 0.48\, d_3$$

FIGURE 5

Correlation between performance change in Experiment I and Experiment II for 15 subjects who participated in both experiments. The variables d_1 and d_3 are defined in the text.

DISCUSSION

Experiment I showed that performance on tasks involving storage and retrieval of information in LTM can be improved with a low dose of physostigmine. Performance on two tests of STM functioning was not affected by physostigmine. On the test of retrieval from LTM physostigmine improved recall but the effect was greater at 80 min after the start of the infusion than it was at 18 min after the start of the infusion. The differential effects at +18 min and +80 min could be due to a difference in drug dose (0.30 mg at +18 min vs. 1.00 mg at +80 min) or they could be due to a change in the memory trace for the list over time. The latter possibility is suggested by Deutsch's studies (Deutsch, 1971; Hamburg, 1967; Wiener and Deutsch, 1968) with animals showing that the effect of a single dose of physostigmine on retrieval is a function of the interval between training and drug administration.

Performance on the verbal learning test occurring 30 min after the start of each infusion was considerably better on the physostigmine day than on the saline day. This result is somewhat ambiguous since storage and retrieval both occurred in the same drug state. Considering the rather small improvement in retrieval following physostigmine, however, it seems reasonable that enhanced recall in this task was primarily a result of an increase in storage into LTM.

A previous study (Davis *et al.*, 1976) showed that either 2 or 3 mg intravenous physostigmine impaired all aspects of memory in normal subjects. Those results, together with the results from the study reported here, indicate that physostigmine has a biphasic effect on cognitive functioning. Low doses tend to produce alertness and enhanced LTM functioning while higher doses produce mental confusion, amnesia and nausea.

The results of Experiment II were less clear. Choline chloride had no effect on average performance but correlational analyses suggested that some subjects may have improved slightly while others were impaired. Performance changes in Experiment II were negatively correlated with performance changes in Experiment I indicating that subjects who were most improved by 1 mg of physostigmine tended to show impairments with 16 g per day of choline.

Retrospective correlations must be interpreted with caution, and firm conclusions about the effects of choline chloride on cognitive functioning can only be drawn after additional studies are done. Nevertheless, it is worthwhile to advance a tentative explanation for these results which can also serve as a guide for subsequent studies of cholinomimetics.

One reasonable explanation assumes that choline, like physostigmine, has biphasic effects on cognitive functioning and that there are individual differences in susceptibility to the effects of both drugs. Susceptibility here refers to the expected magnitude rather than the direction of the drug response. It is not the case that some subjects consistently improve with cholinomimetics while others are consistently impaired. Rather, we assume that subjects who show the greatest improvement at a low dose will show the greatest impairment at a high dose, and subjects who show smaller improvements at a low dose will show smaller impairments at a high dose. If these assumptions are correct then choline will produce a uniform effect only in a narrow low-dose range where improvements can occur and at very high doses where impairments will predominate. By this account the dose used in Experiment II was in the middle range where neither response pattern dominated although subjects most susceptible to the effects of cholinomimetics showed larger effects, primarily impairments. It should be noted here that EEGs recorded from subjects taking 16 g per day of choline were similar to those recorded from subjects receiving a moderately high dose (2 to 2.5 mg) of physostigmine (Pfefferbaum *et al.*, *Electrophysiological Effects of Physostigmine In Humans*, this book). Because of choline's side effects it may be difficult to administer doses much higher than 16 g per day. Even at this dose many subjects experienced nausea, diarrhea and muscle cramps. In a recent uncontrolled clinical trial Boyd *et al.* (1977) gave either 5 or 10 g of choline per day to severely demented patients and noted some improvement in mood and orientation. Further studies are needed to determine whether a quantifiable improvement in cognitive functioning can be produced by choline.

The mechanisms by which cholinomimetic drugs affect performance on memory tasks are not at all clear. On the basis of an extensive series of experiments with animals Deutsch and his colleagues (Deutsch, 1971; Hamburg, 1967; Wiener and Deutsch, 1968; Davis and Yesavage, *Brain Acetylcholine and Disorders of Memory*, this book) have argued that information is stored in memory by changing the conductivity of cholinergic synapses. Performance on subsequent memory tests is assumed to depend upon the level of transmission at these "memory" synapses during retrieval. Drugs that affect transmission at cholinergic synapses will either enhance or decrease performance depending on whether they tend to produce an "optimal" level of transmission. With some additional assumptions about the way synaptic conductivity changes over time a similar theory could account for the results of recent studies of anticholinergics and cholinomimetics in humans. However, the results of these studies are also consistent with other theories involving less restrictive assumptions. As an example, these changes might be due to over-all changes in CNS activity level that are manifest behaviorally as changes in attention or arousal. At present it is not clear whether the effects of physostigmine and choline chloride are specific to situations where associative connections must be formed and utilized in memory or whether many cognitive functions are affected uniformly.

ACKNOWLEDGEMENTS

This research was supported in part by the Medical Research Service of the Veterans Administration and by the National Institute of Mental Health Grants MH-03030, MH-30854 and DA-00854.

RFFERENCES

Anderson, J.R., and Bower, G.H., 1973, "Human Associative Memory," V.H. Winston, New York.

Atkinson, R.C., and Shiffrin, R.M., 1968, Human memory: a proposed system and its control processes, in *"The Psychology of Learning and Motivation: Advances in Research and Theory"* (K.W. Spence, and J.T. Spence, eds.), pp. 89-195, Academic Press, New York.

Atkinson, R.C., and Shiffrin, R.M., 1971, The control of short term memory, *Sci. Am. 224:*82.

Baddeley, A.D., and Hitch, G., 1974, Working memory, in *"The Psychology of Learning and Motivation: Advances in Theory and Research"* (G.H. Bower, ed.), pp. 47-89, Academic Press, New York.

Battig, W.F., and Montague, W.E., 1969, Category norms for verbal items in 56 categories: a replication and extension of the Connecticut category norms, *J. Exp. Psychol. Monograph 80:*1.

Box, G.E.P., and Jenkins, G.M., 1970, "Time-series analysis: forecasting and control," Holden Day, San Francisco.

Boyd, W.D., Graham-White, J., Blackwood, G., Glen, I., and McQueen, J., 1977, Clinical effects of choline in Alzheimer senile dementia, *Lancet 2:*711.

Buschke, H., 1973, Selective reminding for analysis of memory and learning, *J. Verb. Learn. Verb. Behav. 12:*543.

Buschke, H., and Fuld, P.A., 1974, Evaluating storage, retention, and retrieval in disordered memory and learning, *Neurology 24:*1019.

Cohen, E.L., and Wurtman, R.J., 1976, Brain acetylcholine: control by dietary choline, *Science 191:*561.

Davis, K.L., Hollister, L.E., Overall, J., Johnson, A., and Train, K., 1976, Physostigmine: effects on cognition and affect in normal subjects, *Psychopharmacology 51:*23.

Deutsch, J.A., 1971, The cholinergic synapse and the site of memory, *Science 174:*788.

Drachman, D.A., 1977a, Memory and cognitive function in man: does the cholinergic system have a specific role? *Neurology 27:*783.

Drachman, D.A., 1977b, Memory and the cholinergic system, in *"Neurotransmitter Function: Basic and Clinical Aspects"* (W.S. Fields, ed.), pp. 353-372, Symposia Specialists, New York.

Drachman, D.A., and Leavitt, J., 1974, Human memory and the cholinergic system, *Arch. Neurol. 30:*113.

Ghoneim, M.M., and Mewaldt, S.P., 1975, Effects of diazepam and scopolamine on storage, retrieval and organizational processes in memory, *Psychopharmacologia (Berl.) 44:*257.

Ghoneim, M.M., and Mewaldt, S.P., 1977, Studies on human memory: the interactions of diazepam, scopolamine, and physostigmine, *Psychopharmacology 52:*1.

Granacher, R.P., and Baldessarini, R.J., 1975, Physostigmine: its use in acute anticholinergic syndrome with antidepressant and antiparkinson drugs, *Arch. Gen. Psychiatry 32:*375.

Hamburg, M.D., 1967, Retrograde amnesia produced by intraperitoneal injection of physostigmine, *Science 156:*973.

Haubrich, D.R., Wang, P.F.L., Clody, D.E., and Wedeking, P.W., 1975, Increase in rat brain acetylcholine induced by choline or deanol, *Life Sci. 17:*975.

Karczmar, A.G., 1975, Cholinergic influences on behavior, in *"Cholinergic Mechanisms"* (P.G. Waser, ed.), pp. 501-530, Raven Press, New York.

Ketchum, J.S., Sidell, F.R., Cowell, E.B., Aghajanian, G.K., and Hayes, A.H., 1973, Atropine, scopolamine, and ditran: comparative pharmacology and antagonists in man, *Psychopharmacologia (Berl.) 28:*121.

Koelle, G.B., 1975, Anticholinesterase agents, in *"The Pharmacological Basis of Therapeutics"* (L.S. Goodman, and A. Gilman, eds.), pp. 445-466, Macmillan, New York.

Matthies, H., Ott, T., and Kammerer, E., 1975, Cholinergic influences on learning, in *"Cholinergic Mechanisms"* (P.G. Waser, ed.), pp. 493-499, Raven Press, New York.

McGaugh, J.L., 1973, Drug facilitation of learning and memory, in *"Annual Review of Pharmacology"*, pp. 229-241, Annual Reviews, Palo Alto, CA.

Milner, B., 1970, Memory and the medial temporal regions of the brain, in *"Biology of Memory"* (K.H. Pribram, and D.E. Broadbent, eds.), pp. 29-50, Academic Press, New York.

Peters, B.H., and Levin, H.S., 1977, Memory enhancement after physostigmine treatment in the amnesic syndrome, *Arch. Neurol. 34:*215.

Peterson, R.C., 1977, Scopolamine induced learning failures in man, *Psychopharmacology 52:*283.

Postman, L., 1976, Methodology of human learning, in *"Handbook of Learning and Cognitive Processes: Approaches to Human Learning and Motivation"* (W.K. Estes, ed.), pp. 11-70, Lawrence Erlbaum, Hillsdale, N.J.

Safer, D.J., and Allen, R.P., 1971, The central effects of scopolamine in man, *Biol. Psychiatry 3:*347.

Sternberg, S., 1966, High speed scanning in human memory, *Science 153:*652.

Sternberg, S., 1969, Memory scanning: mental processes revealed by reaction-time experiments, *Am. Sci. 57:*421.

Warrington, E.K., and Weiskrantz, L., 1973, An analysis of short-term and long-term memory deficits in man, in *"The Physiological Basis of Memory"* (J.A. Deutsch, ed.), pp. 365-395, Academic Press, New York.
Wiener, N., and Deutsch, J.A., 1968, Temporal aspects of anticholinergic and anticholinesterase-induced amnesia for an appetitive habit, *J. Comp. Physiol. Psychol.* 66:613.

THE TREATMENT OF MEMORY DEFICITS IN THE AGED WITH CHOLINE CHLORIDE

K. L. Davis[1,2], R. C. Mohs[1,2], J. R. Tinklenberg[1,2], L. E. Hollister[1,2], J. A. Yesavage[1,2] and B. S. Kopell[1,2]

[1]Veterans Administration Hospital, 3801 Miranda Avenue, Palo Alto, California 94304

[2]Department of Psychiatry and Behavioral Sciences, Stanford University School of Medicine, Stanford, California 94305

INTRODUCTION

Various lines of evidence suggest that as the brain ages there is a decrement in central cholinergic activity. An age-related decrease in the activity of brain choline acetyltransferase (CAT) in humans has been reported (McGeer and McGeer, 1976). These results parallel animal findings (Hollander and Barrows, 1968; Vernadakis, 1973; Meek *et al.*, 1977). Since CAT has been taken as a marker of cholinergic neurons, these data indicate a loss of cholinergic neurons with increasing age (Kuhar, 1976). Muscarinic receptor binding has also been reported to diminish with age (White *et al.*, 1977). Thus both pre-synaptic and post-synaptic cholinergic degeneration may occur in the process of normal aging. Preliminary studies of patients with Alzheimer's disease have also found decreased CAT activity and muscarinic receptor binding (Davies and Maloney, 1976; Perry *et al.*, 1977; White *et al.*, 1977; Yamamura, personal communication). The extent of these changes in central cholinergic neurons is greater in patients with Alzheimer's disease than normal age matched controls.

Changes in central cholinergic transmission profoundly affect memory function. A subdelirium-producing dose of the anticholinergic agent scopolamine produces a change in long-term memory (LTM) function in normal young people that is indistinguishable from the deficit in normal elderly subjects (Drachman and Leavitt, 1974). Recently this effect has been linked to a specific decrease in cholinergic function, rather than a nonspecific effect of scopolamine (Drachman, 1977). Two studies and one case report indicate that a relatively low dose of physostigmine or arecoline can improve long-term memory function in subjects under age 40 (Peters and Levin, 1977; Davis *et al.*, 1978c; Sitaram *et al.*, 1978). These cholinomimetics improve the aspects of memory that anticholinergic agents impair. On the other hand, a slightly higher dose of physostigmine produces a decrement in LTM functioning. These results indicate that the favorable effect of cholinomimetics on LTM occurs in a narrow dose range.

Taken together, these studies have led to the hypothesis that the deficit in memory function associated with aging, and perhaps Alzheimer's disease, is a result of central cholinergic underactivity. It has been suggested that a long acting central cholinomimetic might improve LTM function in elderly people (Davis and Yamamura, in press). Choline chloride, a drug reported to increase brain acetylcholine levels in rats, might be the desired drug. This paper reports the results of a trial of choline chloride in normal elderly people with mild to moderate LTM impairment.

METHODS

Subjects

All subjects were ambulatory, living in their communities, and had no significant medical illnesses and no overt evidence of cerebrovascular disease. Subjects included seven females and one male. Ages ranged from 64 to 86, with a mean age of 74.5 years. As a screening test for entry into the study, subjects were asked to participate in a recall task. Twenty unassociated items were presented verbally to the subject at a rate of 1 every 2 sec. The subjects were instructed to recall as many items as possible. Subjects' responses were written. Between trials, subjects were reminded of all the words they missed, but no items they correctly recalled. To be accepted into the study, subjects could not recall more than 15 of 20 verbally presented items on the first trial, and never recall 20 items on the 5 succeeding trials. There was no time limit for subjects to recall words between trials. In a separate study, this criteria successfully identified a group of young normal subjects who subsequently were significantly improved in their LTM functioning by administration of physostigmine (Davis *et al.,* 1978c).

All subjects had normal urinalysis, hematocrit, hemoglobin, white count, renal and electrocardiogram (ECG), physical examination, serum glucose, electrolytes and CO_2. Thus, these subjects were relatively healthy, elderly people with the expected age related changes in memory processes. Informed consent was obtained from every subject and the entire study was approved by the Stanford University Committee for the Protection of Human Subjects.

Drug Administration

The study lasted 35 days. Four times daily on days 1-7, subjects received a placebo designed to look and taste like choline chloride. On days 8-14, subjects were given 16 gm of choline chloride per day in four equally divided doses. During days 15-35, subjects received placebo as they had from days 1-7.

Neither subjects nor raters were told when placebo or choline chloride was given. However, while on choline chloride some subjects had a peculiar "fish-like" odor. Subjects were dispensed drug or placebo on days 1, 7, and 14 of the study. In order to augment compliance in taking choline chloride or placebo, subjects returned their bottles of drug on the days they were dispensed new drugs. ECG rhythm strips and blood tests were conducted on days 7, 14 and 35.

Assessment

Memory processes, affective state and global cognitive function were assessed at the end of the first placebo period (day 7), the choline chloride administration (day 14), and at the conclusion of the second placebo period (day 35). LTM function was tested with a task designed to measure retrieval and a task designed to measure the storage of information into LTM. In the paradigm to evaluate retrieval, subjects were verbally presented with a list of 15 definitions of non-related words. Following each definition, subjects were to supply the word defined. At the end of the list, subjects were allowed unlimited time to recall these items in writing. Immediately after this trial, the experimenter informed the subjects of the words the subject had not recalled. Then subjects again attempted to recall the 15 items. Ten minutes later, two more recall trials were conducted, but between these trials subjects were not prompted in the items they could not recall. After another 30 min, another pair of recall trials was completed. Again subjects were not reminded of the words they could not recall. Between each pair of trials, subjects were engaged in other tasks.

The ability of subjects to store information into LTM was evaluated by a modification of the Buschke selective reminding memory task (Buschke, 1973; Buschke and Fuld, 1974). Subjects were verbally presented a list of 20 related items at a rate of 1 per 2 sec, and were asked to recall the items in writing. After 6 min to recall the words, the experimenter reminded the subjects of all the items the subject had not recalled. Subject and experimenter completed six trials in immediate succession. Different but equivalent forms of the retrieval and Buschke task were presented during the three testing days. Varying the material on these tasks prevented subjects from displaying significant practice effects.

Affective state was assessed with a 100 mm mood line. One end of the line was labelled "the happiest I have ever felt," and the opposite end of the line was labelled "the saddest I have ever felt." Subjects were instructed to place a mark on the line corresponding to their present mood. The scale has been found to sensitively reflect changes in affective state produced by alterations in cholinergic activity (Davis et al., 1978a). Six of the eight subjects participated in this aspect of the study. A general measure of the subjects cognitive state and ability to function in the community was obtained by completing the SCAG (Shader et al., 1974). This scale has 19 separate items, each assessed on a seven-point scale. This is a specific geriatric rating scale designed to determine orientation, gross memory function, degree of socialization and the ability to care for oneself.

RESULTS

Table 1 displays the results of the eight subjects on the retrieval task. Comparison of mean scores during each placebo period with the choline chloride period does not indicate any effect of choline chloride on the ability of subjects to retrieve information assumed to be in LTM. However, it should be noted that subject 6, who had the worst performance on this task during the first placebo period, was markedly improved during choline chloride treatment. During the second placebo period he could not recall as many items as he could when receiving choline chloride.

TABLE 1

Effect of Choline Chloride on Retrieval from LTM

Patient Number	Placebo Day 7 Learning Trials		Recall Trials		Recall Trials		Choline Day 14 Learning Trials		Recall Trials		Recall Trials		Placebo Day 35 Learning Trials		Recall Trials		Recall Trials	
1	10	12	11	11	11	12	10	13	12	12	12	12	10	14	14	13	14	13
2	12	10	12	11	11	12	7	11	10	11	12	13	9	14	13	13	12	12
3	9	8	8	8	4	3	4	6	6	4	2	0	3	6	5	7	1	0
4	5	9	9	11	8	9	7	11	7	6	6	7	7	10	8	8	3	7
5	10	10	9	9	9	9	7	10	10	9	7	9	7	9	11	10	8	7
6	4	7	1	1	1	1	5	10	8	7	8	8	6	8	6	7	4	4
7	6	10	7	5	6	5	6	9	6	7	6	7	8	10	8	9	8	8
8	9	12	11	11	10	9	9	12	10	9	10	9	10	15	10	10	11	10
$\bar{X}$	8.10	9.80	8.50	8.40	7.50	7.50	6.90	10.3	8.60	8.10	7.90	8.10	7.50	10.8	9.40	9.60	7.60	7.60
S	2.80	1.75	3.46	3.66	3.59	4.07	1.96	2.12	2.20	2.64	3.40	3.94	2.33	3.24	3.20	2.39	4.63	4.24
$S_{\bar{X}}$	0.99	0.62	1.22	1.30	1.27	1.44	0.69	0.75	0.78	0.93	1.20	1.39	0.82	1.15	1.13	0.84	1.64	1.50

Similar results were found during the Buschke selective reminding task as outlined in Table 2. There were no significant differences between the mean performance of subjects in any phase of the study. Subjects were not able to store more information during choline chloride than placebo treatment.

Table 3 presents the mean scores for six patients on the 100 mm mood line during each of the three phases of the study. Higher scores reflect happier mood. It can be seen that choline chloride had no significant effect on the mean mood scores for the eight subjects.

Table 4 presents the total SCAG score during each phase of the study. Lower scores are associated with better functioning. Mean scores for all eight subjects were not significantly different during choline chloride treatment than while subjects were taking placebo.

DISCUSSION

Choline chloride did not influence the performance of normal elderly people on two tasks of LTM. These results have at least three possible explanations: (1) Choline chloride does not increase central cholinergic activity; (2) Alterations in cholinergic activity cannot be used therapeutically in affecting the memory of people with age related memory changes; (3) The patient population and/or study design was not appropriate to test the efficacy of choline chloride. Each possibility is discussed below.

(1) *Choline chloride does not increase central cholinergic activity:* Although choline chloride has been shown to increase brain levels of acetylcholine, the evidence that it increases central cholinergic activity is indirect (Cohen and Wurtman, 1975; Cohen and Wurtman, 1976; Ulus and Wurtman, 1976). Precursor loading with choline could increase cholinergic activity in the striatum, but not affect levels in brain areas involved in memory. For example, two groups have been unable to demonstrate an effect of choline chloride on acetylcholine levels in any brain section except the striatum (Eckernas, 1977; Hanin et al., 1978). Thus, choline chloride would not be anticipated to improve memory function even in subjects who have diminished cholinergic activity if it does not elevate cholinergic activity in hippocampal cholinergic synapses.

Increased central cholinergic activity can cause some manic patients to become depressed (Janowsky et al., 1973; Davis et al., 1978a). Occasionally, normal subjects, who may have a predisposition to depression, also become depressed after a physostigmine infusion (Davis et al., 1976b). Choline chloride treatment has also been associated with depression in some patients with tardive dyskinesia (Tamminga et al., 1976). Thus, if a subject in this study had become depressed, this response would have been consistent with choline chloride increasing central cholinergic activity, In fact, this did not occur, but the number of patients studied may have been too small to demonstrate this possible effect of choline chloride.

(2) *Alterations in cholinergic activity cannot be used therapeutically to affect memory function in people with age related memory changes:* If this possibility is the explanation for the negative results with choline chloride, the question of whether choline can increase brain cholinergic activity becomes irrelevant. If there is a significant

TABLE 2

Effect of Choline Chloride on Storage Into LTM

Patient Number	Placebo Day 7 Learning Trials		Recall Trials		Recall Trials		Choline Day 14 Learning Trials		Recall Trials		Recall Trials		Placebo Day 35 Learning Trials		Recall Trials		Recall Trials	
1	16	15	17	17	18	19	14	16	19	18	20	18	15	17	18	19	19	17
2	11	15	18	18	18	19	11	11	16	18	19	20	12	14	17	16	16	15
3	10	8	11	8	11	12	10	13	12	11	13	10	8	4	10	10	10	13
4	16	16	15	17	19	19	9	16	17	16	17	16	12	17	17	17	19	19
5	11	13	13	15	17	17	12	17	16	17	15	17	7	12	15	15	16	16
6	12	13	17	17	17	18	10	15	17	18	17	19	13	16	16	17	19	20
7	16	17	18	19	19	19	15	14	16	17	18	19	14	14	16	17	17	16
8	12	18	15	20	19	20	12	16	16	19	17	19	13	18	19	20	20	20
$\bar{X}$	13.0	14.4	15.5	16.4	17.3	17.9	11.6	14.8	16.1	16.8	17.0	17.3	11.8	14.0	16.0	16.4	17.0	17.0
S	2.56	3.11	2.51	2.66	2.53		2.07	1.98	1.96	2.49	2.20	3.20	2.82	4.50	2.73	3.02	3.21	2.51
$S\bar{X}$	0.91	1.10	0.89	1.31	0.94	0.90	0.73	0.70	0.69	0.88	0.78	1.13	1.00	1.59	0.96	1.07	1.13	0.89

TABLE 3

Effect of Choline Chloride on Mood

Mean Mood Line Scores
N = 6

	Placebo Day 7	Choline Day 14	Placebo Day 35
$\overline{X}$	65.50	69.33	72.16
S	16.92	10.36	12.76
$S_{\overline{X}}$	6.92	4.23	5.21

TABLE 4

Effect of Choline Chloride on Cognitive State

Mean SCAG Scores
N = 8

	Placebo Day 7	Choline Day 14	Placebo Day 35
$\overline{X}$	24.00	23.75	20.75
S	4.14	3.84	1.98
$S_{\overline{X}}$	1.46	1.35	0.70

reduction in muscarinic receptor binding in aged individuals, increasing presynaptic levels of acetylcholine would not increase cholinergic activity. This may be the situation in patients with senile dementia (Yamamura, personal communication) and there are preliminary data to support the possibility that with increasing age muscarinic receptor binding decreases (Kuhar, 1976). It is also known that there is a loss of presynaptic cholinergic neurons with increasing age (White *et al.*, 1977). If this loss is extensive, then precursor loading with choline chloride would have a negligible effect on elevating brain acetylcholine levels, and hence on central cholinergic activity.

(3) *The patient population and/or study design was not appropriate to test the efficacy of choline chloride in elderly people with an age related memory loss.* A number of factors support this possibility. The subjects in this study had no major medical problems. All were in excellent health. More than 90% of the subjects who asked to participate were not studied because they had some medical abnormality. Thus, the elderly people who actually participated in this study were quite atypical in that they had very little degenerative disease. If only minor age related changes had also occurred in their central nervous system, they might have an insignificant loss of central cholinergic activity and age related memory changes. Hence, this group of subjects would not be ideally suited to test the effect of choline chloride on LTM functioning in the elderly. In fact, the performance of all but two subjects (3 and 6) was well within the range found in normal young people. It is therefore interesting to note that one of these impaired people (subject 6) was greatly improved on the retrieval task while on choline chloride. Future studies should have a more rigid criteria for excluding people who do not have a real degree of memory impairment. In this way, the so-called "ceiling effect" could be kept to a minimum. On the other hand, future studies might also include people with medical conditions if those conditions would be unaffected by the use of choline chloride.

It is also possible that the dose of choline chloride and its duration of administration were not optimal. Patients with tardive dyskinesia and Huntington's disease who respond to choline chloride usually do not have a significant change in the frequency of their abnormal movements until they have been on high doses of choline chloride for more than 7 days (Davis *et al.*, 1976a). Similarly, in the animal model of tardive dyskinesia, more than a week's ingestion of choline chloride precedes a significant action of the drug (Davis *et al.*, 1978b). This delay in clinical effect was seen despite the acute elevations in brain acetylcholine levels that have been produced in rats following a single intraperitoneal injection of choline chloride (Haubrich *et al.*, 1975; Cohen and Wurtman, 1976). Conceivably a prolonged exposure to choline chloride is a prerequisite for a behavioral change, and the one week period of choline administration in the present study was too short to have affected memory.

The dose of choline chloride could also have adversely affected the outcome of this study. The effects of physostigmine upon LTM functioning have been shown to be exquisitely sensitive to dose. The administration of a low dose of physostigmine improves LTM functioning, but higher doses cause a worsening in subject's performance on tasks of LTM (Davis *et al.*, 1976b; Davis *et al.*, 1978c). There is evidence that the effect of 16 gm of choline chloride per day is more like the effect of physostigmine in a high dose rather than a low dose. The EEG pattern produced in subjects taking 16 gm of choline chloride daily resembles the pattern of a high dose of physostigmine (Pfefferbaum *et al.*, *Electrophysiological Effects of Physostigmine in Humans,* this book). Furthermore, the effects of 16 gm per day of choline chloride to reduce the abnormal involuntary movement frequency of patients with tardive dyskinesia are only matched by a dose of physostigmine that causes a deterioration in LTM functioning. Taken together, these data indicate that a dose considerably below 16 gm/day would be the most likely dose to improve the performance of subjects on tasks of LTM.

Future studies should take into account these factors in testing the effect of choline chloride upon age related changes in memory in elderly people.

ACKNOWLEDGEMENTS

This research was supported by the Medical Research Service of the Veterans Administration, U.S. Public Health Service Grant MH-03030, and the National Institute of Mental Health Specialized Research Grant MH-30854.

REFERENCES

Buschke, H., 1973, Selective reminding for analysis of memory and learning, *J. Verb. Learn. Verb. Behav. 12:*543.

Buschke, H., and Fuld, P.A., 1974, Evaluating storage, retention and retrieval in disordered memory and learning, *Neurology 24:*1019.

Cohen, E.L., and Wurtman, R.J., 1975, Brain acetylcholine: increase after systemic choline administration, *Life Sci. 16:*1095.

Cohen, E.L., and Wurtman, R.J., 1976, Brain acetylcholine control by dietary choline, *Science 191:*561.

Davies, P., and Maloney, A.J.F., 1976, Selective loss of central cholinergic neurons in Alzheimer's disease (letter), *Lancet 2:*1403.

Davis, K.L., and Yamamura, H.I., (in press), Cholinergic underactivity in human memory disorders, *Life Sci.*

Davis, K.L., Hollister, L.E., Barchas, J.D., and Berger, P.A., 1976a, Choline in tardive dyskinesia and Huntington's disease, *Life Sci. 19:*1507.

Davis, K.L., Hollister, L.E., Overall, J., Johnson, A., and Train, K., 1976b, Physostigmine: effects on cognition and affect in normal subjects, *Psychopharmacology 51:*23.

Davis, K.L., Berger, P.A., Hollister, L.E., and De Fraites, E.G., 1978a, Physostigmine in mania, *Arch. Gen. Psychiatry 35(1):*119.

Davis, K.L., Hollister, L.E., Vento, A.L., and Simonton, S.C., 1978b, Choline chloride in animal models of tardive dyskinesia, *Life Sci. 22:*1699.

Davis, K.L., Mohs, R., Tinklenberg, J.R., Pfefferbaum, A., Hollister, L.E., and Kopell, B.S., 1978c, Physostigmine: improvement of long-term memory processes in normal humans, *Science 201:*272.

Drachman, D.A., 1977, Memory and cognitive function in man: does the cholinergic system have a specific role? *Neurology 27:*783.

Drachman, D.A., and Leavitt, J., 1974, Human memory and the cholinergic system. *Arch. Neurol. 30:*113.

Eckernas, S.A., 1977, Plasma choline and cholinergic mechanisms in the brain, *Acta Physiol. Scand. (Suppl.) 449:*1.

Hanin, I., Kopp, U., Zahniser, H.R., Shih, T.M., Spiker, D.G., Merikangas, J.R., Kupfer, D.J., and Foster, F.G., 1978, Acetylcholine and choline in human plasma and red blood cells: a gas chromatograph/mass spectrometric evaluation, in *"Cholinergic Mechanisms and Psychopharmacology"* (D.J. Jenden, ed.), pp. 181-195, Plenum Press, New York.

Haubrich, D.R., Wang, P.F.L., Clody, D.E., and Wedeking, P.W., 1975, Increase in rat brain acetylcholine induced by choline or deanol, *Life Sci. 17:*975.

Hollander, J., and Barrows, C.H., 1968, Enzymatic studies in senescent rodent brains, *J. Gerontol. 23:*174.

Janowsky, D.S., El-Yousef, J.K., and Davis, J.M., 1973, Parasympathetic suppression of manic symptoms by physostigmine, *Arch. Gen. Psychiatry 28:*542.

Kuhar, M.J., 1976, The anatomy of cholinergic neurons, in *"Biology of Cholinergic Function"* (A.M. Goldberg, and I. Hanin, eds.), pp. 3027, Raven Press, New York.

McGeer, E., and McGeer, P.L., 1976, Age changes in the human for some enzymes associated with metabolism of catecholamines, GABA, and acetylcholine, in *"Neurobiology of Aging"* (J.M. Ordee, and R.R. Brizee, eds.), pp. 389, Raven Press, New York.

Meek, J.L., Bertilsson, L., Cheney, D.L., Zsilla, G., and Costa, E., 1977, Aging-induced changes in acetylcholine and serotonin content of discrete brain nuclei, *J. Gerontol.* 32:129.

Perry, E.K., Perry, R.H., Blessed, G., and Tomlinson, B.E., 1977, Necropsy evidence of central cholinergic deficits in senile dementia, *Lancet 1:*189.

Peters, B.H., and Levin, H.S., 1977, Memory enhancement after physostigmine treatment in the amnesic syndrome, *Arch. Neurol. 34(4):*215.

Shader, R.I., Harmatz, J.S., and Salzman, C., 1974, A new scale for clinical assessment in geriatric population: Sandoz Clinical Assessment – Geriatric (SCAG), *J. Am. Geriatr. Soc. XXII 3:*107.

Sitaram, N., Weingartner, H., and Gillin, J.C., 1978, Human serial learning: enhancement with arecoline and choline and impairment with scopolamine, *Science 201:*274.

Tamminga, C., Smith, R.C., Chang, S., Harasti, J.S., and Davis, J.M., 1976, Depression from oral choline (letter), *Lancet 2:*905.

Ulus, I.H., and Wurtman, R.J., 1976, Choline administration: activation of tyrosine hydroxylase in dopaminergic neurons of rat brain, *Science 194:*1060.

Vernadakis, A., 1973, Comparative studies of neurotransmitter substances in the maturing and aging central nervous system of the chicken, *Prog. Brain Res. 40(0):*231.

White, P., Hiley, C.R., Goodhardt, M.J., Carrasco, L.H., Keet, J.P., Williams, I.E.I., and Bowen, D.M., 1977, Neocortical cholinergic neurons in elderly people, *Lancet 1:*668.

THE ELECTROPHYSIOLOGY OF
CHOLINERGIC AGENTS

BRAIN ACETYLCHOLINE AND ANIMAL ELECTROPHYSIOLOGY

A. G. Karczmar

Department of Pharmacology, Loyola University Stritch School of Medicine
2160 South First Avenue, Maywood, Illinois 60153

INTRODUCTION

Aims and Limitations of This Review

This review concerns the relationship between electrophysiological activity of the brain and the central cholinergic system. This dipole may be construed in a sense so broad as to be beyond the space limitations of this article; thus, further defining is necessary. Electrophysiological activity to be reviewed here is generated by neuronal populations rather than single neurons, as it involves cholinergically mediated changes in ongoing electrical activity of neuronal populations referred to as electroencephalograph (EEG), electrocorticogram (ECoG), etc. Another major response of neuronal populations, which is also the subject of this review is the compound potential evoked by peripheral or brain stimulation (EP). On the other hand, while the EEG and ECoG are generated by the summation of individual postsynaptic potentials and related phenomena, the pertinent unitary mechanisms whether concerning noncholinergic or cholinoceptive and cholinergic neurons cannot be reviewed in the present context.

As to the other member of the relationship, the central cholinergic system, some of its characteristics will have to be reviewed, but only in so far as they are pertinent to the relationship in question. Thus, the main mechanisms of synaptic cholinergic transmission will be referred to briefly. Important in the present context is the topography of cholinergic pathways. Indeed, the presence of the cholinergic pathways within certain brain systems such as the reticular formation or the thalamus is particularly pertinent for the generation and control of EEG activity and of EP and thus they will be reviewed at some length.

FUNDAMENTALS OF CENTRAL CHOLINERGIC TRANSMISSION AND PATHWAYS

Characteristics of Synaptic Cholinergic Transmission

As in the periphery, central cholinergic transmission involves cholinergic neurons, the presynaptic nerve cells that synthesize and release acetylcholine (ACh), and the

265

postsynaptic cells which are cholinoceptive, ie, contain cholinergic receptors. The cholinoceptive cells may be also cholinergic and release ACh, or they may be non-cholinergic and release a neurotransmitter other than ACh. These two types of organization correspond respectively to that of the parasympathetic and sympathetic autonomic nervous system, the former includes two successive cholinergic junctions, while in the case of the sympathetic system the cholinergic cell synapses in the ganglia with a catecholamine-releasing neuron. It is assumed frequently that central cholinergic synapses always alternate with non-cholinergic neurons, as proposed by Feldberg and Vogt (1978), analogous to the situation that obtains in the sympathetic autonomic system. Actually, it is difficult to prove that this is so even in the case of such much-studied sites as the nigro-striatal-nigral loop where such an alternation is suspected. In any event, whether via direct couplings with neurons releasing non-ACh neurotransmitters, or indirectly, cholinergic synapses affect most, if not all, neurotransmitter systems (Karczmar, 1978; "Neurochemical and Neurophysiological Interaction Between Cholinergic and Other Bioamine Systems" section of this chapter). It must be also pointed out that whether in the periphery or centrally, cholinoceptive receptors may be present not only on postsynaptic neuronal somas or dendrites but also on the presynaptic nerve terminals of the cholinergic neurons (Nishi, 1974; Szerb, 1975; Giorguieff et al., 1977; Karczmar and Dun, 1978). Thus, cholinergic agonists and antagonists as well as endogenous ACh may modulate their own release.

Enzymatic machinery needed for the function of cholinergic neurons is of importance. The synthesis requires choline acetyltransferase (CAT) and acetylcoenzyme A (AcCoA) as well as the precursor, choline (Fonnum, 1973; Lloyd, 1975). As choline is not synthesized in the cholinergic neuron, a high affinity uptake system is also needed. Diet and several metabolite precursors (Wurtman et al., 1974; Ulus et al., 1977; Wurtman, 1976) are important for the synthesis of both choline and of neuronal ACh. However, to a considerable extent, choline is provided for the uptake by hydrolysis of released ACh (Collier et al., 1977; MacIntosh and Collier, 1976).

The catabolic function is accomplished by the enzymes and isoenzymes of the cholinesterase (ChE) family. Acetylcholinesterase (AChE), an enzyme that hydrolyzes ACh at an extremely high rate, is primarily involved in termination of the synaptic action of ACh both at central and peripheral sites (Koelle, 1963; Usdin, 1970). This is consistent with its pre- and post-synaptic localization. Butyrylcholinesterase (pseudocholinesterase, BuChE) hydrolyzes butyrylcholine quickly, but ACh relatively slowly. Its role is relatively obscure. It is present at certain peripheral and central synaptic sites (Koelle et al., 1977) and in high concentrations in ganglia (Koelle et al., 1977). While less conspicuous in the central nervous system, BuChE may represent up to 20% of total ChE activity of certain brain areas such as the striate (Lloyd, 1975). However, its main central nervous system (CNS) source may be glia or neuroglia. This localization of BuChE may be functionally important as neuroglia responds to ACh. BuChE may also be important when levels of ACh are abnormally high. It is pertinent in this context that such organophosphorus anticholinesterases (antiChE's) as diisopropylphosphofluoridate (diisopropylfluorophosphate; DFP), which evoke profound EEG and other central actions (see "Cortical and Subcortical EEG Actions of Cholinergic Agonists and Anticholinesterases" section of this chapter), are more potent inhibitors of BuChE than of AChE (Usdin, 1970). Other roles for BuChE are suggested as well (Koelle et al., 1977).

Both in the periphery and centrally, ACh produces two types of effects. When applied iontophoretically to the autonomic ganglion cells (Nishi, 1974; Karczmar and Dun, 1978) or to cholinoceptive central neurons (Krnjevic, 1974; 1976), it produces either a prolonged effect with a slow onset of action or a fast, intense response, which is characterized by a minimal latency. At the endplate of the skeletal muscle the fast response occurs almost exclusively. On the basis of pharmacological evaluation of these two effects by means of appropriate cholinomimetic agonists and antagonists, the slow and fast effects are referred to as muscarinic and nicotinic, respectively. Cholinoceptive, muscarinic or nicotinic receptors may be differentiated chemically (De Robertis and Schacht, 1974), and by their differential binding of two ligands: the muscarinic antagonist quinuclidinyl benzilate (QNB) and the nicotinic antagonist a-bungarotoxin (Birdsall et al., 1977).

During both muscarinic and nicotinic central response, the conductance to potassium and sodium are affected (Krnjevic, 1974; 1976). In the case of the central nicotinic response ACh increases the conductance of potassium and sodium (Krnjevic, 1974; 1976) inducing depolarization and decrease in the membrane resistance. The central nicotinic depolarization is analogous to the nicotinic ganglionic or neuromyal excitatory postsynaptic potential, and it gives rise to a spike or neuronal firing. The central muscarinic effect is also excitatory and depolarizing in nature. Both at the ganglia and centrally, this depolarization is not necessarily coupled with decreased resistance. In fact, in the case of central neurons, the membrane resistance may increase (Woody et al., 1974). Krnjevic (1974; 1976) explains this central phenomenon as due to ACh-induced reduction in potassium conductance. Krnjevic (1969; 1974; 1976) pointed out that such a mechanism would have little effect in activating a cell with a very negative resting potential, but would facilitate the neuronal firing in the presence of any excitatory input. To the contrary, the nicotinic response would be primarily synaptic and transmissive in nature.

Certain central, cholinoceptive neurons are capable of still another response to ACh, contrary to the two depolarizing, excitatory responses. The response in question is inhibitory in nature, as first reported by Randic et al. (1964). Generally, but not always, this response is muscarinic as it is blocked by systemic, or local administration of atropine rather than of nicotine or d-tubocurarine. It appears that a direct, inhibitory postsynaptic action of ACh is involved in this phenomenon, rather than a disynaptically- or poly-synaptically-induced release of an inhibitor. Indeed, it could be shown that certain neurons that respond to presynaptic stimulation with inhibition of firing and/or hyperpolarization respond similarly to iontophoretic application of ACh, and that both inhibitions can be blocked by atropine (Phillis and York, 1968). The ionic mechanisms of this inhibition are not known. While it may be suspected that increase in potassium conductance may be involved (as this mechanism underlies cholinergic inhibition at the auricle), such an effect should involve a decrease in resistance which has not been observed at central inhibitory cholinoceptive sites (Krnjevic, 1976). ACh block is not antagonized by blockers of the hyperpolarizing effects of GABA or glycine (Ben-Ari et al., 1976).

Recently an elegant hypothesis was elaborated relating ACh-induced changes to cyclic adenosine $3'$-$5'$-monophosphate (cAMP) and cyclic quanine $3'$-$5'$-monophosphate (cGMP) (Greengard, 1976). It was suggested that the cyclic nucleotides act as second messengers, mediating membrane action of ACh via activation of phosphokinases (Sutherland and Robinson, 1966). Originally, hyperpolarizing an inhibitory mechanism was ascribed by Greengard to a disynaptic circuit of the ganglion (Libet, 1970; Dun *et al.*, 1977a; 1977b; Dun and Karczmar, 1977; 1978; Karczmar and Dun, 1978), the chain of events including ACh, small intensely fluorescent (SIF) interneuron, dopamine and cAMP. As described above, ACh mediated inhibition may not be of hyperpolarizing nature. Greengard (1976) proposed a similar mechanism, mediated by cGMP, for the ganglionic muscarinic and related central responses. The pertinent data are at this time, controversial (Dun and Karczmar, 1977; 1978; Krnjevic and Van Meter, 1976; Krnjevic *et al.*, 1976; Karczmar and Dun, 1978).

It is of interest that comparatively few neurons show only one type of response. Even the classical cholinoceptive site at the spinal interneuron, the Renshaw cell, originally described as purely nicotinic (Eccles *et al.*, 1954), shows a clearly defined muscarinic response. Other nicotinic sites, such as those in the thalamus and the lateral and medial geniculate, exhibit either mixed responses or responses that can be blocked by both atropine and nicotinic antagonists or curaremimetics (Krnjevic, 1974; 1976). In the present context it is of interest that the sites involved in EEG rhythm generating activities such as the medullary, thalamic and midbrain sites, including cholinoceptive neurons of the reticular formation, show frequently inhibitory as well as muscarinic and nicotinic excitatory responses to acetylcholine. Indeed, the presence of both inhibitory and excitatory cholinoceptive sites in the reticular formation may have a bearing on the desynchronizing capacity of the cholinergic system. Of similar significance is the presence of such a dipole in the thalamus, as the latter serves as control for synchronizing activities of the EEG and for gating of sensory transmission, the later being also involved in EEG control (Ben-Ari *et al.*, 1976; "Mechanisms and Sites of Cholinergic Desynchronization" section of this chapter). It is also significant that the neurons of the thalamic nucleus reticularis inhibit thalamic relay cells that are excited by ACh and which are involved in the generation of synchronous EEG patterns.

Cholinergic Pathways

Distribution of Sites of the Components of the Cholinergic System (Choline Acetyltransferase, Acetylcholine and Cholinesterases) and of Acetylcholine Binding and Uptake

To map cholinergic pathways, cholinergic synapses must be identified and their organization within the pathway established. The presence of ACh-containing synaptic vesicles in the nerve terminals combined with demonstration of ACh release from the latter and of its postsynaptic action, constitute sufficient evidence for the presence and localization of central cholinergic synapses, while the cholinergic pathways have to be mapped in conjunction with the localization of the somata of pertinent cholinergic neurons and of their synapses. At present, definite data along the lines indicated cannot be obtained. Central cholinergic synapses cannot be directly demonstrated, and ACh cannot be traced histochemically by techniques such as those employed by the Scandinavian investigators for the mapping of catecholaminergic and serotonergic pathways.

At this time, cholinergic mapping is obtained by the use of several indirect methods. An effective study (Lewis and Shute, 1967) of cholinergic pathways was based on the histochemical procedure for localization of AChE developed by Koelle (1963). Lewis and Shute (1967; Shute, 1975) showed that as AChE is present presynaptically in cholinergic neurons, it disappears distally and accumulates proximally following cuts across the cholinergic axons, and this strategem was employed for tracing the cholinergic pathways. Another methodology involves the measurement of CAT, ACh, and the measurement of ACh turnover. A new methodology permits their quantitative evaluation in separate nuclei or even groups of neurons (Cheney et al., 1976). Additional information comes from the localization by binding, and related techniques, of muscarinic and nicotinic postsynaptic receptors (Kuhar, 1976). Still other information pertains to uptake. Indeed, cholinergic neurons actively take up choline (Kuhar, 1973; 1976). Finally, important pertinent data is based on the presence of cholinoceptive neurons responding to ionto-phoretic application of ACh (Krnjevic, 1969; 1974) and the release of ACh upon stimu-lation of cholinergic structures (Pepeu, 1974). The results from these different methods are generally consistent, i.e., the sites exhibiting cholinoceptivity components of the cholinergic system such as AChE and ACh, and high ACh turnover, overlap (Kuhar, 1976).

Altogether, cholinergic pathways may be briefly described as follows (Shute and Lewis, 1967; Lewis and Shute, 1967; Krnjevic, 1969; Shute and Lewis, 1975; Kuhar, 1976, Butcher, 1977). They originate in the midbrain reticular formation (MRF) and branch into dorsal and ventral components. The ventral tegmental pathway arises from the tip of the MRF and the neurons in the ventral tegmental area and substantia nigra. The ventral pathway innervates supramammilary region, the posterior, dorsal and lateral – but not medial – hypothalamus, lateral preoptic areas, globus pallidus, diagonal band and medial septal nucleus. Tegmental cholinergic area innervates the cerebellum via afferents originating in the dorsal-lateral tegmental nucleus, reticular nuclei and in the nucleus reticularis tegmenti ponti. Some of these areas, including globus pallidus also contain neurons innervating the striate, hypothalamus, some of the limbic nuclei and areas (preoptic area, thalamic nuclei, lateral amygdaloid nucleus, diagonal band of Broca, nucleus accumbens), and the neocortex (Shute and Lewis, 1975). Extensive cholinergic pathways seem to course between amygdaloid complex, preoptic area, stria terminalis and hypothalamus (Ben-Ari et al., 1977). Preoptic area also supplies olfactory tubercle and olfactory bulb. Altogether, cortical areas are cholinergically innervated by cingulate, striatal, olfactory and amygdaloid radiations arising in the areas innervated by the ventral tegmental cholinergic pathway such as the globus pallidus, lateral preoptic area, olfactory tubercle, and amygdaloid nucleus. Thus, the MRF and the ventral tegmental pathway form a diffuse extrapyramidal tegmental-mesencephalic cortical system analogous to the diffuse reticular arousal system (Rinaldi and Himwich, 1955), and the cerebral cortex appears to be rich in cholinergic receptors of both nicotinic and muscarinic type (Kuhar and Yamamura, 1976; Morley et al., 1977).

The dorsal tegmental pathway originates in the MRF and ascends to midbrain tectum and diencephalon, innervating corpora quadrigemina, pretectal area, anterior and medial thalamus with its non-specific nuclei and medial and geniculate bodies, and subcortical visual centers.

The hippocampus is innervated by dense cholinergic neurons of the medial septum and diagonal band constituting septal radiation (Shute and Lewis, 1975; Kuhar, 1976); it seems to contain cholinergic receptors of both muscarinic and nicotinic type (Kuhar and Yamamura, 1976; Morley et al., 1977). Furthermore, noncholinergic hippocampal efferents innervate ventral hippocampal commisure, habenular nuclei, precallosal cells, nucleus accumbens and antero-ventral and dorsal thalamic nuclei which contain cholinergic neurons innervating the rhinencephalon and cingulate cortex, and descending back to ventral, dorsal and deep tegmental nuclei, to the striate (Simke and Saelens, 1977), MRF, the raphe system and hence to interpeduncular areas. Habenula may contain its own cholinergic neurons that innervate interpeduncular nuclei (Lewis and Shute, 1967). This agrees with the fact that among the central nuclei the interpeduncular site exhibits the highest level of CAT as well as cholinoceptivity of muscarinic type (Kuhar and Yamamura, 1976; Kuhar, 1976). The cholinergic septal radiation constitutes then, directly and indirectly, the cholinergic limbic system (Shute, 1975), although both ventral and dorsal tegmental areas contribute, as already described, to the cholinergic limbic system.

Finally, localized cholinergic networks are present in the retina, cortex, hypothalamus and the striate (Pepeu, 1974; Shute and Lewis, 1975; Kuhar, 1976). The areas in question seem to exhibit cholinergic receptors of both muscarinic and nicotinic type (Kuhar and Yamamura, 1976; Morley et al., 1977). Recent evidence suggests that these networks receive cholinergic input from other areas. For instance, the striate may be cholinergically innervated from the brain stem sites such as Raphe nuclei.

Release of Acetylcholine from Brain Sites Upon Chemical, Electrical or Behavioral Stimulation

This subject is of major importance. First, while the release of ACh upon the stimulation of nuclei, cell groups or pathways cannot serve for localization of specific cholinergic synapses, as such stimulation will affect heterogeneous synaptic populations in terms of neurotransmitters. The pertinent evidence indicates the presence and activity of such synapses and helps in evaluating the cholinergic "tone" of a particular pathway. Furthermore, the stimulation of the pathways in question frequently affects the EEG. Hence, the pertinent experiments help relate the EEG phenomena to release of ACh and to the cholinergic system.

The ascending MRF tegmental pathways that correspond to the arousal system (Starzl et al., 1951; Rinaldi and Himwich, 1955) cause liberation of ACh from the cerebral cortex (Pepeu, 1974). This release is spread out over visual, auditory and somatosensory areas. Furthermore, ACh release may be activated by peripheral stimulation, or the stimulation of auditory and visual pathways, and blocked by anesthesia or transection of the reticular formation. Conversely, depression or RF transection increase cortical acetylcholine levels. Appropriate effects upon release and levels of ACh can be obtained by cortical or RF stimulants and depressants, as well as related sleep-wakefulness activity (Maynert et al., 1975). In fact, it is particularly pertinent in the present context that the cortical or subcortical release of ACh is induced by behavioral paradigms relatable to the activation of reticular formation and other brain stem structures, such as behavioral arousal and REM sleep (Pepeu, 1974; Hingtgen and Aprison, 1976; Steriade and Hobson, 1976; Karczmar, 1976; "Role of the Cholinergic System in REM Sleep" section of this chapter).

By the use of push-pull cannulae more detailed evaluation of sites and pathways concerned with the release of ACh may be obtained. Thus, ACh is released locally upon thalamic, septal, striate and hypothalamic stimulation (Pepeu, 1974; Myers, 1974; De Feudis, 1974). This release depends on cholinergic synaptic activity as it is related to the stimulation frequency (Nistri, 1975) and can be blocked by tetrodotoxin (Dudar and Szerb, 1969; Pepeu et al., 1978). Also, ACh is released from the hippocampus (Domino et al., 1977) as well as hippocampal slices, except when the latter were obtained from animals with septal lesions (Szerb, 1977).

It is of interest that cholinergic and anticholinergic drugs that exert potent EEG actions also affect ACh kinetics and release. Nicotine increases ACh release while muscarinic agonists such as oxotremorine and antiChE's decrease it (Pepeu, 1974; Richardson and Szerb, 1974; Bourdois et al., 1974; Szerb, 1977). Finally, atropinics release ACh from brain slices and in situ, and, in consequence, deplete brain ACh (Pepeu, 1974; Szerb, 1977). These results are not readily intelligible. Cholinergic agonists act per definition, on cholinoceptive receptors; these may not be always present on central cholinergic neurons capable of releasing ACh. Thus, it is not self-evident that cholinergic agonists should affect brain release of ACh or its metabolism. In the case of muscarinic agonists and antagonists the pertinent mechanism may concern muscarinic receptors at nerve terminals of cholinergic neurons. Indeed, indirect evidence for their presence at the peripheral synapses is available (Koelle, 1963; Nishi, 1970). Accordingly, Szerb (1977) hypothesized that the muscarinic nerve terminal receptors are concerned with blocking or modulating ACh release. Thus, atropinics could disinhibit ACh release or antagonize the block of ACh release by muscarinic agonists and antiChE's. In fact, Szerb (1977) proposed that endogenous ACh could block its own action. It must be added that in the periphery, it is a moot question whether presynaptic actions of ACh are facilitatory or inhibitory in nature (Nishi, 1970; Koelle, 1969). There are further complications. The decreased release of ACh with oxotremorine is not a universal finding (Guggenheimer and Levinger, 1975). Furthermore, inhibitory pathways to the cortex which include cholinergic synapses act antagonistically with respect to diffuse tegmental systems (Marczynski, 1971; Pepeu, 1974). By blocking this inhibitory system, atropinics could induce or increase cortical release of ACh. As to the nicotinically induced ACh release which cannot be explained by Szerb's hypothesis, this effect may be related to CNS stimulant actions of nicotine and its EEG arousal (vide infra). Thus, nicotinic release of ACh could be analogous to that induced by such CNS stimulants as amphetamine (Pepeu, et al., 1978). Of course, muscarinic drugs exhibit similar actions. Finally, the presence of cholinoceptive receptors on cholinergic neurons was already described.

Acetylcholine Turnover

The activity of a cholinergic neuron may be defined as the rate of impulses that it sends out as related to the release of ACh. This activity may be reflected in the firing rate of its soma or axons and in the parameters of the release of ACh. Neurochemically, this rate may be expressed in terms of ACh turnover. Somewhat simplistically, the turnover is defined as the rate of ACh synthesis or ACh formation per unit time. In actuality, the turnover calculations include several parameters reflecting the dynamics of ACh and choline following a pulse of radioactive choline (Haubrich and Chippendale, 1977; Hanin and Costa, 1976; Jenden, 1977; Cheney and Costa, 1978). It is of particular interest that ACh levels or even ACh release from the nerve terminal do not necessarily reflect ACh turnover and/or the activity of cholinergic neurons. The art of the measurement of ACh turnover is new, and certain theoretical difficulties are not solved as yet. Furthermore, turnover values depend on the method of measurement employed. The present summary refers generally to results obtained by the methods of Costa and Jenden and their associates.

It is particularly pertinent for this review to discuss the turnover effects of cholinergic agonists and antagonists, as well as certain brain stimulants and depressants. Among cholinergic stimulants, cholinomimetics or cholinergic agonists such as oxotremorine and arecoline as well as antiChEs such as physostigmine, increase brain levels of ACh as well as decrease its turnover (Trabucchi *et al.,* 1975; Hanin and Costa, 1976; Cheney and Costa, 1978). This was true both in the case of whole brains and brain parts of mice and rats (Cheney and Costa, 1978). Trabucchi *et al.* (1975a; 1975b) suggested that the occupation of postsynaptic receptors by the agonist or by ACh following its accumulation by antiChEs prevents ACh release and increases its content as well as decreases its utilization and turnover. The effects of cholinergic antagonists on ACh turnover were not measured directly. Cholinergic antagonists generally decrease ACh content and may have variable effects, depending on the drug, on choline uptake. Furthermore, atropine and scopolamine increase release of ACh (Cheney and Costa, 1978). These and other indirect data (Lundholm and Sparf, 1975; Domino and Wilson, 1973) suggest that atropine increases the turnover of ACh while anticholinergic antiparkinsonian drugs may affect the turnover only slightly (Cheney and Costa, 1978).

Among noncholinergic drugs, depressants such as pentobarbital decreased ACh turnover in the whole brain, while they increased ACh levels. The striate and cortex were particularly affected (Cheney and Costa, 1978). Morphine also exerted depressant effects on ACh turnover; its effect on ACh levels is controversial (Karczmar, 1978; Cheney and Costa, 1978). Antipsychotics such as haloperidol and chlorpromazine increased ACh turnover in the striate and nucleus accumbens and decreased it in several other brain parts (Roth and Bunney, 1976; Cheney and Costa, 1978). It is of interest that clozapine, an antipsychotic with potent atropinic activity, decreased ACh turnover only in the globus pallidus and did not affect it anywhere else (Roth and Bunney, 1976; Cheney and Costa, 1978). Finally, dopaminergic agonists increased the levels and decreased the release and turnover of striatal ACh (Guyenet *et al.,* 1975; Roth and Bunney, 1976; Cheney and Costa, 1978).

The neuronal activity and/or ACh turnover must be kept in mind when considering the EEG effects of many drugs referred to in this review. For instance, is the EEG effect of antiChE's and cholinergic agonists to be attributed to the action at the postsynaptic site of accumulated ACh and of the agonist respectively, or to the decreased activity of cholinergic neurons and their decreased turnover? Similarly, is the EEG effect of atropine due to its post-synaptic antimuscarinic action, or to its augmentation of ACh turnover? It must be added in this context that the facilitating action of atropine on ACh release and turnover was attributed to its possible block of a corticopetal cholinergic system which normally blocks the reticulo-cortical pathway (Marczynski, 1971). Similar considerations may be raised in evaluating the interplay between phenothiazines and cholinergic drugs with respect to the EEG: is this interplay generated by the effect of phenothiazines on ACh turnover, or by the electrophysiological interaction between these drugs, not directly related to ACh turnover, at the reticular formation? It must be stressed in this context that ACh turnover as well as the effect of drugs on the latter is site dependent (Cheney and Costa, 1978).

Neurochemical and Neurophysiological Interaction Between Cholinergic and Other Bioamine Systems

It was already stressed (see "Characteristics of Synaptic Cholinergic Transmission" section of this chapter) that cholinergic synapses either alternate with junctions activated by other transmitters or impinge on these junctions across one or several non-cholinergic synapses. At certain sites such as nigro-striatal and locus coeruleus-Raphe nuclei loops, the circuits in question are elucidated to a large extent (Roth and Bunney, 1976; Glowinski and Karczmar, in press a; in press b). In fact, it is clear that the earlier schemes of relatively simple catecholaminergic-cholinergic coupling in the nigro-striate or catecholaminergic-serotonergic coupling in the locus coeruleus-Raphe system must be discarded. For instance, Raphe nuclei also innervate the nigro-striatal loop, and the latter comprises a complex feedback arrangement of serotonergic, dopaminergic, cholinergic and GABAminergic neurons (Roth and Bunney, 1976; Cheramy et al., in press; Glowinski and Karczmar, in press a). Certain sites where such complex, multitransmitter interactions occur must be particularly stressed in the present context. Thus, certain brain stem and midbrain systems participate in the control of sleep-wakefulness and in the related EEG changes. At these sites there is a complex, generally reciprocal interaction between well established serotonergic neurons of Raphe nuclei and the catecholaminergic neurons of the locus coeruleus (Pujol et al., 1978; Pujol, in press) on the one hand, and less well delineated cholinergic neurons, presumably of the pontine tegmentum or related sites, (Jouvet, 1975; Steriade and Hobson, 1976) on the other. Actually, other neurotransmitter systems concerned with special aspects of the sleep-wakefulness dipole such as REM and ponto – occipital – geniculate spikes (see "Role of the Cholinergic System in REM Sleep" section of this chapter), must be also considered (Ruch-Monachon et al., 1976a; 1976b; 1976c), and they may include GABAminergic and histaminergic neurons (Karczmar, 1978).

It must be added that the multitransmitter pontine, brain stem and midbrain systems in question control, besides the sleep-wakefulness dipole and its EEG concomitants, other EEG activities. Other sites involved in EEG synchronization and desynchronization (see "Mechanisms and Sites of Cholinergic Desynchronization" section of this chapter) are the ascending pontine-mesencephalico-cortical reticular formation, the hippocampus and other limbic sites including amygdaloid system, and the striate. These sites are also important in generating or controlling seizures (Maynert et al., 1975). Again, multitransmitter circuitry is concerned. For instance, the hippocampus is innervated by cholinergic, serotonergic and catecholaminergic inputs (Livett, 1973; Palkovits et al., 1974; Jacobowitz, 1978). Furthermore, it becomes apparent that peptidergic and GABAminergic pathways may contribute to some or all of the systems in question (Karczmar and Glowinski, 1978; Glowinski and Karczmar, in press b). Thus, it is not surprising that drugs that affect catecholaminergic systems alter the EEG and related effects of cholinergic drugs (see "Role of the Cholinergic System in REM Sleep" section of this chapter).

One general comment should be made in the present context. The foregoing description contributes to the explanation of the dopaminergic effect, particularly in the striate, on cholinergic neurons and their ACh turnover (see "Acetylcholine Turnover" section of this chapter). In addition serotonergic and noradrenergic agonists and antagonists affect the function of cholinergic neurons at many brain sites (Karczmar, 1976; Roth and Bunney, 1976; Karczmar and Glowinski, 1978). The reverse is also true, and cholinergic agonists and antagonists affect catecholaminergic, serotonergic, and GABA systems (Karczmar, 1976; Karczmar and Glowinski, 1978). Perhaps the most striking is the effect of cholinergic agonists and antiChE's on the serotonergic system as these drugs increase markedly, up to 100%, brain serotonin levels and decrease its turnover (Glisson *et al.*, 1974; Barnes *et al.*, 1975; 1976; in press; Karczmar, 1976). While the circuitry that synaptically couples the two systems was described for the nigro-striatal pathways (Javoy *et al.*, 1978), the marked effect of cholinergic agonists on brain serotonin was demonstrated for other brain sites as well (Glisson *et al.*, 1974; Barnes *et al.*, 1975). Altogether, it appears clear that the effects of cholinergic drugs on the EEG, while frequently appearing to be due to their direct action on cholinergic synapses, may, in fact, depend on other transmitter systems (Garattini *et al.*, 1978; Hokfelt, in press).

EEG AND RELATED ACTIONS OF CHOLINERGIC AGONISTS AND ANTAGONISTS

Cortical and Subcortical EEG Action of Cholinergic Agonists and Anticholinesterases

It is useful to initiate the discussion of the cholinergic EEG with the description of the typical EEG effects of cholinergic agonists and antiChE's, and of the power spectrum analysis of these effects in experimental animals as recorded in our laboratories. Similar effects are exerted by all these drugs in a number of animal species. For description it is convenient to select physostigmine as the representative cholinergic drug. With this short acting agent, the full sequence of events, including the return to control values, can be observed in a relatively short time (1 hr with 0.1 to 0.5 mg/kg doses). When physostigmine is given carefully i.v. (via an indwelling catheter) to a non-anesthetized rabbit protected with a quaternary atropinic, the resting EEG, usually containing waves of mixed frequencies and voltage, is shifted, within a minute of the administration, toward slower frequencies and increased voltage. This is particularly apparent when power spectrum analysis is utilized (Figure 1). Relatively slow frequencies and high voltage patterns appear in all leads, including motor, cortical, thalamic and hippocampal derivations (Van Meter, 1969). Within 2 min of this initial state, EEG desynchronization and fast wave patterns of decreased voltage are noticed in cortical and subcortical leads. A characteristic synchronized pattern, the theta rhythm of 7-12 Hz frequency is noticed, however, in the case of deep hippocampal leads. The power spectrum analysis shows the cortical effects particularly clearly (Figure 2) as the electrogenesis is shifted toward the fast wave end of the spectrum (15-30 Hz) (Fairchild *et al.*, 1975). This effect persists for some 15-20 min with rare intermittent epochs resembling control EEG. Subsequently, more frequent epochs of synchronized EEG intervene and the hippocampal theta waves subside. At about 30 min to 1 hr the record becomes identical with control tracings. It must be emphasized that with these moderate doses of physostigmine the animal shows little or no motor activity. While it may appear sleepy during the first 2 min following the administration of physostigmine, subsequently it shows some signs of behavioral alertness such as sniffing and head motions.

With increasing doses of physostigmine (0.7-1.0 mg/kg), hypersynchronous fast wave spikes and bursts appear 5-10 min following the drug administration, particularly in the leads derived from amygdala, hippocampus, motor cortex and globus pallidus, this change generally being noticed first in amygdala. Some restlessness, rolling about, vocalizing and indications of aggressive behavior may be noticed at this time in some

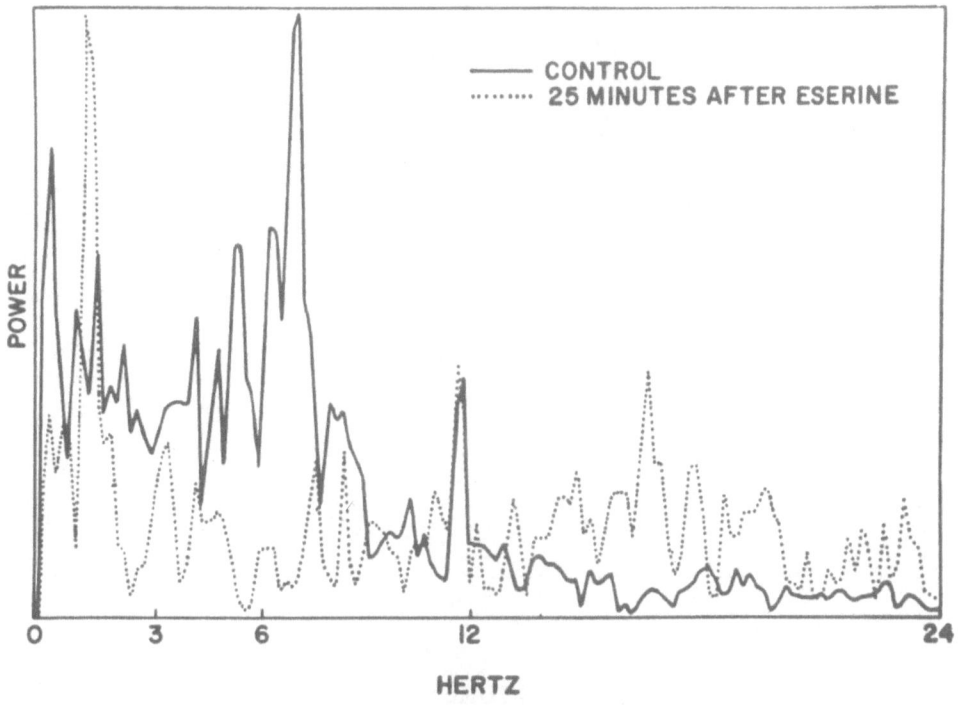

FIGURE 1

Early effect of physostigmine (eserine) on the cortical EEG of the rabbit. The graphs represent power spectrum analysis; the power (ordinates) is expressed in arbitrary units with respect to frequency per second (Hertz units, abscissae). Power constitutes a voltage-frequency derivation at the given frequency and represents essentially relative contribution of various wave frequencies to the EEG. The recording was obtained in unanesthetized animals. Bipolar recording; surface silver ball electrodes were applied to anterior motor cortex. Power spectrum analysis shows the shift of preponderant frequencies to low frequencies, 2 min after administration of 0.1 mg/kg, i.v., of physostigmine (Van Meter and Karczmar, unpublished data).

animal species, ie, the cat (Bokums and Elliott, 1968). At the end of this time period, high voltage hypersynchronous waves and spikes appear in all leads resulting in generalized EEG seizure activity as well as overt motor convulsions. Unless lethal doses of physostigmine (> 1mg/kg) are administered (Van Meter et al., 1978), the EEG seizure and the behavioral concomitants of this state subside and in due time normal EEG and behavior are restored. It must be noted that similar effects arise also with intracarotid, intraventricular or intracerebral administration. 25-50 mcgm (total dose) of physostigmine, administered via the carotid, induces the sequence of slow and then fast desynchronized EEG pattern, while doses of 100 mcg cause, in addition, convulsive behavior and EEG seizures.

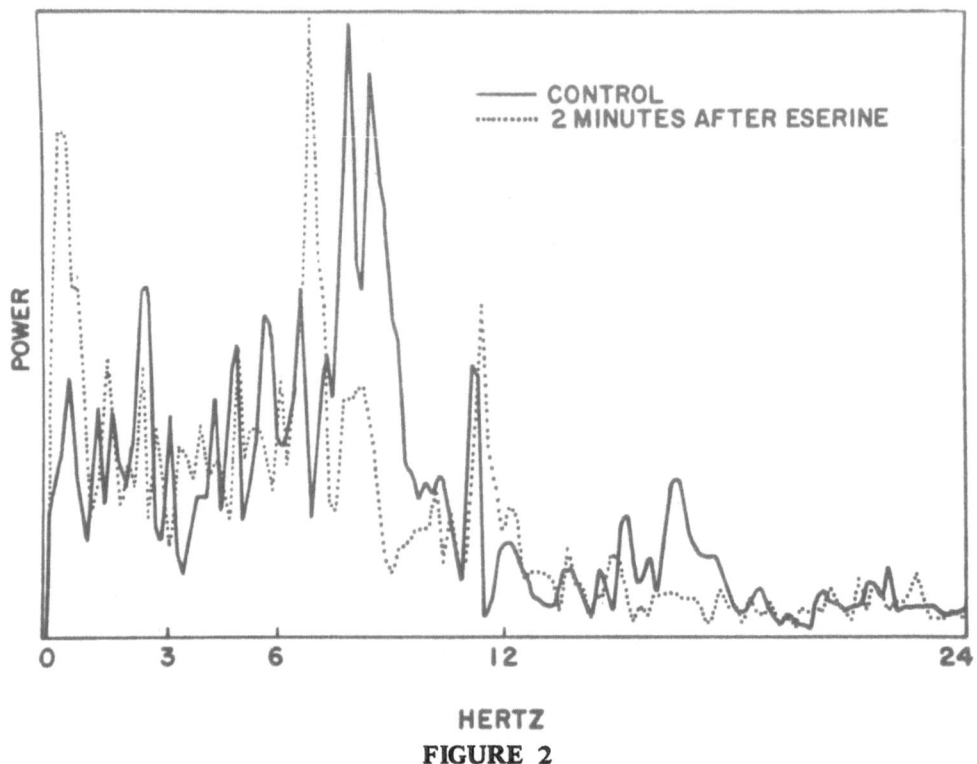

POWER

CONTROL
········· 2 MINUTES AFTER ESERINE

0   3   6   I 2   24

HERTZ

FIGURE 2

Late effect of physostigmine (eserine) on the cortical EEG of the rabbit. Power spectrum analysis was carried out 25 min after the administration of physostigmine, 0.1 mg/kg, i.v. Note marked shift of frequency to 12-24 Hz side of the spectrum. The rabbit is different from the animal illustrated in Figure 1 (Van Meter and Karczmar, unpublished data).

Of the EEG responses described, the desynchronized EEG was most widely demonstrated by most investigators with cholinergic agonists and antiChE's, beginning with the observations of Bonnet and Bremer (1937) and of Moruzzi (1939). For other references to these early investigations see Miller *et al.*, 1940; Bremer and Chatonnet, 1949; Bradley and Elkes, 1953; 1957; Bovet *et al.*, 1957; Holmstedt, 1959; Machne and Unna, 1963; Votava, 1967; Karczmar, 1967; 1970a; 1970b; Schmitt, 1972. The studies quoted generally concerned physostigmine and ACh (given intracarotidally) (Kinaldi and Himwich, 1955; Longo, 1962), and the effects in question were obtained either in encephale isole preparations, after midbrain or pontine sections, or in intact animals (Karczmar, 1967). Essentially similar effects were described earlier for such organophosphorus compounds as diisopropylphosphofluoridate (diisopropylfluorophosphate, DFP) (Wescoe *et al.*, 1948; Essig *et al.*, 1950). Subsequently, both nicotinic and muscarinic (such as oxotremorine) agonists were found to exert similar action (Everett, 1964; Levy and Michel-Ber, 1967; Domino *et al.*, 1967; Yamamoto *et al.*, 1967; Ban and Hojo, 1971). Additional similar findings continue to be described till this day (Van Meter *et al.*, 1978). Particularly frequent in Western, Japanese and USSR literature is the reference to desynchronizing actions, in animals as well as in man, of pesticidal organophosphorus antiChEs, the war gas congeners (Dura *et al.*, 1975; Rieger and Okonek, 1975a; 1975b; Khinkova *et al.*, 1975; Desi *et al.*, 1975; Osumi *et al.*, 1975; Roshchina, 1976; Korsak and Sato, 1977). It must be added that with large doses of the compounds in question — including antiChE and nicotinic and muscarinic drugs — convulsant EEG activity was also evoked (Van Meter *et al.*, 1978; Phan *et al.*, 1974; "EEG Seizures" section in this chapter).

An important point must be clarified in this context. In the case of many investigations cited, the cholinergic agonists or antiChE's were administered systemically. Thus given, these compounds produce a wide gamut of peripheral effects that include actions on blood pressure, smooth and skeletal muscle, blood flow, glands and, presumably, sensory systems (Karczmar *et al.*, 1963; Karczmar, 1967). Therefore, rather than inducing EEG effects directly and centrally, the cholinergic compounds may have produced these actions indirectly via concomitant peripheral phenomena. However, the compounds in question exerted similar effects when administered intraventricularly or into the brain. Furthermore, while tertiary atropinics such as atropine and scopolamine antagonized the EEG actions of cholinergic agonists, systemically administered quaternary anticholinergics, such as quaternary atropinics, ganglionic blockers or muscle relaxants, which are essentially incapable of crossing the blood-brain barrier, did not block or even attenuate the EEG effects of cholinergic agonists (Bokums and Elliott, 1968; Van Meter *et al.*, 1978), although they could do so when administered into the brain or the ventricles (Longo, 1966; Wills, 1970). Thus it appears clear that EEG actions of cholinergic agonists are due to their central actions, independent of their route of administration.

The early, essentially visual determination of the desynchronizing action of cholinergic agonists and antiChE's was confirmed subsequently by means of either semiquantitative methods (Bokums and Elliott, 1968), Drohocki's voltage integrator (Pierre and Cahn, 1957), or sophisticated power spectrum analysis (Montplaisir and and Sazie, 1973; Fairchild *et al.*, 1975; Montplaisir, 1975; Losey, 1977). Altogether, the phenomenon of cholinergically induced ECoG desynchronization, flattening and increased incidence of high frequency patterns, and of hippocampal theta waves is well established and documented for several animal species, including man.

Are these effects due to the cholinomimetic action exerted on or via the reticular formation? Certain data seem to support this contention. For instance, localized injection of ACh, carbachol and physostigmine with or without ACh into the brain stem and pontine or bulbar reticular formation produced occasionally (Cordeau *et al.*, 1959; 1963) or regularly (Endroczi *et al.*, 1963a; 1963b; Yamaguchi *et al.*, 1963; 1964; Kostowski, 1971; McKenna *et al.*, 1974; Amatruda *et al.*, 1975; Steriade and Hobson, 1976; Smialowski, 1977) EEG desynchronization. In particular, this effect was obtained with the administration of cholinergic agonists onto the giant cells of the pontine reticular formation (gigantocellular tegmental field or FTG of Berman, 1968; Steriade and Hobson, 1976). It is important, as described later in detail, that in many instances EEG desynchronization induced by cholinergic agony at the brain stem was coupled with paradoxical sleep. Similar effects arose when ACh or carbachol were injected in the areas that can be construed as parts of the diffuse reticular system (medullary-mesendiencephalic cortical) (Rinaldi and Himwich, 1955) such as the hypothalamus (Myers, 1974). This is true in the case of birds as well (Macphail, 1969; Marley and Seller, 1972).

On the other hand, antiChE's, ACh and related substances such as oxotremorine, pilocarpine and arecoline induced EEG arousal even when the reticular formation was sectioned at the midbrain level (Karczmar, 1967). Nicotine was similarly effective in cerveau isole preparation (Floris et al., 1963). This indicates that cholinergic agonists arouse the EEG even in the absence, at least partial, of the reticular formation. Furthermore, cholinergic agonists evoke EEG desynchronization when administered into sites not considered as components of the ascending reticular system, even if the latter is equated, with some latitude with Himwich's diffuse system. For instance, ACh and/or carbachol caused desynchronization when injected into rhinencephalon including olfactory bulb (Penaloza-Rojas and Zeidenweber, 1965; Myers, 1974) and mesencephalic grey (Baxter, 1969). In fact, application of cholinergic agonists to a number of limbic sites induced EEG desynchronization (Hernandez-Peon, 1962; 1965; Steriade and Hobson, 1976). It must be emphasized however that sometimes slow EEG patterns were observed. (see "Cholinergic System and Slow Sleep" section of this chapter). Furthermore, these particular EEG findings must be evaluated jointly with their behavioral concomitants, ie, with the phenomena of sleep. This point will be returned to later.

Finally, as known for some 40 years, patterns resembling desynchronization can be obtained when ACh is applied directly to the cortex (Sjostrand, 1937; Obrador, 1947; Machne and Unna, 1963; Karczmar, 1967), or to isolated or semi-isolated cortex (Echlin and McDonald, 1954; Morrel, 1967; Echlin, 1975). However, as EEG patterns of isolated cortex differ from those of intact cortex, it is difficult to decide whether or not cholinergic agonists affect wave frequency so as to produce what may be referred to as desynchrony. Thus, at least some cholinergic drugs seem to exhibit potent desynchronizing activities on neuronal populations which are not under the control of reticular formation.

It is of interest in this context to establish whether or not the nicotinic and muscarinic agonists differ with regard to the EEG action. Given systemically, nicotine frequently induced desynchronization, particularly when given in low doses (Longo et al., 1954; Longo, 1962; Domino et al., 1967; Longo et al., 1967; Guha and Pradhan, 1976). Given systemically in large doses or intraventricularly, nicotine may also cause behavioral depression and EEG synchronization (Stadnicki and Schaeppi, 1972). Furthermore, several investigators observed biphasic action of nicotine, initial EEG desynchronization being followed by synchronization (Stumpf et al., 1967). Guha and Pradhan (1976) suggested that the first phase of action of nicotine may be cholinergic in nature while the second phase depends on its indirect effect via the noradrenergic neurons. Guha and Pradhan also suggested that the first desynchronizing phase of action of nicotine depends on muscarinic receptors, thus being homologous with actions of antiChE's and oxotremorine. It must be stressed however that while most of EEG and other central actions of nicotine are readily blocked by antinicotinic or curaremimetic substances such as dihydro-β-erythroidine (Domino et al., 1967; Domino, 1968; Maynert et al., 1975), the capacity of scopolamine or atropine to do so is controversial (Domino et al., 1967; Guha and Pradham, 1976). It is generally agreed however, that muscarinic antagonists block EEG desynchronization due to arecoline, pilocarpine (Kawamura and Domino, 1969) or antiChE's. Altogether, the analysis of EEG actions of nicotinic and muscarinic cholinergic agonists by means of lesion techniques (Kawamura and Domino, 1969) led Domino to propose that the nicotinic receptors involved in EEG desynchrony are located in the midbrain reticular formation, whereas muscarinic receptors involved in this effect embrace, in addition, the mesencephalico-cortical arousal system.

The potent, characteristic desynchronizing action of cholinergic agonists deserves attention and emphasis. This action is, in many instances, more potent on a mg per kg basis than that of such desynchronizing agents as amphetaminics (Longo and Silvestrini, 1957; Longo, 1962). Conversely, anticholinergics exert very extreme synchronizing actions (Longo, 1966). A very special illustration of the desynchronizing action of anti-ChE's and cholinergic agonists is their effect on just about any paradigm capable of inducing synchronization. Thus, given systemically, cholinergic agonists produce desynchronization in drowsy or sleeping animals exhibiting slow sleep or in animals exhibiting slow rhythms at the moment of rewarded response in the course of operant conditioning (Marczynski and Burns, 1976). These drugs are also effective in antagonizing, in animals and in man, synchrony or hypersynchrony induced not only by atropinics and related drugs such as tricyclic antidepressants but also by anesthetics, phenothiazines and butyrophenones, and barbiturates (Karczmar, in press).

Effects of Atropinics, Curaremimetics and Related Drugs

It must be stated first that when anticholinergic drugs are administered systemically, only tertiary or lipid soluble compounds that cross the brain barrier may affect the EEG, or EEG changes evoked by CNS-active drugs. Thus, quaternary atropinic antispasmodics generally do not effect the EEG unless given intraventricularly or intracerebrally, although a few exceptions to this generalization were described in the literature. Similarly, tertiary but not quaternary anticholinergics antagonize or modify central actions of antiChE's, cholinergic agonists and of certain other drugs.

The action of atropine and scopolamine upon the EEG is well known (Longo, 1958; 1962; 1966). Atropinized cats, rabbits, rats, monkeys or apes, and man display high voltage slow wave EEG activity intermingled at random with high voltage spikes (Marczynski, 1971). This activity is present in several leads in a form so pronounced that Longo (1958; 1962; 1966) deems the term "synchronized" insufficient as applied to the atropine pattern and prefers to describe this rhythm as hypersynchronous. This effect occurs whether the animal or man is asleep, awake or aroused; the hippocampal theta rhythm exhibited normally by aroused animals is also affected by atropine. This visually observed effect may be readily confirmed by means of power-spectrum analysis (Fairchild et al., 1975). Furthermore, atropinics block or attenuate the EEG arousal normally observed in response to sensory or electrical stimulation of the reticular formation as well as cholinergic desynchrony induced by muscarinic agonists (Rinaldi and Himwich, 1955; Bradley and Elkes, 1957; Longo, 1966).

It is of interest that the EEG pattern induced by atropinics and their block of arousal is not accompanied by behavioral depression or sleep. Occasionally, excitement and aggression and frequently, confusional states are observed in animals or man (Karczmar, 1977; 1978). This should not be as surprising as it seems to appear to some investigators. Indeed, behavioral depression should not be expected from drugs that induce hypersynchrony rather than synchrony. In fact, the rhythm in question differs in power-spectrum analysis from that of slow sleep, and the concomitant behavior may be termed confusional (Longo, 1966; Karczmar, 1978). It is of further interest that EEG and behavioral consequences of atropinic drugs resemble those due, in man or animals, to the consequences of the overdosage with tricyclic antidepressants, which are well known to exhibit a high degree of atropinic activity (Karczmar, in press). This toxicity of the tricyclics as well as that arising in man or animals from atropine over-dosage is referred to as anticholinergic coma and both states can be antagonized by physostigmine and other antiChEs or cholinergic agonists.

It is of interest in the present context to discuss EEG action of another anticholin-ergic drug, the antinicotinic d-tubocurarine. As already indicated, this quaternary drug exhibits little or no central actions when given systemically. However, it exerts marked effects when applied to cortical surface or injected intracerebrally or intraventrically. Surprisingly, under these conditions it caused spike and high-voltage seizure activity. These effects were obtained by many investigators. When tubocurarine was given sub-cortically, the seizures seemed to originate in the hippocampus, reticular formation or the thalamus (Kumagai et al., 1962a; 1962b; Feldberg and Fleischhauer, 1963; Myers, 1974). Several authors suggested that this effect of d-tubocurarine depends on its block of cholinergic inhibitory action and resulting disinhibition (Banerjee et al., 1970) or on its antagonism of GABA (Hill et al., 1972). It is difficult to accept these explanations as drugs that are not cholinergic blockers also induce, when applied to the cortex or given intracerebrally, seizures or spiking. This is true for convulsants such as pentylenetetrazol or strychnine (Banerjee et al., 1970; Myers, 1974). Furthermore, a similar effect is exerted by cholinergic agonists including bis-quaternary depolarizers (Tan, 1977), and, to complicate the matter further, local anesthetics (Myers, 1974). As the latter drugs exhibit local irritant action (Luduena and Hoppe, 1952), and as such irritants as alumina are routine means of inducing local epileptic foci, it is tempting to ascribe the seizure activity of curarine to its irritant properties. It is of interest in this context that the tertiary curaremimetic, dihydro-β-erythroidine, or a curare congener gallamine did not induce seizures on local application (Baker and Benedict, 1968). On the other hand, dihydro-β-erythroidine, and other antinicotinic curaremimetics (given systemically) blocked nicotine induced seizures (Longo et al., 1954; Stone et al., 1958; Yamamoto and Domino, 1967).

Behavioral Correlates of EEG Effects of Cholinergic Agonists

The desynchronizing action of cholinergic agonists must be commented upon in the context of its behavioral correlates. The EEG action in question resembles, at least superficially, the EEG activation arising from the sensory stimulation of the reticular formation (Moruzzi and Magoun, 1949), as well as the EEG activation due to adrenergic substances (Marczynski, 1967; Myers, 1974) or to amphetamine. As reticularly or amphetamine-mediated EEG desynchronization is accompanied by behavioral arousal (Moruzzi and Magoun, 1949; Longo, 1966; Marczynski, 1967), the latter could be expected to also accompany cholinergically mediated desynchronization. Yet, as pointed out as early as in 1952 by Wikler, this is not the case. In fact, behavioral and motor depression rather than behavioral arousal seem frequently to be induced by systemic, intraventricular or intracerebral administration of cholinergic agonists, and Wikler (1952) coined the term "divorce" to describe the apparent dissociation between the EEG and behavioral effects of cholinergic agonists. To elucidate Wikler's concept, certain behavioral aspects of the central cholinergic action must be adduced. Indeed, the EEG desynchron-ization induced by cholinergic drugs may represent a specific behavior, which should be differentiated from alertness and wakefulness as well as from depression. Two states are particularly pertinent: the Alert Non-Mobile Behavior (ANMB) (Karczmar, 1977), also referred to as "immobility reflex" or "animal hypnosis" (Klemm, 1976), and its concomitant, the hippocampal theta waves; and the Rapid Eye Movement (REM) or paradoxical sleep.

Cholinergic Induction of Theta Waves and Its Behavioral Correlates

The appearance of theta waves is a characteristic concomitant of cholinergic desynchronization originating mainly in the hippocampus (Brucke and Stumpf, 1957; Longo, 1966; Longo and Loizzo, 1973; Radil-Weiss, 1974; Karczmar et al., 1970). Cholinergically induced theta waves exhibit a frequency varying from 6-12 Hz. Their amplitude, when recorded by means of implanted electrodes, amounts to at least 500 μv. The appearance of the theta waves is particularly clearcut in rabbits (Longo, 1962), although it is also present in other species. It may be less pronounced in man in the leads that can be expected to show this rhythm.

According to some investigators, there are two types of theta waves, or rhythmical slow activity (RSA) (Vanderwolf, 1975; Klemm, 1976), only one of which may be related to cholinergic desynchronization and behavioral arrest. This particular RSA is regular and relatively slow, ranging in frequency from 4-7 Hz. It is accompanied by motor immobility, particularly in response to sensory stimulation. This immobility is coupled in animals with several signs of alertness such as head motion, sniffing, face washing, scratching and chewing. The eyes remain wide open (Irmi, 1974a; 1974b; Coleman and Lindsley, 1975; Irmi, 1977). This syndrome is called type II behavior (Vanderwolf, 1975) or Alert Non-Mobile Behavior (ANMB) (Karczmar, 1977).

On the other hand, several investigators also describe an RSA which is irregular, ranging in frequency from 7-14 Hz, accompanied by type I behavior, ie, mobility, voluntary motor activity such as walking or swimming, changes of posture and manipulation of objects by means of paws or muzzle (Kramis et al., 1975; Vanderwolf, 1975; Whishaw et al., 1976). These investigators claim that while type II syndrome is generated by cholinergic agonists and blocked by atropinics which also block the concomitant EEG desynchronization, the type I syndrome is not blocked by atropine or scopolamine. They claim also that the slow and fast RSA's and the associated behavioral syndromes are initiated by two different generators, the CA-1 and the granule cells respectively (Kramis et al., 1975). Also, the frequency of the RSA may depend on the perceptual content of the stimulus and hippocampal input-output relationships (Klemm, 1976). Several lines of evidence are inconsistent with the concept of differential cholinergic action on the two RSA's. Cholinergics seem to affect all the hippocampal cells studied (Krnjevic, 1974) and exert generalized hippocampal actions (Vosu and Wise, 1975). Furthermore, Teitelbaum et al. (1975) associated the fast theta pattern with forced running and demonstrated that it was very similar to that induced by physostigmine. Both theta responses were blocked by atropinics and both were abolished by lesions of the medial septal nucleus (Petsche, 1962; Karczmar, 1977).

Although, it is the impression of this investigator that cholinergic agonists induce a single syndrome which consists of ANMB, EEG desynchronization, and RSA of relatively wide (4-12 Hz or 14 Hz) frequency range. In fact, RSA or theta rhythms associated with paradoxical (REM) sleep (see below) are also blocked by atropinics (Usui et al., 1977). Thus, Wikler's (1952) phenomenon may simply concern a specific syndrome rather than a divorce between EEG and behavioral phenomena. This view is reinforced by the fact that, when quantified by means of power spectrum analysis (Fairchild et al., 1975), cholinergic EEG desynchrony is not identical with that which accompanies behavioral arousal.

Role of the Cholinergic System in REM Sleep

Another interpretation of Wikler's (1952) divorce phenomenon may be posited. In 1971, Karczmar emphasized that the effect of cholinergic agonists on EEG and behavior may be related to REM sleep. Indeed, under certain circumstances, antiChE drugs and cholinergic agonists induce paradoxical sleep and all of its concomitants (theta waves, lowered EMG, PGO spikes and REM). Thus, following pontine and related lesions, or upon their application to the tegmental, pontine (and perhaps striate) sites, antiChE's and cholinergic agonists were capable of inducing REM sleep (George *et al.*, 1964; Pompeiano, 1967; Matsuzaki *et al.*, 1968; Matsuzaki, 1968; 1969; Barnes and Pompeiano, 1970; Magherini *et al.*, 1971; Kingsley and Barnes, 1973; Hobson, 1974; Hall and Keane, 1975). The most detailed examination of the REM sleep induction by brain stem application of a cholinergic agonist, carbachol, was carried out by Hobson and his colleagues (Steriade and Hobson, 1976). Carbachol was particularly effective when injected onto the FTG field of Berman (Amatruda *et al.*, 1975; McKenna *et al.*, 1974). In addition, one of the most faithful pharmacological models of REM sleep is provided when antiChEs are administered to rabbits following treatment with reserpine (Karczmar *et al.*, 1970). Consequently, Karczmar (1971; 1975; 1977) stressed the significance of the cholinergic system for REM sleep. It should be added that reserpine alone produces some symptoms of REM sleep in the cat, ie, PGO spikes (Brooks and Gershon, 1972; Brooks *et al.*, 1972). That the cholinergic system is implicated in REM sleep is also indicated by the fact that REM sleep is accompanied by increased cortical release of ACh (Jasper and Tessier, 1971; Gadea-Ciria *et al.*, 1973). In addition, cholinergic agonists, including nicotine (Domino and Yamamoto, 1965; Jewett and Norton, 1966) and antiChEs, facilitate and enhance duration and frequency of REM sleep episodes in animals and in man (Karczmar, 1967; Sitaram *et al.*, 1976; Karczmar, 1978; in press), while atropinics, and particularly those tricyclic antidepressants which exhibit marked atropinic potency (Kupfer and Edwards, 1978; Karczmar, 1978; in press), exhibit opposite properties.

This and additional evidence (Steriade and Hobson, 1976) strongly inculpates the cholinergic system of the brain stem in the control of REM sleep. Accordingly, in 1976 Steriade and Hobson concluded in their interesting and detailed review that REM sleep involves as "the executive elements . . . the pontine . . . giant cells of the reticular formation (FTG)." They suggest that these neurons are cholinoceptive and cholinergic (see "Characteristics of Synaptic Cholinergic Transmission" section of this chapter), and that they control EEG desynchronization as well as the characteristic phasic events of the paradoxical sleep such as REM, pontogeniculate occipital spikes (PGO) and muscle relaxation (Magherini *et al.*, 1972). That these phenomena, particularly REM, depend on cholinergic activity of brain stem sites was documented in the studies of Pompeiano and his associates (Magherini *et al.*, 1971; Mergner *et al.*, 1976).

The views of Steriade and Hobson (1976) and Karczmar (1975; 1977) as to the importance of the cholinergic components of the REM sleep should be compared with those of Jouvet (1972; 1975; Pujol *et al.*, 1978; in press). While Jouvet and his colleagues emphasized that atropine prevents the occurrence of REM sleep (Jouvet, 1961; 1967), they stress the concept that REM sleep depends mainly on the activity of the locus coeruleus and of its ascending noradrenergic pathways, whereas slow wave sleep (SWS) involves Raphe nuclei and the ascending serotonergic system. Furthermore, Jouvet and Pujol (Pujol *et al.*, 1978; Pujol, in press) emphasized that the REM-SWS cycle depends on the reciprocal feedbacks existing between Raphe nuclei and locus coeruleus. The views of Jouvet and Hobson may not be irreconcilable as Jouvet (1967; 1972) himself presented evidence as to the role of cholinergic system in the REM sleep. Furthermore, some data suggest that there is a relationship between dorsal Raphe nucleus, locus coeruleus and FTG cells (Jalfre *et al.*, 1974; Steriade and Hobson, 1976). In fact, cholinergic inner-vation or involvement in the function of dorsal Raphe nuclei was amply documented (Palkovits and Jacobowitz, 1974; Cheney *et al.*, 1975). There are, however, some dis-cordant data. For instance, when perfused directly into the dorsal Raphe nucleus, ACh increased or induced EEG synchrony (Key and Krzywoskinski, 1977). Some investigators (Ruch-Monachon *et al.*, 1976a; 1976b; 1976c; 1976d; 1976e) envisage that additional neurotransmitters such as GABA and even histamine participate in the control of REM sleep and its phasic (such as PGO spikes) events (Jacobs *et al.*, 1972; Drucker-Colin 1976; Karczmar, 1978).

One point should be emphasized. As interpreted by Steriade and Hobson (1976) the results of Karczmar *et al.* (1970) demonstrate that "the stimulation of a hypnogenic cholinergic system . . . by eserine (physostigmine) . . . leads to . . . D sleep . . . after removal of a suppressive amine influence . . . by reserpine", the "suppressive influence" in question being the catecholaminergic wakefulness (Karczmar, 1975; 1978). The additional implications of these findings are that antiChEs may induce EEG desynchrony (Van Meter and Karczmar, 1971), even in the absence of catecholamines, and that contrary to Jouvet's conceptualization, REM sleep does not require norepinephrine (Jalowiec *et al.*, 1973; Drucker-Colin, 1976).

Cholinergic System and Slow Sleep

So far, desynchronizing and REM sleep and theta pattern-inducing effects of cholin-ergic agonists have been stressed. A disconcerting point must be added at this time: a synchronizing, SWS sleep-inducing hypnogenic cholinergic system may be also present. The circuitry involved differs from the brain stem circuits generating REM sleep as it originates at pontine level and comprises ascending and descending limbs, the latter coinciding with Nauta's (1958) limbic midbrain circuit and including the lateral pre-optic area of the basal forebrain (Sterman and Clemente, 1962; Marczynski, 1967. Rojas-Ramirez and Drucker-Colin, 1973; Steriade and Hobson, 1976). The electrical or cholinergic (Hernandez-Peon and Chavez-Ibarra, 1963; Velluti and Hernandez-Peon, 1963; Hernandez-Peon, 1965) stimulation of these sites induced SWS sleep, while lesions in this area induce sleeplessness (Marczynski, 1967; Karczmar, 1967; Karczmar, 1975; 1976; Steriade and Hobson, 1976; Drucker-Colin, 1976; Karczmar, 1978). It should be added that, under certain circumstances, antiChEs and cholinergic agonists given into the vertebral artery may induce SWS (Haranath *et al.*, 1977). When given i.v. they cause biphasic actions, the early effect which precedes the desynchronizing action exhibiting SWS characteristics (Figure 1) (Van Meter *et al.*, 1978; Van Meter, 1969). It must be stressed, however, that not all investigators could duplicate the results of Hernandez-Peon (Hernandez-Peon *et al.*, 1963; Cordeau *et al.*, 1963; Babb *et al.*, 1973) and that Hernandez-Peon himself (1962; 1965) found that ACh may induce REM sleep when applied at some of the sites described above. Sometimes, the effect was biphasic, SWS preceding the REM sleep.

Mechanisms and Sites of Cholinergic Desynchronization

It was already pointed out that cholinergic EEG desynchronization may not depend on, or be due to, the cholinergic activation of midbrain or diffuse reticular formation. That this is so is suggested in part by the ability of cholinergic agonists to cause cortical desynchrony after lesions or division of the reticular formation or when applied outside of the latter (see "Cortical and Subcortical EEG Actions of Cholinergic Agonists and Anticholinesterase" section of this chapter).

Cholinergic desynchrony could be, however, due to cholinergic action at sites or mechanisms not directly related to the reticular formation. Several such sites and mechanisms may be involved. The thalamico-cortico-cerebellar system should be mentioned first in this context. This system is involved in a synchronizing evoked cortical response referred to as recruitment. This continous waxing and waning, slow (4-6 Hz) rhythm may be generated by low-rate stimulation of non-specific thalamic nuclei (Dempsey and Morison, 1941; 1942), or of certain cerebellar nuclei, which may be coupled with the thalamic recruitment mechanism via the anterior thalamic nucleus (Sasaki et al., 1972a; 1972b; 1975). The recruitment pattern may be related to spontaneous synchronized EEG rhythms such as alpha waves and sleep spindles (Andersen and Andersson, 1968).

It is of great interest in the present context that this synchronous rhythm is readily blocked by cholinergic agonists and antiChE's (Longo and Silvestrini, 1957; Van Meter and Karczmar, 1971) and that drugs that desynchronize the EEG via their stimulation of the reticular formation are not as effective in this respect. Thus, the classical EEG desynchronizer, amphetamine, is a less potent antagonist of recruitment than antiChEs (Longo, 1962; Karczmar, 1971; 1977).

The analysis of the neurochemical basis of the cholinergic antagonism of recruitment has afforded a demonstration that this action cannot be solely responsible for the cholinergic desynchronization, also that catecholamines are not necessary for cholinergic desynchrony. The antirecruitment effect of the cholinergics depends on the availability of catecholamines, most likely of norepinephrine, as the depletion of catecholamines by reserpine or by a-methyl-p-tyrosine (a-MPT), as well as a-blockers, has been shown to prevent the antirecruitment action of antiChEs. In contrast, the restoration of catecholamines, following a-MPT or reserpine by means of DOPA, reinstates the effectiveness of antiChEs (Van Meter, 1969; Van Meter and Karczmar, 1971). Yet, when the antirecruitment effect of antiChEs was prevented by catecholamine block or depletion, with a concomitant slowing of the EEG and blockade of the reticular arousal mechanisms, antiChEs and cholinergic agonists still readily induced EEG desynchronization (Van Meter and Karczmar, 1971).

Another synchronizing system that should be considered in the present context is the "caudate loop" (Buchwald et al., 1961a; 1961b; 1961c). Indeed, slow-rate stimulation of the caudate induces cortical spindling and related synchronized patterns, as well as appropriate behavioral symptomatology (Monnier et al., 1960; Knott et al., 1960; Buchwald et al., 1961a; 1961b; 1961c), and these phenomena may be antagonized by electrical or sensory stimulation of the reticular formation. Unfortunately, the action of cholinergics on caudate-induced spindling has not been investigated sufficiently (Herz and Ziegelgansberger, 1968). The application of ACh to the caudate (Langlois and Poissart,

1969) induced cortical "spindling" which, however, differed from sleep spindles, as well as what appeared to be a background of fast EEG activity. Similarly, our own preliminary data indicate that cortical spindling induced by caudate stimulation is attenuated by antiChEs (Van Meter, unpublished data; Figure 3). Finally, antiChEs and muscarinic agonists depress intra- and inter-caudate responses (Koller and Berry, 1976).

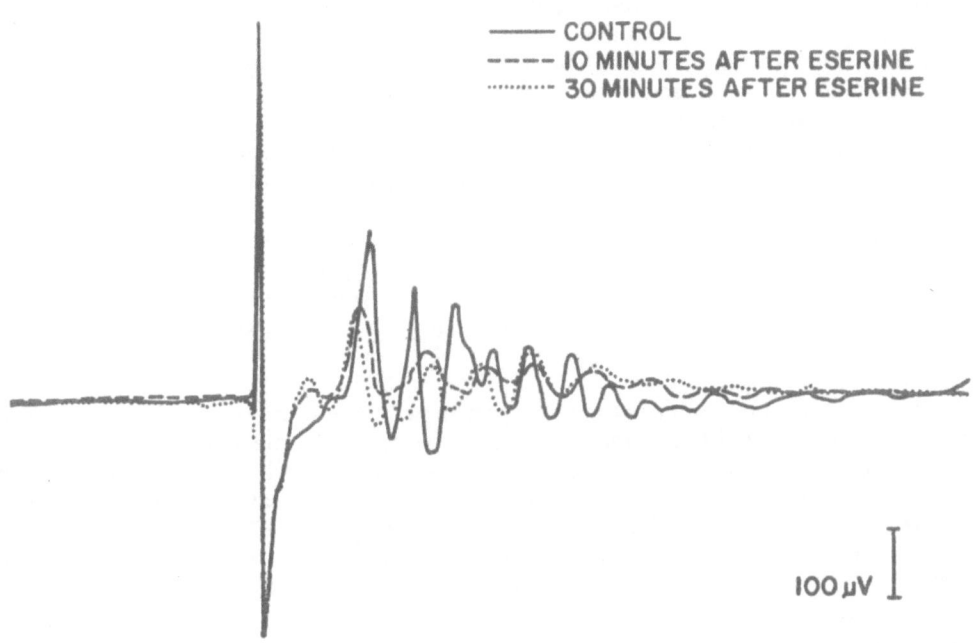

— CONTROL
- - - - 10 MINUTES AFTER ESERINE
·········· 30 MINUTES AFTER ESERINE

100 μV

FIGURE 3

Effect of physostigmine on caudato-cortical spindle. The tracings represent computerized 2 sec analysis of spindles by signal averaging method. Recording taken from anterior sigmoid gyrus; supermaximal shock was applied to the caudate. Cat *in situ* preparation; physostigmine, 0.1 mg/kg, was administered i.v. Note the progressive attenuation of spindles 10 min and 25 min following physostigmine, as well as some shift of polarity and of phase (Van Meter and Karczmar, unpublished data).

Still another synchronizing system is readily affected by cholinergic agonists and antagonists. At this time this system is more readily defined behaviorally than morphologically. The synchronization in question is referred to as post-reinforcement synchronization (PRS) (Clemente *et al.*, 1964; Buchwald *et al.*, 1964; Sterman and Wyrwicka, 1967; Marczynski *et al.*, 1968). PRS is a light-dependent response occurring over the occipital primary and secondary visual projections upon presentation of a palatable and appropriate reward in an environmental situation which is completely familiar to the animal. It is of interest that similar synchrony may occur in man upon occurrence of pleasurable emotional stimuli, "hedonic hypersynchrony" (Maulsby, 1971). Another point of interest in the present context is that PRS may be considered as resulting from transient but powerful suppression of ARAS (Marczynski and Burns, 1976). PRS is readily blocked by very small doses of physostigmine or nicotine, but, to obscure matters further, it is also prevented by antimuscarinic substances (Marczynski, 1969; Marczynski, 1971; Marczynski and Burns, 1976).

It was originally thought that PRS depends on a cholinergic synchronizing thalamico-cortical system; this might explain the anti-PRS action of atropinics. Normally, this system is in balance with another cholinergic system, which constitutes a component of the reticular formation and which contributes to, or facilitates the reticular desyn-chronization (Marczynski, 1971). Modifications of this proposal were proposed recently (Marczynski and Burns, 1976). Atropine may also block PRS by incapacitating the animal from carrying out reward-contingent activities (Marczynski and Burns, 1976).

There are other synchronizing systems that may contribute to cholinergic desyn-chronizations; for instance, slow rate stimulation of specific thalamic nuclei induces cortical augmentation, a synchronous, slow evoked response. Unfortunately, the effects of cholinergic and anticholinergic drugs on augmentation and other pertinent evoked responses were not investigated.

One final general comment may be pertinent in the present context. It was men-tioned above with regard to several synchronizing systems and mechanisms that they may be considered as forming a dipole with the arousal systems such as those represented by the reticular formation. For instance, the stimulation of the latter antagonizes recruit-ment (Monnier et al., 1960; Purpura et al., 1966; Purpura, 1974; Sasaki et al., 1976), augmentation (Purpura, 1974), caudate loop-induced spindling (Monnier et al., 1960), and the PRS (Marczynski and Burns, 1976). Potentials evoked by appropriate sensory stimulation in the auditory, somatosensory and visual areas should be also mentioned in this context, as they represent global responses that require synchronization of post-synaptic neuronal populations for their appearance. However, the effects of reticular stimulation upon these evoked responses are variable and not easy to summarize. This is due partially to the mixed, inhibitory-facilitatory role that is exerted upon these potentials by the reticular formation (Bremer, 1960). Furthermore, the effect of reticular arousal and of drugs depends on the form and phase of these compound potentials (Guha and Pradhan, 1976). However, it may be generalized that desynchronizing action on the field potential of a given neuronal population tends to decrease its evoked potential. It is of interest then that cholinergic agonists frequently diminished evoked responses as reported since the forties, whether these drugs were applied topically (Chatfield and Dempsey, 1942) or systemically (Bremer and Chatonnet, 1949). While many discordant data were also presented (Borbely, 1973), a depressant effect of cholinergic agonists and antiChEs continues to be reported (Schmidt and Wolf, 1972; Montplaisir and Sazie, 1973; Rump et al., 1974; Guha and Pradhan, 1976). Again, caution must be exerted in the interpretation of the data as the cholinergic agonists may affect sensory evoked potential, not necessarily via their desynchronizing action but by their analgesic effects (Koehn and Karczmar, 1978).

Altogether, it may be suggested that cholinergics attenuate the evoked responses. It may be also emphasized that while they may do so via activating the reticular forma-tion, thus mimicking the effect of reticular arousal on evoked potentials, this effect may be localized (Chatfield and Dempsey, 1942; Chatfield and Lord, 1955; Ben-Ari et al., 1976) and directed at electrogenic activities of neuronal populations (Karczmar, 1974a; 1974b; 1975).

Altogether, the evidence seems to favor the concept that cholinergic agonists and antiChEs exhibit a basic and characteristic desynchronizing effect that seems to depend in part only on their activating action on reticular formation. The cholinergic system seems to be able to block a number of synchronizing mechanisms including those that may operate on the level of restricted neuronal populations (see "General Interpretation of the Functional Role of the Central Cholinergic System with Respect to EEG Patterns" section of this chapter).

EEG Seizures

It was already pointed out that, following desynchronization cholinergic agonists and antiChEs induce EEG seizures and motor convulsions (petit and grand mal), when administered systemically in large doses (Stone, 1957; Bokums and Elliott, 1968; Machne and Unna, 1963; Wills, 1970; Phan et al., 1974; Myers, 1974; Maynert et al., 1975; Van Meter et al., 1978). Whether or not muscarinic and nicotinic agonists are equally effective in this respect is a matter of some controversy (Molnar et al., 1967; Phan et al., 1974). It is of interest that with antiChEs of both carbamate and organophosphorus type convulsions could be due not only to the accumulation of ACh, but also to a direct cholinomimetic effect of these drugs (Van Meter et al., 1978). Similar effects were also recorded following topical application of cholinergic agonists onto localized brain structures such as the motor cortex (Machne and Unna, 1963; Crawford et al., 1966; Ferguson and Jasper, 1971; Myers, 1974; Ferguson and Cornblath, 1975; Tan, 1977), or parts of the limbic brain: thalamic nuclei (Babb et al., 1973); hippocampus (MacLean et al., 1955; Baker and Benedict, 1968); amygdala (Vosu and Wise, 1975). A particularly pertinent study was that of Ferguson and Jasper (1971) as they found that neostigmine-ACh superfusion of undercut cat cortex caused massive depolarization of deep-lying pyramidal cells which extended to their apical dendrites, as well as rhythmic oscillations at 8-20 Hz originating in superficial cortical layers (Rech and Domino, 1960; Maiti and Domino, 1961).

All these data may be interpreted as indicating that the hyperactivity of brain cholinergic systems is epileptogenic in nature as are ACh and cholinergic agonists. Several additional lines of evidence point in the same direction. For instance, antiChEs synergize with strychnine (Baker, 1965; Baker and Benedict, 1968; Karczmar, 1974b) and lower the electroconvulsive shock (ECS) threshold. Furthermore, experimentally induced epileptic foci showed increase activity of AChE (Pope et al., 1947; Guerrero-Figuera et al., 1964), and Tower and McEachern (1949) found detectable levels of ACh in the CSF fluid of epileptic patients. Third, strains of mice susceptible to audiogenic or posture-dependent seizures may exhibit high levels of brain ACh (Naruse et al., 1960; Takahashi et al., 1961; Kurokawa et al., 1963; Pryor, 1968). Similarly, it was stressed that young animals from the convulsive strains are less prone to seizures and have lower ACh levels than the older mice (Naruse et al., 1960; Schlesinger et al., 1965; Fink, 1966; Reeves, 1966; Sobotka, 1969). Additionally, Naruse et al., (1960) attributed the onset of spontaneous seizures to conversion of bound (stable) to free (labile) form of ACh (Sobotka, 1969). Fourth, drugs such as methionine sulfoxamine that increase brain ACh levels by mechanisms other than antiChE action induce seizures (Karczmar *et al.*, 1973). However, methionine sulfoxamine affects other systems than cholinergic transmission such as gabaminergic transmission (Sellinger *et al.*, 1972). Finally, under certain circumstances atropinics may act as anticonvulsants (Wolff, 1956; Tripod, 1957; Chen *et al.*, 1968; Greer and Alpern, 1977). It is also of interest that benzodiazepine anticonvulsants are effective to a certain extent in attenuating cholinergically induced seizures (Lipp, 1972; 1973; 1974).

On the other hand, some data do not seem consistent with the concept of cholinergic facilitation of seizure activity. For instance, cholinergic agonists antagonized and shortened repetitive cortical discharges elicited by electrical stimulation from isolated slabs (Vazques and Kripp, 1973) or by cobalt implants *in situ* (Hoover *et al.*, 1977). Conversely, blockers of ACh synthesis produced seizures in untreated animals (Slater, 1968), or facilitated cobalt-induced epilepsy (Hoover *et al.*, 1977). Furthermore, atropinics produced seizures when applied to cerebral cortex (Daniels and Spehlman, 1973) and facilitated or increased the duration of early repetitive discharge that follows the electrical stimulation of chronically isolated cortical slabs. Altogether, it is as easy to find references to epileptogenic (Vas *et al.*, 1969; Minvielle *et al.*, 1954; Hanigan *et al.*, 1970; Karczmar *et al.*, 1973) as to antiepileptogenic action of atropinic substances.

ACh dynamics should be also considered in the context of the postulated proconvulsive function of the cholinergic system. Strychnine, pentylenetetrazol or ECS-induced convulsions seem to decrease ACh levels in the whole brain and in brain parts (Loewi, 1937; Richter and Crossland, 1949; Naruse *et al.*, 1960; Fink, 1966; Essman, 1972; Karczmar *et al.*, 1973; Svenneby and Roberts, 1974; Longoni *et al.*, 1976; Pedata *et al.*, 1976) and increase ACh efflux, particularly from the cortex (Beleslin *et al.*, 1965; Celesia and Jasper, 1966; Hemsworth and Neal, 1968; Gardner and Webster, 1977). Occasionally, CAT and/or ACh levels increase rapidly following seizures (Karczmar *et al.*, 1973; Longoni *et al.*, 1976). These findings may indicate that turnover of ACh is increased during or after seizures, as indicated by the data of Karczmar *et al.*, (1973) using a rather unorthodox method for the turnover measurement. All this evidence may suggest that ECS and related seizures were caused by release of ACh and its action upon strategic cholinoceptive sites (Gardner and Webster, 1977). On the other hand, it may be speculated that in these experiments, ACh was mobilized and its turnover increased in the course of an attempt by the central cholinergic system to prevent seizures (Karczmar, 1974b). Two specific mechanisms may be theoretically activated during such a homeostatic process. First, the cholinergic system may be responsible for reflex inhibition of motoneurons via cholinoceptive interneurons which may activate inhibiting circuitry directed either at the motoneurons (Kubota *et al.*, 1968; Kidokoro *et al.*, 1968; Iwata *et al.*, 1971) or at the afferent nerve terminals (Nicoll, 1975). Similar mechanisms may be present at the relays of primary afferent pathways in the somesthetic cortex, caudate, and thalamus (Frazier and Boyarski, 1967). Altogether, cholinergic interneurons may activate inhibitory circuitry involving inhibitory amino-acids (Nishi *et al.*, 1974; Nicoll, 1975). At the spinal and cortical and subcortical level, these effects would be antagonistic to the induction of spinal tetanic convulsions and cortical clonic or epileptoid seizures.

Second, desynchronization phenomena should be considered in this context. EEG desynchronization may act antagonistically to certain forms of seizures, as the latter "are rarely detectable during wakefulness or desynchronized sleep." On the other hand, slow-wave sleep and synchronized EEG activate certain epileptic foci (Maynert et al., 1975). Similarly, cholinergic drugs, as potent and specific dysrhythmic agents, may act as anticonvulsants. In fact, as seizures constitute "hypersynchronous" phenomenon (Gastaut and Fischer-Williams, 1959, Ward et al., 1969), this hypersynchrony should be mitigated by desynchronizing tendencies.

Several lines of evidence may indirectly support this contention. Some of the pertinent evidence was already quoted (Slater, 1968; Vazques and Kripp, 1973; Hoover et al., 1977). Furthermore, in some experiments in animals and in man, small doses of physostigmine reduced seizures whether endogenous, induced by pentylenetetrazol or overbreathing, while atropinics caused, on occasion, opposite effects (Williams and Russell, 1941; Longo and Silvestrini, 1957; Ikonomoff, 1970; Karczmar, 1974b; Maynert et al., 1975; Karczmar, 1976). In this context, it may be suggested that convulsive activity arising upon topical or systemic administration of cholinomimetics or antiChEs may be interpreted as due not to cholinergic activation, but to the contrary, to the block of cholinergic synapses resulting from depolarization (Ferguson and Jasper, 1971) and/or densensitization concomitant with large concentrations of cholinomimetics or accumulation of ACh.

Altogether, it is fair to state that the situation is far from being resolved. Perhaps the major difficulty with the concept of antiepileptic properties of the cholinergic system concerns the action of atropinics. While on the basis of the speculation presented here atropinics should induce or at least facilitate convulsions, and while such phenomena are observed sometimes with atropinics, atropinics frequently exhibit anticonvulsive properties in man and animals (Wolff, 1956). Furthermore, there is no record of occurrence of frank convulsions with the very large doses of atropine used in "atropine coma therapy" which acquired wide popularity in the treatment of depression (Karczmar, in press). It must be remembered that the processes underlying seizures are multitransmitter in nature (Mikrotvorskaa, 1968; Maynert et al., 1975; Karczmar, 1978) and that they involve several circuits. The contribution of catecholaminergic, serotonergic and gabaminergic systems is well recognized. It is of interest, for instance, that the catecholaminergic blockers or depletors which decrease the convulsive threshold were shown in certain instances to facilitate or induce convulsions following treatment with muscarinic agonists (Phan et al., 1974). Thus, the net effect of a cholinergic agonist or antagonist on seizures may be vectoral and depend on conditions in question.

EPILOGUE

General Interpretation of the Functional Role of the Central Cholinergic System with Respect to EEG Patterns

It is apparent from the foregoing that the central cholinergic system plays a conspicuous part in the control of the rhythms of electrical activity of the brain and that the cholinergic agonists and antagonists readily affect that activity. The pertinent actions of cholinergic agonists include EEG desynchronization and its behavioral concomitants such as ANMB, as well as, under certain conditions, EEG synchrony, sleep, particularly its REM phase, and, finally, EEG seizures and motor convulsions.

The story relevant to seizures is quite complex. It was pointed out that cholinergic agonists exhibit clear-cut anticonvulsive actions (see "EEG Seizures" section of this chapter). Yet, this effect appears paradoxical in view of the equally clear-cut seizure-inducing actions of cholinergic agonists and antiChEs, and of the fact that cholinergic synapses abound at such sites as the hippocampus (see "Cholinergic Pathways" section of this chapter), an area that seems to serve readily as one of the epileptogenic foci. To reconcile these opposing lines of evidence it may be speculated that locally applied high concentrations of cholinomimetics or ACh, which accumulates following the adminis-tration of antiChEs, block cholinergic synapses which otherwise would exert anti-convulsive influences. Such a synaptic block due to prolonged depolarization and sub-sequent desensitization was amply demonstrated for the periphery (Karczmar, 1967). The anticonvulsive function of the cholinergic system and of the effects of cholinergic agonists may derive from two sources. First, cholinergic interneurons activate central inhibitions acting both pre- and postsynaptically (see "EEG Seizures" section of this chapter; Nishi et al., 1974; Iwata et al., 1971; Nicoll, 1975). Second, it was emphasized that desynchronization and seizure hypersynchrony (Gastaut and Fischer-Williams, 1959) may constitute a dipole (Maynert et al., 1975). Thus, potent desynchronizing action of cholinergic agonists may act antagonistically with respect to seizures. It should be added, however, that this concept of the role of anticonvulsives of the cholinergic system is probably a minority opinion (Karczmar, 1974a; 1974b; Maynert et al., 1975), even though much recent evidence (Hoover et al., 1977) appears to support it.

This leads us then to cholinergic desynchronization, and, more generally, to the conspicuous actions of cholinergic agonists and antagonists on the EEG rhythms. It was already emphasized that cholinergic desynchronization need not depend on either the reticular formation, even when the latter is comprehended in its extended form of diffuse ascending reticulo-thalamico-cortical system (see "Cholinergic Pathways" and "Cortical and Subcortical EEG Actions of Cholinergic Agonists and Anticholinesterases" sections of this chapter; Rinaldi and Himwich, 1955), or cholinergic antagonism of the several synchronizing systems present in the brain (see "Effects of Atropinics, Curaremimetics and Related Drugs" section of this chapter). It may be speculated that cholinergic synapses are concerned with throwing out of phase postsynaptic potentials of neuronal popula-tions wherever the latter generate synchronous slow potentials. This may be accomplished by cholinergic activation of inhibitions, which was already suggested to underlie the cholinergic effect on EEG seizures. This role of cholinergic synapses can be demon-strated for both peripheral and central circuitries.

Indeed, at the autonomic ganglia, cholinergic neurons liberate, via an interneuron, an inhibitory transmitter; this mechanism was clearly demonstrated for the sympathetic ganglia (Libet, 1970; Dun and Karczmar, 1978) and appears plausible at certain para-sympathetic circuits (Karczmar and Dun, 1978). Analogous mechanisms may be wide-spread in the CNS; the classical example is the spinal circuit involving the Renshaw cell (Eccles et al., 1954). Other sites such as the striate (Roth and Bunney, 1976) possibly utilize similar mechanisms for the conversion of excitation into inhibition (Eccles, 1973). In addition, cholinergic involvement with neurotransmitters such as GABA and dopamine, which exhibit central inhibitory effects, was widely demonstrated neurochemically for a multitude of brain sites (see "Neurochemical and Neurophysiological Interaction Between Cholinergic and Other Bioamine Systems" section of this chapter). It should be added that cholinergic neurons may also induce inhibitions directly, without acting via an inhibitory interneuron (see "Characteristics of Synaptic Cholinergic Transmission" section of this chapter; Phillis and York, 1968; Ben-Ari et al., 1976).

That switching inhibitions into excitatory pathways leads to changes in activity patterns of the latter is very likely. This was shown with respect to the participation of inhibitory interneurons in autonomic sympathetic transmission (Dun and Karczmar, 1978) and was recently suggested for the cholinergic "gating" mechanisms of thalamic sensory transmission (Ben-Ari et al., 1976). In fact, certain mathematical models clearly demonstrate the effectiveness of such mechanisms for inducing cyclic desynchronizations into the synchronized flow of sigals emitted by cell populations (Eccles, 1973; Karczmar, unpublished data). It is of interest that earlier similar mechanisms were inculpated in cyclic synchronizations such as those involved in recruitment and alpha rhythms, and in their alteration with desynchronizations (Andersen and Andersson, 1968).

It may be added that this speculative mechanism is consistent with the desynchronizing action of cholinergic agonists not only on the EEG, but also on the EP's (see "Mechanisms and Sites of Cholinergic Desynchronization" section of this chapter). Furthermore, it is in keeping with the topography, distribution and character of cholinergic pathways (see "Cholinergic Pathways" section of this chapter). Contrary to serotonergic and catecholaminergic pathways (Livett, 1973) cholinergic pathways are composed frequently of short axonal circuits or even localized networks; because of this, their ubiquity and their involvement with several inhibitory neurotransmitters, cholinergic synapses seem ideally cast for acting as desynchronizers of the EEG patterns. It may not be wise to attempt to make an hypothesis work for all occasions. Yet, it appears obvious that such a role is consistent with the significance of the cholinergic system for EEG rhythms generally, and thus may account for cholinergic synchrony that is encountered under certain conditions (see "Behavioral Correlates of EEG Effects of Cholinergic Agonists" section of this chapter).

Clinical Exploitation of EEG and Related Actions of Cholinergic Drugs

In view of the ubiquity of the cholinergic pathways and their marked presence (see "Cholinergic Pathways" section of this chapter) within the relay, sensory, motor and limbic systems and systems important for homeostatic and autonomic activities, it is not astonishing that the cholinergic system participates in a wide gamut of behaviors and functions, varying from appetitive and thermoregulating functions to aggression and learning (Myers, 1974; Karczmar, 1975; 1976; Hingtgen and Aprison, 1976; Karczmar, 1977; 1978). Conversely, cholinergic agonists and antagonists affect the behaviors in question.

Perhaps because of this very ubiquity of the cholinergic pathways it is not easy to employ these drugs therapeutically without incurring nonspecific effects and side actions, and their uses for specific CNS diseases are relatively limited and novel (Karczmar, in press). Such uses, at least on an experimental level, are on the increase and include neurologic and psychiatric applications. It is particularly pertinent in the present context to list briefly therapeutic uses of cholinergic agonists and antagonists in mental and related disease before commenting on those particular uses that are described at length by others in this book and that relate more specifically to the EEG effects of these drugs.

These uses have included the employment of large doses of atropine for atropine coma therapy in obsessive neuroses and schizophrenia characterized by anxiety, tension and agitation and in the manic phase of manic-depressive psychosis, as well as of smaller doses of atropine in postpsychotic depression. More recently physostigmine has been used in manic states, in certain schizophrenic conditions, in geriatric memory disturbances, and, finally, in anticholinergic delirium resulting from overdose with atropine or with antidepressants exhibiting potent anticholinergic activities and with atropinic tricyclics (such as amitryptyline) in schizoaffective and related depressive disorders (Karczmar, in press). In some of these conditions, cholinomimetic drugs and acetylcholine precursors (choline and deanol) may be employed besides physostigmine.

Special comment is pertinent for atropine coma therapy, the use of atropinic tricyclic antidepressants in sleep disorders and the employment of physostigmine in manic, hyperkinetic and schizophrenic states, since characteristic EEG changes and certain concomitant phenomena already reviewed in this article occur in these cases.

With respect to the use of physostigmine in certain mental conditions it should be recalled that physostigmine produces in animals an interesting state of EEG and mental alertness combined with ANMB (see "Cholinergic Induction of Theta Waves and Its Behavioral Correlates" section of this chapter). Should the mechanism of action of physostigmine in manic and related diseases of man be homologous to its ANMB action in animals, its therapeutic usefulness may not be due to improvement of a cholinergic defect which was proposed by some investigators to exist in these and related conditions (Klawans et al., 1976), but to a symptomological effect. Indeed, arrest of motor behavior which is not combined with depression would be symptomatically important and, in fact, might activate a feedback mechanism perceived by the patient as beneficial. It must be added however, that Pfefferbaum et al. ("Electrophysiological Effects of Physostigmine in Humans" chapter, this volume) noticed an EEG slowing in his patients treated with physostigmine; such slowing and synchrony may be noticed also in animals (see "Cholinergic System and Slow Sleep" section of this chapter) and may reflect an ameliorative effect not related to the induction of ANMB.

The use of tricyclic antidepressants in certain depressive states relates to REM sleep in the context here (see "Role of the Cholinergic System in REM Sleep" section of this chapter). Kupfer and Edwards (1978) demonstrated that shortened latency and high frequency of occurrence of REM sleep, and deficiency of slow wave or delta (Stage IV) sleep characterizes primary unipolar depression and schizoaffective state; they advocated therefore, the use of tricyclic antidepressants endowed with particularly high atropinic potency in an effort to attenuate REM sleep activity which might be clinically beneficial. That atropinics attenuate REM sleep in animals, physostigmine having an opposite effect in animals and man (Sitaram et al., 1976) is well known; the role of REM sleep in mental health and disease can be only conjectured at present, and the benefit of its curtailment in depressed states cannot be readily predicted.

Similarly, atropine coma therapy should be considered in the light of atropinic effects on the EEG (see "Effects of Atropinics, Curaremimetics and Related Drugs" section of this chapter). While patients undergoing atropine coma therapy exhibit characteristic high voltage and hypersynchronous slow EEG similar to that induced in animals by large doses of atropine and related drugs in animals, the mechanism of the therapeutic

effectiveness of this treatment cannot be readily ascertained. Atropinic EEG is characteristic of confusional mental state; it relates to the block of conditioning and learning, and
of memory processes (Longo, 1958; Longo and Loizzo, 1973); this amnesic effect is
similar to that which obtains following ECS treatment. Furthermore, the latter may
sometimes lead to hypersynchrony. Paradoxically, under these circumstances atropine
may normalize the EEG and induce desynchronization (Fink, 1966). Perhaps the common
mechanism of atropine and ECS treatment is the temporary reversible block of integrative
function of the brain, which is in keeping with speculations presented above. It must
be added however, that atropine coma and ECS therapy are indicated for apparently
different forms of depressive illness (Lynch and Anderson, 1976).

Altogether, we appear to witness the onset of the era of therapeutic use of cholinergic and anticholinergic drugs for mental and geriatric disease; the earlier complaint of
this author (Karczmar, 1967) that the potential of these drugs for CNS therapy is not
exploited is progressively answered. Physostigmine has as its drawbacks its short duration
of action, unreliability of absorption upon oral administration, and limited specificity of
its CNS effects. The efficacy of acetylcholine precursors and deanol is not proven
and/or marked (Ulus *et al.*, 1977). There is no doubt that the initial success achieved
particularly with physostigmine will lead to the development of drugs more reliable
and effective in a number of mental and geriatric defects. No less interesting is the use
of these drugs as tools in exploration of brain functions, particularly in the context of
their EEG effects and the significance of these effects for the understanding of the
phenomena of neuronal integration.

ACKNOWLEDGEMENTS

Published and unpublished investigations carried out in these laboratories and
referred to in this paper were supported in part by the National Institutes of Health
Grant NSO6455, and GM77, and the VA Grant 4830.

REFERENCES

Amatruda III, T.T., Black, D.A., McKenna, T.M., McCarley, R.W., and Hobson, J.A.,
1975, Sleep cycle control and cholinergic mechanisms; differential effects of carbachol
injections at pontine brain stem sites, *Brain Res. 98:*501.

Andersen, P., and Andersson, S.A., 1968, *"Physiological Basis of Alpha Rhythm,"* Appleton-
Century-Crofts, New York.

Babb, T.L., Babb, M., Mahnke, J.H., and Verseano, M., 1973, The action of cholinergic
agents on the electrical activity of the non-specific nuclei of the thalamus, *Int. J.
Neurol. 8:*198.

Ban, T., and Hojo, M., 1971, A comparative study of the effects of antiparkinsonian
drugs on oxotremorine-induced EEG and muscular activities, *Psychopharmacologia
(Berl.) 14:*1.

Banerjee, U., Feldberg, W., and Flynn, V.P., 1970, Microinjections of tubocurarine,
leptazol, strychnine and picrotoxin into the cerebral cortex of anaesthesized cats,
*Br. J. Pharmacol. 40:*6.

Baker, W.W., 1965, Tremorine suppression of hippocampal strychnine foci, *Arch. Int.
Pharmacodyn. Ther. 155:*273.

Baker, W.W., and Benedict, F., 1968, Analysis of local discharges induced by intrahippocampal microinjection of carbachol or diisopropylfluorophosphate (DFP), *Int. J. Neuropharmacol. 7:*135.

Barnes, C.D., and Pompeiano, O., 1970, A brain stem cholinergic system activated by vestibular volleys, *Neuropharmacology 9:*391.

Barnes, L., Karczmar, A.G., and Ingerson, A., 1975, Effects of DFP on brain serotonin, *Pharmacology 17:*180.

Barnes, L., Karczmar, A.G., and Ingerson, A., 1976, Serotonin and acetylcholine of rabbit brain following DFP, *Pharmacology 18:*202.

Barnes, L., Koehn, G., and Karczmar, A.G., in press, Effects of diisopropylphosphofluoridate (DFP) on pain threshold and and serotonin, *Proceedings of the Seventh International Congress of Pharmacology, Abstracts.*

Baxter, B.L., 1969, Induction of both emotional behavior and a novel form of REM sleep by chemical stimulation applied to cat mesencephalon, *Exp. Neurol. 23:*220.

Beleslin, D., Polak, R.L., and Sproull, D.H., 1965, The effect of leptazol and strychnine on the acetylcholine release from the cat brain, *J. Physiol. (Lond.) 181:*308.

Ben-Ari, Y., Dingledine, R., Kanazawa, I., and Kelly, J.S., 1976, Inhibitory effects of acetylcholine on neurones in the feline nucleus reticularis thalami, *J. Physiol. (Lond.) 261:*647.

Ben-Ari, Y., Zigmond, R.E., Shute, C.C.D., and Lewis, P.R., 1977, Regional distribution of choline acetyltransferase and acetylcholinesterase within the amygdaloid complex and stria terminalis system, *Brain Res. 120:*435.

Birdsall, N.J.M., Burgeu, A.S.V., and Hulme, E.C., 1977, Correlation between the binding properties and pharmacological responses of muscarinic receptors, in *"Cholinergic Mechanisms and Psychopharmacology",* (D.J. Jenden, ed.), pp. 25-33, Plenum Press, New York.

Bokums, J.A., and Elliott, H.W., 1968, Effects of physostigmine on electrical activity of the cat brain, *Pharmacology 1:*98.

Bonnet, V., and Bremer, F., 1937, Action du potassium, du calcium et de l'acetylcholine sur les activites electriques, spontanees et provoquees, de l'ecorce cerebrale, *C.R. Soc. Biol. 136:*1271.

Borbely, A.A., 1973, *"Pharmacological Modifications of Evoked Brain Potentials",* Hans Huber, Bern.

Bourdois, P.S., Mitchell, J.F., Somogyi, G.T., and Berle, J.C., 1974, The output per stimulus of acetylcholine from cerebral cortical slices in the presence or absence of cholinesterase inhibition, *Br. J. Pharmacol. 52:*509.

Bovet, D., Longo, V.G., and Silvestrini, B., 1957, Les methodes d'investigations electrophysiologiques dans l'etude des medicaments tranquillisants, in *"Internatl. Symp. on Psychotropic. Drug",* (S. Garattini and V. Ghetti, eds.), pp. 193-206, Elsevier, Amsterdam.

Bradley, P.B., and Elkes, J., 1953, The effect of atropine, hyoscyamine, physostigmine, and neostigmine on the electrical activity of the brain of the conscious cat, *J. Physiol. (Lond.) 120:*14P.

Bradley, P.B., and Elkes, J., 1957, The effects of some drugs on the electrical activity of the brain, *Brain 88:*77.

Bremer, F., 1960, Neurophysiological mechanism in cerebral arousal, in *"The Nature of Sleep",* (G.E. Wolstenholm and M. O'Connor, eds.), pp. 30-50, Little Brown & Co., Boston.

Bremer, F., and Chatonnet, J., 1949, Acetylcholine et cortex cerebrale, *Arch. Int. Physiol. Biochim. 57:*106.

Brooks, D.C., and Gershon, M.D., 1972, An analysis of the effect of reserpine upon ponto-geniculo-occipital wave activity in the cat, *Neuropharmacology 11:*449.

Brooks, D.C., Gershon, M.D., and Simon, R.P., 1972, Brain stem serotonin depletion and ponto-geniculo-occipital wave activity in the cat treated with reserpine, *Neuropharmacology 11:*511.

Brucke, F.T., and Stumpf, C., 1957, The pharmacology of "arousal reactions" in *"Internatl. Symp. on Psychotropic Drugs",* (S. Garattini and V. Ghetti, eds.), pp. 319-324, Elsevier, Amsterdam.

Buchwald, N.A., Jeuser, G., Wyers, E.J., and Lauprecht, C.W., 1961a, The "caudate spindle". III. Inhibition of high frequency stimulation of subcortical structures, *Electroencephalogr. Clin. Neurophysiol. 13:*525.

Buchwald, N.A., Wyers, E.J., Lauprecht, C.W., and Jeuser, G., 1961b, The "caudate spindle". IV. A behavioral index of caudate-induced inhibition, *Electroencephalogr. Clin. Neurophysiol. 13:*531.

Buchwald, N.A., Wyers, E.J., Okuma, T., and Jeuser, G., 1961c, The "caudate spindle". I. Electrophysiological properties, *Electroencephalogr. Clin. Neurophysiol. 13:*509.

Buchwald, N.A., Horwath, F.E., Wyers, E.J., and Wakefield, C., 1964, Electroencephalogram rhythm correlated with milk reinforcement in cats, *Nature (Lond.) 201:*830.

Butcher, L.L., 1977, Recent advances in histochemical techniques for the study of central cholinergic mechanisms, in *"Cholinergic Mechanisms and Psychopharmacology",* (D.J. Jenden, ed.), pp. 93-124, Plenum Press, New York.

Celesia, G.C., and Jasper, H.H., 1966, Acetylcholine released from cerebral cortex in relation to state of activation, *Neurology 16:*1053.

Chatfield, P.O., and Dempsey, E.W., 1942, Some effects of prostigmine and acetylcholine on cerebral potentials, *Am. J. Physiol. 135:*633.

Chatfield, P.O., and Lord, J.T., 1955, Effects of atropine, prostigmine and acetylcholine on evoked cortical potentials, *Electroencephalogr. Clin. Neurophysiol. 7:*553.

Chen, G., Ensor, C.R., and Bohner, B., 1968, Studies of drug effects on electrically-induced extensor seizures and clinical implications, *Arch. Int. Pharmacodyn. Ther. 172:*183.

Cheney, D.L., and Costa, E., 1978, Biochemical pharmacology of cholinergic neurons, in *"Psychopharmacology – A Generation of Progress",* (M.A. Lipton, A. DiMascio, K.F. Killam, eds.), pp. 283-291, Raven Press, New York.

Cheney, D.L., LeFevre, H.F., and Racagni, G., 1975, Choline acetyltransferase activity and mass fragmentographic measurement of acetylcholine in specific nuclei and tracts of rat brain, *Neuropharmacology 14:*801.

Cheney, D.L., Racagni, E., and Costa, E., 1976, Appendix II: Distribution of acetylcholine and choline acetyltransferase in specific nuclei and tracts of rat brain, in *"Biology of Cholinergic Function",* (A.M. Goldberg and I. Hanin, eds.), pp. 655-660, Raven Press, New York.

Cheramy, A., Nieoullon, A., and Glowinski, J., in press, Role of various nigral afferents on the activity of the nigrostriatal dopaminergic pathways, in *"Interdependence of Neurotransmitter Systems in the CNS"* (J. Glowinski and A.G. Karczmar, eds.), 7th International Congress of Pharmacology, Pergamon Press, Oxford.

Clemente, D.C., Sterman, M.B., and Wyrwicka, W., 1964, Post-reinforcement EEG synchronization during alimentary behavior, *Electroencephalogr. Clin. Neurophysiol. 16:*355.

Coleman, J.C., and Lindsley, D.B., 1975, Hippocampal correlates of free behavior and behavior induced by stimulation of two hypothalamic-hippocampal systems in the cat, *Exp. Neurol. 49:*506.

Collier, B., Ilson, D., and Lovet, S., 1977, Factors affecting choline uptake by ganglia and the relationship between choline uptake and acetylcholine synthesis, in *"Cholinergic Mechanisms and Psychopharmacology"* (D.J. Jenden, ed.), pp. 457-464, Plenum Press, New York.

Cordeau, J.D., and Mancia, M., 1959, Evidence for the existence of an electroencephalographic synchronization mechanism originating in the lower brain stem, *Electroencephalogr. Clin. Neurophysiol. 11:*551.

Cordeau, J.D., Moreau, A., Beaulnes, A., and Lanrin, C., 1963, EEG and behavioral changes following microinjections of acetylcholine and adrenaline in the brain stem of cats, *Arch. Ital. 101:*30.

Crawford, J.M., Curtis, D.R., Voorhoens, P.E., and Wilson, V.J., 1966, Acetylcholine sensitivity of cerebellar neurons in the cat, *J. Physiol. (Lond.) 186:*139.

Daniels, J.C., and Spehlman, R., 1973, The convulsant effects of topically applied atropine, *Electroencephalogr. Clin. Neurophysiol. 34:*83.

De Feudis, F.W., 1974, *"Central Cholinergic Synapses and Behaviour,"* Academic Press, London.

Dempsey, F.W., and Morison, R.S., 1941, The production of rhythmically recurrent cortical potentials after localized thalamic stimulation, *Am. J. Physiol. 135:*293.

Dempsey, E.W., and Morison, R.S., 1942, The interaction of certain spontaneous and induced cortical potentials, *Am. J. Physiol. 135:*301.

De Robertis, E., and Schacht, J., 1974, *"Neurochemistry of Cholinergic Receptors,"* Raven Press, New York.

Desi, I., Dura, G., Gonczi, L., Kneffel, Z., Strohmayer, A., and Szabo, Z., 1975, Toxicity of malathion to mammals, aquatic organisms and tissue culture cells, *Arch. Environ. Contam. Toxicol. 34:*410.

Domino, E.F., 1968, Cholinergic mechanisms and the EEG, *Electroencephalogr. Clin. Neurophysiol. 24:*292.

Domino, E.F., and Wilson, A.E., 1973, Enhanced utilization of brain acetylcholine during morphine withdrawal in the rat, *Nature 243:*285.

Domino, E.F., and Yamamoto, K., 1965, Nicotine effect on the sleep cycle of the cat, *Science 150:*631.

Domino, E.F., Dren, A.T., and Yamamoto, K.I., 1967, Pharmacologic evidence for cholinergic mechanisms in neocortical and limbic activating systems, *Prog. Brain Res. 27:*337.

Domino, E.F., Bartolini, A., Kawamura, H., 1977, Effects of reticular stimulation, d-amphetamine and scopolamine on acetylcholine release from the hippocampus of brainstem transected cats, *Arch. Int. Pharmacodyn. Ther. 225(2):*294.

Dudar, J.D., and Szerb, J.C., 1969, The effect of topically applied atropine on resting and evoked cortical acetylcholine release, *J. Physiol. (Lond.) 203:*741.

Dun, N.J., and Karczmar, A.G., 1977, A comparison of the effect of theophylline and cyclic adenosine 3'5'-monophosphate on the superior cervical ganglion of the rabbit by means of the sucrose-gap method, *J. Pharmacol. Exp. Ther. 202:*89.

Dun, N.J., and Karczmar, A.G., 1978, Involvement of an interneuron in the generation of the slow inhibitory postsynaptic potential in mammalian sympathetic ganglia, *Proc. Natl. Acad. Sci. USA 75:*4029.

Dun, N.J., Kaibara, K., and Karczmar, A.G., 1977a, Direct postsynaptic membrane effect of dibutyryl cyclic GMP on mammalian sympathetic neurons, *Neuropharmacology 16:*715.

Dun, N.J., Kaibara, K., and Karczmar, A.G., 1977b, Dopamine and adenosine 3'5'-mono-phosphate responses of single mammalian sympathetic neurons, *Science 197*:778.

Dura, G., Illes, I., Major, M., and Goenczi, C., 1975, Neurophysiological investigations with an organic phosphate compound, *Acta. Physiol. Acad. Sci. Hung. 44*:313.

Eccles, J.C., 1973, *"The Understanding of the Brain,"* McGraw Hill Co., New York.

Eccles, J.C., Fatt, P., and Koketsu, K., 1954, Cholinergic and inhibitory synapses in a pathway from motor-axon collaterals to motoneurons, *J. Physiol. (Lond.) 126*:524.

Echlin, F.A., 1975, Time course of development of supersensitivity to topical acetyl-choline in partially isolated cortex, *Electroencephalogr. Clin. Neurophysiol. 38*:225.

Echlin, F.A., and McDonald, J., 1954, The supersensitivity of chronically isolated cere-bral cortex as a mechanisms in focal cortical epilepsy, *Trans. Am. Neurol. Assoc. 79*:75.

Endroczi, E., Schreiberg, G., and Lissak, K., 1963a, The role of central nervous activating and inhibitory structures in the control of pituitary-adrenocortical function. Effects of intracerebral cholinergic and adrenergic stimulation, *Acta Physiol. Acad. Sci. Hung. 24*:211.

Endroczi, E., Hartmann, G., and Lissak, K., 1963b, Effect of intracerebrally adminis-tered cholinergic and adrenergic drugs on neocortical and archicortical electrical activity, *Acta Physiol. Acad. Sci. Hung. 24*:199.

Essig, C.F., Hampson, J.L., Bales, P.D., Willis, A., and Himwich, H.E., 1950, Effect of panparnit on brain wave changes induced by DFP, *Science 111*:38.

Essman, W.B., 1972, Neurochemical changes in ECS and ECT, *Semin. Psychiatry 4*:67.

Everett, G.M., 1974, Pharmacological studies of oxotremorine, in *"Biochemical and Neurophysiological Correlates of Centrally Acting Drugs"* (E. Trabucchi, R. Paoletti, and N. Canal., eds.), pp. 69-74, Pergamon Press, Oxford.

Fairchild, M.D., Jenden, D.J., and Mickey, M.R., 1975, An application of long-term frequency analysis in measuring drug-specific alterations in the EEG of the cat, *Elec-troencephalogr. Clin. Neurophysiol. 38*:337.

Feldberg, W., and Fleishhauer, K., 1963, The hippocampus as the site of origin of the seizure discharge produced by tubocurarine acting from the cerebral ventricles, *J. Physiol. (Lond.) 168*:435.

Feldberg, W., and Vogt, M., 1948, Acetylcholine synthesis in different regions of the central nervous system, *J. Physiol. (Lond.) 107*:373.

Ferguson, J.H., and Cornblath, D.R., 1975, Acetylcholine epilepsy: relationship of sur-face concentration, chronicity of denervation, and focus size, *Exp. Neurol. 46*:302.

Ferguson, J.H., and Jasper, H.H., 1971, Laminar DC studies of acetylcholine-activated epileptiform discharge in cerebral cortex, *Electroencephalogr. Clin. Neurophysiol. 30*:377.

Fink, M., 1966, Cholinergic aspects of convulsive therapy, *J. Nerv. Ment. Dis. 24*:475.

Floris, V., Morocutti, G., and Ayala, G.F., 1963, Azione della nicotina sulla attivita bioelettrica della corteccia, del talamo e dell' ippocampo nel cogniglio. Sull 'azione di "arousal" e convulsivante primitiva sulle strutture ippocampo-talamiche, *Boll. Soc. Ital. Biol. Sper. 38*:407.

Fonnum, F., 1973, Recent developments in biochemical investigations of cholinergic transmission, *Brain Res. 62*:495.

Frazier, D.T., and Boyarski, L.L., 1967, Cholinergic properties of the relay functions of the primary afferent pathways, *J. Pharmacol. Exp. Ther. 156*:1.

Gadea-Ciria, M., Stadler, H., Lloyd, K.G., and Bartholini, G., 1973, Acetylcholine release within the cat striatum during the sleep-wakefulness cycle, *Nature 243*:518.

Gardner, C.R., and Webster, R.A., 1977, Convulsant-anticonvulsant interactions on seizure activity and cortical acetylcholine release, *Eur. J. Pharmacol. 42*:247.

Garrattini, S., Pujol, J.F., and Samanin, R., 1978, *"Interactions Between Putative Neurotransmitters in the Brain,"* Raven Press, New York.

Gastaut, H., and Fischer-Williams, M., 1959, The physiopathology of epileptic seizures, in *"Handbook of Physiology Sect. I: Neurophysiology"* (J. Fields, ed.), pp. 329-363.

George, R., Haslett, W.L., and Jenden, D.J., 1964, A cholinergic mechanism in the brain stem reticular formation: Induction of paradoxical sleep, *Int. J. Neuropharmacol. 3:*541.

Giorguieff, M.F., Le Floc'H, M.L., Glowinski, J., and Besson, M.J., 1977, Involvement of cholinergic presynaptic receptors of nicotinic and muscarinic types in the control of the spontaneous release of dopamine from striatal dopaminergic terminals in the rat, *J. Pharmacol. Exp. Ther. 200:*535.

Glisson, S.N., Karczmar, A.G., and Barnes, L., 1974, Effects of DFP on acetylcholine, cholinesterase and catecholamines of several rabbit brain parts, *Neuropharmacol. 13:*623.

Glowinski, J., and Karczmar, A.G., in press a, Interdependence of neurotransmitter systems in the CNS, in *"Proceedings of the Seventh International Congress of Pharmacology"* (J. Glowinski, and A.G. Karczmar, eds.), Pergamon Press, Oxford.

Glowinski, J., and Karczmar, A.G., in press b, Concluding remarks on the symposium: Interdependence of neurotransmitter systems in the CNS, in *"Proceedings of the Seventh International Congress of Pharmacology"* (J. Glowinski, and A.G. Karczmar, eds.), Pergamon Press, Oxford.

Greer, C.A., and Alpern, H.P., 1977, Mediation of myoclonic seizures by dopamine and clonic seizures by acetylcholine and GABA, *Life Sci. 21:*385.

Guerrero-Figueroa, R., Verster, F., DeB., Barros, A., and Heath, R.C., 1964, Cholinergic mechanisms in subcortical mirror focus and effects of topical application of γ-aminobutyric acid and acetylcholine, *Epilepsia 5:*140.

Guggenheimer, E.H., and Levinger, I.M., 1975, The effect of oxotremorine on the acetylcholine output from the CSF containing spaces, *Experientia 31:*88.

Guha, D., and Pradhan, S.N., 1976, Effects of nicotine on EEG and evoked potentials and their interactions with autonomic drugs, *Neuropharmacology 15:*225.

Guyenet, P., Agid, Y., Javoy, F., Beaujouan, J.C., Rossier, J., and Glowinski, J., 1975, Effects of dopaminergic receptor agonists and antagonists on the activity of the neostriatal cholinergic system, *Brain Res. 84:*227.

Hall, R.C., and Keane, P.E., 1975, Dopaminergic and cholinergic interactions in the caudate nucleus in relation to the induction of sleep in the cat, *Br. J. Pharmacol. 54:*247.

Hanigan, W.C., Scudder, C.L., and Karczmar, A.G., 1970, Adrenergic, serotonergic and cholinergic systems and electroconvulsive seizures in mice, *Fed. Proc. 29:*486.

Hanin, I., and Costa, E., 1976, Approaches used to estimate brain acetylcholine turnover rate *in vivo;* effects of drugs on brain acetylcholine turnover rate, in *"Biology of Cholinergic Function"* (A.M. Goldberg, and I. Hanin, eds.), pp. 355-377, Raven Press, New York.

Haranath, P.S.R.K., Indira, G., and Krishnamurthy, A., 1977, Effects of cholinomimetic drugs and their antagonists injected into vertebral artery of unanaesthetized dogs, *Pharmacol. Biochem. Behav. 6:*259.

Hemsworth, B.A., and Neal, M.J., 1968, The effect of central stimulant drugs on the release of acetylcholine from the cerebral cortex, *Br. J. Pharmacol. 32:*543.

Hernandez-Peon, R., 1962, Sleep induced by localized or chemical stimulation of the forebrain, *Electroencephalogr. Clin. Neurophysiol. 14:*423.

Hernandez-Peon, R., 1965, Central neurohumoral transmission in sleep and wakefulness, in *"Progress in Brain Research, Sleep Mechanisms"* (K. Akert, C. Bally, and J.P. Schade, eds.), pp. 96-116, Elsevier, Amsterdam.

Hernandez-Peon, R., and Chavez-Ibarra, G., 1963, Sleep induced by electrical or chemical stimulation of the forebrain, *Electroencephalogr. Clin. Neurophysiol. (Suppl.) 24:*188.

Hernandez-Peon, R., Chavez-Ibarra, G., Morgane, P.J., and Timo-Iaria, C., 1963, Limbic cholinergic pathways involved in sleep and behaviour, *Exp. Neurol. 8:*93.

Herz, A., and Zieglgansberger, W., 1968, The influence of microelectrophoretically applied biogenic amines, cholinomimetics and procaine on synaptic excitation in the corpus striatum, *Int. J. Neuropharmacol. 7:*221.

Hill, R.C., Simmonds, M.A., and Straughan, D.W., 1972, Convulsive properties of d-tubocurarine and cortical inhibition, *Nature 240:*51.

Hingtgen, J.N., and Aprison, M.H., 1976, Behavioral and environmental aspects of the cholinergic system, in *"Biology of Cholinergic Function"* (A.M. Goldberg, and I. Hanin, eds.), pp. 515-566, Raven Press, New York.

Hobson, J.A., 1974, The cellular basis of sleep cycle control, in *"Advances in Sleep Research"* (E.D. Weitzman, ed.), pp. 217-250, Spectrum, New York.

Hokfelt, T., in press, Interdependence of neurotransmitter systems, anatomical basis, in *"Interdependence of Neurotransmitter Systems in the CNS"* (J. Glowinski and A.G. Karczmar, eds.), Pergamon Press, Oxford.

Holmstedt, B., 1959, Pharmacology of organophosphorus anticholinesterase agents, *Pharmacol. Rev. 11:*567.

Hoover, D.B., Craig, C.R., and Colasanti, B.K., 1977, Cholinergic involvement in cobalt-induced epilepsy in the rat, *Exp. Brain Res. 29:*501.

Ikonomoff, S.I., 1970, Anticholinesterase drugs and epileptic seizures, *Br. J. Psychiatry 177:*679.

Irmi, S.F., 1974a, Correlation between spontaneous behavior and cortical or hippocampal EEG in rats — dissociation after physostigmine, *Acta. Nerv. Super. (Prague) 16:*48.

Irmi, S.F., 1974b, Effects of scopolamine on EEG of cortex and hippocampus during spontaneous behavior in rat, *Acta. Nerv. Super. (Prague) 16:*220.

Irmi, S.F., 1977, Cortical and hippocampal EEG during spontaneous behavior in rats: Normal conditions and anticholinergic drugs proceedings, *Acta. Nerv. Super. (Prague) 19:*145.

Iwata, N., Sakai, Y., and Deguchi, T., 1971, Effects of physostigmine on the inhibition of trigeminal motoneurons by cutaneous impulses in the cat, *Exp. Brain Res. 13:*519.

Jacobowitz, D.M., 1978, Histochemical and micropunch analysis of aminergic and cholinergic pathways in the brain, in *"Interrelationship Between Various Neurotransmitter Systems"* (A.G. Karczmar, and J. Glowinski, eds.), Pergamon Press (in press).

Jacobs, B.L., Henriksen, S.J., and Dement, W.C., 1972, Neurochemical bases of the PGO waves, *Brain Res. 58:*157.

Jalfre, M., Ruch-Monachon, M.A., and Haefely, W., 1974, Methods for assessing the interaction of agents with 5-hydroxytryptamine neurone and receptors in the brain, in *"Advances in Biochemistry and Psychopharmacology"* (E. Costa, and P. Greengard, eds.), pp. 121-134, Raven Press, New York.

Jalowiec, J.E., Morgane, P.J., Stern, W.C., Zolovick, A.J., and Panksepp, J., 1973, Effects of midbrain tegmental lesions on sleep and regional brain serotonin and norepinephrine levels in cats, *Exp. Neurol. 41:*670.

Jasper, H.H., and Tessier, J., 1971, Acetylcholine liberation from cerebral cortex during paradoxical (REM) sleep, *Science 172:*601.

Javoy, F., Euvrard, C., Bockaert, J., and Glowinski, J., 1978, Action of "gabaminergic" and "serotonergic" drugs on the activity of striatal cholinergic interneurons, in *"Inter-relationship Between Various Neurotransmitter Systems"* (A.G. Karczmar, and J. Glowinski, eds.), Pergamon Press, (in press).

Jenden, D.J., 1977, Estimation of acetylcholine and the dynamics of its metabolism, in *"Cholinergic Mechanisms and Psychopharmacology"* (D.J. Jenden, ed.), pp. 139-162, Plenum Press, New York.

Jewett, R.E., and Norton, S., 1966, Effects of some stimulant and depressant drugs on sleep cycles of cats, *Exp. Neurol. 15:*463.

Jouvet, M., 1961, Telencephalic and rhombencephalic sleep in the cat, in *"The Nature of Sleep"* (G.E.W. Wolstenholme, and M. O'Conner, eds.), pp. 188-208, J. & A. Churchill, London.

Jouvet, M., 1967, Neurophysiology of the states of sleep, in *"The Neurosciences, A Study Program"* (G.C. Quarton, T. Melnechuk, and F.U. Schmitt, eds.), pp. 529-544, University Press, New York.

Jouvet, M., 1972, Some monoaminergic mechanisms controlling sleep and waking, in *"Brain and Human Behavior"* (A.G. Karczmar, and J.C. Eccles, eds.), pp. 131-160, Springer-Verlag, Berlin.

Jouvet, M., 1975, Cholinergic mechanisms and sleep, in *"Cholinergic Mechanisms"* (P. Waser, ed.), pp. 455-476, Raven Press, New York.

Karczmar, A.G., 1967, Pharmacologic, toxicologic and therapeutic properties of anti-cholinesterase agents, in *"Physiological Pharmacology"* (W.S. Root, and F.G. Hofman, eds.), pp. 163-322, Academic Press, New York.

Karczmar, A.G., 1970a, Central cholinergic pathways and their behavioral implications, in *"Principles of Psychopharmacology"* (W.G. Clark, and J. del Giudice, eds.), pp. 57-86, Academic Press, New York.

Karczmar, A.G., 1970b, History of the research with anticholinergic agents, in *"Anti-cholinesterase Agents"* (A.G. Karczmar, ed.), pp. 1-44, International Encyclopedia of Pharmacology and Therapeutics, Vol. 1, Section 13, Pergamon Press, Inc., Oxford.

Karczmar, A.G., 1971, Possible mechanisms underlying the so-called "Divorce" phenomena of EEG desynchronizing actions of anticholinesterases, Presented at the Regional Midwest EEG Meeting, April 1971, Hines, V.A. Hospital.

Karczmar, A.G., 1974a, The chemical coding via the cholinergic system: its organization and behavioral implications, in *"Neurochemical Coding of Brain Function"* (R.D. Myers, and R.R. Drucker-Colin, eds.), pp. 399-418, Adv. in Behav. Biol. Vol. 10, Plenum Press, New York.

Karczmar, A.G., 1974b, Brain acetylcholine and seizures, in *"Psychobiology of Convulsive Therapy"* (M. Fink, S. Kety, J. McGaugh, and T.A. Williams, eds.), pp. 251-270, V.H. Winston, Washington, D.C.

Karczmar, A.G., 1975, Cholinergic influences on behavior, in *"Cholinergic Mechanisms"* (P.G. Waser, ed.), pp. 501-529, Raven Press, New York.

Karczmar, A.G., 1976, Central actions of acetylcholine, cholinomimetics, and related drugs, in *"Biology of Cholinergic Function"* (A.M. Goldberg, and I. Hanin, eds.), pp. 395-449, Raven Press, New York.

Karczmar, A.G., 1977, Exploitable aspects of central cholinergic function, particularly with respect to the EEG, motor, analgesic and mental functions, in *"Cholinergic Mechanisms and Psychopharmacology"* (D.J. Jenden, ed.), pp. 679-708, Plenum Press, New York.

Karczmar, A.G., 1978, Multitransmitter mechanisms underlying selected function, particularly aggression, learning and sexual behavior, in *"Interdependence Between Various Neurotransmitter Systems"* (A.G. Karczmar, and J. Glowinski, eds.), pp. 581-608, Pergamon Press, Oxford.

Karczmar, A.G., in press, Mechanisms and clinical uses of peripherally and centrally acting cholinergic and anticholinergic drugs, *Drug Therapy.*

Karczmar, A.G., and Dun, N.J., 1978, Cholinergic synapses: Physiological, pharmacological and behavioral considerations, in *"Psychopharmacology: A Generation of Progress"* (M.A. Lipton, A. DiMascio, and K.F. Killam, eds.), pp. 293-305, Raven Press, New York.

Karczmar, A.G., and Glowinski, J., 1978, Interrelationships between various neurotransmitter systems, in *Neuropsychopharmacology Proceedings of the Tenth Congress CINP* (P. Deniker, C. Radouco-Thomas, and A. Villeneuve, eds.), Pergamon Press, Oxford.

Karczmar, A.G., Blachut, K., Ridlon, S., Gothelf, B., and Awad, O., 1963, Pharmacological actions in various neuroeffectors of single and combined administration of EPN and Malathion, *Int. J. Neuropharmacol.* 2:163.

Karczmar, A.G., Longo, V.G., *et al.*, 1970, Pharmacological model of paradoxical sleep: the role of cholinergic and monoamine systems, *Physiol. Behav.* 5:175.

Karczmar, A.G., Scudder, C.L., and Richardson, D.L., 1973, Interdisciplinary approach to the study of behavior in related mice types, in *"Neurosciences Research"* (I. Kopin, ed.), pp. 159-244, Academic Press, New York.

Kawamura, H., and Domino, E.F., 1969, Differential actions of m and n cholinergic agonists on the brainstem activating system, *Int. J. Neuropharmacol.* 8:105.

Key, B.J., and Krzywoskinski, L., 1977, Electrocortical changes induced by the perfusion of noradrenaline, acetylcholine and their antagonists directly into the dorsal raphe nucleus of the cat, *Br. J. Pharmacol.* 61:297.

Khinkova, L., Kaloianova, F., Dimov, S., and Atsev, E., 1975, Comparative study of the changes in the EEG and cholinesterase activity in experimental dipterex poisoning, *Probl. Khig.* 1:39.

Kidokoro, Y., Kubota, K., Shuto, S., and Sumino, R., 1968, Possible interneurons responsible for reflex inhibition of motoneurons of jaw-closing muscles from inferior dental nerve, *J. Neurophysiol.* 31:709.

Kingsley, R.E., and Barnes, C.B., 1973, Olivo-cochlear inhibition during physostigmine-induced activity in pontal reticular formation in decerebrate cat, *Exp. Neurol.* 40:43.

Klawans, H.A., Westheimer, R., and Goetz, C.G., 1976, A pharmacological model of the pathophysiology of schizophrenia, *Dis. Nerv. Syst.* 36:267.

Klemm, W.R., 1976, Physiological and behavioral significance of hippocampal rhythmic, slow activity ("Theta rhythm"), *Prog. Neurobiol.* 6:23.

Knott, J.R., Ingram, W.R., and Correll, P.E., 1960, Some effects of subcortical stimulation on the bar pressing response, *Arch. Neurol.* 2:476.

Koehn, G.L., and Karczmar, A.G., 1978, Effect of diisopropylphosphofluoridate on analgesia and motor behavior in the rat, *Prog. Neuropsychopharmacol.* 2:169.

Koelle, G.B., 1963, Cytological distributions and physiological functions of cholinesterases, in *"Handbuch der Experimentellen Pharmakologie, Ergazungswk, Cholinesterases and Anticholinesterase Agents, Vol. 15"* (G.B. Koelle, ed.), pp. 189-298, Springer-Verlag, Berlin.

Koelle, G.B., 1969, Significance of acetylcholinesterase in central synaptic transmission, *Fed. Proc.* 28:95.

Koelle, G.B., Koelle, W.A., Smyrl, E.G., Davis, R., and Nagle, A.F., 1977, Histochemical and pharmacological evidence of the function of butyrylcholinesterase, in *"Cholinergic Mechanisms and Psychopharmacology"* (D. J. Jenden, ed.), pp. 125-138, Plenum Press, New York.

Koller, W.C., and Berry, C.A., 1976, Modification of evoked responses in the caudate nucleus by cholinergic agents, *Neuropharmacology 15:*233.

Korsak, R.J., and Sato, M.M., 1977, Effects of chronic organophosphate pesticide exposure on the central nervous system, *Clin. Toxicol. 11:*83.

Kostowski, W., 1971, Effects of some cholinergic and anticholinergic drugs injected intracerebrally to the midline pontine area, *Neuropharmacology 10:*595.

Kramis, R., Vanderwolf, C.H., and Bland, B.H., 1975, Two types of hippocampal rhythmical slow activity in both rabbit and the rat: relations to behavior and effects of atropine, diethyl ether, urethane, and pentobarbital, *Exp. Neurol. 49:*58.

Krnjevic, K., 1969, Central cholinergic pathways, in *"Central Cholinergic Transmission and its Behavioral Aspects"* (A.G. Karczmar, ed.), *Fed. Proc. 28:*115.

Krnjevic, K., 1974, Chemical nature of synaptic transmission in vertebrates, *Physiol. Rev. 54:*418.

Krnjevic, K., 1976, Acetylcholine receptors in vertebrate CNS, in *"Handbook of Psychopharmacology"* (L.L. Iversen, S.D. Iversen, and S.H. Snyder, eds.), pp. 97-125, Plenum Press, New York.

Krnjevic, K., and Van Meter, W.G., 1976, Cyclic nucleotides in spinal cells, *Can. J. Physiol. Pharmacol. 54:*416.

Krnjevic, K., Puil, E., and Werman, R., 1976, Is cyclic guanosine monophosphate the internal "second messenger" for cholinergic actions on central neurons? *Can. J. Physiol. Pharmacol. 54:*172.

Kubota, K., Kidokoro, Y., and Suzuki, J., 1968, Postsynaptic inhibition of trigeminal and lumbar motoneurons from the superficial radial nerve of the cat, *Jpn. J. Physiol. 18:*198.

Kuhar, M.J., 1973, Neurotransmitter uptake: a tool in identifying neurotransmitter-specific pathways, *Life Sci. 13:*1623.

Kuhar, M.J., 1976, The anatomy of cholinergic neurons, in *"Biology of Cholinergic Function"* (A.M. Goldberg, and I. Hanin, eds.), pp. 3-27, Raven Press, New York.

Kuhar, M.J., and Yamamura, H.I., 1976, Localization of cholinergic muscarinic receptors in rat brain by light microscopic radioautography, *Brain Res. 110:*229.

Kumagai, H., Sakai, F., and Otsuka, Y., 1962a, EEG responses to subcortical microinjection of d-tubocurarine chloride and other drugs in cats, *Arch. Int. Pharmacodyn. Ther. 139:*588.

Kumagai, H., Sakai, F., and Otsuka, Y., 1962b, Analysis of central effect of d-tubocurarine chloride in the cat, *Int. J. Neuropharmacol. 1:*157.

Kupfer, D.J., and Edwards, D.J., 1978, Multitransmitter mechanisms and treatment of affective disease, in *"Interrelationship Between Various Neurotransmitter Systems"* (A.G. Karczmar, and J. Glowinski, eds.), Pergamon Press, Oxford (in press).

Kurokawa, M., Machiyama, Y., and Kato, M., 1963, Distribution of acetylcholine in the brain during various states of activity, *J. Neurochem. 10:*341.

Langlois, J.M., and Poussart, Y., 1969, Electrocortical activity following cholinergic stimulation of the caudate nucleus in the cat, *Brain Res. 15:*581.

Levy, J., and Michel-Ber, E., 1967, Contribution a l'etude des cholinergiques et cholinolytiques centraux et perpheriques. II. Activites cholinergiques centrales de l'oxotremorine, *Therapie 22:*87.

Lewis, P.R., and Shute, C.C.D., 1967, The cholinergic limbic system: projections to hippocampal formation, medial cortex, nuclei of the ascending cholinergic reticular system, and the subfornical organs and supra-optic crest, *Brain 90:*521.

Libet, B., 1970, Generation of slow inhibitory and excitatory postsynaptic potentials, *Fed. Proc. 29:*1945.

Lipp, J.A., 1972, Effect of diazepam upon soman-induced seizure activity and convulsions, *EEG Clin. Neurophysiol. 32:*557.

Lipp, J.A., 1973, Effect of benzodiazepine derivatives on soman-induced seizure activity and convulsions in the monkey, *Arch. Int. Pharmacodyn. Ther. 202:*244.

Lipp, J.A., 1974, Effect of small doses of clonazepam upon soman-induced seizure activity and convulsions, *Arch. Int. Pharmacodyn. Ther. 210:*49.

Livett, B.G., 1973, Histochemical visualization of peripheral and central adrenergic neurons, *Br. Med. Bull. 29:*93.

Lloyd, K.G., 1975, Special chemistry of the basal ganglia. 2. Distribution of acetylcholine, choline acetyltransferase and acetylcholinesterase, *Pharmacol. Ther. (b) 1:*49.

Loewi, O., 1937, Strychninerregung und Acetylcholingehalt des Zentralnervensystems, *Naturwiss 25:*526.

Longo, V.G., 1958, Effects of scopolamine and atropine on electroencephalorganic and behavioral reactions due to hypothalamic stimulation, *J. Pharmacol. Exp. Ther. 116:*198.

Longo, V.G., 1962, *"Electroencephalograhic Atlas for Pharmacological Research,"* Elsevier, Amsterdam.

Longo, V.G., 1966, Mechanisms of the behavioral and electroencephalographic effects of atropine and related compounds, *Pharmacol. Rev. 18:*965.

Longo, V.G., and Loizzo, A., 1973, Effects of drugs on hippocampal O-rhythm. Possible relationships to learning and memory processes, in *"Brain, Nerves and Synapses"* (F.E. Bloom, and G.H. Acheson, eds.), pp. 46-54, Karger, Basel.

Longo, V.G., and Silvestrini, G., 1957, Action of eserine and amphetamine on the electrical activity of rabbit brain, *J. Pharmacol. Exp. Ther. 120:*160.

Longo, V.G., Von Berger, G.P., and Bouvet, D., 1954, Action of nicotine and of the "ganglioplegiques centraux" on the electrical activity of the brain, *J. Pharmacol. Exp. Ther. 111:*349.

Longo, V.G., Giunta, F., *et al.,* 1967, Effect of nicotine on the electroencephalogram of the rabbit, *Ann. NY Acad. Sci. 142:*159-169.

Longoni, R., Mulas, A., Oderfeld-Novak, B., Marconcini, I., and Pepeu, G., 1976, Effect of single and repeated electroshock applications on brain acetyltransferase activity in the rat, *Neuropharmacology 15:*283.

Losey, N.A., 1977, Effect of arecoline, phenamine and ethimizol on the distribution of electroencephalographic frequency characteristics, *Farmakol. Toksikol. 40:*389.

Luduena, F.P., and Hoppe, J.O., 1952, Local anesthetic activity, toxicity and irritancy of 2-alkoxy analogs of procaine and tetracaine, *J. Pharmacol. Exp. Ther. 104:*40.

Lundholm, B., and Sparf, B., 1975, The effect of atropine on the turnover of acetylcholine in the mouse brain, *Eur. J. Pharmacol. 32(02):*287.

Lynch, H.D., and Anderson, M.H., 1976, Atropine coma therapy in psychiatry: clinical observations over a 20 year period and a review of the literature, *Dis. Nerv. Syst. 30:*648.

Machne, K., and Unna, K.R.W., 1963, Actions at the central nervous system, in *"Handbuch der Experimentellen Pharmakologie, Erganzungswk, Vol. 15"* (G.B. Koelle, ed.), pp. 679-700, Springer-Verlag, Berlin.

MacIntosh, F.C., and Collier, B., 1976, Neurochemistry of cholinergic terminals, in *"Handbuck der Experimentellen Pharmakologie, Erganzungswk, Neuromuscular Junction, Vol. 42"* (E. Jaimis, ed.), pp. 99-228, Springer-Verlag, Berlin.

MacLean, P.D., Flanigan, S., Flynn, J.P., Kim, C., and Stevens, J.R., 1955, Hippocampal function: tentative correlations of conditioning, EEG, drug and radioautographic studies, *Yale J. Biol. Med. 23:*389.

Macphail, E.M., 1969, Cholinergic stimulation of dove diencephalon: A comparative study, *Physiol. Behav. 4:*655.

Magherini, P.C., Pompeiano, O., and Thoden, U., 1971, The neurochemical basis of REM sleep: A cholinergic mechanism responsible for rhythmic activation of the vestibulo-occulomotor system, *Brain Res. 35:*565.

Magherini, P.C., Pompeiano, O., Thoden, U., 1972, Cholinergic mechanisms related to REM sleep. I. Rhythmic activity of the vestibulo-oculomotor system induced by an anticholinesterase in the decerebrate cat, *Arch. Int. Biol. 110:*234.

Maiti, A., and Domino, E.F., 1961, Effects of methylated xanthines on the neuronally isolated cerebral cortex, *Exp. Neurol. 3:*18.

Marczynski, T.J., 1967, Topical application of drugs to subcortical brain structures and related aspects of electrical stimulation, *Ergebn. d. Physiol. Biol. Chem. Exp. Pharmakol. 59:*86.

Marczynski, T.J., 1969, Invited discussion: postreinforcement synchronization and the cholinergic system, in *"Symposium on Central Cholinergic Transmission and Its Behavioral Aspects"* (A.G. Karczmar, ed.), *Fed. Proc. 28:*132.

Marczynski, T.J., 1971, Cholinergic mechanism determines the occurrence of reward contingent positive variation (RCPV) in cat, *Brain Res. 28:*71.

Marczynski, T.J., and Burns, L.L., 1976, Reward contingent positive variation (RCPV) and post-reinforcement EEG synchronization (PRS) in the cat: Physiological aspects, the effects of morphine and LSD-25, and a new interpretation of cholinergic mechanisms, *Gen. Pharmacol. 7:*211.

Marczynski, T.J., Rosen, A.J., and Hackett, J.T., 1968, Postreinforcement electrocortical synchronization and facilitation of cortical auditory potentials in appetitive instrumental conditioning, *Electroencephalogr. Clin. Neurophysiol. 24:*227.

Marley, E., and Seller, T.J., 1972, Effects of muscarine given into the brain of fowls, *Br. J. Pharmacol. 44:*413.

Maulsby, R.L., 1971, An illustration of emotionally evoked theta rhythm in infancy: Hedonic hypersynchrony, *Electroencephalogr. Clin. Neurophysiol. 31:*157.

Maynert, E.W., Marczynski, T.J., and Browning, R.A., 1975, The role of the neurotransmitters in the epilepsies, *Adv. Neurol. 13:*79.

McKenna, T., McCarley, R.W., Amatruda, T., Black, D., and Hobson, J.A., 1974, Effects of carbachol at pontine sites yielding long duration desynchronized sleep episodes, in *"Sleep Research"* (M.H. Chase, W.C. Stern, and P.L. Walter, eds.), BIS/BRI, Los Angeles.

Mergner, T., Magherini, P.C., and Pompeiano, O., 1976, Temporal distribution of rapid eye movements and related monophasic potentials in the brain stem following injection of an anticholinesterase, *Arch. Int. Biol. 114:*75.

Miller, R.F., Stavraky, G.W., and Woonton, G.A., 1940, Effects of eserine, acetylcholine and atropine on the electrocorticogram, *J. Neurophysiol. 3:*131.

Minvielle, J., Cadilhac, J., and Passouant, M., 1954, Action of atropine on epileptics, *Electroencephalogr. Clin. Neurophysiol. 6:*162.

Mirotvorskaia, G.N., 1968, Neurochemistry of epilepsy, *Nevropatol. Psikhiatr. 68:*609.

Monnier, M., Kalberer, M., and Krupp, P., 1960, Functional antagonism between diffuse reticular and intralaminary recruiting projections in the medial thalamus, *Exp. Neurol.* 2:271.

Montplaisir, J.Y., 1975, Cholinergic mechanisms involved in cortical activation during arousal, *Electroencephalogr. Clin. Neurophysiol. 38:*263.

Montplaisir, J.Y., and Sazie, E., 1973, Effects of eserine and scopolamine on neuronal after-discharges of the auditory cortex, *Electroencephalogr. Clin. Neurophysiol. 35:* 311.

Morrell, F., 1967, Electrical signs of sensory coding, in *"The Neurosciences"* (J.C. Quarton, T. Melnechuk, and F.O. Schmitt, eds.), pp. 452-468, Rockfeller Press, New York.

Moruzzi, G., 1939, Contribution a l'electrophysiologie du cortex moteur: Facilitation, apres discharge et epilepsie corticales, *Arch. Internatl. Physiol. 49:*33.

Moruzzi, G., and Magoun, H.W., 1949, Brain stem reticular formation and activation of the EEG, *Electroencephalogr. Clin. Neurophysiol. 1:*455.

Myers, R.D., 1974, *"Handbook of Drug and Chemical Stimulation of the Brain,"* Reinhold, New York.

Naruse, H., Kato, M., Kurokawa, M., Haba, R., and Yabe, T., 1960, Metabolic defects in a convulsive strain of mouse, *J. Neurochem. 5:*359.

Nauta, W.J.H., 1958, Hippocampal projections and related neural pathways to the midbrain in the cat, *Brain 81:*319.

Nicoll, R.A., 1975, The action of acetylcholine antagonists on amino acid responses in the frog spinal cord, *Br. J. Pharmacol. 55:*449.

Nishi, S., 1970, Cholinergic and adrenergic receptors at sympathetic preganglionic nerve terminals, *Fed. Proc. 29:*1457.

Nishi, S., 1974, Ganglionic transmission, in *"The Peripheral Nervous System"* (J.I. Hubbard, ed.), pp. 225-255, Plenum Press, New York.

Nishi, S., Minota, S., and Karczmar, A.G., 1974, Primary afferent neurones: the ionic mechanism of GABA-mediated depolarization, *Neuropharmacology 13:*215.

Nistri, A., 1975, The effect of electrical stimulation and drugs on the release of acetylcholine from the frog spinal cord, *Naunyn Schmiedebergs Arch. Pharmacol. 293:* 269.

Obrador, S., 1947, Hiperexcitabilidad de neurones motoras producida por aislamiento de areas de la corteza cerebral, *Rev. Clin. Esp. 25:*171.

Osumi, Y., Fujiwara, H., Oishi, R., and Takaori, S., 1975, Central cholinergic activation by chlorfenvinphos, and organophosphate in the rat, *Jpn. J. Pharmacol. 25:*47.

Palkovits, M., and Jacobowitz, D.M., 1974, Topographic atlas of catecholamine and acetylcholinesterase-containing neurons in the rat brain. II. Hindbrain (mesencephalon, rhombencephalon), *J. Comp. Neurol. 157:*29.

Palkovits, M., Richardson, J.S., and Jacobowitz, D.M., 1974, A histochemical study of ventral tegmental acetylcholinesterases-containing pathway following destructive lesions, *Brain Res. 81:*183.

Pedata, F., Mulas, A., Pepeu, I.M., and Pepeu, G., 1976, Changes in regional brain acetylcholine levels during drug-induced convulsions, *Eur. J. Pharmacol. 40:*329.

Penaloza-Rojas, J.H., and Zeidenweber, J., 1965, Local and EEG effects of adrenaline and acetylcholine application within the olfactory bulb, *Electroencephalogr. Clin. Neurophysiol. 19:*88.

Pepeu, G., 1974, The release of acetylcholine from the brain: An approach to the study of the central cholinergic mechanisms, in *"Progress in Neurobiology"* (G.A. Kerkut, and J.W. Phillis, eds.), pp. 257-288, Pergamon Press, Oxford.

Pepeu, G., Nistri, A., and Mantovani, P., 1978, Influence of different putative neurotransmitters on ACh release from the brain and spinal cord, in *"Interrelationships Between Various Neurotransmitter Systems"* (A.G. Karczmar, and J. Glowinski, eds.), Pergamon Press, (in press).

Petsche, H., 1962, Practical problems of localization by the EEG, *Electroencephalogr. Clin. Neurophysiol. 14:*791.

Phan, D.V., Bite, A., and Gyorgy, L., 1974, Oxotremorine on behavior and EEG of reserpine – pretreated rats, *Acta Physiol. Acad. Sci. Hung. 45:*131.

Pierre, R., and Cahn, J., 1957, Considerations sur l 'utilite en electrophysiologe et en pharmacologie de l'evaluation quantitative de l'EEG. Quelques examples, in *"International Symposium on Psychotropic Drugs"* (S. Garattini, and V. Ghetti, eds.), pp. 299-300, Elsevier, Amsterdam.

Phillis, J.W., and York, D.H., 1968, Pharmacological studies on a cholinergic inhibition in the cerebral cortex, *Brain Res. 10:*297.

Pompeiano, O., 1967, The neurophysiological mechanisms of the postural and motor events during desynchronized sleep, *Res. Publ. Assoc. Res. Nerv. Ment. Dis. 45:*351.

Pope, A., Morris, A.A., Jasper, H., Elliot, K.A.C., and Penfield, W., 1947, Histochemical and action potentials studies on epileptogenic areas of cerebral cortex in man and the monkey, *Res. Publ. Assoc. Res. Nerv. Ment. Dis. 26:*218.

Pryor, G.T., 1968, Postnatal development of cholinesterase, acetylcholinesterase, aromatic l-amino acid decarboxylase and monoamine oxidase in C57B116 and DBA2 mice, *Life Sci. 7:*867.

Pujol, J.F., in press, Reciprocal interactions between serotonergic neurons and noradrenergic neurons originating from the locus coeruleus in the CNS, in *"Interdependence of Neurotransmitter Systems in the CNS"* (J. Glowinski, and A.G. Karczmar, eds.), Pergamon Press, Oxford.

Pujol, J.F., Keane, P.E., and Jouvet, M., 1978, Importance of interactions between transmitter systems in relation to regulation of the sleep-waking cycle, in *"Interrelationships Between Various Neurotransmitter Systems"* (A.G. Karczmar, and J. Glowinski, eds.), Pergamon Press, (in press).

Purpura, D.P., 1974, Intracellular studies of thalamic synaptic mechanisms in evoked synchronization and desynchronization of electrocortical activity, in *"Basic Sleep Mechanisms"* (O. Petre-Quadens, and J.D. Schlag, eds.), pp. 99-125, Academic Press, New York.

Purpura, D.P., Frygyesi, T.L., McMurty, J.G., and Scarf, T., 1966, Synaptic mechanisms in thalamic regulation of cerebello-cortical projection activity, in *"Thalamus"* (D.P. Purpura, and M.D. Yahr, eds.), pp. 153-170, Columbia University Press, New York.

Radil-Weiss, T., 1974, Power spectral density of hippocampal theta activity during rhombencephalic sleep, after physostigmine administration and during orienting reaction, *Act. Nerv. Super. (Praha) 16:*126.

Randic, M., Sminoff, R., and Straughan, D.W., 1964, Acetylcholine depression of cortical neurones, *Exp. Neurol. 9:*236.

Rech, R.H., and Domino, E.F., 1960, Effects of various drugs on activity of the neuronally isolated cerebral cortex, *Exp. Neurol. 2:*364.

Reeves, C., 1966, Cholinergic synaptic transmission and its relationship to behavior, *Psychol. Bull. 65:*321.

Richardson, I.W., and Szerb, J.C., 1974, The release of labelled acetylcholine and choline from cerebral cortical slices stimulated electrically, *Br. J. Pharmacol. 52:*499.

Richter, D., and Crossland, J., 1949, Variation in acetylcholine content of the brain with physiological state, *Am. J. Physiol. 159*:247.

Rieger, H., Okonek, S., 1975a, Proceedings: The EEG in alkylphosphate poisoning (anticholinesterase insecticides), *Electroencephalogr. Clin. Neurophysiol. 39*:555.

Rieger, H., and Okonek, S., 1975b, EEG in intoxication by cholinesterase inhibitors (organo-phosphate insecticides), *Rev. Electroencephalogr. Neurophysiol. Clin. 5*: 98.

Rinaldi, R., and Himwich, H., 1955, Cholinergic mechanisms involved in function of mesodiencephalic activating system, *Arch. Neurol. Psychiatry 73*:394.

Rojas-Ramirez, J.A., and Drucker-Colin, R.R., 1973, Sleep induced by spinal cord cholinergic stimulation, *Int. J. Neurosci. 5*:215.

Roshchina, L.F., 1976, Electroencephalographic analysis of the central action of pyrazidol, *Farmakol. Toksikol. 39*:397.

Roth, R.H., and Bunney, B.S., 1976, Interaction of cholinergic neurons with other chemically defined neuronal systems in the CNS, in *"Biology of Cholinergic Function"* (A.M. Goldberg, and I. Hanin, eds.), pp. 379-394, Raven Press, New York.

Ruch-Monachon, M.A., Jalfre, M., and Haefely, W., 1976a, Drugs and PGO waves in the lateral geniculate body of the curarized cat. I. PGO waves activity induced by RO4-1284 and by b-chlorophenylalanine (PCPA) as a basis for neuropharmacological studies, *Arch. Int. Pharmacodyn. Ther. 219*:205.

Ruch-Monachon, M.A., Jalfre, M., and Haefely, W., 1976b, Drugs and PGO waves in the lateral geniculate body of the curarized cat. II. PGO wave activity and brain 5-hydroxytryptamine, *Arch. Int. Pharmacodyn. Ther. 219*:269.

Ruch-Monachon, M.A., Jalfre, M., and Haefely, W., 1976c, Drugs and PGO waves in the lateral geniculate of the curarized cat. III PGO wave activity and brain catecholamines, *Arch. Int. Pharmacodyn. Ther. 219*:287.

Ruch-Monachon, M.A., Jalfre, M., and Haefely, W., 1976d, Drugs and PGO waves in the lateral geniculate body of the curarized cat. IV The effects of acetylcholine, GABA and benzodiazepines on PGO wave activity, *Arch. Int. Pharmacodyn. Ther. 219*:308.

Ruch-Monachon, M.A., Jalfre, M., and Haefely, W., 1976e, Drugs and PGO waves in the lateral geniculate body of the curarized cat. V Miscellaneous compounds. Synopsis of the role of central neurotransmitters of PGO wave activity, *Arch. Int. Pharmacodyn. Ther. 219*:326.

Rump, S., Rabsztyn, T., and Kopec, J., 1974, Effects of cholinesterase inhibition on the visual evoked potentials in the rabbit and their modification with various drugs, *Act. Nerv. Super. (Praha) 16*:224.

Sasaki, K., Kawaguchi, S., Matsuda, Y., and Mizuno, N., 1972a, Electrophysiological studies on cerebello-cerebral projections in the cat, *Exp. Brain Res. 16*:75.

Sasaki, K., Matsuda, Y., Kawaguchi, S., and Mizuno, N., 1972b, On the cerebello-thalamo-cerebral pathway for the parietal cortex, *Exp. Brain Res. 16*:89.

Sasaki, K., Matsuda, Y., Oka, H., and Mizuno, N., 1975, Thalamo-cortical projections for recruiting responses and spindling-like responses in the parietal cortex, *Exp. Brain Res. 22*:87.

Sasaki, K., Shimono, T., Oka, H., Yamamoto, T., and Matsuda, Y., 1976, Effects of stimulation of the midbrain reticular formation upon thalamo-cortical neurones responsible for cortical recruiting responses, *Exp. Brain Res. 26*:261.

Schlesinger, K., Boggan, W., and Freedman, D., 1965, Genetics of audiogenic seizures. I. Relation to brain serotonin and norepinephrine in mice, *Life Sci. 4*:2345.

Schmidt, J., and Wolf, H., 1972, Influence of atropine and cholinesterase inhibitors on brain potentials caused by dental pulp stimulation, *Acta Biol. Med. Ger. 29*:723.

Schmitt, H., 1972, Actions centrales des substances parasympathomimetiques, in *"Le Systeme Cholinergique"* (G.G. Nahas, J.C. Salamagne, P. Viars, and G. Vourc'L, eds.), pp. 181-228, Librairie Arnette, Paris.

Sellinger, O.Z., Azcurra, J.M., Ohlsson, W.G., Kohl, H.H., and Zand, R., 1972, Neurochemical correlates of drug-induced seizures: selective inhibition of cerebral protein synthesis by methionine sulfoximine, *Fed. Proc. 31:*160.

Shute, C.C.D., 1975, Chemical transmitter systems in the brain, *Mod. Trends Neurol. 6:*183.

Shute, C.C.D., and Lewis, P.R., 1975, Cholinergic pathways 1. Histochemical localization, *Pharmacol. Ther. 1:*79.

Simke, J.P., and Saelens, J.K., 1977, Evidence for a cholinergic fiber tract connecting the thalamus with the head of the striatum of the rat, *Brain Res. 126(3):*487.

Sitaram, N., Wyatt, R.J., Dawson, S., and Gillin, J.C., 1976, REM sleep induction by physostigmine infusion during sleep, *Science 191:*1281.

Sjostrand, T., 1937, Potential changes in the cerebral cortex arising from cellular activity and the transmission of impulses in the white matter, *J. Physiol. (Lond.) 90:*41.

Slater, P., 1968, The effects of triethylcholine and hemicholinium-3 on the acetylcholine content of rat brain, *Int. J. Neuropharmacol. 7:*421.

Smialowski, A., 1977, Comparison of effects of the intrahippocampal 5-hydroxytryptamine and acetylcholine on EEG and behavior of rabbits, *Act. Nerv. Super. (Praha) 19(2):*156.

Sobotka, T.J., 1969, *"Studies on Acetylcholine Levels in Mouse Brain,"* Doctoral thesis, Loyola University, Chicago.

Stadnicki, S.W., and Schaeppi, U., 1972, Nicotine changes in EEG and behavior after intravenous infusion in awake unrestrained cats, *Arch. Int. Pharmacodyn. Ther. 197:*72.

Starzl, T.E., Taylor, C.W., and Magoun, H.W., 1951, Ascending conduction in the reticular activating system with special reference to the diencephalon, *J. Neurophysiol. 14:*461.

Steriade, M., and Hobson, J.A., 1976, A neuronal activity during the sleep-waking cycle, *Prog. Neurobiol. 6:*155.

Sterman, M.B., and Clemente, C.B., 1962, Forebrain inhibitory mechanisms. Sleep patterns induced by basal forebrain stimulation in the behaving cat, *Exp. Neurol. 6:*103.

Sterman, M.B., and Wyrwicka, W., 1967, EEG correlates of sleep: evidence for separate forebrain substrates, *Brain Res. 6:*143.

Stone, C.A., Meckelnberg, K.L., and Torchiana, M.A., 1958, Antagonism of nicotine-induced convulsions by ganglionic blocking agents, *Arch. Int. Pharmacodyn. Ther. 117:*419.

Stumpf, C., and Gogolak, G., 1967, Actions of nicotine upon the limbic system, *Ann. NY Acad. Sci. 142:*143.

Sutherland, E.W., and Robinson, G.A., 1966, The role of cyclic $3',5'$-AMP in responses to catecholamines and other hormones, *Pharmacol. Rev. 18:*145.

Svenneby, G., and Roberts, E., 1974, Elevated acetylcholine contents in mouse brain after treatment with bicuculline and picrotoxin, *J. Neurochem. 23:*275.

Szerb, J.C., 1975, The release of acetylcholine from cerebral cortical slices in the presence or absence of an anticholinesterase, in *"Cholinergic Mechanisms"* (P.G. Waser, ed.), pp. 213-216, Raven Press, New York.

Szerb, J.C., 1977, Characterization of presynaptic muscarinic receptors in central cholinergic neurons, in *"Cholinergic Mechanisms and Psychopharmacology"* (D.J. Jenden, ed.), pp. 49-60, Plenum Press, New York.

Takahashi, R., Nasu, T., Tamura, T., and Kariya, T., 1961, Relationship of ammonia and acetylcholine levels to brain excitability, *J. Neurochem. 7:*103.

Tan, U., 1977, Electrocorticographic changes induced by topically applied succinylcholine and biperiden, *Electroencephalogr. Clin. Neurophysiol. 42:*252.

Teitelbaum, H., Lee, J.F., and Johannessen, J.N., 1975, Behaviorally evoked hippocampal theta waves: a cholinergic response, *Science 188:*1114.

Tower, D.B., and McEachern, D., 1949, Acetylcholine and neuronal activity. II. Acetylcholine and cholinesterase activity in the cerebrospinal fluids of patients with epilepsy, *Can. J. Res. 27:*120.

Trabucchi, M., Cheney, D.L., Hanin, I., and Costa, E., 1975a, Application of principles of steady-state kinetics to the estimation of brain acetylcholine turnover rate: Effects of oxotremorine and physostigmine, *J. Pharmacol. Exp. Ther. 194:*57.

Trabucchi, M., Cheney, D.L., Racagni, C., and Costa, E., 1975b, *In vivo* inhibition of striatal acetylcholine turnover by L-DOPA, apomorphine and (+)-amphetamine, *Brain Res. 85:*130.

Tripod, J., 1957, Characterisation generale des effets pharmacodynamiques de substances psychotropiques, in *"Psychotropic Drugs"* (S. Garattini, and V. Ghetti, eds.), pp. 437-447, Elsevier, Amsterdam.

Ulus, I.H., Wurtman, R.J., Scally, M.C., and Hirsch, M.J., 1977, Effect of choline on cholinergic function, in *"Cholinergic Mechanisms and Psychopharmacology"* (D.J. Jenden, ed.), pp. 525-538, Plenum Press, New York.

Usdin, E., 1970, Reactions of cholinesterases with substrates, inhibitors and reactivators, in *"Anticholinesterase Agents"* (A.G. Karczmar, ed.), pp. 47-354, International Encyclopedia of Pharmacology & Therapeutics, Vol. 1, Section 13, Pergamon Press, Oxford.

Van Meter, W.G., 1969, *"Central Nervous System Responses to Anticholinesterase in Rabbits: Evidence for a Non-inhibitory Action and for an Adrenergic Link,"* Ph.D. Thesis, Loyola University, Chicago.

Van Meter, W.G., and Karczmar, A.G., 1971, An effect of physostigmine on the central nervous system of rabbits, related to brain levels of norepinephrine, *Neuropharmacology 10:*379.

Van Meter, W.G., Karczmar, A.G., and Fiscus, R.R., 1978, CNS effects of anticholinesterases in the presence of inhibited cholinesterases, *Arch. Int. Pharmacodyn. Ther. 23:*249.

Vanderwolf, G.H., 1975, Neocortical and hippocampal activation in relation to behavior: Effects of atropine, phenothiazines and amphetamine, *J. Comp. Physiol. Psychol. 88:*300.

Vas, C.J., Delgado, J.M.R., and Glasser, G., 1969, Effect of anticholinergic drugs on epileptic activity from amygdala and frontal cortex, *Neurology 19:*234.

Vazquez, A.J., and Krip, G., 1973, Evidence for an inhibitory role for acetylcholine, catecholamines, and serotonin on the cerebral cortex, in *"Chemical Modulation of Brain Function"* (H.C. Sabelli, ed.), Raven Press, New York.

Velluti, R., and Hernandez-Peon, R., 1963, Atropine blockade within a cholinergic hyponogenic circuit, *Exp. Neurol. 8:*20.

Vosu, H., and Wise, R.A., 1975, Cholinergic seizure kindling in the rat: Comparison of caudate, amygdala and hippocampus, *Behav. Biol. 13:*419.

Votava, Z., 1967, Pharmacology of the central cholinergic synapses, *Ann. Rev. Pharmacol.* 7:223.

Ward, A.A., Jasper, H.J., and Pope, A., 1969, Clinical and experimental challenges of the epilepsies, in *"Basic Mechanism of the Epilepsies"* (H. J. Jasper, A.A. Ward, and A. Pope, eds.), pp. 1-12, Little Brown, Boston.

Wescoe, W.C., Green, R.E., McNamara, B.P., and Krop, S., 1948, The influence of atropine and scopolamine on the central effects of DFP, *J. Pharmacol. Exp. Ther. 92:* 63.

Whishaw, I.Q., Robinson, T.E., and Schallert, T., 1976, Intraventricular anticholinergics do not block cholinergic hippocampal RSA or neocortical desynchronization in the rabbit or rat, *Pharmacol. Biochem. Behav. 5:*275.

Wikler, A., 1952, Pharmacologic dissociation of behavior and EEG sleep patterns in dogs: Morphine n-allyl normorphine and atropine, *Proc. Soc. Exp. Biol. Med. 79:*261.

Williams, D., and Russell, W.R., 1941, Action of eserine and prostigmine on epileptic cerebral discharges, *Lancet 1:*476.

Wills, J.H., 1970, Toxicity of anticholinesterases and treatment of poisoning, in *"Anticholinesterase Agents"* (A.G. Karczmar, ed.), pp. 355-469, Internatl. Encyclop. Pharmacol. Therap, Vol. 1, Section 13, Pergamon Press, Oxford.

Wolff, V.H., 1956, Die Behandlung Zerebraler Anfalle mit Scopolamine. Ein Betrag zur Klinik des "Synkopalin" Syndroms, *Dtsch. Med. Wochenschr. 81:*1358.

Woody, C.D., Carpenter, D.O., Grieu, E., Knispel, J.D., Crow, T.J., and Black-Cleworth, P., 1974, Prolonged increases in resistance of neurons in cat motor cortex following extracellular iontophoretic application of acetylcholine (ACh) and intracellular current injection, *Fed. Proc. 33:*399.

Wurtman, R.J., Larin, F., Mostafapour, S., and Fernstrom, J.D., 1974, Brain catechol synthesis: Control by brain tyrosine concentration, *Science 185:*183.

Wurtman, R.J., 1976, Control of neurotransmitter synthesis by precursor availability and food consumption, in *"Subcellular Mechanisms in Reproductive Neuroendocrinology"* (F. Naftolin, ed.), pp. 149-166, Elsevier, Amsterdam.

Yamaguchi, N., Marczynski, T.J., and Ling, G.M., 1963, The effects of electrical and chemical stimulation of the preoptic region and some nonspecific thalamic nuclei in unrestrained, waking animals, *Electroencephalogr. Clin. Neurophysiol. 15:*154.

Yamaguchi, N., Ling, G.M., and Marczynski, T.J., 1964, The effects of chemical stimulation of the preoptic region, nucleus centralis medialis or brain stem reticular formation with regard to sleep and wakefulness, *Recent Adv. Biol. Psychiatry 6:*9.

Yamamoto, K.I., and Domino, E.F., 1967, Cholinergic agonist-antagonist interactions on neocortical and limbic EEG activation, *Int. J. Neuropharmacol. 6:*357.

ACETYLCHOLINE: POSSIBLE INVOLVEMENT IN SLEEP AND ANALGESIA

N. Sitaram[1] and J. C. Gillin[1,2]

[1]Biological Psychiatry Branch, The National Institute of Mental Health, NIH, Bethesda, Maryland 20014

[2]Laboratory of Clinical Psychopharmacology, The National Institute of Mental Health, St. Elizabeths Hospital, Washington, D.C. 20032

INTRODUCTION

Sleep and analgesia are two of the most prominent physiological functions in which acetylcholine (ACh) may play a role. This chapter is intended as a review of past and present research implicating the cholinergic systems in these activities.

ACETYLCHOLINE AND SLEEP

The sleep-waking cycle of man and the mammals consists of nonREM sleep and REM (Rapid Eye Movement) sleep (also known as D-sleep or paradoxical sleep). Non-REM sleep in man is further divided into Stages I to IV, based on EEG patterns. Stages III and IV are known as Delta sleep and usually occur early in the night in young adults; these stages normally disappear in late middle age. Growth hormone concentrations in peripheral blood increase in temporal association with Delta sleep in young people but disappear in middle age (Carlson et al., 1972). In the normal adult, REM sleep occupies 20-25% of total sleep time and consists of three to six separate REM periods at intervals of approximately 90 min. Dreaming is closely, although not exclusively, associated with REM sleep. The duration of nonREM sleep between the onset of sleep and the first REM period is known as the REM latency and averages about 90 min in normal adult nocturnal sleep. The REM latency may be markedly shortened in primary depression (Kupfer and Foster, 1972; Kupfer, 1976; Gillin et al., in press, b), in some schizophrenic patients (Gulevich et al., 1967; Stern et al., 1969, Jus et al., 1973), in narcolepsy (Zarcone, 1973), during the recovery period after REM sleep deprivation (Dement, 1960), and in "phase shift" and nap experiments when subjects sleep during their normal late morning hours (Weitzman et al., 1970; Karacan et al., 1970). REM latency may also be extremely short in infants (Roffwarg et al., 1966) and unusually long during childhood and preadolescence (Feinberg, 1974) as compared with adults.

Despite considerable research over the past 70 years, the biochemical bases of the sleep-wakefulness cycle remain elusive (Jouvet, 1972; Wyatt, 1972; Hobson, *et al.*, 1976; Drucker-Colin and Spanis, 1976; Holman *et al.*, 1975; Mendelson *et al.*, 1977; Gillin *et al.*, in press, a). Various investigators have suggested that serotonin (Jouvet, 1972) or "sleep factors" (Pieron, 1913; Pappenheimer *et al.*, 1975; Nagasaki *et al.*, 1974; Monnier *et al.*, 1977) are responsible for initiating and maintaining sleep. Furthermore, wakefulness or EEG desynchronization may be maintained by neurons containing dopamine and norepinephrine. The evidence for and against these hypotheses is still controversial.

Various neurochemical mechanisms have also been proposed to modulate REM sleep. These include hypotheses that (1) serotonin, or a metabolite, "primes" and "triggers" REM sleep once nonREM sleep starts; (2) norepinephrine neurons in the caudal locus coeruleus mediate EMG suppression and in the medial locus coeruleus mediate both phasic and tonic ascending components of REM sleep; (3) a subpopulation of norepinephrine-containing neurons in locus coeruleus ("D-off" cells, so-called because they fire more slowly during REM or D sleep) inhibit REM sleep (Hobson *et al.*, 1976); (4) dopamine inhibits REM sleep (Post *et al.*, in press); and (5) ACh facilitates or maintains REM sleep (see reviews by Jouvet, 1975; Hobson *et al.*, 1976; Gillin *et al.*, in press, c). Again, there is controversy about certain of these hypotheses. Jones *et al.*, (1977), for example, have reported that lesions of the locus coeruleus did not alter the total amount of REM sleep or wakefulness.

In the following sections, we shall review some data indicating a role for ACh in wakefulness and in initiating REM sleep. As Jouvet (1975) has emphasized in his review of cholinergic mechanisms in sleep, our understanding has been hampered by the absence of precise mapping of cholinergic pathways in the brain. Not only are lesioning and stimulation techniques impossible, but the interconnections between cholinergic neurons and other neuronal systems are poorly understood.

Cholinergic Changes Correlated With the States of Consciousness

The concentration of ACh has been reported to increase during REM sleep in cortical cups in the cat (Jasper and Tessier, 1971), in the effluent of a push-pull cannula in cat striatum (Gadea-Ciria, *et al.*, 1973), and in the ventricles of the dog (Haranath and Venkatakrishna-Bhatt, 1973). These findings suggest that cholinergic neurons are active during physiological and psychological arousal, which occurs during both wakefulness and REM sleep. Although the ACh concentration was higher during REM than wakefulness in the striatum (Gadea-Ciria *et al.*, 1973), these data, as well as those of the other two studies, fail to establish whether cholinergic neurons play a specific role in the initiation or maintenance of REM sleep. An increased concentration of ACh could be a nonspecific consequence of increased cerebral blood flow, increased general neuronal activity, or increased brain temperature, all of which occur in arousal.

In an old study, prior to the discovery of nonREM and REM sleep, Richter and Crossland (1949) reported that the ACh concentration of rat whole brain increased in sleep. More recently, the concentration of piperidine, an alicyclic amine with nicotine-like actions on the brain, has been reported to increase during dormancy in mice (Stepita-Klavco *et al.*, 1974) and snails (Dolezalova, *et al.*, 1974). Aside from replicating these findings with EEG recordings of sleep and waking, it is important in future studies to correlate the concentrations of piperidine with wakefulness, nonREM sleep, and REM sleep.

Based on data from single cell recordings in head-restrained cats, Hobson and his colleagues (1976) have proposed that neurons within the fastigial tegmental gigantocellular field (FTG) may be the "executive" cells for REM sleep. They report that these cells fire specifically and selectively during REM sleep, especially in association with eye movements. These investigators believe these cells are both cholinoreceptive and cholinergic. Furthermore, they postulate that these cells interact reciprocally with cells in the locus coeruleus or, possibly, the raphe to produce the nonREM-REM cycle. The FTG neurons are seen as facilitory to REM sleep, to themselves, and to certain cells within the locus coeruleus (the "D-off" cells). The "D-off cells" are seen as inhibitory to REM sleep, to themselves, and to the cells within the FTG. As further evidence for this hypothesis, local administration of the cholinomimetic, carbachol, prolonged REM periods when placed in the FTG and, though less clear, may have inhibited REM sleep when placed in the locus coeruleus (Amatruda et al., 1975).

Current questions facing this model include: (1) the previously mentioned study by Jones et al., (1977), reporting little effect on sleep of bilateral lesions of locus coeruleus; (2) the lack of precise evidence confirming the assumption that the FTG is both cholinoreceptive and cholinergic; and (3) the report of Siegel and McGinty (1977), based on single cell recordings from freely mobile cats, that FTG firing is correlated with specific patterns of motor activation rather than for REM sleep. Further evidence will be required before we can resolve these controversies and judge the value of the elegant model proposed by Hobson and his colleagues (1976).

Previous Pharmacological Studies of ACh and Sleep

The intracerebral administration of cholinomimetic agents has been reported to produce REM-onset sleep, prolonged REM periods, or selected components of REM sleep, such as EEG activation, EMG suppression, or pontine-geniculate-occipital (PGO) spikes. In some of the first studies of this type, Hernandez-Peon and his colleagues reported that crystals of ACh induced sleep, leading rapidly to REM sleep, when placed in "limbic midbrain and forebrain" sites; in a few cases, narcoleptic and cataplectic-like phenomena were elicited from pyriform cortical sites (Hernandez-Peon, 1965; Hernandez-Peon et al., 1963; 1967; Mazzuchelli-O'Flaherty, et al., 1967).

George et al., (1964) reported two types of response to microinjections of either oxotremorine or carbachol into caudal and oral reticular nuclei of the pontomesencephalic reticular formation. The first response was indistinguishable physiologically from REM sleep (EEG activation, REM's, hippocampal theta, EMG suppression, miotic pupils) except that it was of greater duration; in the second response, the cats showed EEG activation and EMG suppression; in neither type of response could EMG suppression be blocked by auditory, tactile, or reticular stimulation.

Baxter (1969) reported that crystalline carbachol produced prolonged episodes of REM-like sleep about 9-14 min after placement in the mesencephalic central grey, possibly with diffusion into the ventricular system. As in the REM-like state observed by George et al., (1964), that produced by Baxter was characterized by complete lack of arousal to strong external stimulation; Baxter reported, for example, unresponsiveness to surgical incision. Following microinjections of carbachol into the pontine reticular formation near the central grey at the level of the inferior colliculus, possibly identical to the sites studied by George et al., (1964), Mitler and Dement (1974) reported only cataplectic-like effects (EEG activation, EMG suppression, nystagmoid movement together with PGO spikes) rather than authentic REM periods. As mentioned previously, Amatruda et al., (1975) reported that microinjections of carbachol into the FTG produced dose dependent prolonged but variable REM sleep-like effects (EEG activation, EMG suppression within or without REM's, PGO spikes, and hippocampal theta).

Systemic administration of cholinergic agonists or cholinesterase inhibitors have also been reported to induce REM sleep or to prolong REM sleep periods in cats. More-over, cholinergic antagonists have been reported to inhibit REM sleep. Studying the chronic mesencephalic or pontine cat, Jouvet (1962) observed increased duration of REM periods after physostigmine and complete absence of REM sleep after atropine. Likewise, Karczmar et al., (1970) induced REM sleep in the awake cat, rabbit, or rat with physostigmine only if it had been reserpinized or pretreated with the catecholamine synthesis blocker, alpha-methyl-paratyrosine (AMPT). These REM periods were also unusually long, and they could be prevented by pretreatment with atropine. In an effort to localize the brain stem sites responsible for PGO spikes and REM's of REM sleep, Matsuzaki (1969) studied the effect of various lesions on physostigmine-induced REM phenomena; he concluded that REM sleep depended upon the whole pons but that caudal portions played a dominant role in PGO spikes and REM's. Magherreni et al., (1971) found that physostigmine produced REM's, possible PGO spikes, and loss of decerebrate rigidity in cats which had been transected at precollicular or retrocollicular levels. Atropine prevented these effects when administered prior to physostigmine and reversed them afterwards. In a follow-up study, Sequin et al., (1973) reported that com-plete lesions of the vestibular complex prevented physostigmine-induced REM's and loss of decerebrate rigidity.

Both nicotinic and muscarinic cholinergic agents have been reported to affect REM sleep in animals. Domino et al., (1968) reported both increased wakefulness and "fast-wave sleep" (EEG desynchronization, hippocampal theta and EMG atonia) with physo-stigmine and pilocarpine (a muscarinic agonist). These effects were antagonized by systemic atropine but were unaffected by methylatropine (which fails to cross the blood brain barrier) or by the nicotinic blockers, trimethidium and mecamylamine. Domino and Yamamoto (1965) also observed that small doses of nicotine given intravenously to sleeping cats produced behavioral arousal followed by slow-wave sleep and within 15 to 30 min "fast-wave" sleep (EEG desynchronization). Since "fast-wave sleep" was defined by EEG criterion alone, it is unclear as to whether it was identical to conventional REM sleep. Jewett and Norton (1966) also reported that nicotine increased "activated" sleep at low doses (50, 100 μg/kg s.c.) in cats but decreased it at high doses (200 μg/kg s.c.). Again, the data of Jewett and Norton (1966) are difficult to interpret since "activated sleep" was defined by EEG desynchronization criterion alone and, moveover, the authors reported *increased* EMG time with all doses of nicotine. Eye movements were not moni-tored either by Domino et al., (1968) or by Jewett and Norton (1966). Another agent possessing nicotinic effects, piperidine, was also reported to induce REM sleep in cats (Drucker-Colin and Giacobini, 1975; Kase and Miyata, 1976). Nixon and Karnovsky (1977), however, reported a decrease of REM sleep after intraventricular injection of piperidine to rats.

Reduction of REM sleep has been reported following intraventricular administration of hemicholinium, which blocks synaptic uptake of choline and synthesis of ACh (Hazra, 1970; Domino et al., 1968).

Acute administration of scopolamine, a centrally active muscarinic receptor blocker, significantly prolonged REM latency and reduced total REM time (Sagales et al., 1969). Atropine, which is less active centrally, had inconsistent effects on sleep (Toyoda et al., 1966). When scopolamine was administered nightly for three nights, however, it produced less and less effects with each administration; a REM rebound occurred on withdrawal (Sagales et al., 1976). Whether this loss of response reflects tolerance or the competing effect of REM deprivation cannot be determined. In this regard, it is noteworthy that George et al., (1964) found that animals, demonstrating motor inhibitory effects to intracerebrally administered carbachol or oxotremorine, became refractory for several days to additional injections, suggesting possible tolerance. Mitler and Dement (1974), however, observed effects persisting for as long as 48 hr after a single brain stem injection of carbachol; they suggested that the seeming tolerance could reflect enduring effects of a single injection.

In summary, the bulk of the evidence supports the view that cholinergic mechanisms facilitate REM sleep, its components (cortical activation, EMG suppression, etc.), and wakefulness. While the evidence showing that anticholinergic agents inhibit REM sleep is strong, some of the evidence favoring cholinergic induction of REM sleep, however, has remained unconvincing. Not all of the studies used controls, making it impossible, therefore, to determine whether observed REM periods were induced experimentally or whether they occurred spontaneously. The REM-like states attributed to cholinomimetic agents were often abnormal in their duration, in their response to external stimulation (sound, light, pain), and in their physiological appearance. These states often could be elicited only in abnormal preparations, i.e., brain stem transected or reserpinized animals. For these reasons, we decided to further investigate the role of cholinergic systems in the sleep-wakefulness cycle.

Current Cholinergic Sleep Studies in Man

In our initial studies, we administered physostigmine intravenously to normal volunteers while they were asleep (Sitaram et al., 1976, 1977a; Gillin et al., in press, c). The studies were approved by the Human Research Review Committee and subjects gave informed consent. They were pretreated with methscopolamine (0.5 mg IM) before bedtime in order to reduce peripheral side effects of physostigmine. Physostigmine was administered through a ten-foot polyethylene tubing which was connected to an intra-catheter or scalp vein needle in the subject's forearm.

Figure 1 shows the results obtained with administration of physostigmine under three different conditions: bolus infusion of 0.5 mg 35 min after sleep onset, bolus infusion of 0.5 mg five min after sleep onset, and slow infusion (over one hr) of 1.0 mg beginning 35 min after sleep onset. In all three conditions, physostigmine hastened the onset of REM sleep as compared with nights when the subject received placebo infusions. When the bolus infusion at 35 min was compared with that at five min, however, the latency from the infusion until the first REM period was significantly shorter ($p < .05$) with the former (11±2 min) than with the latter (52±10). The one-hr slow infusion also shortened the duration of the second nonREM period, probably because physostigmine continued to be infused during the first portion. In none of the three experiments was the duration of the first REM period affected, not even during the slow infusion when the infusion continued beyond the end of the REM period. Moreover, in all three experiments, once the first REM period was advanced, the succeeding REM period moved forward as well. That is, the administration of physostigmine appeared to advance the ultradian clock governing the nonREM-REM cycle.

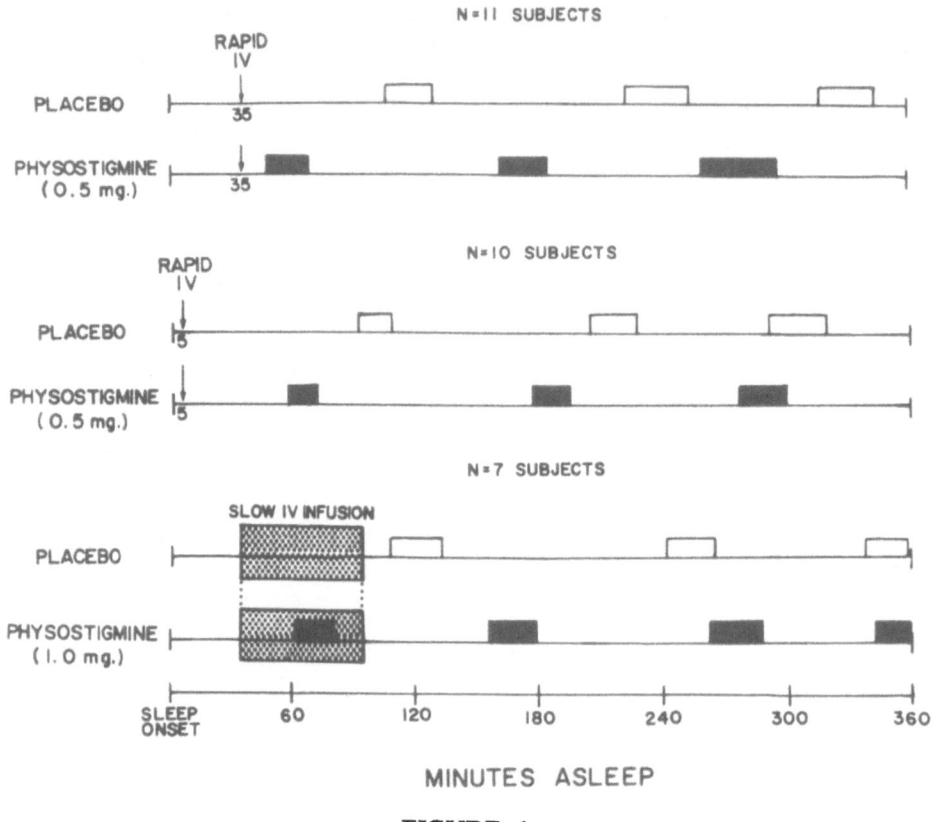

FIGURE 1

Physostigmine Resets REM Sleep (Ultradian) Rhythm in Man

Administration of physostigmine by either rapid bolus or slow intravenous (IV) infusion induces REM sleep and advances onset of subsequent REM periods without altering the duration of individual REM periods.

When physostigmine was administered by bolus infusion at REM onset or in the second nonREM period, the same dose which induced REM earlier in the night awoke the subjects (Sitaram *et al.*, 1977a). This observation reemphasizes the role that cholinergic mechanisms play in arousal. A low dose of physostigmine (0.25 mg), however, did induce REM when administered during the second nonREM sleep period (Sitaram *et al.*, 1977a).

More recently, we have acquired preliminary data on the effects of arecoline on sleep in normal volunteers. Arecoline is a direct muscarinic agonist in low doses. Intravenous administration of arecoline (1.5 mg) induces the onset of REM sleep (Sitaram *et al.*, 1978). The early results of these studies confirm and extend the findings with physostigmine. Not only has a second cholinomimetic agent been found to advance REM onset without altering REM duration, but the effect appears to occur with specific muscarinic stimulation. The role of the nicotinic effects of ACh in sleep awaits future investigation in man.

In the physostigmine-induced REM periods mentioned above, the EEG patterns, eye movements and EMG suppression appeared normal. These observations did not, however, answer the question, "Are the subjects dreaming in these experimentally induced REM periods?" To address this question, we conducted a study in which we awoke subjects from a physostigmine-induced REM period and questioned them about dreaming (Sitaram *et al.*, 1978). On both control and physostigmine nights, bolus infusions of physostigmine (0.5 mg) were administered 35 min after sleep onset and subjects were awakened 20 min later, i.e., about 7-8 min after the onset of REM sleep on physostigmine nights. Dreaming was reported on eight of the nine nights when physostigmine induced REM and on two of seven nights after awakening in nonREM sleep following a placebo infusion ($p < .01$ Fisher exact test). When physostigmine and placebo were administered 10 min after sleep onset and subjects were awakened 20 min later (in nonREM sleep in both conditions), there was no evidence that physostigmine-induced dreaming. Subjects were also awakened from spontaneously occurring REM periods; when asked to compare dreams from physostigmine-induced and spontaneous REM periods, subjects rated them as similar in terms of bizarreness, vividness, and the certainty they felt that they were dreaming. These results suggest that normal dreaming occurs during physostigmine-induced REM sleep but that physostigmine (at these doses, at least) does not induce dreaming in the absence of REM sleep.

The demonstration that physostigmine can produce both dreaming and REM sleep may be related to reports of excessive dreaming and nightmares among victims of anticholinesterase poisoning (Gershon and Shaw, 1961; Grob and Harvey, 1958). There is also a brief abstract reporting narcoleptic-like symptoms in a patient following organophosphorus poisoning (Taneda and Hara, 1975).

Discussion of Cholinergic Mechanisms in Sleep-Wakefulness

Evidence from human and animal studies, summarized above, strongly suggests a role for cholinergic mechanisms in wakefulness and in the induction of REM sleep. No convincing evidence currently exists that cholinergic mechanisms alone prolong the duration of individual REM periods in normal man. Although prolonged REM-like episodes have been produced in animals following intracerebral administration of cholinomimetic drugs, it is not clear that these are true REM periods. Physostigmine can, however, produce arousal or REM sleep in man, depending upon dose and time of administration.

Systemic administration of physostigmine or other cholinomimetic agents does not seem sufficient to induce sleep onset REM sleep in the intact and awake animal or man. These agents can cause sleep onset REM periods, however, in cats which have been reserpinized or transected in brain stem. Thus, a balance of forces governs REM onset. Such a model has been proposed by Hobson and his colleagues. It is consistent with our data that physostigmine induces REM sleep and L-DOPA (Gillin *et al.*, 1973) delays REM sleep when either is infused during nonREM sleep.

In this regard, it is well to remember that several other drugs have been reported to induce or increase REM sleep: 5-hydroxytryptophan (Wyatt, 1972), reserpine (Hartmann and Cravens, 1973), LSD (Torda, 1968), the alpha-adrenergic receptor blockers phenoxybenzamine (Hartmann and Zwilling, 1976) and thymoxamine (Oswald *et al.*, 1975), alpha-methylpara-tyrosine (Wyatt, 1972), and nicotinamide (Robinson *et al.*, 1977). The ultimate goal, therefore, is understanding the integration of diverse neuronal systems, cholinergic as well as others, in the regulation of behavior and the states of consciousness.

These observations suggest that a simple cholinergic hypothesis will not be able to account for the sleep onset REM periods which have been described in narcolepsy, depression, and other conditions. If excessive cholinergic activity does play a role in the sleep-onset REM period, other mechanisms, possibly catecholaminergic depletion, must also be operative. Nevertheless, the EEG sleep characteristics of primary depression — shortened REM latency, fragmented sleep, reduced total time asleep — are compatible with the hypothesis that cholinergic activity is increased in depression, possibly in combination with reduced activity in catecholamine systems (Janowsky *et al.*, 1972). Increased cholinergic activity might be able to induce all three of these EEG sleep abnormalities. It should be noted, however, that no evidence currently exists on whether tolerance develops to prolonged administration of cholinesterase inhibitors.

Understanding REM sleep will be child's play compared to understanding dreams. We now have the outline for the neurochemistry of dreaming, but not of dreams. We know something about what controls when a person dreams or if he dreams at all, but little about what he dreams. Even the phenomenology of dreams is so complex as to defy current understanding. How do we experience the visions, colors, sounds, smells and tastes of dreams? The sense of motion and flying? The mirth, fear, and passion? How is this sensation the expression of an integrated story with a plot which may go on for many min? Is the dream the improvisation of a jazz combo, made up as the musicians play along, or is it a set piece, written before the performance, but embellished as it is played according to the mood and circumstances of the musicians? The recurrent dream could be an example of the latter, the dream about the radio program heard at the sleeper's bedside could be an example of the former. How are we to square a physiological theory of dreaming with the apparent reality that dream-like mentation can be found not only in REM sleep but, occasionally, in nonREM sleep, at sleep onset, and even in daydreams? Is REM sleep physiology necessary for dream psychology?

ACETYLCHOLINE AND ANALGESIA

Among the putative neurotransmitters in the brain, the role of ACh in the mediation of nociceptive (pain) mechanisms is of special interest for several reasons: (1) The neuroanatomical pathways outlined by Casey (1973) for pain perception (i.e., the brainstem reticular formation, medial and intralaminar thalamic nuclei, hypothalamus, septal nucleus, and medial forebrain area) bears a close resemblance to the ascending cholinergic reticular system of Shute and Lewis (1967). (2) Although controversial, there is some evidence that cholinergic agents raise pain thresholds (i.e., produce analgesia) in several species of animals and in man. (3) Another line of evidence points to a possible interaction between opiates and ACh at both neurochemical and behavioral levels. Cholinergic and anticholinergic agents influence the analgesic potency of morphine and other opiates. Conversely, opiate antagonists block or attenuate ACh-induced analgesia. In the following sections we review the literature to evaluate some of the evidence and controversies surrounding the role of ACh in pain mechanisms. The reader is also referred to Karczmar (1975, 1976) for previous excellent reviews of this area.

Analgesic Activity of Cholinergic and Anticholinergic Drugs

The early observation of Pellandra (1933) that the anticholinesterase, physostigmine, may increase the threshold for pain caused by radiant heat to the forehead of human subjects led to the speculation that ACh may modulate pain mechanisms. A host of investigations has been carried out in several species using a vast array of cholinergic and anticholinergic drugs. In Table 1 we have attempted to organize the studies according to the species studied and the drug administered. We have included only reports where the authors present quantitative data on some clearly defined pain measure. The presence of significant analgesic activity is indicated by + and the absence of analgesia or a decrease of pain threshold (hyperalgesia) indicated by the − sign. Since most studies do not differentiate between absence of analgesia and hyperalgesia produced by drugs, our review is limited to a discussion of only whether analgesia was present or not. The notations P, A and N refer to whether the drug potentiated, antagonized or had no effect on opiate analgesia. In this section we will consider only the analgesic activity of the cholinergic and anticholinergic drugs; their interaction with opiates is discussed in another section of this chapter.

The following methodological issues must be borne in mind while interpreting the results from Table 1.

(1) In most animal studies, the procedures used to measure pain threshold (e.g. tail flick test) are somewhat reflexive in nature. Since cholinomimetics produce cataplexy in mice (Zetler, 1968) and also depress spinal reflexes (Tang and Yim, 1963), one must rule out the effects of the drug on motor tonicity before concluding that analgesia is produced.

(2) In higher doses cholinomimetics produce behavioral depression and decrease in motor activity. Inasmuch as pain threshold measurement in animals depends upon a motor response (e.g. flicking the tail, writhing, vocalization, etc.) data obtained after using high doses must be interpreted cautiously. For example, Pert (1975) reported analgesic activity for physostigmine in monkeys but this occurred at the dose of 0.1 mg/kg which also produced profound debilitation. A lower but physiological dose (0.05 mg/kg)

TABLE 1

THE EFFECT OF CHOLINERGIC AND ANTICHOLINERGIC DRUGS ON ANALGESIA

Author and Year of Publication	Species Used	Experimental Procedure	Cholinomimetics							Anticholinesterase Agents			Anticholinergics			
			Carbachol	Oxotremorine	Arecoline	Tremorine	RS 86	Pilocarpine	Acetylcholine	Physostigmine	Neostigmine	DFP	Atropine	Benztropine	Scopolamine	Methyl Benactyzine
Pellandra (1933)	Man	Radiant heat								+	P		-A		–	
Slaughter and Munsell (1940)	Man	*								+	+P				-A	
Floodmark (1945)	Man	Radiant heat to forehead									+P		–			
Christensen (1948)	Man	Radiant heat to forehead									–					
Andrews (1942)	Man	Radiant heat to forehead									P		-A			
Abaza (1952)	Man	Tibial														
Dundee (1961)	Man	Pressure														
Migdal (1963)	Man	Post-operative pain ratings (See text)								+				+	+	
Sitaram (1977b)	Man				-N					-N					+P[7]	
Houser and Houser (1973)	Primate	Electric shock						–			–	-N				
Pert (1975); Pert and Maxey (1975)	Primate	Electric shock						–			P[1]					
Slaughter et al., (1940)	Cat	Tail squeeze						-P			-P					
Saxena (1958)	Rats	Tail clip						+							–	
Houser and Vanhart (1973)	Rats	Electric shock (grid)														
Dahlstrom (1975)	Rats	Electric shock to tail											-N			
Chen (1958)	Mice	Tail clip				+										
Lenke (1958)	Mice	Tail clip				+										
Herz (1962)	Mice	Tail clip														
Loew (1964)	Mice	Tail clip			+		+									
Harris (1969)	Mice	Tail flick		+P												
Leslie (1969)	Mice	Electric shock		+[3]						+P						

TABLE 1 (CONTINUED)

THE EFFECT OF CHOLINERGIC AND ANTICHOLINERGIC DRUGS ON ANALGESIA

Author and Year of Publication	Species Used	Experimental Procedure	Carbachol	Oxotremorine	Arecoline	Tremorine	RS 86	Pilocarpine	Acetylcholine	Physostigmine	Neostigmine	DFP	Atropine	Benztropine	Scopolamine	Methyl Benactyzine
Ireson (1970)	Mice	Electric shock +phenylbenzoquinone writhing test		+P						+P					—	
VanEich (1971)	Mice	Hot plate								+	—					
Pleuvy (1971)	Mice	Hot plate		+						+P	P					
Cox (1972)	Mice	Hot plate		+		+					P					
Bhargave (1972)	Mice	Tail flick										P				
Kamat (1972)	Mice	Hot plate				—		—								
		Electric shock	—													
Pedigo (1975)	Mice	Tail flick							+P[4]	P						
		Tail flick+ phenylquinone writhing														
Mudgill (1974)	Mice	Tail flick														
Dewey (1975)	Mice	Writhing test														
Takemori (1975)	Mice	Tail flick							-[5]	-[5]			-A			
Denisenko (1965)	Rabbit	Thermal stimulus		+[2]	+[2]		+[2]			P			P			
Metys (1969)	Mice, rat rabbit	Hot plate tail flick, electric shock	+[2]	+[2]	+[2]					P	—		P			
DeJong (1954)	Guinea pigs	Thermal stimulus		+[8]					-[5] +[6]							
Nistri (1974)	Frog	Thermal stimulus											P			P

TABLE 1 (CONTINUED)

NOTES:

+ Indicates presence of significant antinociceptive activity
P Indicates potentiation of opiate analgesia
− Indicates absence of analgesia or hyperalgesia
A = Antagonism of opiate analgesia
N = No effect on opiate analgesia

*Patients suffering from different painful diseases were used. Analgesic action of 8 mg morphine + 0.5 mg neostigmine was subjectively estimated to be equal to 15 mg morphine. RS 86 = Spiro-(N′ -methyl piperidyl 4′) N ethyl succinimid, a synthetic cholinomimetic (Sandoz)

1   0.165 mg/kg IV had analgesic effect but animal was sick and may not have responded to tail squeeze. 0.085 mg/kg IV had no effect.

2   Oxotremorine, arecoline and RS 86 were injected subcutaneously. Carbachol, arecoline and oxotremorine were injected intraventrically and intracerebrally into septum, mesencephalic reticular formation and hypothalamus which produced analgesia but injections into caudate nucleus or hippocampus did not.

3   Oxotremorine given subcutaneously to mice was reported to be 3,000 times more potent than morphine.

4   The analgesic effect of intraventricular acetylcholine was potentiated by intraventricular neostigmine, blocked by intraperitoneal atropine but not atropine methylnitrate. Not blocked by intraperitoneal mecamylamine.

5   Intraventricular route of administration.

6   Writhing was produced by intraperitoneal p-phenylquinone and acetylcholine. Analgesia induced by intraventricular injection of only the S(+) isomer of Beta methyl substituted acetylcholine (β-CH$_3$ ACh). The S(−) isomer of β-CH$_3$ ACh and alpha methyl ACh was ineffective.

7   In a follow-up study Pert and Maxey (1975) found that tolerance to morphine analgesia attenuated response to scopolamine but tolerance to scopolamine had no effect in morphine analgesia.

8   It is of interest that in the frog a subcutaneous dose of oxotremorine but not morphine induced marked analgesic effect though both drugs increased brain acetylcholine.

had no analgesic effect. In Table 1 we have included only studies where effects from physiological doses are reported.

(3) Although animal studies have generally controlled for placebo and order effects, none of the human studies (except for Sitaram et al., 1977b) used statistical comparisons with double blind placebo administration. Furthermore, the procedure used by Pellandra (1933), Slaughter and Munsell (1940a), Floodmark and Wramner (1945) and Christensen and Gross (1948) to measure pain threshold is by the method of ascending limits; i.e., radiant heat was applied to subject's forehead for as long as it was required for him to subjectively register pain. This method may confound pain threshold with the subject's biases. He need merely stop the ascent early to avoid any uncomfortable sensations. Anticipatory responses may also occur. It was, therefore, ambiguous whether changes produced by the cholinergic agents resulted primarily from changes in motivation, anticipatory anxiety, or attention.

The 35 studies reviewed in Table 1 contain observations of ten different cholinergic (i.e. cholinomimetic and anticholinesterases) and four anticholinergic agents on the pain threshold of several species of animals. As is readily apparent, there is little consensus among investigators about the analgesic activity of the drugs. If one considered all the ten cholinergic drugs together, there are 41 observations of which 25 show positive analgesic effect and 16 show absence of any analgesia. With anticholinergics, except for three observations, the results of the rest of the nine studies are in the predicted direction, i.e., absence of any analgesic effect. This suggests that the pharmacological evidence for the role of ACh in modulating pain mechanisms is far from convincing. In spite of this, after a closer look at Table 1, the following broad trends emerge which deserve further discussion.

Species Differences

It is possible that various species differ in their responses to cholinergic and anticholinergic drugs. The two primate studies (Pert 1975; Houser and Houser, 1973) indicate that arecoline, pilocarpine, physostigmine and neostigmine have no analgesic effect but scopolamine does. With rats, however, Houser and Vanhart (1973) reported analgesic activity with pilocarpine but not scopolamine. Within rodents (rats and mice), out of a total of 30 observations of different cholinergic agents, 21 (i.e., about two-thirds) of the studies show positive analgesic effect. The nine negative results, however, include two studies using neostigmine (Saxena, 1958; Pleuvy and Tobias, 1971; on rats and mice, respectively) and another negative study by Kamat et al., (1972) using intraperitoneal administration of carbachol in mice. Neither neostigmine nor carbachol cross the blood brain barrier when administered parenterally and their lack of effect may merely indicate that peripheral cholinergic mechanisms do not play a role in nociception. Excluding the above three studies, we end up with 27 trials of centrally active cholinergic agents in rodents of which 21 trials resulted in significant analgesia. The negative findings using parenteral administration of pilocarpine (Saxena, 1958; Kamat et al., 1972), tremorine (Kamat et al., 1972) and intraventricular ACh and physostigmine (Mudgill et al., 1974) must, however, be taken seriously and cast some doubt on the role of ACh in pain mechanisms on rodents. With respect to anticholinergic drug effects on rodents, all four studies using atropine and scopolamine showed an absence of analgesia or hyperalgesia (Houser and Vanhart, 1973; Dahlstrom et al., 1975; VanEich and Bock, 1971; and

Takemori *et al.*, 1975). Studies by Metys *et al.*, (1969) on rabbits indicate that intra-ventricular cholinomimetics increase pain threshold as in rodents. An intriguing finding by Nistri *et al.*, (1974) suggests that frogs show analgesic response to oxotremorine but not morphine, although both drugs increase brain ACh.

In humans, three out of three studies with physostigmine and two out of three studies with neostigmine indicate significant analgesia. As discussed earlier, human studies using subjective evaluation of radiant-heat pain, tibial pressure and postoperative pain ratings are confounded by methodological problems. The paucity of controlled, double-blind studies in humans is especially surprising considering the wide clinical use of morphine and scopolamine to induce the amnesic-analgesic state called "twilight-sleep" in obstetric practice.

Having these considerations in mind, we recently studied the effect of physostig-mine in normal human volunteers (Sitaram *et al.*, 1977b). Fourteen normal volunteers (ten men and four women) participated in a double-blind placebo-controlled experiment consisting of one adaptation ("throw away") and two experimental sessions. They were pretreated with an intramuscular injection of 0.5 mg methscopolamine prior to both experimental sessions to protect them from peripheral cholinergic effects of physostig-mine. Forty-five minutes following methscopolamine they received an intramuscular dose of either physostigmine (0.5 mg) or placebo. Electrical stimulation (1 msec biphasic pulse) was provided by a concentric electrode (Tursky and Watson, 1964) connected to a digitally controlled constant current stimulator and placed on the dorsal surface of the left forearm. Shocks were administered at 2.5 second intervals with random order of intensity (ranging from 1 to 31 milliamps) and subjects were asked to rate each shock on a four point scale: 1=barely noticeable; 2=distinct but not uncomfortable; 3=unpleasant; 4=painful. The response to electrical stimuli was analyzed using signal detec-tion techniques (Clark, 1974) whereby two pain measures were obtained: (1) a response criterion for the distinct/unpleasant dichotomy (i.e., ratings 2 or below and 3 or above) by finding the stimulus intensity for which the least overlap between ratings 2 and 3 occurred. (2) Error rate, which is the percent of total responses that were in error (ratings of 3 or 4 for stimuli actually below criterion milliamperage and ratings of 2 or 1 for stimuli above criterion). Figure 2 illustrates the method of computing the criterion and error rate for a typical subject. Average evoked responses (AER) from EEG electrodes placed on the vertex and right ear were also recorded after stimulation at four intensity levels.

Our results indicated that the criterion for categories distinct/unpleasant was significantly higher for physostigmine (17.8 mA) than placebo (16.2 mA; paired t-test $p < .05$ two-tailed). The error rate was 10.2% and 8% respectively, which did not differ significantly, indicating good reliability of the criterion measure. The AER amplitude for the P100 component was also reduced significantly after physostigmine (1.81 micro-volts) compared to placebo (2.39 microvolts; $F=5.69$ $p < .05$). This effect was most pronounced for higher intensity stimuli. The AER effect on P100 is consistent with earlier reports by Buchsbaum (1975) associating individual differences in pain tolerance between normal subjects with P100 amplitude/intensity slopes. Another study on audio-analgesia by Lavine *et al.*, (1976) also reports that subjects who were relatively more pain tolerant show greater reduction of P100 component. As in the Buchsbaum (1975) and Lavine *et al.*, (1976) studies, pain tolerance induced by physostigmine was associated

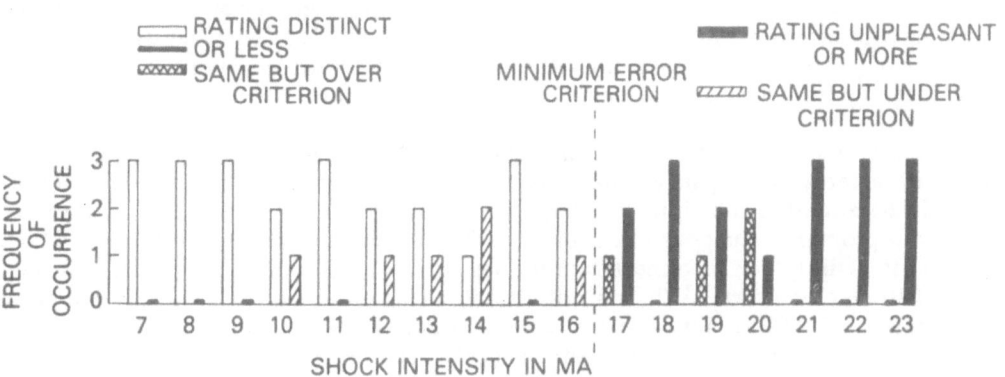

FIGURE 2

Pain Rating Procedure

Data from a typical subject (for a portion of the total shock range) is illustrated to show means of calculating minimum error criterion. In this case 16.5 mA is the empirical "criterion" dividing the "distinct" and "unpleasant" categories with the least overlap or "errors." The number of errors is indicated by striped or crosshatched bars. After administration of physostigmine 0.5 mg IV to 14 normal volunteers (see text and Sitaram *et al.*, 1977b) minimum error criterion was increased from 16.7 mA (on placebo) to 17.8 mA (physostigmine) demonstrating a significant analgesic effect.

with low AER amplitude, especially at the higher stimulus intensities. These data indicate that central cholinergic mechanisms may play a role in the modulation of pain and arousal systems in humans.

Thus in summary it appears that pharmacological enhancement of brain ACh is associated with analgesia in the rodent, rabbit and man. In nonhuman primates the opposite holds true; blockade of central cholinergic action induces analgesia and cholinomimetics have no effect. Adequate data on other species are not available. Whether this represents a genuine species-specific difference in the neurohumoral coding of pain or an experimental artifact is not clear.

Comparative Role of Cholinergic "Muscarinic" and "Nicotinic"
Receptors in Pain Mechanisms

The suggestion that the hypothesized cholinergic modulation of pain may result from selective stimulation of cholinergic "muscarinic" as opposed to "nicotinic" receptors comes from investigators such as Metys *et al.*, (1969) and Leslie (1969) who reported extremely potent analgesic activity for oxotremorine, a well-known central muscarinic agent. Leslie (1969) calculated the equimolar potency of subcutaneous oxotremorine in mice to be 3000 times that of morphine and the effect of oxotremorine was antagonized by antimuscarinic agents such as atropine and scopolamine but not by an antinicotinic agent such as mecamylamine. Pert (1975) also reported that both the nicotinic agonist (nicotine) and nicotinic antagonists (mecamylamine and hexamethonium) had no effect on pain thresholds in monkeys. Another study which deals with this issue is that of Pedigo *et al.*, (1975) who report that the analgesic effect of intraventricular ACh was antagonized by intraperitoneal atropine but not mecamylamine.

By far the most elegant and convincing data regarding the relative role of muscarinic and nicotinic receptors in pain mechanisms comes from Dewey *et al.*, (1975). They report that only *beta* methyl substituted ACh (β-CH$_3$ ACh), which has specific affinity for muscarinic receptors, has analgesic effect in mice. The *alpha* methyl substituted ACh which has specific affinity for nicotine receptors has no analgesic effect. Moreover, it is only the S(+) isomer of β-CH$_3$ ACh and not the S(-) isomer which resembles the preferred conformation of ACh as reported by Canepa *et al.*, (1966) and this strikingly parallels the reported presence and absence of analgesic activity of the S(+) and S(-) isomer respectively.

Acetylcholine and Opiates: Neurochemical and Analgesic Interactions

The relationship between ACh and morphine has been a subject of a great deal of investigation and speculation since the early report by Bernheim and Bernheim (1936) that morphine inhibited the rate of hydrolysis of ACh by brain precipitates. Slaughter *et al.*, (1940a; 1940b) and others (see Table 1) reported that, indeed, several cholinergic drugs, such as ACh, oxotremorine, pilocarpine, physostigmine and neostigmine, potentiated morphine analgesia. Anticholinergics in turn antagonized the effect of morphine. Conversely, morphine was found to modify ACh content, release and turnover (see below). Several investigators have also attempted to determine the relationship (if any) between the opiate-induced changes in brain ACh and its analgesic actions. Although the exact interrelationships and mechanisms of action are poorly understood, several interesting leads have emerged suggesting an ACh-opiate synergism on the mediation of pain. In the following review we will examine data for and against such a synergism at both neurochemical and behavioral levels. The recent discovery of the opiate receptor (Pert and Snyder, 1973) and morphine-like endogenous peptides, enkephalin (Hughes *et al.*, 1975) and endorphins (Li *et al.*, 1976), have significantly advanced our knowledge of pain mechanisms. Any hypothesized role for a neurotransmitter such as ACh in modulating pain must necessarily take into account interactions that it may have with opiates and opiate-like endogenous peptides.

Although we will concentrate on the relationship of opiates to ACh, it must be borne in mind that the literature contains many reports of the modification of morphine analgesia by drugs affecting serotonergic and catecholaminergic activity (Takemori *et al.*, 1975; Price and Fibiger, 1975; Dahlstrom *et al.*, 1975). We will, however, examine only data pertaining to ACh. The data are presented in Table 2 and, in order to avoid unnecessary repetition, the following text will serve only to selectively highlight and expand on some salient points.

The Effect of Opiates on Acetylcholine Neurochemistry

The original speculations by Bernheim and Bernheim (1936) and Slaughter *et al.*, (1940a; 1940b) that the analgesic action of morphine was due to its anticholinesterase activity were effectively refuted by Young et al., (1956) who were unable to find any correlation between anticholinesterase activity and analgesic potency of a large series of opiate compounds. A similar fate befell the notion that morphine and other opiates produced analgesia by increasing brain ACh content (see Table 2).

Reports that morphine and related agonists prevented the release of ACh from guinea pig ileum and from cerebral cortex has generated a great deal of interest. Furthermore, Crossland (1970) found that after acute morphine administration there was a decrease of ACh release, an increase of "total ACh pool," but a decrease of its "free ACh" component. During development of tolerance after chronic morphine treatment, the "free ACh" fraction increased to return to normal levels but could not be released due to morphine-induced blockade of ACh release. Upon withdrawal, or induction of abstinence syndrome by an antagonist like naloxone, there is an "explosive" release of the "free ACh" fraction. Alternately, Pinski et al., (1973) have hypothesized development of supersensitive ACh receptors (secondary to ACh-release blockade during chronic morphine treatment) to explain the intense parasympathetic activation seen during withdrawal. An interesting study by Jhamandas and Sutak (1976) suggests that the site of ACh-release inhibiting action of morphine may be at the level of the medial thalamus and reticular formation. Raphe-lesioning blocked both the analgesic and the ACh-release inhibiting action of morphine, indicating a link between serotonin, ACh and opiates (Garau et al., 1975).

Although the above evidence strongly supports an inhibitory role for opiates in cortical release of ACh, the question still remains: does this have anything to do with opiate analgesia? It is interesting that although work on the effect of narcotics on ACh has been in progress since 1957, very few investigators have attempted to meaningfully correlate the neurochemical and analgesic effects of morphine. Lewis (1949) did report that the peak of analgesia was associated with the peak of morphine-induced depression and ACh-release inhibition in the rat. Domino and coworkers (Domino, 1975; Labrecque and Domino, 1974; Matthews et al., 1973; Domino and Wilson, 1973), however, reject a "simplistic morphine ACh antirelease hypothesis." Their data indicate that morphine analgesia considerably outlasts its antagonism of ACh release (about 90 min in the rat) and the hemicholinium induced ACh depletion (peak effect in 30 min).

Another recently developed technique involves estimation of ACh turnover by measuring the turnover rate of tracer amounts of labelled phosphorylcholine in animals sacrificed by microwave irradiation. Zsilla et al., (1976) found that ACh turnover was decreased in specific brain areas by analgesic narcotics, whereas a nonanalgesic stereoisomer of viminol R_2 failed to affect ACh turnover. Similarly, Moroni et al., (1977) recently reported that only β-endorphin (corresponding to fragment 61-91 of β-Lipotropin (β-LPH) produces analgesia and reduced ACh turnover in rat cortex, hippocampus, nucleus accumbens and globus pallidus; a-endorphin (61-76 fragment of β-Lipotropin) which has no analgesic activity has no effect on ACh turnover either. These reports are important in that they show that opiates and endorphin influence ACh turnover. Any further speculation by the authors on the relationship between ACh turnover effects and analgesia is preliminary at best.

TABLE 2

ACETYLCHOLINE AND OPIATE ANALGESIA

The Effect of Opiates on:	Species Studied and Methods	Findings and Conclusions
ACh Content Herken et al., (1957) Giarman and Pepeu (1962) Maynert (1967) Howes et al., (1969)	Rats, mice. ACh levels by bioassay or gas chromatography (G.C.).	Morphine and other agonists increase ACh levels but no correlation between ACh increase and analgesic potency could be demonstrated (Howes et al., 1969). Furthermore, narcotic antagonists such as nalaxone, with no analgesic activity, also increased brain ACh content.
ACh Release (peripheral nervous system) Schaumann (1957) Paton (1957) Kosterlitz (1968) Waterfield and Kosterlitz (1975)	Guinea pig ileum. ACh release evoked by low intensity electrical stimulation.	Morphine and related agonists prevented evoked release of ACh. Naloxone increased evoked ACh release.
ACh Release (central nervous system) Beani et al., (1968) Mitchell (1963) Beleslin and Polak (1965) Jhamandas et al., (1971)	Rabbit Cat Cat Cat	Morphine decreased ACh output from cerebral cortex.

TABLE 2 (CONTINUED)

The Effect of Opiates on:	Species Studied and Methods	Findings and Conclusions
ACh Release (con't.) (central nervous system)		
Yaksh and Yamamura (1975) Labrecque and Domino (1974) Mathews *et al.*, (1973)	Mid pontine pretrigeminal transected cat. Mid pontine pretrigeminal transected cat. Pretrigeminal rat.	Morphine prevented ACh release from caudate nucleus. Antagonized by naloxone. Morphine and nalorphine (i.p.) decreased cortical ACh release. Above effects reversed by naloxone. Time course of morphine analgesia outlasted and is dissociable from the ACh antirelease effect (90 min).
Jhamandas and Sutak (1976)	Rat, intact and medial thalamus lesioned. Electrical stimulation of medial thalamus and reticular formation.	Morphine (2.5 mg IV) inhibited cortical ACh release. Subsequent IV injection but not topical application of naloxone reversed morphine effect. Naloxone by itself had no effect on ACh output. Medial thalamus lesion abolished above morphine and naloxone effects. Low dose of naloxone (0.1 mg/kg) and naltrexone facilitated ACh release evoked by electrical stimulation of thalamus and reticular formation. The above effect of naloxone was greater in morphine dependent than in naive rats.
Garau *et al.*, (1975)	Rat, raphe lesioned.	Raphe lesions prevented both morphine analgesia and ACh antirelease effects. These 5HT and ACh systems may interact in producing opiate analgesia.

TABLE 2 (CONTINUED)

Species Studied and Methods	Findings and Conclusions
The Effect of Opiates on:	
ACh Content and Release During Chronic Morphine Administration	
Crossland and Slater (1968) Crossland (1970) Mice, chronic morphine treatment to produce tolerance and addiction.	Crossland and associates found an increase of total "ACh pool" and decrease in ACh release after acute morphine administration; however, the "free" fraction of pool was reduced. After chronic administration, the total "bound" and "free" ACh levels returned to normal (premorphine) values. Crossland hypothesizes that morphine tolerance is due to the return to normal levels of "free" ACh after initial reduction and during withdrawal this "free" ACh is liberated explosively.
Hemicholinium (HC-3) Induced ACh Depletion	
Domino and Wilson (1973) Rat intraventricular injection of HC-3 and i.p. injection of narcotic agonists and antagonists given simultaneously. Brain ACh levels measured 30 min later by frog rectus bioassay and G.C. methods.	Narcotic agonists antagonize HC-3 induced ACh depletion. Above antagonism closely paralleled their analgesic potency in the following order: Heroin > Levarphanol > Methadone > Phenazocine > morphine > codeine > meperidine. Naloxone and nalorphine but not cyclazocine and pentazocine antagonized morphine induced anti-ACh depletion after HC-3.

TABLE 2 (CONTINUED)

	Species Studied and Methods	Findings and Conclusions
The Effect of Opiates on:		
ACh Turnover		
Zsilla et al., (1976)	Rats infused with phosphoryl [CH_3 ^{14}C] choline for 6 min killed by microwave irradiation.	Analgesic doses (ED_{50} of morphine, meperidine, viminol R_2 and azidomorphine decreased ACh turnover in cortex and hippocampus but not in striatum. Antagonized by naltrexone. Viminol S_2 a nonanalgesic stereoisomer of viminol R_2 failed to affect ACh turnover.
Moroni et al., (1977)	Rat injected intraventricularly with α- and β-endorphin. Tail flick test used to measure analgesia.	Analgesic doses of β-endorphin decreased ACh turnover in cortex, hippocampus, nucleus accumbens and globus pallidus but not in nucleus caudatus. Antagonized by naltrexone. In contrast α-endorphin failed to cause analgesia or to influence ACh turnover.
The Effect of Opiate Antagonists on:		
ACh Analgesia		
Pedigo et al., (1975)	Mice. Tail flick test and phenylquinone writhing test.	Analgesia produced by intraventricular ACh (ED_{50}=7.3 μg) was blocked by five narcotic antagonists, naltrexone, naloxone, cyclazo-

TABLE 2 (CONTINUED)

The Effect of Opiate Antagonists on:

Species Studied and Methods	Findings and Conclusions
ACh Analgesia (con't.)	cine, *nalorphine* and *pentazocine* in the same rank order of potency in which they antagonized morphine analgesia. Stereospecificity was shown with cyclazocine and pentazocine whose L-isomers blocked morphine but not ACh analgesia, and the D-isomers blocked ACh but not morphine analgesia.
Harris (1969) — Mice. Tail flick test.	Physostigmine and oxotremorine-induced analgesia were partially blocked by naloxone. Large doses of naloxone (10 mg/kg) were, however, required for complete blockage. Repeated (X5) injections of oxotremorine produced tolerance to same extent as seen with morphine. No cross tolerance between oxotremorine and morphine was seen, however.

The Effect of Cholinergic and Anticholinergic Drugs on:

Species Studied and Methods	Findings and Conclusions
Opiate Analgesia	
See Table 1	See Table 1

TABLE 2 (CONTINUED)

The Effect of Cholinergic and Anticholinergic Drugs on:

	Species Studied and Methods	Findings and Conclusions
Morphine Withdrawal Syndrome		
Pinski et al., (1973)	Rat injected i.p. twice daily with morphine in increasing doses of 20 mg/kg to 600 mg/kg over 21 days.	Withdrawal syndrome reduced by i.p. *choline chloride* 100 mg/kg during withdrawal period. Mecamylamine or mecamylamine-atropine mixture did not influence withdrawal. Authors suggest development of ACh supersensitivity during morphine habituation.
Morphine Abstinence Syndrome Induced by Opiate Antagonists		
Grumbach (1969)	Rat	Pretreatment with atropine increased and physostigmine decreased abstinence syndrome (hyperirritability) induced by *lavallorphan.*
Jhamandas and Dickinson (1973)	Rat, morphine i.p. injections for 24 days or more from 20 mg/kg to 300 mg/kg. Naloxone given 4 hr after last dose.	Pretreatment with anticholinergics (atropine and mecamylamine) and physostigmine intensified abstinence syndrome induced by *naloxone.*
Collier et al., (1972)	Rat, dependence induced by a single s.c. dose of 150 mg/kg in a sustained release suspension	Pretreatment with atropine, para-chlorphenylalanine or indomethacin suppressed various components of

TABLE 2 (CONTINUED)

The Effect of Cholinergic and Anticholinergic Drugs on:	Species Studied and Methods	Findings and Conclusions
Morphine Abstinence Syndrome Induced by Opiate Antagonists (con't.)	and 24 hr later abstinence precipitated by naloxone.	abstinence syndrome. Authors suggest multipartite basis for morphine dependence with ACh, 5HT and prostaglandin playing a role.
Way *et al.*, (1975)	Withdrawal induced by naloxone on morphine-dependent mice.	DFP and physostigmine prevent naloxone induced withdrawal reaction. Atropine, hemicholinium and other ACh antagonists exacerbate reaction. Way *et al.*, (1975) hypothesized a dopamine-dependent mechanism as they observed that dopamine levels increased after naloxone and this was antagonized by physostigmine.

The Effect of Opiate Antagonists on ACh Induced Analgesia

As indicated on Table 2, Dewey et al., (1975) showed that ACh analgesia was blocked by narcotic antagonists in the same order of potency in which they antagonized morphine analgesia. Another interesting finding was the stereospecificity effect as shown by the fact that *Dextro* isomer of cyclazocine and pentazocine blocked morphine but not ACh analgesia, while the *Levo* isomers modified ACh but not morphine analgesia.

The Effect of Cholinergic and Anticholinergic Agents on Opiate Analgesia and Morphine Withdrawal and Abstinence Syndromes

These studies are summarized in Table 1 (effect on opiate analgesia) and Table 2. As indicated in Table 1, the majority of studies report that cholinergic agents potentiated (P) and anticholinergic drugs antagonized (A) morphine analgesia. With respect to the role of these drugs in modifying morphine withdrawal or abstinence syndromes, it is apparent from even a cursory glance at the data summarized in Table 2, that there is little or no consensus between various investigators. No firm conclusions can be drawn regarding the role of ACh in the morphine withdrawal syndrome.

In summary, what is the weight of the evidence supporting a role for ACh in pain mechanisms? Our review of the literature suggests that at least in rodents, and probably in humans too, cholinergic drugs have analgesic effects and potentiate opiate analgesia. There also appear to be several well-documented actions of opiates on ACh metabolism in the brain. Whether these actions are related to opiate analgesia or not has not been sufficiently investigated.

DISCUSSION

The evidence, presented in this chapter, suggest various ways in which cholinergic mechanisms are involved in the regulation of sleep-wakefulness and analgesia. Not only may cholinergic mechanisms produce wakefulness, but they appear to regulate the timing of REM periods. Cholinergic agonists, such as physostigmine and arecoline, induce REM sleep and shorten the interval between REM periods, whereas cholinergic antagonists, such as scopolamine, delay the onset of REM sleep. Cholinomimetic drugs may have analgesic effects by themselves, may potentiate opiate analgesia, and cholinergic mechanisms may be metabolically altered by opiates.

At first blush, it may seem strange to discuss such divergent topics as sleep and analgesia within the same chapter. But be that as it may, this book is testimony to many functions in which ACh plays an important role, and in this chapter we could well have discussed other functions as well, such as memory or neuroendocrinology. While in our everyday world we tend to focus narrowly on one or two roles played by a specific neurotransmitter, we should not forget that each transmitter may play many parts. Furthermore, a transmitter may alter diverse functions by controlling underlying factors, such as the level of cortical activation. Whether or not this is the case in terms of sleep and analgesia is unknown at this time. For that matter, little is known about analgesia during natural states of sleep and whether or not subjective pain thresholds differ during wakefulness, nonREM, and REM sleep.

REFERENCES

Abaza, A., and Gregoire, M., 1952, Potentiation of analgesic effect of opiates by combination with prostigmine, *Presse. Med. 60:*331.

Amatruda, T.T., Black, D.A., McKenna, T.M., McCarley, R.W., and Hobson, J.A., 1975, Sleep cycle control and cholinergic mechanisms: differential effects of carbachol at pontine brain stem sites, *Brain Res. 98:*501.

Andrews, H.L., 1942, The effect of morphine and prostigmine methylsulfate on measurement of pain threshold, *JAMA 120:*525.

Baxter, B.L., 1969, Induction of both emotional behavior and a novel form of REM sleep by chemical stimulation applied to cat mesencephalon, *Exp. Neurol. 23:*220.

Beani, L., Bianchi, C., Santinoceto, L., and Marchetti, P., 1968, The cerebral acetylcholine release in conscious rabbits with semi-permanently implanted epidural cups, *Int. J. Neuropharmacol. 7:*469.

Beleslin, D., and Polak, R.L., 1965, Depression by morphine and chloralose of acetylcholine release from the cat's brain, *J. Physiol. (Lond.) 117:*411.

Bernheim, F., and Bernheim, M.L.C., 1936, Action of drugs on choline esterase of the brain, *J. Pharmacol. Exp. Ther. 57:*427.

Bhargave, U.N., and Way, E.L., 1972, Anticholinesterase inhibition and morphine effects in morphine tolerant and dependent mice, *J. Pharmacol. Exp. Ther. 183:*31.

Buchsbaum, M.S., 1975, Average evoked response augmenting/reducing in schizophrenia and affective disorders, in *"Biology of the Major Psychoses"* (D.X. Freedman, ed.), pp. 129-141, Raven Press, New York.

Canepa, F.G., Pauling, P., and Sorum, H., 1966, Structure of acetylcholine and other substrates of cholinergic systems, *Nature 210:*907.

Carlson, H.E., Gillin, J.C., Gorden, P., and Snyder, F., 1972, Absence of sleep related growth hormone peaks in aged normal subjects and in acromegaly, *J. Clin. Endocrinol. Metab. 34:*1102.

Casey, K.L., 1973, Pain: a current view of neural mechanisms, *Am. Sci. 61:*194.

Chen, G., 1958, The antitremorine effect of some drugs as determined by Haffner's method of testing analgesia in mice, *J. Pharmacol. Exp. Ther. 124:*73.

Christensen, E.M., and Gross, E.G., 1948, Analgesic effects in human subjects of morphine, meperidine and methadone, *JAMA 137:*594.

Clark, W.C., 1974, Pain sensitivity and the report of pain, *Anesthesiology 10:*272.

Collier, H.O.J., Francis, D.L., and Schneider, C., 1972, Modification of morphine withdrawal by drug interacting with humoral mechanisms: some contradictions and their interpretation, *Nature 237:*220.

Cox, B., and Tha, S., 1972, The antinociceptive activities of oxotremorine, physostigmine and dyflos, *J. Pharm. Pharmacol. 24:*547.

Crossland, J., 1970, Neurohumoral substances and drug abstinence syndromes, Abst. VII Conger. C.I.N.P., Prague p. 94.

Crossland, J., and Slater, P., 1968, The effect of some drugs on the "free" and "bound" acetylcholine of rat brain, *Br. J. Pharmacol. Chemother. 33:*42.

Dahlstrom, B., Paalzow, G., and Paalzow, L., 1975, A pharmacokinetic approach to morphine analgesia and its relation to regional turnover of rat brain catecholamines, *Life Sci. 17:*11.

DeJong, D.K., 1954, Remarks on the mechanism of analgesic action of morphine, *Acta Physiol. Pharmacol. Neer. 3:*164.

Dement, W., 1960, The effect of dream deprivation, *Science 131:*1705.

Denisenko, P.P., 1965, Pharmacological blocking of central cholinoreactive systems and the possibilities of its therapeutic applications, in *"Pharmacology of Cholinergic and Adrenergic Transmission"* (G.B. Koelle, W.W. Douglas, A. Carlson, and V. Trcka, eds.) pp. 147-152, Macmillan, New York.

Dewey, W.L., Cocolas, G., Daves, E., and Harris, L.S., 1975, Stereospecificity of intraventricularly administered acetylmethylcholine antinociception, *Life Sci. 17:*9.

Dolezalova, H., Stepita-Klavco, M., and Farringather, R., 1974, The accumulation of piperidine in the control ganglia of dormant snails, *Brain Res. 72:*115.

Domino, E.F., 1975, Role of central cholinergic mechanisms in the specific actions of narcotic agonists, in *"Cholinergic Mechanisms"* (P.G. Waser, ed.), pp. 433-453, Raven Press, New York.

Domino, E.F., and Wilson, A.E., 1973, Effects of narcotic analgesic agonists and antagonists on rat brain acetylcholine, *J. Pharmacol. Exp. Ther. 184:*18.

Domino, E.F., and Yamamoto, K., 1965, Nicotine: effect on the sleep cycle of the cat, *Science 150:*637.

Domino, E.F., Yamamoto, K., and Dren, A.T., 1968, Role of cholinergic mechanisms in states of wakefulness and sleep, in *"Anticholinergic Drugs and Brain Function in Animals and Man, Prog. Brain Res. Vol. 28"* (P.B. Bradley, and M. Fink, eds.), pp. 113-133, Elsevier, Amsterdam.

Drucker-Colin, R.R., and Giacobini, E., 1975, Sleep inducing effect of piperidine, *Brain Res. 88:*186.

Drucker-Colin, R.R., and Spanis, C.W., 1976, Is there a sleep transmitter?, *Prog. Neurobiol. 6:*1.

Dundee, J.W., Nicholl, R.M., and Moore, J., 1961, Alteration in response to somatic pain associated with anaesthesia: VIII, the effect of atropine and hyoscine, *Br. J. Anaesth. 33:*565.

Feinberg, I., 1974, Changes in sleep cycle patterns with age, *J. Psychiatry Res. 10:*283.

Floodmark, S., and Wramner, T., 1945, The analgetic action of morphine, eserine and prostigmine studied by a modified Hardy-Wolff-Goodell method, *Acta. Physiol. Scand. 9:*88.

Gadea-Ciria, M., Stadler, H., Lloyd, K., and Bartholini, G., 1973, Acetylcholine release within the cat striatum during the sleep-wakefulness cycle, *Nature 243:*518.

Garau, L., Mulas, M.L., and Pepeu, G., 1975, The influence of raphe-lesions on the effect of morphine on nociceptive and cortical ACh output, *Neuropharmacology 14:*259.

George, R., Haslett, W.L., and Jenden, D.J., 1964, A cholinergic mechanism in the brain stem reticular formation: induction of paradoxical sleep, *Int. J. Neuropharmacol. 3:*541.

Gershon, S., and Shaw, F., 1961, Psychiatric sequelae of chronic exposure to organophosphate insecticides, *Lancet I:*1371.

Giarman, N.F., and Pepeu, G., 1962, Drug induced changes in brain acetylcholine, *Br. J. Pharmac. Chemother. 19:*226.

Gillin, J.C., Post, R.M., Wyatt, R.J., Goodwin, F.K., Snyder, F., and Bunney, W.E., Jr., 1973, REM inhibitory effect of L-DOPA infusion during human sleep, *Electroencephalogr. Clin. Neurophysiol. 35:*181.

Gillin, J.C., Mendelson, W.B., Sitaram, N., and Wyatt, R.J., in press (a), The neuropharmacology of sleep and wakefulness, *Ann. Rev. Pharmacol. Toxicol.*

Gillin, J.C., Duncan, W.C., Pettigrew, K.D., Frankel, B.L., and Snyder, F., in press (b), Successful separation of depressed, normal, and insomniac subjects by EEG sleep data, *Arch. Gen. Psychiatry.*

Gillin, J.C., Sitaram, N., Mendelson, W.B., and Wyatt, R.J., in press (c), Physostigmine alters onset but not duration of REM sleep in man, *Psychopharmacology.*

Grob, P., and Harvey, J.C., 1958, Effects in man of the anticholinesterase compound sarin (isopropyl-methylphosphoro-fluoridate), *J. Clin. Invest. 37:*350.

Grumbach, L., 1969, The effect of cholinergic and cholinergic blocking drugs on the abstinence syndrome in the rat, *Fed. Proc. 28:*262.

Gulevich, G., Dement, W.C., and Zarcone, V., 1967, All night sleep recordings of chronic schizophrenics in remission, *Compr. Psychiatry 8:*141.

Haranath, P.S.R.K., and Venkatakrishna-Bhatt, H., 1973, Release of acetylcholine from perfused cerebral ventricles in unanaesthetized dogs during waking and sleep, *Jpn. J. of Physiol. 23:*241.

Harris, L., 1969, Central neurohumoral systems involved in narcotic agonists and antagonists, *Fed. Proc. 29:*28.

Hartmann, E., and Cravens, J., 1973, The effects of long-term administration of psychotropic drugs on human sleep: II the effects of reserpine, *Psychopharmacologia 33:*169.

Hartmann, E., and Zwilling, G., 1976, The effect of alpha and beta adrenergic receptor blockers on sleep in the rat, *Pharmacol. Biochem. Behav. 5:*135.

Hazra, J., 1970, Effect of hemicholinium-3 on slow wave and paradoxical sleep of cat, *Eur. J. Pharmacol. 11:*395.

Herken, H., Maibauer, D., and Muller, S., 1957, Acetylcholingehalt des Gehirns und Analgesie nach Einwirkung von Morphin und einigen 3-Oxymorphinanen, *Arch. Exp. Path. Pharmak. 230:*313.

Hernandez-Peon, R., 1965, A cholinergic hypogenic limbic forebrain-hindbrain circuit, in *"Neurophysiologie des etats de sommeil"* (M. Jouvet, ed.), pp. 63-88, C.N.R.S., Lyon.

Hernandez-Peon, R., Chavez-Ibana, G., Morgane, P.J., and Timo-Iaria, C., 1963, Limbic cholinergic pathways involved in sleep and emotional behavior, *Exp. Neurol. 8:*93.

Hernandez-Peon, R., O'Flaherty, J.J., and Mazzuchelli-O'Flaherty, A.C., 1967, Sleep and other behavioral effects induced by acetylcholinic stimulation of basal temporal cortex and striate structures, *Brain Res. 4:*243.

Herz, A., 1962, Wirkungen des arecolins auf das zentralnervensysten, *Arch. Exp. Pathol. Pharmakol. 242:*414.

Hobson, J.A., McCarley, R.W., and McKenna, T.M., 1976, Cellular evidence bearing on the pontine brain stem hypothesis of desynchronized sleep control, *Prog. Neurobiol. 6:*155.

Holman, R.B., Elliott, G.R., and Barchas, J., 1975, Neuroregulators and sleep mechanisms, *Ann. Rev. Med. 26:*499.

Houser, V.P., and Houser, F.L., 1973, The alteration of aversive thresholds with cholinergic and adrenergic agents, *Pharmacol. Biochem. Behav. 1:*433.

Houser, V.P., and Vanhart, D.A., 1973, The effect of scopolamine and pilocarpine upon the aversive threshold of the rat, *Pharmacol. Biochem. Behav. 1:*427.

Howes, J.F., Harris, L.S., Dewey, W.L., and Voydd, C., 1969, Brain acetylcholine levels and inhibition of the tail-flick reflex in mice, *J. Pharmacol. Exp. Ther. 169:*23.

Hughes, J., Smith, T., Morgan, B., and Fothergill, L., 1975, Purification and properties of enkephalin — the possible endogenous ligand for the morphine receptor, *Life Sci. 16:*1753.

Ireson, J.D., 1970, A comparison of the antinociceptive actions of cholinomimetic and morphine like drugs, *Br. J. Pharmacol. 40:*92.

Janowsky, D.C., El-Yousef, M.K., Davis, J.M., and Sekerke, H.J., 1972, A cholinergic-adrenergic hypothesis of mania and depression, *Lancet 2(7778):*632.

Jasper, H.H., and Tessier, J., 1971, Acetylcholine liberation from cerebral cortex during paradoxical (REM) sleep, *Science 172:*601.

Jewett, R.E., and Norton, S., 1966, Effects of some stimulant and depressant drugs on sleep cycles of cat, *Exp. Neurol. 15:*463.

Jhamandas, K., and Dickinson, G., 1973, Modification of methadone abstinence in mice by acetylcholine antagonists, *Nature 245:*219.

Jhamandas, K., and Sutak, M., 1976, Morphine-naloxone interaction in the cerebral cholinergic system: the influence of subcortical lesioning and electrical stimulation, *Br. J. Pharmacol. 58:*101.

Jhamandas, K., Phillis, J.W., and Pinski, C., 1971, Effect of narcotic analgesics and antagonists on the *in vivo* release of acetylcholine from the cerebral cortex of the cat, *Br. J. Pharmacol. 43:*53.

Jones, B.E., Harper, S.T., and Halaris, A.E., 1977, Effects of locus coeruleus lesion upon cerebral monoamine content, sleep-wakefulness states, and the response to amphetamine in the cat, *Brain Res. 124:*473.

Jouvet, M., 1962, Recherches sur les structures nerveuses et les mechanismes responsables des differentes phases du sommeil physiologique, *Arch. Ital. Biol. 100:*125.

Jouvet, M., 1972, The role of monoamines and acetylcholine-containing neurons in the regulation of the sleep-waking cycle, *Ergeb. Physical. 64:*166.

Jouvet, M., 1975, Cholinergic mechanisms and sleep, in *"Cholinergic Mechanisms"* (P.G. Waser, ed.), pp. 455-476, Raven Press, New York.

Jus, K., Bouchard, M., Jus, A.K., Villeneuve, A., and Lachance, R., 1973, Sleep EEG studies in untreated long-term schizophrenic patients, *Arch. Gen. Psychiatry 29:*386.

Kamat, U., Pradhan, R., and Sheth, U., 1972, Potentiation of a non-narcotic analgesic, dipyrone, by cholinomimetic drugs, *Psychopharmacologia (Berl.) 23:*180.

Karacan, I., Williams, R.L., Finley, W.W., and Hursch, C.J., 1970, The effects of naps on nocturnal sleep: influence on the need for Stage 1 REM and Stage 4 sleep, *Biol. Psychiatry 2:*391.

Karczmar, A.G., 1975, Cholinergic influences on behavior, in *"Cholinergic Mechanisms"* (P.G. Waser, ed.), pp. 501-529, Raven Press, New York.

Karczmar, A.G., 1976, Central actions of acetylcholine, cholinomimetics and related drugs, in *"Biology of Cholinergic Function"* (A.M. Goldberg and I. Hanin, eds.), pp. 395-449, Raven Press, New York.

Karczmar, A.G., Longo, V.G., and Scott de Carolis, A., 1970, A pharmacological model of paradoxical sleep: the role of cholinergic and monoamine systems, *Physiol. Behav. 5:*175.

Kase, Y., and Miyata, T., 1976, Neurobiology of piperidine: its relevance to CNS function, *Adv. Biochem. Psychopharmacol. 15:*5.

Kosterlitz, H.W., and Watt, A.J., 1968, Kinetic parameters of narcotic agonists and antagonists with particular reference to N-allylnoroxy morphine (naloxone), *Br. J. Pharmacol. Chemother. 33:*266.

Kupfer, D.J., 1976, REM latency: a psychobiologic marker for primary depressive disease, *Biol. Psychiatry 11:*159.

Kupfer, D.J., and Foster, F.G., 1972, Interval between onset of sleep and rapid eye movement sleep as an indicator of depression, *Lancet 2:*648.

Labrecque, G., and Domino, E.F., 1974, Tolerance to and physical dependence on morphine: relation to neocortical acetylcholine release in the cat, *J. Pharmacol. Exp. Ther. 191:*189.

Lavine, R., Buchsbaum, M.S., and Poncy, M., 1976, Auditory analgesia: somatosensory evoked response and subjective pain rating assessment, *Psychophysiology 13:*140.

Lenke, D., 1958, Narkosepotenzierende and analgetische wirkung von 1.4 dipyrrolido 2 butin, *Arch. Exp. Pathol. Pharmacol. 234:*35.

Leslie, G.B., 1969, The effect of antiparkinsonian drugs on oxotremorine-induced analgesia in mice, *J. Pharm. Pharmacol. 21:*248.

Lewis, J.R., 1949, The development of tolerance in rats to some new synthetic analgesics, *J. Pharmacol. Exp. Ther. 96:*31.

Li, C.H., Lamaire, S., Yamashiro, D., and Doneen, B.A., 1976, The synthesis and opiate activity of β-endorphin, *Biochem. Biophys. Res. Commun. 71:*19.

Loew, D., and Taeschler, M., 1964, Uber die analgetische wirkung von RS 86 einem cholinomimeticum mit zentraler wirkungskomponente, *Helv. Physiol. Pharmacol. Acta. 22c:*80.

Magherini, P.C., Pompeiano, O., and Thoden, U., 1971, The neurochemical basis of REM sleep: a cholinergic mechanism responsible for rhythmic activation of the vestibulo-oculomotor system, *Brain Res. 35:*565.

Matthews, J.D., Labrecque, G., and Domino, E.F., 1973, Effect of morphine, nalorphine and naloxone on neocortical release of ACh in the rat, *Psychopharmacologia 29:*113.

Matsuzaki, M., 1969, Differential effects of sodium butyrate and physostigmine upon the activities of para-sleep in acute brain stem preparations, *Brain Res. 13:*247.

Maynert, E.W., 1967, Effects of morphine on acetylcholine and certain other neurotransmitters, *Arch. Biol. Med. Exp. (Santiago) 4:*36.

Mazzuchelli-O'Flaherty, A.L., O'Flaherty, J.J., and Hernandez-Peon, R., 1967, Sleep and other behavioral responses induced by acetylcholinic stimulation of frontal and mesial cortex, *Brain Res. 4:*268.

Mendelson, W.B., Gillin, J.C., and Wyatt, R.J., 1977, *"Human Sleep and its Disorders,"* Plenum Press, New York.

Metys, J., Wagner, N., Metysova, J., and Herz, A., 1969, Studies on the central antinociceptive action of cholinomimetic agents, *Int. J. Neuropharmacol. 8:*413.

Migdal, W., and Frumin, J.J., 1963, Amnesic and analgesic effects in man of centrally acting anticholinergics, *Fed. Proc. 22:*188.

Mitchell, J.F., 1963, The spontaneous and evoked release of acetylcholine from the cerebral cortex, *J. Physiol. 165:*98.

Mitler, M.M., and Dement, W.C., 1974, Cataplectic-like behavior in cats after microinjection of carbachol in pontine reticular formation, *Brain Res. 68:*335.

Monnier, M., Dudler, L., Gaechter, R., Maier, P.F., Tobler, H.J., and Schoenenberger, G.A., 1977, The delta sleep inducing peptide (DSIP). Comparative properties of the original and synthetic nonapeptide, *Experientia 33:*548.

Moroni, F., Cheney, D.L., and Costa, E., 1977, β-Endorphin inhibits ACh turnover in nuclei of rat brain, *Nature 267:*267.

Mudgill, L., Friedhoff, A.J., and Tobey, J., 1974, Effect of intraventricular administration of epinephrine, norepinephrine, dopamine, acetylcholine and physostigmine on morphine analgesia in mice, *Arch. Int. Pharmacodyn. 210:*85.

Nagasaki, H., Iriki, M., Inoue, S., and Uchizono, K., 1974, The presence of sleep-promoting material in the brain of sleep deprived rats, *Proc. Japan. Acad. 50:*241.

Nistri, A., Pepeu, G., Cammelli, E., Spina, L., and DeBellis, A.M., 1974, Effect of morphine in brain and spinal acetylcholine levels and nociceptive threshold in the frog, *Brain Res. 80:*199.

Nixon, R.A., and Karnovsky, M.L., 1977, Uptake and metabolism of intraventricularly administered piperidine and its effects on sleep and wakefulness in the rat, *Brain Res.* *134:*501.

Oswald, I., Thacore, V.R., Adam, K., Brezinova, V., and Burack, R., 1975, Alpha-adrenergic receptor blockage increases human REM sleep, *Br. J. Clin. Pharmacol. 2:* 107.

Pappenheimer, J.R., Koski, G., Fencl, V., Karnovsky, I., and Krueger, J., 1975, Extraction of sleep-promoting Factor S from cerebrospinal fluid and from brains of sleep-deprived animals, *J. Neurophysiol. 38:*1299.

Paton, W.D.M., 1957, The action of morphine and related substances on contraction and on acetylcholine output of coaxially stimulated guinea pig ileum, *Br. J. Pharmacol. 12:*119.

Pedigo, N.W., Dewey, W.L., and Harris, L.S., 1975, Determination and characterization of the antinociceptive activity of intraventricularly administered acetylcholine in mice, *J. Pharmacol. Exp. Ther. 193:*845.

Pellandra, C.L., 1933, La geneserine-morphine adjuvant de l'anesthesia generale, *Lyon. Med. 151:*653.

Pert, A., 1975, The cholinergic system and nociception in the primate: interactions with morphine, *Psychopharmacologia (Berl.) 44:*131.

Pert A., and Maxey, G., 1975, Asymmetrical cross-tolerance between morphine and scopolamine induced antinociception in the primate: differential sites of action, *Psychopharmacologia (Berl.) 44:*139.

Pert, C.B., and Snyder, S.H., 1973, Opiate receptor: demonstration in nervous tissue, *Science 179:*1011.

Pieron, H., 1913, *"Le probleme physiologique du sommeil,"* Masson, Paris.

Pinski, C., Fredrickson, R.C.A., and Vasquez, A.J., 1973, Morphine withdrawal syndrome responses to cholinergic antagonists and to a partial cholinergic agonist, *Nature 242:* 59.

Pleuvy, B.J., and Tobias, M.A., 1971, Comparison of the antinociceptive activities of physostigmine, oxotremorine and morphine in the mouse, *Br. J. Pharmacol. 43:*706.

Post, R.M., Gerner, R.H., Carman, J.S., Gillin, J.C., Jimerson, D.C., Goodwin, F.K., and Bunney, W.E., Jr., in press, Effects of a dopamine agonist Piribedil in depressed patients: relationship of pretreatment HVA to antidepressant response, *Arch. Gen. Psychiatry.*

Price, M.T.C., and Fibiger, H.C., 1975, Ascending catecholamine systems and morphine analgesia, *Brain Res. 99:*189.

Richter, D., and Crossland, J., 1949, Variation in acetylcholine content of the brain with physiological state, *Am. J. Physiol. 159:*247.

Robinson, C.R., Pegram, G.V., Hyde, P.R., Beaton, J.M., and Smythies, J.R., 1977, The effects of nicotinamide upon sleep in humans, *Biol. Psychiatry 12:*139.

Roffwarg, H.P., Muzio, J.N., and Dement, W.C., 1966, Ontogenetic development of the human sleep-dream cycle, *Science 152:*604.

Sagales, T., Erill, S., and Domino, E.F., 1969, Differential effects of scopolamine and chlorpromazine on REM and NREM sleep in normal male subjects, *Clin. Pharmacol. Ther. 10:*522.

Sagales, T., Erill, S., and Domino, E.F., 1976, Effects of repeated doses of scopolamine on the electroencephalographic stages of sleep in normal volunteers, *Clin. Pharmacol. Ther. 18:*727.

Saxena, P.N., 1958, Mechanism of cholinergic potentiation of morphine analgesia, *Indian J. Med. Res. 46:*653.

Schaumann, W., 1957, Inhibition by morphine of the release of acetylcholine from the intestine of the guinea pig, *Br. J. Pharmacol. 12:*115.

Sequin, J.J., Magherini, P.C., and Pompeiano, D., 1973, Cholinergic mechanisms related to REM sleep III. Tonic and phasic inhibition of monosynaptic reflexes induced by an anticholinesterase in the decerebrate cat, *Arch. Ital. Biol. III:*1.

Shute, C.C.D., and Lewis, P.R., 1967, The ascending cholinergic reticular system: neocortical, olfactory and subcortical projections, *Brain 90:*520.

Siegel, J.M., and McGinty, D.J., 1977, Pontine reticular formation neurons: relationship of discharge to motor activity, *Science 196:*678.

Sitaram, N., Wyatt, R.J., Dawson, S., and Gillin, J.C., 1976, REM sleep induction by physostigmine infusion during sleep, *Science 191:*1281.

Sitaram, N., Mendelson, W.B., Wyatt, R.J., and Gillin, J.C., 1977a, The time-dependent induction of REM sleep and arousal by physostigmine infusion during normal human sleep, *Brain Res. 122:*562.

Sitaram, N., Buchsbaum, M.S., and Gillin, J.C., 1977b, Physostigmine analgesia and somatosensory evoked responses in man, *Eur. J. Pharmacol. 42:*285.

Sitaram, N., Moore, A., and Gillin, J.C., 1978, Cholinergic induction of dreaming in man (submitted).

Slaughter, D., and Munsell, D.W., 1940, Some new aspects of morphine action effects on pain, *J. Pharmacol. Exp. Ther. 68:*104.

Slaughter, D., Parsons, J.C., and Munal, H.D., 1940, New clinical aspects of the analgesic action of morphine, *JAMA 115:*2058.

Stepita-Klavco, M., Dolezalova, H., and Fairweather, R., 1974, Piperidine increase in the brain of dormant mice, *Science 183:*536.

Stern, M., Fram, D., Wyatt, R.J., Grinspoon, L., and Tursky, B., 1969, All-night sleep studies of acute schizophrenics, *Arch. Gen. Psychiatry 20:*470.

Takemori, A.E., Cankat, T.F., and Ichiro, Y., 1975, Differential effects of morphine analgesia and naloxone antagonism by biogenic amine modifiers, *Life Sci. 17:*21.

Taneda, M., and Hara, T., 1975, Narcoleptic-like symptoms in organophosphorous poisoning, a case report, *Shinkef: Brain and Nerve 27:*211.

Tang, A.H., and Yim, G.K.W., 1963, The effects of arecoline on spinal reflexes of the cat, *Int. J. Neuropharmacol. 4:*309.

Torda, C., 1968, Contribution to serotonin theory of dreaming (LSD infusion) *N.Y. State J. Med. 68:*1135.

Toyoda, J., Sasaki, K., and Kurihara, M., 1966, A polygraphic study on the effect of atropine on human nocturnal sleep, *Folia Psychiatry Neurol. Jpn. 20:*275.

Tursky, B., and Watson, P.D., 1964, Controlled physical and subjective intensities of electric shock, *Psychophysiology 1:*151.

VanEich, A., and Bock, J., 1971, Comparisons of analgesic cholinomimetic, anticholinergic and sympathomimetic drugs by means of the hot plate test, *Arch. Int. Pharmacodyn. Ther. 189:*384.

Waterfield, A., and Kosterlitz, H.W., 1975, Stereospecific increase by narcotic antagonists of evoked acetylcholine output in guinea pig ileum, *Life Scie. 16:*1787.

Way, F.L., Iwamoto, E.T., Bhargava, H.N., and Loh, H.H., 1975, Adaptive cholinergic dopaminergic responses in morphine dependence, in *"Advances in Biochemical Psychopharmacology, Vol. 13: Neurobiological Mechanisms of Adaptation and Behavior"* (A.J. Mandell, ed.), pp. 169-184, Raven Press, New York.

Weitzman, E.D., Kripke, D.F., Goldmacher, D., McGregor, P., and Nogeire, C., 1970, Acute reversal of the sleep-waking cycle in man, *Arch. Neurol. 22:*483.

Wyatt, R.J., 1972, The serotonin-catecholamine dream bicycle: a clinical study, *Biol. Psychiatry 5:*33.

Yaksh, T.L., and Yamamura, H., 1975, Blockade by morphine of acetylcholine release from the caudate nucleus in mid-pontine pretrigeminal cat, *Brain Res. 83:*520.

Young, D.C., Ploeg, R.A.V., Featherstone, R.M., and Gross, E.G., 1956, The interrelationships among the central peripheral and anticholinesterase effect of some morphinan derivatives, *J. Pharmacol. 114:*33.

Zarcone, V., 1973, Narcolepsy, *N. Engl. J. Med. 288:*1156.

Zetler, G., 1968, Cataleptic state and hypothemia in mice caused by central cholinergic stimulation and antagonized by anticholinergic and antidepressant drugs, *Int. J. Neuropharmacol. 7:*325.

Zsilla, G., Cheney, D.L., Racagni, G., and Costa, E., 1976, Correlation between analgesia and the decrease of acetylcholine turnover rate in cortex and hippocampus elicited by morphine, meperidine, Viminol R_2 and Azidomorphine, *J. Pharmacol. Exp. Ther. 199:*662.

ELECTROPHYSIOLOGICAL EFFECTS OF PHYSOSTIGMINE IN HUMANS

A. Pfefferbaum[1,2], K. L. Davis[1,2], C. L. Coulter[1], R. C. Mohs[1,2] and B. S. Kopell[1,2]

[1] Veterans Administration Hospital, 3801 Miranda Avenue, Palo Alto, California 94304

[2] Department of Psychiatry and Behavioral Sciences, Stanford University School of Medicine, Stanford, California 94305

INTRODUCTION

Single cell and depth recording of CNS electrical activity in animals is a valuable technique for assessing the activity of neurotransmitters and psychopharmacologic agents. In humans, however, these invasive techniques are rarely possible. While the electrical activity of the brain can be observed from scalp electrodes, there is considerable attenuation of specificity. Nonetheless, the scalp recorded EEG has proved to be of value in the evaluation of psychoactive compounds. In general, it is reasonable to look for EEG changes accompanying the administration of agents that produce behavioral effects. The reported behavioral and affective changes induced by the cholinesterase inhibitor physostigmine have concomitant neurophysiologic changes which might be reflected in the EEG. Demonstration of neurophysiologic alterations caused by this compound may lead to more information about the specificity of action of physostigmine and the reflection of central cholinergic activity in the EEG.

The effects of physostigmine on the EEG of animals is extensively reviewed by Karczmar (see Karczmar chapter, this book). A detailed study by Van Meter and Karczmar (1971) illustrates the effects on animals. Physostigmine was administered to unanesthesized rabbits restrained with a head holder. EEG was recorded from implanted electrodes in anterior and posterior motor cortices, lenticular nucleus, olfactory area, midbrain reticular substance and dorsal hippocampus. Thalamocortical recruitment was evoked by electrical stimulation of anterior midline nuclei of the thalamus. Animals were pre-treated with atropine methyl-nitrate to protect the peripheral cardiovascular responses. Physostigmine, 100-150 μg/kg i.v., was given to animals with and without reserpine and/or alpha methyl paratyrosine (a-MPT) pre-treatment. The intravenous administration of physostigmine was followed by 2 min of slow wave sleep and then a continuous desynchronized EEG pattern. This desynchrony occurred at 5 min post drug and lasted for about 5 min.

345

Full thalamocortical recruitment was attenuated during the period of maximal desynchrony even when suprathreshold stimuli were applied. The recruitment response and the EEG tracings resumed pre-drug characteristics 30-40 min after drug administration. In the reserpine and a-MPT treated (catecholamine depleted) animals, physostigmine induced EEG desynchrony but failed to attenuate recruitment. The addition of L-DOPA restored the capacity of physostigmine to attenuate recruitment in the catecholamine depleted animals. These results were illustrated with tracings of bipolar recordings from motor cortex to occipital cortex or basal olfactory area.

There have been a few reports of the effects of cholinesterase inhibitors and cholinergic agents on the human EEG. One of the earliest studies was done by Grob et al., (1974). They administered daily intramuscular injections (1 to 2 mg per day) of the anticholinesterase compound diisopropylfluorosphosphate (DFP) for several days. This resulted in "increased electrical activity of the brain" in 17 of 23 subjects. This increased EEG activity included "greater variations in potential," an increase in beta activity, increased rhythmic "irregularities," and the intermittent appearance of high voltage slow waves (3 to 6 Hz), which were most marked in the frontal leads and were exacerbated by hyperventilation. Intravenous administration of atropine (1.2 mg) to subjects who had received DFP and exhibited the EEG changes resulted in an inhibition of the DFP effects on the EEG. This included an immediate decrease in irregularities of rhythm, a decrease in beta activity, an increase in alpha activity, and a decrease in the appearance of the abnormal slow waves (both before and during hyperventilation).

Rowntree et al., (1950) gave 2 mg of DFP intramuscularly for 7 days to nine manic-depressives and thirteen schizophrenics; an additional four schizophrenic patients received daily injections for an average of 37 days with an average total dose of 43 mg. Ten normal subjects were also given daily DFP injections, but most of them could receive no more than 7 mg total because of the severity of drug induced systemic symptoms. EEG recordings were made with a bipolar electrode configuration at frontal, central, temporal, and occipital locations while the subjects were recumbent in a lighted room. EEG recordings were characterized as "early" if they were taken within 24 hr of the last injection and "late" if taken more than 24 hr after the last injection. The early records produced a generalized lowering of EEG amplitude with a diminution in the amount and spread of alpha activity. Half the cases demonstrated the intermittent appearance of low voltage slow activity in the theta range (4 to 7 Hz). The late records revealed an increase in amplitude as compared to the original record with increased dominance and spread of alpha activity. There was also an increase in slow activity (2 to 7 Hz). The frequency of the alpha rhythm decreased as much as 2 Hz in the majority of records in both the early and late recordings. Both recording times also produced increased instability with hyperventilation.

Lesny and Vojta (1960) gave .15 to .35 mg of eserine (physostigmine) via subcutaneous injection to 71 children, 6 to 15 years of age, and to 12 adults, all of whom had a seizure disorder but normal pre-drug EEG. EEG was recorded for a ½ hr after the injection of eserine. There were no systemic side effects and pulse rate never slowed more than four beats per minute. Twenty of the 71 children revealed spike and wave patterns after eserine, 17 had a "shift to the slow side" (slowing of the basic frequency), and 15 had the appearance of episodic synchronous slow activity. These changes usually occurred from 20 to 30 min post injection. Similar eserine injections in 18 normal children (no history of epilepsy) produced no changes in 14 and slowing of the basic rhythm in 4. The normal subjects were also reported to have a "hypersynchronization of the dominant activity as a regular response to the injection of eserine." In the 12 adult patients, one revealed spike and wave patterns, four showed rhythmic slow activity after eserine administration, three had a shift to the slow side, and four had no change.

In another study (Pfeiffer *et al.*, 1963) 20 male volunteers were administered intravenous doses of deanol (the metabolic precursor of choline — 1 mg/kg), choline (1 mg/kg), dl-amphetamine (.1 mg/kg), or .9 percent saline. EEG was recorded and analyzed with a Drohocki integrator which estimates the electrical energy content of the EEG. With this apparatus, a burst of alpha will cause an increase in output from the integrator, whereas the decrease in EEG energy seen with arousal (high frequency, low voltage EEG) will produce a decrease in output from the integrator. Deanol injection was followed by a 10 min latent period and then "a significant stimulant effect compared to control levels ($p < .05$)." Amphetamine had a similar effect and choline had no effect. Oral deanol and amphetamine produced similar effects but at longer latencies after administration than the intravenous route. Oral choline produced no significant changes as measured with the EEG integrator.

In a study investigating the effects of physostigmine on sleep, Sitaram *et al.*, (1976) gave seven normal volunteers .5 mg physostigmine i.v. prior to the first REM (rapid eye movement) period of the night. This resulted in a significant decrease in the latency of the first REM period when compared to a night in which a placebo infusion was given. There was no significant difference in the length of this REM period or in the eye movement density (amount of eye movement activity) during the REM period. When physostigmine infusions were given during REM periods, the subjects woke up significantly more often than when given placebo. It was proposed that non-REM to REM to awake forms a continuum of increasing levels of arousal and that cholinergic mechanisms are involved in shifting the level of arousal from lower to higher on this continuum.

Sitaram *et al.*, (1977) gave 14 normal subjects .5 mg physostigmine i.v. followed 20 min later by testing for pain sensitivity and tolerance. In addition, cortical evoked potentials were recorded for somatosensory stimuli of four different intensities. The positive component of the somatosensory evoked response occurring at about 100 msec post stimulation (P100) was significantly smaller after physostigmine treatment than after placebo.

Reiger and Okonek (1975) reported on 70 EEGs which were recorded during different stages of organophosphate poisoning from anticholinesterase insecticides in 17 patients. In the deepest coma, during which there was no blood cholinesterase activity, the EEG was relatively flat, containing alpha and beta frequencies which did not respond to stimuli. No slow waves were present, and the EEG was described as desynchronized. At a higher level of consciousness, characterized clinically by coma and stupor but still with no blood cholinesterase activity, the EEG was described as having "dominant" delta activity. At the clinical level of somnolence, with some recovery of cholinesterase activity, the EEG had unstable alpha rhythm associated with generalized or frontal-temporal slow waves.

These studies present some inconsistencies. They can be divided into those with findings of abnormal frontal slow wave activity which might be seen as a decreased level of arousal or a depressant effect, and those studies with findings of low amplitude, high frequency EEG activity which is seen with activation and increased arousal. These inconsistencies might be attributed to the dosage range (quite low to toxic), clinical diagnostic factors, and EEG assessment and quantitation techniques.

The study reported below was carried out because it was felt that the effects of physostigmine on the normal human EEG had not been definitively demonstrated. In addition, there was the hope that the EEG responses might resemble those of the animal work which produced a model sensitive to both cholinergic and dopaminergic influences and allowed the definition of contributions of each to neurophysiologic responses.

METHODS

The compromise between safety and the desire to look at the acute effects of physostigmine resulted in the use of a multi-injection technique. This allowed the observation of the EEG immediately after each injection of a small amount of drug, and then for a longer period after the build up by several injections.

The protocol employed a placebo-drug-placebo single blind design completed in one session, consisting of three series of injections: the first condition involving the injection of saline; the second the injection of physostigmine; and the third, again, saline. The drug (or saline) was given in .5 mg or ½ cc boluses at 5 min intervals.

Seventeen paid subjects participated in the study after giving informed consent. They were male volunteers 21-30 years of age. Four subjects received only 0.5 mg of physostigmine (one 0.5 mg injection), four received a total of 1.5 mg of physostigmine (three 0.5 mg injections), and nine received 2.5 mg of physostigmine (five 0.5 mg injections). Four of the subjects who received 2.5 mg of physostigmine were also pre-treated with prochlorperazine (10 mg p.o.) prior to the EEG recording session in order to block the nausea and vomiting that occurs with high doses of physostigmine.

The EEG was recorded in discrete 5 min periods. Each period consisted of 2.5 min with eyes closed and 2.5 min with eyes open while the subject was reading. Between periods the subject was asked to blink several times before beginning the procedure again. Injections were given between these 5 min periods. This routine was employed in order to maintain the subjects in a fairly uniform state of arousal and specifically to avoid their going to sleep.

Table 1 outlines the experimental protocol. The subjects arrived in the laboratory at 7:30 a.m., having fasted for 8 hr and were given 12 oz of fruit juice as a breakfast. All were pre-treated with 0.5 mg methscopolamine subcutaneously to block the peripheral cholinergic effects of physostigmine. EEG recordings were begun after the methscopolamine had produced a tachycardia of 100 beats/min.

After a 15 min baseline recording, a ½ cc injection of saline was given at 5 min intervals until the entire dosage had been administered. After the last injection, eight continuous periods (totalling 40 min) of EEG were recorded. The EEG technician entered the recording booth briefly every 10 min to check for drowsiness or any drug side effects. This 40 min period was followed by a 5 min break, during which the subject was free to

TABLE 1

Protocol for Subjects Receiving 1.5 mg

Subject arrives: receives standard breakfast

Methscopolamine .5 cc subcutaneously

Start saline i.v.

Tachycardia criterion of 100 beats/min

First Saline Injection Series

EEG baseline recording: 15 min
.5 mg saline injection #1
EEG recording: 5 min
.5 mg saline injection #2

EEG recording: 5 min
.5 mg saline injection #3
EEG recording: 40 min

Physostigmine Injection Series

EEG baseline recording: 5 min
.5 mg physostigmine injection #1
EEG recording: 5 min
.5 mg physostigmine injection #2

EEG recording: 5 min
.5 mg physostigmine
injection #3
EEG recording: 40 min

Second Saline Injection Series

EEG baseline recording: 5 min
.5 mg saline injection #1
EEG recording: 5 min
.5 mg saline injection #2

EEG recording: 5 min
.5 mg saline injection #3
EEG recording: 40 min

move around. After a second 5 min baseline recording, this procedure was repeated using physostigmine injections, and EEG recordings were made in the same manner. The procedure was performed a third time with saline injections.

The EEG was recorded from frontal and occipital electrode placements with platinum pins referenced to linked mastoid disc electrodes. Electrocardiogram (EKG) and electrooculogram (EOG) were also recorded. The EEG was amplified 10K with amplifiers set at a nominal bandpass of 1-30 Hz (3dB points of 6 dB/octave rolloff curves). The EEG was constantly monitored on paper and simultaneously recorded on a seven-channel FM tape recorder. The raw EEG was later entered into a PDP-11/40 computer in discrete epochs. The analysis only included the eyes closed epochs as these were the most artifact-free. After editing out any sections showing movement or large eye blink artifact, 1.5 to 2.5 min of "clean" EEG from each "eyes closed" epoch was entered. These epochs were than subjected to fast Fourier analysis, which resulted in a power spectrum with ¼ Hz resolution for 0 to 32 Hz components. This procedure yielded separate EEG power spectra for recordings taken every 5 min.

The Fourier analysis provides a mathematical description of the EEG. It quantifies the amount of activity (amplitude) of the EEG at each frequency, resulting in a description of the contribution (power) of each frequency to the overall EEG. This provides information about the total absolute EEG activity (total power) and the relative contribution of any frequency component. The results are usually presented as a power spectrum graph over a range of frequencies (see Figure 1).

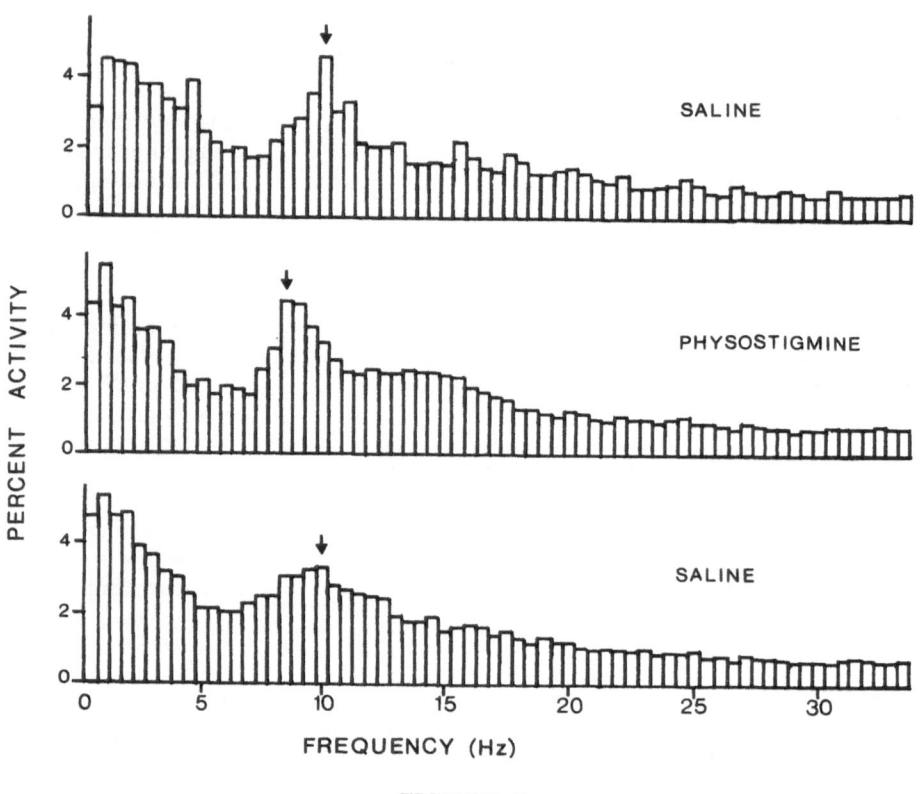

FIGURE 1

EEG power spectra for one subject from recordings made after administration of 2.5 mg of saline, physostigmine, and saline. Arrows pointing to peak alpha frequency in each condition indicate slowing after physostigmine administration.

Spectral analysis produces an excessively detailed mathematical description of the EEG. In order to make this large amount of information more manageable, the data were collapsed into a measure of the total power of the EEG, and the percentage contribution to the total power of the 0-4 Hz (delta), 4-8 Hz (theta), 8-12 Hz (alpha) and 12-30 Hz (beta) frequency components. Percentage of the total power was used because it provides a more stable measure than the absolute power of each of the frequencies in the normal resting EEG (Matousek, 1973).

In addition to the spectral total power measure and the percent contribution of the four frequency bands, a determination was made of the dominant frequency of the alpha activity as measured at the occiput. This was accomplished by determining the frequency between 8 and 12 Hz (in ¼ Hz resolution) which contained the largest amount of power. This measure was labelled the "peak alpha frequency."

RESULTS

The protocol, recording techniques, and data analysis were the same for all groups of subjects, with the exception of fewer injections at the lower doses. In none of these 17 subjects were there obvious visible changes in the raw EEG data such as have been reported with the implanted electrode animal studies. The subjects who received .5 mg could not distinguish physostigmine from placebo. The 1.5 and 2.5 mg dose, however, did produce subjective effects. These included dizziness, diaphoresis, difficulty with reading, and nausea. Some subjects vomited. Prochlorperazine pre-treatment significantly attenuated the nausea and vomiting produced by 2.5 mg of physostigmine.

The data were collected in 5-min discrete epochs. The statistical analysis for acute drug effects utilized these 5-min epochs after each drug injection. The 40 min after the last injection of each series were treated as two 20-min epochs for analysis purposes.

The two groups receiving 2.5 mg of physostigmine (five without and four with prochlorperazine pre-treatment) were initially analyzed as separate groups. There were no significant group or drug by group effects. Therefore, the two were combined for subsequent analysis and treated as one dosage group.

Figure 2 illustrates the most salient EEG changes found in the frontal lead for the nine subjects receiving 2.5 mg. This figure presents the mean (N=9) percentage activity for each of the four frequency bands at successive 5 min intervals during the protocol. It can be seen that the percent of delta activity began to increase after the third physostigmine injection, returning during the second 20 min period to the levels found during the first placebo run. There was a corresponding decrease in the percent of beta activity.

Acute Effects

The acute effects of physostigmine were determined by analyzing three epochs after the beginning of the injection series for each of the three treatments (saline, physostigmine, and saline). For the subjects who received 2.5 mg, this provided samples immediately after the dose totalled .5 mg, 1.5 mg, and 2.5 mg of physostigmine or saline. For the 1.5 mg subjects, the samples were taken after .5 and 1.5 mg total dose; the third sample was taken at the time the 2.5 mg group would have received the last injection. Similarly,

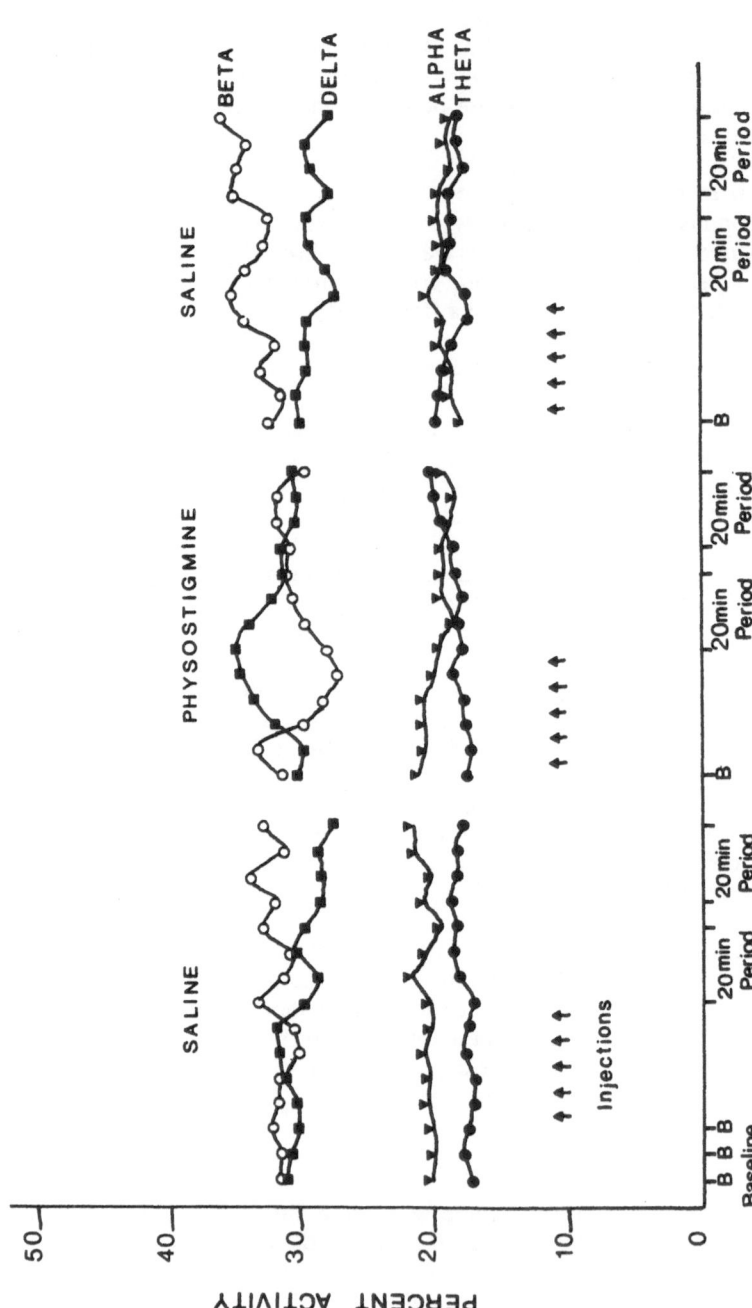

Mean percent activity of delta, theta, alpha, and beta in frontal lead for nine subjects receiving 2.5 mg of saline, physostigmine, and saline. Points represent data collected at 5 min intervals during the three treatment conditions.

the .5 mg group had the second and third samples taken at the time the other groups received the 1.5 and 2.5 mg cumulative dose.

Three-way analyses of variance (dose group x drug x time) were performed for frontal and occipital leads for each frequency band for all 17 subjects. Two-way analyses were performed for each dose group separately. Table 2 presents these results.

The overall analysis of variance for all 17 subjects produced a significant drug main effect for frontally recorded delta and beta activity and occipitally recorded delta activity. There was an increase in the percentage of delta activity and a corresponding decrease in the percentage of beta activity. The amount of alpha was unaffected. The significant drug effects for theta activity in both frontal and occipital leads, and the significant drug by time interaction in the occiput were caused by an increase in the percent of theta activity occurring 20-40 min after drug administration and persisting into the post-injection epochs of the second placebo administration. These effects, which also occurred in the group receiving 2.5 mg, are therefore actually "late" effects and are discussed below.

When the three dose groups were analyzed separately, the 2.5 mg group showed a significant drug effect for delta activity in the frontal lead. A significant drug x time effect for delta activity in both frontal and occipital leads indicated that the delta activity increased with increasing dose. There were significant corresponding decreases in beta activity (see Figure 2). The drug main effects and the drug x time interactions were most prominent in the 2.5 mg group, less so for the 1.5 mg group and essentially non-existent for the .5 mg group.

Though few acute drug effects were found for the groups receiving 1.5 and 0.5 mg, a number of time effects reached statistical significance. The 1.5 mg group showed a significant time effect for the percent of theta activity in the occipital lead; theta activity increased across all three injection series, with the highest percentages occurring during the second set of saline injections. For subjects receiving 0.5 mg of physostigmine, the percentage of alpha activity showed a significant increase during each injection series in both frontal and occipital leads. In addition, the amount of occipitally recorded beta activity for this group showed a significant decrease in each of the three treatments.

Table 2 presented the effects found during and shortly after the injection series. The more immediate effects of the different dosages were examined by comparing the data collected in the epoch immediately following the injection of a given dose. All 17 subjects received the first .5 mg injection; 13 received at least 1.5 mg, and 9 received all 2.5 mg. This provided 17 observations at .5 mg, 13 observations at 1.5 mg and 9 observations at 2.5 mg. Analyses of variance were performed for each frequency band for the frontal and occipital leads. Both the increase in delta activity and the corresponding decrease in beta in the frontal lead did not occur until 1.5 mg was given (drug effect $p < .001$ for delta; $p < .01$ for beta) and persisted for the 2.5 mg dose (drug effect $p < .001$ for delta; $p < .01$ for beta). The occipital lead showed the same increase in percent delta at the 1.5 mg dose (drug effect $p < .05$) and 2.5 mg dose (drug effect $p < .05$). However, the corresponding pattern of decrease in percent beta activity was not apparent in the occipital lead.

TABLE 2

F Ratios and Significance Levels from Anovas for Acute Effects

		Frontal				Occipital			
		Total (N=17)	2.5 mg (N=9)	1.5 mg (N=4)	0.5 mg (N=4)	Total (N=17)	2.5 mg (N=9)	1.5 mg (N=4)	0.5 mg (N=4)
Total Power	D	1.98	1.58	1.20	1.65	2.03	0.75	2.23	3.56
	T	0.14	0.89	1.51	1.03	0.35	0.57	0.22	0.32
	DT	2.23	2.35	1.49	0.66	1.23	1.63	1.19	0.13
	DTG	0.61				0.64			
% Delta	D	10.14***	6.34**	1.36*	2.14	4.71*	1.58	4.10	1.00
	T	1.10	1.79	0.76	0.19	1.72	0.31	4.69	2.13
	DT	3.14*	3.85*	4.33*	0.93	1.42	4.86**	1.42	1.17
	DTG	2.08				2.22*			
% Theta	D	6.63**	4.25*	2.63	1.23	3.64*	4.68*	0.98	0.36
	T	0.21	0.62	2.30	1.28	2.95	0.35	11.05*	0.07
	DT	1.01	1.45	1.06	0.42	3.19*	1.99	0.85	1.02
	DTG	0.78				0.30			
% Alpha	D	0.29	0.46	0.21	0.84	2.27	0.72	1.51	0.79
	T	0.21	0.25	0.78	7.74*	1.61	0.66	3.87	6.11*
	DT	0.95	0.98	1.48	1.17	0.07	0.85	0.35	0.47
	DTG	1.07				0.64			
% Beta	D	9.71**	12.87***	4.91	0.34	2.03	0.26	2.90	1.82
	T	0.19	2.44	2.30	1.88	0.05	0.55	0.09	5.89*
	DT	0.38	2.91*	0.56	0.74	0.86	2.75*	1.10	2.58
	DTG	1.58				1.89			

*p < .05 – **p < .01 – ***p < .001

Late Effects

After the total dose of saline or physostigmine was administered, EEG recording continued for 40 min. The late effects were defined as changes occurring during this 40 min time period. The EEG power spectra calculated for the epochs collected during the first half of this period (four 5-min epochs) were collapsed across time to yield a single power spectrum for the first 20 min time period. The data recorded from 20 to 40 min after the last injection were treated in the same fashion. Thus there were two late measures for each subject for each injection series.

The results of three-way analyses of variance (dosage group x drug treatment x time) using all 17 subjects are presented in Table 3. There was a significant increase in total power in frontal and occipital leads for both 20 min epochs (drug effect $p < .05$) following the physostigmine injections. This overall total power increase can probably be accounted for by the increases seen in delta and theta activity; however, when these frequency bands were considered independently, many of the increases failed to meet the .05 level of significance. This pattern occurred in both the frontal and occipital leads. In addition, a significant time effect was found for frontally recorded delta activity; it tended to decrease from the first to the second 20 min period after each injection series.

When dose groups were analyzed separately (see Table 3), there was a significant drug x time effect for the percent of theta activity for the 2.5 mg subjects in both the frontal and occipital recording ($p < .05$) which was not present in the other two doses. This effect was produced by an increase in theta activity occurring 20 to 40 min after the last physostigmine injection. The 1.5 mg subjects showed a significant drug x time effect for delta activity ($p < .05$).

The analysis of variance also revealed a few significant effects due to time per se. The 2.5 mg group showed an increase in frontal delta activity, and a decrease in occipital theta activity, during the 40 min period following each of the three treatments. In addition, the 1.5 mg group revealed a significant increase in the percent of beta activity in the frontal lead during the 40 min period after each injection series.

The primary synchronous EEG activity is the 10 Hz alpha rhythm which can best be seen and measured at the occiput. The peak alpha frequency provided a quantification of the slowing of this synchronous activity caused by physostigmine. The 2.5 mg group demonstrated a significant ($p < .05$) slowing in the peak alpha frequency measure (see Figures 1 and 3). The first saline run for the 2.5 mg group had a mean peak alpha frequency of 9.9 Hz, the post physostigmine frequency was 9.5 Hz and the second saline run returned to 9.6 Hz. The two lower dosage groups did not demonstrate this effect.

DISCUSSION

Physostigmine administration resulted in a decrease in the frequency of the resting synchronous activity of the brain (decrease in peak alpha frequency) and an increase in the amount of slow frequency activity (delta and theta) with a concomitant decrease in high frequency activity (beta). These results appear to be dose related; they are not present after .5 mg, but become apparent after 1.5 mg and still more prominent after

TABLE 3

F Ratios and Significance Levels from ANOVAs for Late Effects

		Frontal				Occipital		
		Total (N=17)	2.5 mg (N=9)	1.5 mg (N=4)	0.5 mg (N=4)	Total (N=17)	2.5 mg (N=9)	1.5 mg (N=4)	0.5 mg (N=4)
Total Power	D	4.44*	3.58	1.59	3.81	5.29*	3.92*	3.69	6.05*
	T	1.55	0.04	5.54	2.03	0.23	1.30	0.10	6.57
	DT	0.78	2.27	1.44	0.47	0.10	1.56	3.90	0.34
	DTG	1.01				2.13			
% Delta	D	3.84*	2.31	3.12	1.51	3.19	2.10	3.76	0.55
	T	6.92*	9.13*	4.96	0.06	1.38	0.71	4.20	0.53
	DT	6.09**	2.27	5.36*	1.48	1.59	0.34	4.13	0.12
	DTG	2.74*				0.74			
% Theta	D	3.32	0.80	2.91	1.76	3.19	2.64	1.39	0.29
	T	1.51	1.47	0.91	0.32	4.51	5.66*	1.48	0.10
	DT	1.28	6.01*	0.86	0.18	1.36	4.14*	0.47	0.06
	DTG	2.03				0.89			
% Alpha	D	0.82	1.17	2.57	0.52	0.50	0.24	0.88	0.57
	T	0.06	0.23	0.00	6.20	1.08	1.50	0.08	0.40
	DT	0.24	1.83	1.37	0.17	1.70	1.91	0.53	0.15
	DTG	1.38				0.24			
% Beta	D	2.38	3.46	1.34	0.61	0.18	0.00	0.25	0.23
	T	1.31	3.37	13.50*	0.59	1.59	2.12	0.30	1.26
	DT	2.22	0.50	3.44	0.84	0.24	1.14	0.69	0.26
	DTG	2.70				0.52			

*$p < .05$ – **$p < .01$

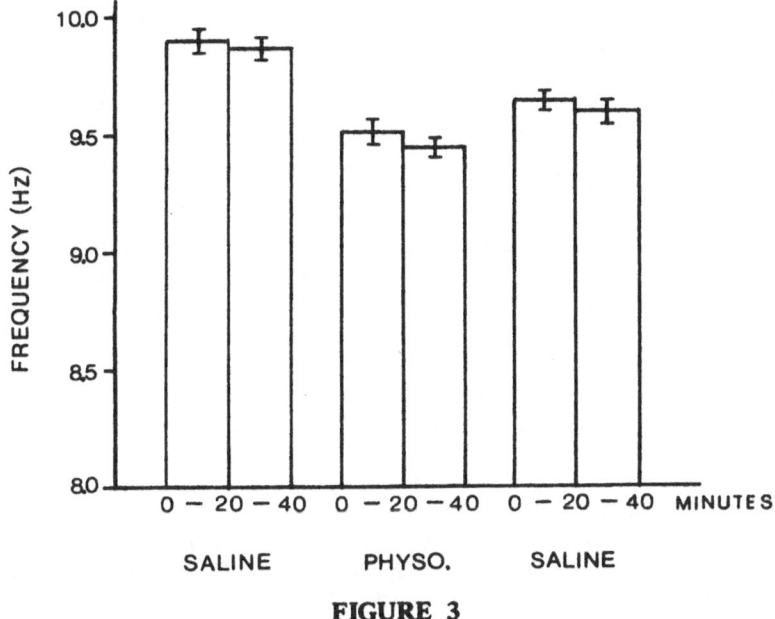

FIGURE 3

Mean (N=9) peak alpha frequency as measured from occipital lead shows decrease for subjects receiving 2.5 mg physostigmine. First bar in each condition represents data collected for the nine subjects during the 20 min period following the fifth injection. Second bar represents data collected 20-40 min after fifth injection.

2.5 mg of physostigmine. This is consistent with the clinical reports of stuporous states produced by organophospate poisoning (Reiger and Okonek, 1975) during which the EEG revealed unstable alpha rhythm and generalized slowing. Animal studies have also demonstrated late (20-25 min post injection) facilitation of theta activity (Karczmar, 1977), and this same trend is seen in the data presented here. The general picture, therefore, might be interpreted as one of EEG slowing. This generalized slowing is seen in a variety of toxic states (Romano and Engel, 1944). In addition, high doses of physostigmine also can cause a generalized stress response, in which case many secondary systems are activated (Davis *et al.*, 1977a, 1977b). Thus the data presented here cannot be offered as a purely cholinergic effect.

The experimental sessions in this study involved 2½ to 3½ hr of recording time. When recording the EEG for such long periods of time, it is difficult to keep the subjects at a constant level of arousal. This becomes a particular problem in drug studies, since the effects of drowsiness or fatigue on the EEG may confound or mask the drug effect. Considerable effort was made in this study to maintain the subjects in a stable waking state. The fact that few significant time effects occurred suggests that this attempt was fairly successful. Time effects occurring in the 40 min period following each injection series were in the direction of higher levels of arousal (decreased delta, increased beta), indicating that the subjects were not becoming drowsy during these periods. In addition, time effects were more evident in the 0.5 mg group, perhaps because there were few drug effects to obscure the time dependent changes. This group showed time effects for epochs recorded immediately after saline or drug injections, and the changes are indicative of a more relaxed state (increased alpha, decreased beta) which may have resulted when subjects did not perceive the anticipated drug side effects. The significant time effects occurring for the percent of theta activity are more complicated, and may have resulted partially from a late drug-related increase in theta activity which continued into the second placebo administration.

The Sitaram et al., (1976) study, which demonstrated that .5 mg of physostigmine caused a shortened REM latency and increased awakening during sleep was interpreted as demonstration of an "arousing effect" caused by physostigmine. The analogous effect in the waking EEG might be expected to be an increase in high and a decrease in low frequency activity (the "activated EEG"). This was not seen in the data produced by this study. Several explanations could be offered for the failure to find this effect. Larger doses were given in this study over a shorter time than in the sleep experiment. The subjects were relatively activated to start with, making further activation less likely. Furthermore, attempts were made to control arousal level whereas this is not the case with the sleeping subjects. Finally, the waking state might have significantly different foci of EEG regulation than the sleeping state. The sleep study did not present any data suggesting that there were qualitative changes in the EEG characteristics within a given sleep state but rather that the dream and waking regulators were activated.

The dramatic effects seen in animals were also not apparent. These studies (e.g. Van Meter and Karczmar, 1971), however, employed implanted electrodes; therefore, they were able to measure activity at specific loci which might not be reflected as dramatically in scalp recordings. In addition, the doses used were considerably greater than those employed in this study. For instance, in Van Meter and Karczmar (1971), the equivalent mg/kg dose used in rabbits would require that 8 mg be given to our subjects in a single bolus.

The findings of slowing of the dominant frequency and the increase in low frequency activity demonstrated by spectral analysis must be interpreted with caution. There were not observable delta and theta waves in the raw EEG as are seen in some pathologic states, but rather the power at these frequencies was increased when the EEG was subjected to mathematical analysis. There is some evidence that activity in this low frequency range does occur in normal individuals. For instance, time locked averaging reveals phenomena such as the Contingent Negative Variation (CNV) with a period of 1 sec or longer, or the P300 with a frequency of 2 Hz. A major source of slow frequency activity contamination can be from eye movements. Indeed, many of the changes reported for the EEG leads could also be seen in the eye lead. The source of the changes is unclear because bipolar eye lead recordings also contain large EEG contaminants, including the higher frequency activity such as alpha. The slowing of the alpha frequency and the increase in delta activity with concomitant decrease in beta activity was prominent in the occipital recordings as well as the frontal ones, and the influence of eye movements on the EEG is minimal at the occiput.

A 1 mg i.v. dose of physostigmine, administered over 60 min, has been shown to enhance certain aspects of cognitive performance (Davis et al., 1978). The most comparable dose in the present study was the single .5 mg i.v. bolus, which produced only slight EEG effects; much larger doses were necessary to produce significant EEG changes as measured by spectral analysis techniques. These changes seen at the higher doses are indicative of a toxic effect, and it has been found that cognitive functioning deteriorates at doses of 1.5 mg or higher (Davis *et al.*, 1976). Other EEG techniques may be more sensitive than spectral analysis to the neurophysiological changes produced by low close cholinergic stimulation. Certain evoked potential components, such as the CNV and the P300, have been shown to be correlated with cognitive performance. Application of these simultaneously recorded cognitive and electrophysiologic measures may prove more useful in illuminating the neurophysiologic changes associated with the memory enhancing dose of physostigmine.

ACKNOWLEDGEMENTS

This research was supported by the Medical Research Service of the Veterans Administration, NIDA Research Grant DA-00854 and by NIMH Specialized Research Center Grant MH-30854.

REFERENCES

Davis, B.M., Davis, K.L., and Berger, P.A., 1977a, Cholinergic effects on neuroendocrine function, VI World Congress of Psychiatry: Honolulu, Hawaii, August.

Davis, K.L., Hollister, L.E., Overall, J., Johnson, A., and Train, K., 1976, Physostigmine: effects on cognition and affect in normal subjects, *Psychopharmacology 51:*23.

Davis, K.L., Hollister, L.E., Goodwin, F.K., and Gordon, E.K., 1977b, Neurotransmitter metabolites in the cerebrospinal fluid of man following physostigmine, *Life Sci. 21:* 933.

Davis, K.L., Mohs, R.C., Tinklenberg, J.R., Pfefferbaum, A., Hollister, L.E., and Kopell, B.S., 1978, Physostigmine: improvement of long-term memory processes in normal humans, *Science* (in press).

Grob, D., Harvey, A.M., Langworthy, O.R., and Lilienthal, Jr., J.L., 1947, The administration of diisopropylfluorophosphate (DFP) to man. III. Effect on the central nervous system with special reference to the electrical activity of the brain, *Bull. John Hopkins Hospital 81:*257.

Karczmar, A.G., 1977, Exploitable aspects of central cholinergic functions particularly with respect to the EEG, motor, analgesic, and mental functions, in *Cholinergic Mechanisms and Psychopharmacology*, (D. Jenden, ed.), Plenum Press, New York.

Lesny, I., and Vojta, V., 1960, Eserine activation of the EEG in children, *Electroenceph. Clin. Neurophys. 12:*742.

Matousek, M., (Ed.), 1973, Frequency and correlation analysis, Part A of *Handbook of Electroencephalography and Clinical Neurophysiology* (A. Remond, ed.), Volume 5: evaluation of bioelectrical data from brain, nerve and muscle, section II (M.A.B. Brazier, and D.A. Walker, eds.), p. 61, Elsevier/North Holland, Amsterdam.

Pfeiffer, C.C., Goldstein, L., Munoz, C., Murphree, H.B., and Jenny, E.H., 1963, Quantitative comparisons of the electroencephalographic stimulant effects of deanol, choline, and amphetamine, *Clin. Pharm. Therapeutics 4:*461.

Reiger, H., and Okonek, S., 1975, The EEG in alkylphosphate poisoning (anticholinesterase insecticides), *Electroenceph. Clin. Neurophys. 39:*555.

Romano, J., and Engel, G.L., 1944, Studies of delerium. I. Electroencephalographic data, *Arch. Neurol. Psychiat. 51:*356.

Rowntree, D.W., Nevin, S., and Wilson, A., 1950, The effects of diisopropylfluorophos-phonate in schizophrenia and manic depressive psychosis, *J. Neurol. Neurosurg. Psychiat. 13:*47.

Sitaram, M., Wyatt, R.J., Dawson, S., and Gillin, J.C., 1976, REM sleep induction by physostigmine during sleep, *Science 191:*1281.

Sitaram, N., Buchsbaum, M.S., and Gillin, J.D., 1977, Physostigmine analgesia and somatosensory evoked responses in man, *European Journal of Pharmacology 42:*285.

Van Meter, W.G., and Karczmar, A.G., 1971, An effect of physostigmine on the central nervous system of rabbits, related to brain levels of norepinephrine, *Neuropharmacology 10:*379.

ELECTROPHYSIOLOGICAL EFFECTS OF CHOLINE CHLORIDE IN ELDERLY SUBJECTS

A. Pfefferbaum[1,2], K. L. Davis[1,2], C. L. Coulter[1], R. C. Mohs[1,2] and B. S. Kopell[1,2]

[1] Laboratory of Clinical Psychopharmacology and Psychophysiology, Veterans Administration Hospital, 3801 Miranda Avenue, Palo Alto, California 94304

[2] Department of Psychiatry and Behavioral Sciences, Stanford University School of Medicine, Stanford, California 94305

INTRODUCTION

Cholinergic mechanisms have been shown to function in normal memory storage and retrieval processes, and have also been implicated in age-related memory loss. Cholinergic agonists, such as physostigmine, have been shown to improve certain aspects of long-term memory in humans (Davis *et al.*, 1978). Choline chloride, a precursor of acetylcholine, was reported to produce some behavior improvement in patients suffering from Alzheimer's disease (Boyd *et al.*, 1977). In contrast, anticholinergics, such as scopolamine, induce cognitive impairments (Sitaram *et al.*, 1978) similar to the cognitive deficits seen in patients with senile dementia (Drachman and Leavitt, 1974). It has been suggested that the long-term administration of cholinergic agents might benefit patients with age-related memory impairments. Recently choline chloride was administered to a group of elderly subjects with mild to moderate memory loss in order to assess the effect of choline on memory functioning (Mohs *et al.*, 1978). This chapter reports preliminary results of electrophysiological testing performed on this same group of subjects. The aim of the study was to investigate the effect of choline on the human electroencephalogram (EEG) and to relate these findings to any cognitive changes that might result from the use of this drug.

Electroencephalographic measurements provide a useful adjunct in evaluating the CNS effects of psychopharmacologic agents. The frequency composition of spontaneous EEG activity reflects changes brought on by altered levels of arousal and is a sensitive indicator of drug-induced electrophysiological changes (Fink, 1963). EEG evoked responses can be obtained during the performance of specific cognitive tasks. These measures provide a neurophysiological reflection of cognitive and perceptual processes and can be correlated with behavioral responses, such as reaction time.

361

In animal studies, the administration of cholinomimetics has typically resulted in the appearance of a desynchronized EEG pattern consisting of low voltage, fast activity (Karczmar, 1977). These effects indicate EEG arousal or activation. Results have been less consistent in human studies. A stimulant or desynchronizing effect has been reported for i.v. doses of deanol, a precursor of choline (Pfeiffer et al., 1963), and for i.v. doses of choline, although a large range of *oral* doses of choline had no effect on the EEG (Goldstein and Beck, 1965). Daily injections of the anticholinesterase compound diisopropylfluorophosphate (DFP) produced greater variations in potential and an increase of fast (beta) activity, in conjunction with the appearance of abnormal slow wave activity (Grob et al., 1947). A generalized slowing of the EEG, or an increase in slow wave activity has been reported following the administration of DFP (Rowntree et al., 1950) and physostigmine (Lesny and Votja, 1960), and after accidental poisoning with anticholinesterase insecticides (Reiger and Okonek, 1975). The same slowing effect was seen in this laboratory when normal volunteers were administered i.v. injections of physostigmine (Pfefferbaum et al., *Electrophysiological Effects of Physostigmine In Humans,* this book). Due to differences in subject populations, drugs used, dosage range, and EEG assessment techniques, these studies are difficult to compare, and do not yield a clear picture of the effects of cholinergic stimulation on the human EEG. The investigations reported in this chapter were undertaken in an attempt to elucidate the effects of choline on the human EEG by using a variety of EEG quantification and analysis techniques, and to relate these to behavioral and cognitive measures.

METHODS

Experiment I

Subjects and Design

Subjects were one male and five female volunteers aged 60-82 (mean age = 70.5 years). All potential subjects underwent a screening process to eliminate those with significant mental or physical illness, including cardiovascular disease or seizure disorder. Approximately 50 potential subjects did not participate in the study because of physical illness. In addition, subjects were screened with the use of a long-term memory task (Davis et al., 1978), and only those subjects who demonstrated some room for memory improvement were selected for participation in the study. These screening procedures resulted in a group of subjects who were exceptionally healthy for their age group and who also had mild to moderate memory impairment. However, none of the subjects showed a severe loss of memory and all were ambulatory, self-sufficient members of their communities.

The experimental protocol consisted of a placebo-choline-placebo, single blind design. EEG testing was performed in each of the three treatment conditions. The first placebo period lasted for one week, during which the subjects took a placebo designed to look and taste like choline. EEG testing occurred on day 6 of this week. Subjects then received 16 gm/day of choline (4 gm, 4 times a day) for one week, with EEG testing again occurring on day 6. A two-week placebo washout period followed the week of choline administration, with testing performed at the end of this period.

Testing

Two EEG measures were employed: 1) spontaneous waking EEG recordings were obtained in order to analyze the frequency composition of the EEG; and 2) a Contingent Negative Variation (CNV) paradigm involving a constant-foreperiod reaction-time task was used to elicit reaction times and EEG event-related potentials.

Recordings of spontaneous resting EEG were made while subjects were sitting in a sound-attenuated chamber. Two-min periods of reading were alternated with two-min periods during which the subject sat quietly with eyes closed, until 10-15 min of EEG were recorded. The EEG was recorded from frontal and occipital electrode placements with AG/AgCl disc electrodes referenced to linked ears. Electrooculogram (EOG) was recorded with electrodes pasted above and below the right eye. An electrode on the forehead served as a ground. EEG was amplified 10K and EOG was amplified 2K with amplifiers set at a nominal bandpass of 1-30 Hz (3 dB points of 6 dB/octave rolloff curves). EEG was recorded on a six-channel FM tape recorder. Movement and eye-blink artifact made the reading periods unsuitable for analysis. For this reason only the sections recorded while subjects sat with their eyes closed were analyzed. After editing out eye movement and muscle artifact, 2-3 min of raw EEG from each testing day were entered into a PDP-11/40 computer for fast Fourier analysis.

The fast Fourier (or spectral) analysis provides a detailed mathematical description of the EEG. It quantifies the amount of activity or amplitude at each frequency, resulting in a measure of the contribution (or power) of each frequency component to the total EEG activity. This produced a power spectrum for each sample of EEG with ¼ Hz resolution for the 0-30 Hz components. Pfefferbaum *et al., Electrophysiological Effects of Physostigmine In Humans,* this book, provides a more detailed description of this procedure (see also Matousek, 1973). Most EEG research of this sort reports activity for specified "bands" or sections of the frequency range rather than small (single cycle or less) frequency components. Accordingly, the data were collapsed into measures of the percentage contribution of the 0-4 Hz (delta), 4-8 Hz (theta), 8-12 Hz (alpha), and 12-30 Hz (beta) frequency bands. In addition, a determination was made of the dominant frequency of the occipital alpha activity by identifying the frequency between 8-12 Hz (in ¼ Hz resolution) containing the largest amount of power. This peak alpha frequency measure provides a generalized indication of EEG slowing or activation. One-way analyses of variance were performed for the peak alpha frequency measure, and for the percentage of delta, theta, alpha, and beta activity.

The CNV is a slow, surface-negative, cortical potential that can be recorded from scalp electrodes during the anticipation of certain motor or sensory activities. The development of this slow DC shift depends on the association or contingency of two successive stimuli, and has been related to expectancy, motivation, attention, and arousal (Tecce, 1972). Typically, the CNV is elicited in an experimental paradigm involving a constant-foreperiod reaction-time task, in which a warning signal (S1) is followed after a constant interval by an imperative stimulus (S2) requiring a motor response. The CNV develops over frontal and central cortical areas during the "anticipatory" interval between S1 and S2.

Figure 1 presents a CNV obtained by averaging 32 trials recorded from a subject in this study. The top tracing shows vertical eye movements, with eyeblink activity occurring after S2. The lower tracing shows averaged EEG activity. The peaks occurring 100-400 msec after S1 represent the cortical evoked response to the light flash. Approximately 500 msec after S1, the negative shift of the CNV becomes evident, reaching maximum negativity around S2, and then gradually returning to baseline.

In this experiment, the S1 consisted of a 10-msec light flash (0.85 log foot-lamberts) produced by a PDP-12-controlled Iconix light driver and four fluorescent bulbs installed in a box. One side of the box was made of neutral density glass 31 cm x 36 cm and situated 4 ft from the subject. Each light flash was followed after 1500 msec by the S2, a computer-generated 70 dB sound pressure level (SPL) 1-msec square-wave click, delivered through stereo headphones. Inter-trial intervals (S1 to S1) of 6, 8, 10, and 12 sec were distributed randomly throughout the run. These were used in order to minimize the anticipation of the S1, and to prevent the formation of a CNV prior to S1 onset. The subjects sat in a dimly-lit, sound-attenuated chamber, and were instructed that the light flash was the warning signal, and to press a button as quickly as possible after hearing the click. EEG and EOG were recorded in the same manner as in the spontaneous EEG recording, with the exception that the amplifiers were set at a high frequency bandpass of 100 Hz, and with a 10-sec time constant in order to transmit the slow DC shifts. EEG obtained from the central (Cz) lead and EOG were sampled on-line by a PDP-12 analogue-to-digital converter every 4 msec (250 Hz) for 4000 msec following S1. EEG, EOG, and reaction time (RT) were stored for each S1-S2 sequence for a total of 32 trials.

The amplitude of the CNV was determined by measuring the area under the curve from baseline for activity occurring 1300-1500 msec after S1 onset for each trials. Trials in which eye movements were large enough to saturate the analogue-to-digital converter were not analyzed. The percentage of eye movement activity reflected in the EEG was calculated for each subject, and these were used to subtract eye movement activity from the remaining trials. Trials for which there was no reaction time, and those with reaction times longer than 1000 msec were not used in the analysis.

One-way analyses of variance were performed separately for CNV amplitude and reaction time.

The relationship between CNV amplitude and reaction time was assessed by correlating the CNV amplitude of each trial with the RT of that trial. Single trials from all subjects were combined, and the CNV-RT correlation was determined for the entire group for each day of testing.

RESULTS

Five of the six subjects experienced effects while taking choline chloride. These included vomiting, diarrhea, and dizziness. These side effects were of mild to moderate intensity and generally subsided after a day or two; however, two subjects (not included in this analysis) experienced more severe side effects and withdrew from the study.

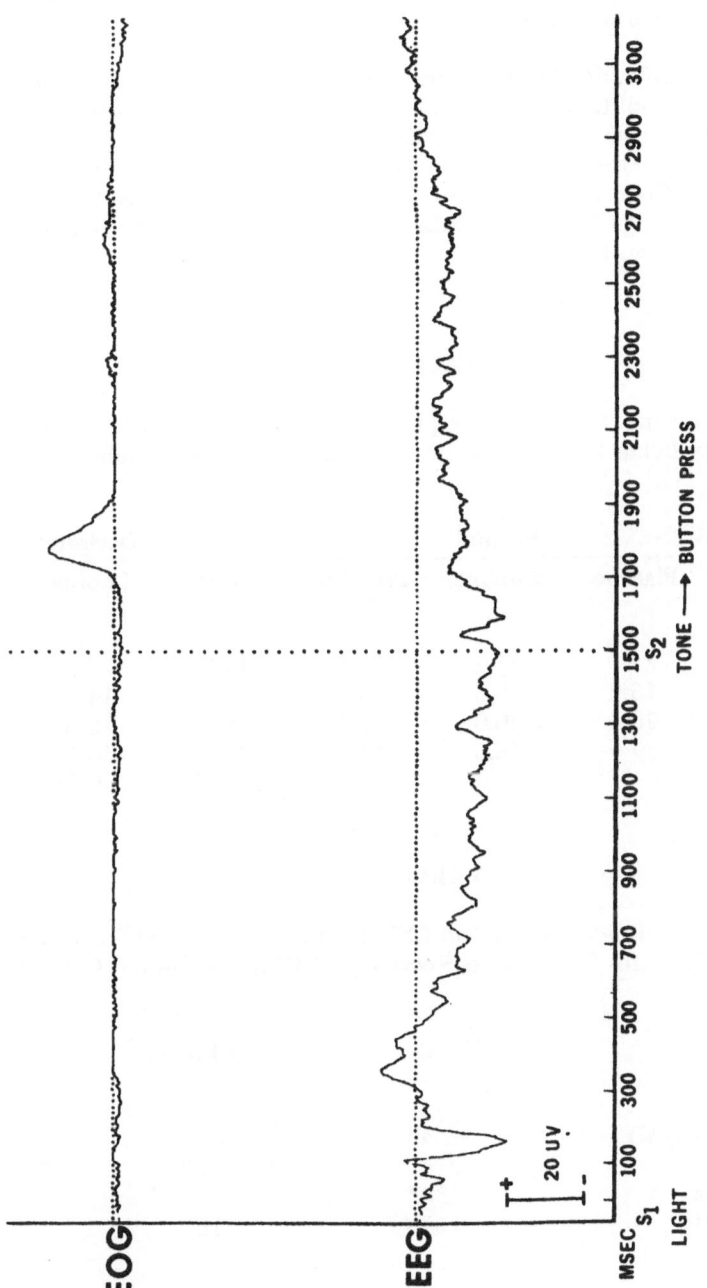

FIGURE 1

Averaged CNV and vertical EOG based on 32 trials.

No significant drug effects were found for the peak alpha frequency measure, or for the percentage of delta, theta, alpha, or beta activity. Table 1 presents group means for these variables for each testing day for frontal and occipital leads.

Neither CNV amplitude nor RT showed significant drug effects. Table 2 shows group means for CNV amplitude and RT, in addition to CNV-RT correlation coefficients. A change was noted in the CNV-RT correlations. Data from the first placebo period produced a significant negative correlation between CNV amplitude and RT. That is, larger negative shifts (CNVs) during the S1-S2 interval were associated with faster RTs. This correlation was not significant during the choline period, but returned to a significant level during the second placebo period.

TABLE 1

Means from Each Testing Day for Peak Alpha Frequency and Percentage of Activity In Four Frequency Bands for Six Subjects Receiving 16 GM/Day Choline Chloride

	Frontal			Occipital		
	Placebo	Choline	Placebo	Placebo	Choline	Placebo
Percentage delta	24.0	25.2	22.4	17.8	20.2	17.6
Percentage theta	16.2	16.6	16.2	13.8	14.4	14.0
Percentage alpha	20.4	20.0	21.4	28.2	26.6	27.8
Percentage beta	39.6	38.6	40.0	39.9	38.7	40.5
Peak a frequency	—	—	—	9.38	9.38	9.33

TABLE 2

Means CNV Amplitude and RT and CNV-RT Correlation Coefficients and Number of Trials for Six Subjects Receiving 16 GM/Day Choline Chloride

	Placebo	Choline	Placebo
Mean CNV amplitude (μV)	-12.4	-15.4	-15.5
Mean RT (msec)	214	227	217
CNV-RT correlations, r =	.230*	.131[n.s.]	.215*
Total number of trials	163	180	162

* $p < .01$

In order to test whether these changes were statistically significant, a z' transform was performed (Edwards, 1967). None of the correlations for the 3 days were found to be significantly different from the others.

Experiment II

The lack of measureable EEG changes in this group of subjects suggested that a longer period of time on the drug might be needed to reveal CNS changes produced by choline. In addition, it was thought that the occurrence of side effects might confound or interfere with the EEG and behavioral responses being measured. It was decided to study a second group of subjects who received the drug over a longer period of time at a lower dosage level.

Five subjects, all female, aged 62-79 (mean age = 67.8 years) participated in this section of the study. One week of placebo was followed by three weeks of choline administration. This was followed by a three-week placebo washout period. Subjects received 8 gm/day of choline (2 gm, 4 times a day). EEG testing was performed during the first placebo period, the first and third weeks of choline, and the last (third) week of the placebo washout period. Subject selection and screening procedures, EEG testing, and data analysis were the same as for the first group of subjects. None of the subjects reported side effects while in this study.

As in the first group of subjects, no changes were found in peak alpha frequency or in the percentage of activity in the 4 frequency bands. Table 3 presents group means for this data for each testing day.

TABLE 3

Means from Each Testing Day for Peak Alpha Frequency and Percentage of Activity In Four Frequency Bands for Five Subjects Receiving 8 GM/Day Choline Chloride

	Frontal				Occipital			
	Placebo	Choline Week 1	Choline Week 3	Placebo	Placebo	Choline Week 1	Choline Week 3	Placebo
Percentage delta	26.7	24.3	24.8	26.3	17.6	17.4	17.6	18.6
Percentage theta	14.0	14.3	14.5	14.4	12.8	12.7	13.3	13.0
Percentage alpha	18.9	19.4	19.0	18.8	23.7	24.8	23.7	25.2
Percentage beta	40.4	42.0	41.8	40.4	46.0	45.0	45.1	43.2
Peak α frequency	—	—	—	—	9.40	9.45	9.25	8.85

No changes were found in CNV amplitude or in RT. Table 4 presents group means for RT and CNV amplitude, in addition to CNV-RT correlation coefficients for each testing day. The CNV-RT correlations showed a pattern similar to that seen in the first group of subjects. A significant correlation was found during the first placebo period. This correlation was lower, though still statistically significant, after the first week of choline. At the end of the third choline week, the correlation was nonsignficant, but again returned to a statistically significant level after the three-week placebo washout period. A z' transform performed on these coefficients revealed a significant difference between the first placebo week and the third choline week ($p < .05$). No other significant differences between the correlations were found.

TABLE 4

Means CNV Amplitude and RT, and CNV-RT Correlation Coefficients and Number of Trials for Five Subjects Receiving 8 GM/Day Choline Chloride

	Placebo	Choline Week 1	Choline Week 3	Placebo
Mean CNV amplitude (μV)	-12.1	-13.4	-12.4	-9.6
Mean RT (msec)	278	245	237	239
CNV-RT correlations, r =	.395***	.194*	.178[n.s.]	.259**
Total number of trials	141	142	143	142

* $p < .05$
** $p < .01$
*** $p < .001$

DISCUSSION

In the present study, oral doses of choline chloride produced no changes in the frequency composition of spontaneous EEG activity. CNV amplitude and reaction time were also unchanged. It should be noted that no cognitive or memory changes were found in these patients (Mohs et al., 1978). This lack of a measurable EEG response may be due to a number of factors. Oral administration may be an inappropriate route for this drug. Pfeiffer et al., (1963) also found no EEG effect of oral choline but changes were reported after i.v. administration (Goldstein and Beck, 1965).

Group sizes were small in this study, and it is possible that significant changes would be more apparent in a larger sample population. There is evidence of considerable individual variation in the response to cholinergic compounds (Davis et al., 1978; Sitaram et al., 1978), in which case it might be necessary to run a large number of subjects in order to identify response patterns.

Choline did alter the relationship between CNV amplitude and reaction time. These two measures generally show low negative correlations (Tecce, 1972). In this study, the significant negative CNV-RT correlations obtained during placebo dropped to non-significant levels during choline administration. After a placebo washout period, the correlations again reached statistical significance. This pattern appeared in both dose groups.

The significance of CNV-RT correlations is unclear. A number of experimental manipulations can cause a dissociation between these two measures (Tecce, 1972). Although both CNV and reaction time are considered to reflect attention, arousal, and motivation, it is possible for one to change without affecting the other. The dissociation found for CNV and RT during choline was not due to measurable changes in either CNV or RT, so the cause of these lower correlations is unclear.

These correlational findings indicate that choline does have some effect on neuro-physiological processes. The lack of measurable EEG alterations in this study, however, and the absence of memory changes in the cognitive project (Mohs et al., 1978) suggest that choline chloride may be an inappropriate compound for investigating the central cholinergic system. It is possible that the doses of choline used in this study were too low to produce significant changes in cholinergic activity. The occurrence of side effects, however, will make it difficult to use higher doses. More promising results have been found with other cholinomimetics, such as physostigmine. At this time, however, a long-acting cholinomimetic appropriate for use with human subjects is not available.

ACKNOWLEDGEMENTS

This research was supported in part by the Medical Research Service of the Veterans Administration and by the National Institute of Mental Health Grant MH-30854 and the National Institute of Drug Abuse Research Grant DA-99854.

REFERENCES

Boyd, W.D., Graham-White, J., Blackwood, G., Glen, I., and McQueen, J., 1977, Clinical effects of choline in Alzheimer senile dementia, *Lancet 2:*711.

Davis, K.L., Mohs, R.C., Tinklenberg, J.R., Pfefferbaum, A., Hollister, L.E., and Kopell, B.S., 1978, Physostigmine: improvement of long-term memory processes in normal humans, *Science* (in press).

Drachman, D.A., Leavitt, J., 1974, Human memory and the cholinergic system, *Arch. Neurol. 30:*113.

Edwards, A.L., 1967, *Statistical Methods,* Holt, Rinehart and Winston, New York.

Fink, M., 1963, Quantitative electroencephalography in human psychopharmacology II: drug patterns, in *EEG and Behavior,* (G. Glaser, ed.), pp. 177, Basic Books, New York.

Goldstein, L., and Beck, R.A., 1965, Amplitude analysis of the electroencephalogram, *Int. Rev. Neurobiol. 8:*265.

Grob, D., Harvey, A.M., Langworthy, O.R., and Lilienthal, J.L., Jr., 1947, The administration of diisopropylfluorophosphate (DFP) to man, III. Effect on the central nervous system with special reference to the electrical activity of the brain, *Bull. Johns Hopkins Hospital 81:*257.

Karczmar, A.G., 1977, Exploitable aspects of central cholinergic functions particularly with respect to the EEG, motor, analgesic, and mental functions, in *Cholinergic Mechanisms and Psychopharmacology*, (D. Jenden, ed.), p. 679, Plenum Press, New York.

Lesny, I., and Vojta, V., 1960, Eserine activation of the EEG in children, *Electroenceph. Clin. Neurophysiol. 12:*742.

Matousek, M., (Ed.), 1973, Frequency and correlation analysis, Part A of *Handbook of Electroencephalography and Clinical Neurophysiology* (A. Remond, ed.), Volume 5: Evaluation of bioelectrical data from brain, nerve, and muscle, Section II (M.A.B. Brazier, and D.A. Walker, eds.), p. 61, Elsevier/North Holland, Amsterdam.

Mohs, R.C., Davis, K.L., Tinklenberg, J.R., Hollister, L.E., Yesavage, J.A., and Kopell, B.S., 1978, Choline chloride treatment of memory deficits in the elderly, (Submitted for publication).

Pfeiffer, C.A., Goldstein, L., Munoz, C., Murphree, H.B., and Jenny, E.J., 1963, Quantitative comparisons of the electroencephalographic stimulant effects of deanol, choline, and amphetamine, *Clin. Pharm. Therapeutics 4:*461.

Reiger, H., and Okonek, S., 1975, The EEG in alkylphosphate poisoning (anticholinesterase insecticides), *Electroenceph. Clin. Neurophysiol. 39:*555.

Rowntree, D.W., Nevin, S., and Wilson, A., 1950, The effects of diisopropylfluorophosphonate in schizophrenia and manic depressive psychosis, *J. Neurol. Neurosurg. Psychiat. 13:*47.

Sitaram, N., Weingartner, H., and Gillin, J.C., 1978, Human serial learning: Enhancement with arecoline and impairment with scopolamine correlated with performance on placebo, *Science* (in press).

Tecce, J.J., 1971, Contingent negative variation and individual differences, *Arch. Gen. Psychiat. 24:*1.

Tecce, J.J., 1972, Contigent negative variation (CNV) and psychological processes in man, *Psychol. Bull. 77:*73.

INTERACTIONS OF BRAIN ACETYLCHOLINE AND OTHER NEUROTRANSMITTERS

THE ROLE OF CHOLINERGIC AND DOPAMINERGIC INTERACTIONS IN DISEASES OF THE CENTRAL NERVOUS SYSTEM

M. H. Van Woert

Departments of Pharmacology and Neurology, Mt. Sinai School of Medicine, City University of New York, New York, N.Y. 10029

INTRODUCTION

Multiple neurons, each of which release different chemicals at their nerve terminals, synapse in the central nervous system (CNS), and pathological changes in the metabolism of one neurotransmitter can alter the release of transmitters from other neurons in the circuit. The most thoroughly investigated example of this phenomenon is the synaptic interaction of nigro-striatal dopaminergic neurons with intrastriatal cholinergic nerve cells. Different types of abnormalities of this pathway have been implicated as causally related to movement disorders such as Parkinson's disease, Huntington's chorea and tardive dyskinesias. Dysfunction of dopaminergic-cholinergic synapses in the limbic system may be relevant to an understanding of the pathophysiology of certain psychiatric disorders. The purpose of this chapter is to summarize our knowledge of the central dopaminergic and cholinergic interactions which may be abnormal in certain types of psychoses and movement disorders.

EXTRAPYRAMIDAL SYSTEM

Neuroanatomy and Neurochemistry

A dopaminergic neuronal pathway with cell bodies in the zona compacta of the substantia nigra projects to the striatum (caudate and putamen) (Figure 1). Dopamine (DA), released from these nigro-striatal nerve terminals, has been found to inhibit the neuronal discharge frequency of some neurons in the striatum and facilitate others (Bloom *et al.*, 1965; McLennan and York, 1967; Connor, 1970). The released DA reacts with receptor sites on the post synaptic neurons. There appears to be at least two topographically, pharmacologically and functionally distinct types of DA-sensitive sites in the striatum: an inhibition mediating DA receptor and an excitation-mediating DA receptor (Cools *et al.*, 1975). It has been possible to further define the characteristics of DA receptors by measuring the binding of radioactively labelled DA and haloperidol to those receptors. These studies reveal that dopaminergic receptors can exist in two states or perhaps in two separate forms, one with a high affinity for ^{3}H DA (agonist) and another with a high affinity for ^{3}H haloperidol (antagonist) (Creese *et al.*, 1975).

Some but not all of the DA receptors in the striatum are linked with DA-sensitive adenylate cyclase (Clement-Cormier *et al.*, 1974). Dopamine stimulates adenylate cyclase activity which increases adenosine $3'$ $5'$ monophosphate (cyclic AMP) formation; cyclic AMP is believed to mediate the depolarization or hyperpolarization of these particular neurons (Greengard, 1974). Apparently other neurons respond to DA by a mechanism which is unrelated to cyclic AMP. At present the relationship of these different types of DA receptors to synapses involved in various neurological and psychiatric disorders is not clear.

Most of the neurons intrinsic to the striatum are either cholinergic or GABAergic (see Figure 1). Cholinergic cell bodies, axons and nerve endings have been visualized in the striatum of the rat using an immunohistochemical localization technique for choline acetyltransferase (McGeer *et al.*, 1975). Dopamine receptors are thought to be present on the dendrites and cell bodies. of the striatal cholinergic and/or GABAergic neurons. The cholinergic intrastriatal neurons are particularly responsive to DA released by the nigrostriatal nerve terminals. DA receptor agonists and antagonists alter the synthesis and release of acetylcholine (ACh) from these intrastriatal neurons. Initially, chronic administration of L-DOPA was observed to increase whole rat brain ACh concentration (Sethy and Van Woert, 1973a). Subsequently DA receptor agonists (apomorphine, amphetamine, trivastal, L-DOPA + the peripheral decarboxylase inhibitor, carbidopa) were found to increase ACh in the striatum of the rat brain presumably by inhibiting the neuronal discharge frequency and release of ACh from the intrastriatal cholinergic neurons (Sethy and Van Woert, 1974a; Sethy and Van Woert, 1974b; Consolo *et al.*, 1974). Dopamine receptor blocking agents (phenothiazines and butyrophenones) have the opposite effects on striatal ACh. Dopamine receptor blocking agents also have been shown to increase the turnover (Trabucchi *et al.*, 1974) and release (Stadler *et al.*, 1973) of ACh in the striatum. The DA-induced changes in the activity of the striatal cholinergic neurons may be mediated through cyclic AMP since the intraventricular administration of dibutyryl cyclic AMP prior to chlorpromazine administration prevented the decrease in striatal ACh concentration (Harris *et al.*, 1977).

There are cholinergic neuronal projections into the striatum from the cerebral cortex (Mitchell, 1963) and from the thalamus (Simke and Saelens, 1977). These projections may be predominantly stimulatory since ACh infused locally increases the activity of some caudate neurons; this effect is reduced by microiontophoretically applied DA (Salmoiraghi *et al.*, 1965) suggesting that functionally antagonistic cholinergic and dopaminergic receptor sites might exist on the same striatal neuron. Striatal DA-ACh balance is regulated by several feedback mechanisms. Blockade of DA receptors by chlorpromazine and butyrophenones increases the discharge frequency and DA turnover in the nigrostriatal neurons (Anden *et al.*, 1969; Nyback and Sedvall, 1969), whereas DA agonists induce feedback inhibition of these neurons (Nyback *et al.*, 1970; Bunney *et al.*, 1973). These effects of DA agonists and antagonists on the nigrostriatal neurons are mediated by one or more striatonigral pathways. A cholinergic feedback projection from the striatum to the substantia nigra, which regulates the activity of the nigrostriatal pathway, has been postulated. This striatonigral cholinergic projection may be stimulatory since cholinergic drugs such as oxotremorine, physostigmine and pilocarpine increase

DA synthesis in the striatum whereas ACh receptor blockers like atropine reduce striatal DA turnover (O'Keefe *et al.*, 1970; Anden and Bedard, 1971; Bowers and Roth, 1972).

It has also been postulated that some of the intrastriatal cholinergic neurons also contribute to the regulation of the nigrostriatal dopaminergic neurons. Recent work has shown that ACh enhances the release of DA from rat striatal slices presumably by stimulating cholinergic presynaptic receptors of both nicotinic and muscarinic types on dopaminergic nerve terminals (Giorguieff *et al.*, 1977).

There is also an inhibitory feedback pathway, originating in the caudate nucleus and terminating in the substantia nigra which is mediated by gamma-aminobutyric acid (GABA) (Kim *et al.*, 1971; Kataoka *et al.*, 1974; Feltz, 1971). Electrical stimulation of the caudate nucleus inhibits the discharge frequency of the nigrostriatal neurons; this effect is blocked by GABA receptor blocking agents (Precht and Yoshida, 1971). There is also experimental evidence suggesting an additional inhibitory GABAergic feedback pathway arising from the globus pallidus and terminating in the substantia nigra (Hattori *et al.*, 1973). Recently it has been observed that GABAergic neurons may also directly influence dopaminergic nerve terminals within the caudate nucleus (Cheramy *et al.*, 1977). Intrastriatal neurons may release GABA which reacts with GABAergic receptors localized on nigrostriatal nerve terminals and inhibit DA release. Therefore GABAergic feedback inhibition of striatal DA release is localized at both the nigrostriatal cell body and nerve terminal. GABA also is the neurotransmitter of neurons projecting from the striatum to the globus pallidus.

Our understanding of the neurochemistry of this region of the brain is far from complete. Preliminary observations indicate that DA and ACh metabolism in the substantia nigra and striatum are influenced by multiple other putative neurotransmitters. For example, neurons containing substance P (Hokfelt *et al.*, 1975; Duffy *et al.*, 1975) and serotonin (Palkovits *et al.*, 1974a; Dray *et al.*, 1976) have been identified in the substantia nigra, but the synaptic interactions of these neurons have not yet been well defined. Conrad *et al.*, (1974) suggest that a serotoninergic neuronal pathway projects from the B8 raphe region to the substantia nigra. Lesions of B8 area decrease striatal ACh synthesis suggesting that the B8 serotoninergic projection stimulates nigrostriatal neurons, which in turn inhibit cholinergic neurons (Butcher *et al.*, 1976).

In summary, DA released from nigrostriatal neurons regulates ACh synthesis and release in the striatum. There are also intrinsic and extrinsic feedback mechanisms, many still poorly understood, which modulate this DA-ACh interaction. The next section will attempt to relate our limited understanding of this region of the brain to the pathogenesis of Parkinson's disease, tardive dyskinesias and Huntington's chorea.

PARKINSON'S DISEASE

The major symptoms of parkinsonism consist of akinesia, rigidity, resting tremor, and loss of postural reflexes. Although most cases are idiopathic, some of the etiologies of parkinsonism are known, eg. postencephalitis, neuroleptic drug therapy (eg. reserpine, phenothiazines, butyrophenones) and chronic manganese poisoning. The major breakthrough in our understanding of the pathogenesis of Parkinson's disease occurred in 1960 when Hornykiewicz found that the concentration of DA was markedly decreased in the striatum and globus pallidus in the brains of parkinsonian patients (Ehringer and Horny-kiewicz, 1960). Subsequently, it was discovered that the enzymes necessary for DA synthesis, tyrosine hydroxylase and dopa decarboxylase, were also decreased in parkin-sonian brains (Lloyd *et al.*, 1973). The deficiency in brain DA synthesis is attributed to the degeneration of nigrostriatal dopaminergic neurons which is the most consistent pathological finding in this disease. These findings led to the successful therapy of Parkin-son's disease with L-DOPA, the precursor of DA (Barbeau, 1961; Birkmayer and Horny-kiewicz, 1961; Cotzias *et al.*, 1967) and more recently with the DA receptor agonist bromocriptine, (Calne *et al.*, 1974). Presumably the anti-parkinsonian action of L-DOPA is due to its decarboxylation to form DA which stimulates DA receptor sites.

In drug-induced parkinsonism, akinesia, rigidity and tremor are due to the blockade of DA receptors in the striatum by neuroleptic drugs such as phenothiazines and butyrophenones (van Rossum, 1966). The net effect in idiopathic and drug-induced parkinsonism is a deficiency of DA at the receptor sites in the striatum. Since DA inhibits ACh synthesis and release in the striatum, a hyperfunctioning striatal cholinergic system should exist in parkinsonism, and in fact this is the case. Therefore anticholinergic drugs are also potent anti-parkinsonian agents. In fact, antimuscarinic drugs are the treatment of choice for drug-induced parkinsonism (Sheppard and Merlis, 1967). The neuroleptic drugs which have minimal or no parkinsonian side effects (eg. clozapine, thioridazine) have very potent antimuscarinic actions and thereby counteract the extrapyramidal side effects of DA receptor blockade in the striatum (Miller and Hilley, 1974).

There is now a very extensive literature supporting the hypothesis that parkinsonian symptoms are related to excessive cholinergic and/or deficient dopaminergic activity in the striatum. Extrapyramidal tremor has been induced in animals by creating an imbalance of ACh-DA levels in the striatum. For example, direct injection of cholinergic agents (ACh, carbachol, oxotremorine) into the caudate nuclei of cats produces tremor which is due to stimulation of muscarinic ACh receptors (Baker *et al.*, 1969). This tremor was diminished by intracaudate injection of DA as well as muscarinic receptor blocking agents. Nashold (1959) performed a similar experiment in humans. He injected ACh directly into the globus pallidus of parkinsonian patients during stereotaxic procedures and observed an increase in tremor, whereas injection of anticholinergic drugs into the same area reduced the tremor.

Intraperitoneal injection of oxotremorine, a cholinergic agonist, as well as physostig-mine, a cholinesterase inhibitor, also produces tremor in animals and there is a correlation between the increase in brain ACh and the tremors; the tremors and elevated ACh levels are inhibited by antimuscarinic agents like atropine or agents that interfere with ACh synthesis, eg. hemicholinium-3 and triethylcholine (Sethy and Van Woert, 1973b; Cho *et al.*, 1962; Holmstedt and Lundgren, 1966).

Phenothiazines (which block DA receptors) and reserpine (which depletes brain DA) increase the tremorigenic potency of physostigmine in the rat (Ambani and Van Woert, 1972). Similarly, physostigmine aggravates parkinsonian neurological signs in dogs whose catecholamine-containing neurons were destroyed by intracisternal injections of 6-hydroxydopamine (Van Woert *et al.*, 1972). L-DOPA inhibits the tremorigenic action of physostigmine in animals pretreated with either 6-hydroxydopamine or phenothiazines (Ambani and Van Woert, 1972; Van Woert *et al.*, 1972). As previously described, striatal ACh turnover is controlled by nigrostriatal dopaminergic input. Nigrostriatal degeneration or blockade of DA receptor sites by neuroleptic drugs increases ACh turnover which may be responsible for parkinsonian symptoms, particularly tremor. Further elevation of striatal ACh, such as by administration of physostigmine which inhibits ACh breakdown, increases the severity of the parkinsonian symptoms.

Similar investigations can be carried out in patients with parkinsonism. Intravenous injections of 1 mg of physostigmine aggravate tremor and rigidity in idiopathic and drug-induced parkinsonism but has no effect in normal subjects (Duvoisin, 1967; Weintraub and Van Woert, 1971; Ambani *et al.*, 1973). L-DOPA blocks the tremorigenic action of physostigmine in idiopathic Parkinson's disease, just as it does in the dog pretreated with intracisternal 6-hydroxydopamine.

Since the activities of choline acetyltransferase and cholinesterase are normal in the parkinsonian brain (McGeer and McGeer, 1971), the most reasonable interpretation is that the DA deficiency produces a functional change in striatal ACh metabolism in Parkinson's disease. The decreased input of DA into the striatum due to either degeneration of the nigrostriatal pathway in idiopathic Parkinson's disease or blockade of DA receptors by neuroleptic drugs sensitizes humans to the tremorigenic action of physostigmine. In other words, the pharmacologically demonstrated functional hyperactivity of the cholinergic system is secondary to DA deficiency in parkinsonism.

TARDIVE DYSKINESIAS AND HUNTINGTON'S CHOREA

These two neurological disorders consist of hyperactive involuntary movements which have gross similarities in appearance. There is considerable data from animal and human pharmacological studies that abnormal DA-ACh interactions must be involved in the pathophysiology of these hyperactive involuntary movements. Beneficial clinical responses to DA antagonists and ACh agonists in both disorders suggest that an excessive dopaminergic activity and a depressed cholinergic activity, presumably in the striatum, exist in both tardive dyskinesias and Huntington's chorea.

Tardive Dyskinesias

The involuntary movements found in tardive dyskinesias usually involve predominantly the face, mouth, lips and tongue. There may be grimacing, lip smacking, protruding and twisting tongue movements commonly called the buccolingualmasticatory syndrome. Choreo-athetoid movements of the trunk and extremities may also be present. Tardive dyskinesias are a complication of long-term neuroleptic drug therapy, most frequently phenothiazines and butyrophenones. Although tardive dyskinesias may subside months after discontinuing neuroleptic drug therapy, they frequently can be persistent and irreversible. Typically tardive dyskinesias are aggravated, or first appear, after the reduction or discontinuance of a neuroleptic drug.

Neuroleptic drugs block striatal DA receptors producing a chemical form of denervation. Tardive dyskinesias are thought to be caused by a supersensitivity of striatal DA receptors secondary to this chemical denervation. Dopamine receptor supersensitivity has been demonstrated in numerous animal models after chronic administration of neuroleptic drugs or lesions of the nigrostriatal pathway (Klawans and Rubovits, 1972a; Fjalland and Möller-Nielsen, 1974; Tarsy and Baldessarini, 1974; Moore and Thornburg,

1975; Von Voigtlander et al., 1975; Sayers et al., 1975). The postsynaptic DA receptors in the corpus striatum become supersensitive to DA agonists after prolonged removal of their normal stimulation. Stereotyped oral movements, analogous to human orofacial dyskinesia, can be produced in rodents by injection of large doses of drugs which enhance striatal dopaminergic activity (eg. amphetamine, methylphenidate, apomorphine).

Rubovits and Klawans (1972) demonstrated that these stereotyped oral movements would occur in guinea pigs after much lower doses of amphetamine if the animals were pretreated for several weeks with chlorpromazine. Presumably the oral dyskinesias result from amphetamine-induced stimulation of striatal DA receptors made supersensitive by chronic chlorpromazine administration. Fjalland and Möller-Nielsen (1974) observed that following chronic administration of haloperidol, methylphenidate-induced gnawing occurred at lower doses than required in control mice. Dyskinesias can be produced in monkeys by pretreatment with 6-hydroxydopamine followed by administration of small doses of L-DOPA, or just by giving large doses of L-DOPA alone (Ng et al., 1973).

Dopamine receptor supersensitivity could be due to an increased number of DA receptors. This hypothesis is supported by some recent studies of Creese et al., (1977). They observed that ^{3}H haloperidol binding to rat striatal DA receptors increased in rats following lesions of the nigrostriatal DA pathway. This increased number of DA receptors could account for the behavioral supersensitivity to DA agonists which results from the lesion. A similar increase in striatal DA sites, assayed using ^{3}H haloperidol, can be demonstrated in rats after chronic treatment with the neuroleptic drugs haloperidol, fluphenazine and reserpine (Burt et al., 1977).

In patients, drugs which enhance brain DA activity (amphetamine, methylphenidate, L-DOPA) exacerbate tardive dyskinesias (Klawans and McKendall, 1971; Marsden et al., 1975) providing further evidence that tardive dyskinesias are due to DA hyperactivity. L-DOPA dyskinesias which are similar in appearance to tardive dyskinesias occur in parkinsonian patients treated with large doses of L-DOPA. L-DOPA dyskinesias do not occur in non-parkinsonian patients (Barbeau et al., 1971) suggesting that denervation supersensitivity of the striatal DA receptors due to nigrostriatal degeneration in Parkinson's disease may be an essential requirement. Dopamine supersensitivity in tardive dyskinesias would explain why a reduction in the dose of a neuroleptic drug worsens symptoms while a dose increase temporarily reverses motor abnormalities. Although tardive dyskinesias may improve if the neuroleptic drug is increased this therapeutic approach is risky since it perpetuates the pathophysiological mechanisms which produced tardive dyskinesia in the first place. Other therapeutic agents such as reserpine and tetrabenazine, which deplete brain DA, improve tardive dyskinesias and have been useful therapeutic agents for some patients (Sato et al., 1971; Kazamatsuri et al., 1972). Alpha methyl-paratyrosine (AMPT), which reduces DA by inhibiting its synthesis, also ameliorates tardive dyskinesias (Gerlach et al., 1974).

From the previous discussion of the neurochemistry of the striatum one might infer that increased striatal dopaminergic activity secondary to supersensitive striatal DA receptors would produce an inhibition of striatal ACh synthesis and release. There is some direct evidence consistent with that corollary in both animal and human studies. The DA agonist, apomorphine, induces turning away from the side of a unilateral lesion of the substantia nigra in rats, by directly stimulating supersensitive striatal DA receptors on the side of the lesion (Ungerstedt, 1971). Apomorphine-induced turning, in unilateral nigrostriatal lesioned animals, is inhibited by the cholinomimetic agent oxotremorine (Kelly and Miller, 1974). Striatal cholinergic stimulation by oxotremorine may balance or antagonize dopaminergic hyperactivity on the side of the lesion in this situation. Furthermore, in an animal model of tardive dyskinesia induced in guinea pigs by intrastriatal injection of DA, cholinergic agents such as physostigmine abolished dyskinetic oral movements (Costall and Naylor, 1975). These findings are consistent with the clinical observation that anticholinergic drugs exacerbate or may rarely even induce tardive dyskinesia (Gerlach et al., 1974; Klawans and Rubovits, 1974; Birket-Smith, 1974).

The most recent promising therapeutic approach to tardive dyskinesias has been the attempt to treat them with drugs that increase the levels of ACh in the striatum. The results have been encouraging. Initially, physostigmine, an anticholinesterase which increases brain ACh, was tried with early reports of improvement in tardive dyskinesias by some investigators (Gerlach et al., 1974; Klawans and Rubovits, 1974; Fann et al., 1975a) but not by others (Tarsy et al., 1974). Next precursors of ACh were tested. 2-dimethylaminoethanol (deanol, Deaner), the immediate precursor of choline (DuVigneaud et al., 1946) was reported to improve tardive dyskinesias by some investigators (Casey and Denney, 1974; Miller et al., 1974; Fann et al., 1975b; DeSilva and Huang, 1975) but not by others (Davis et al., 1977; Escobar and Kemp, 1975; Klawans et al., 1975). Deanol crosses the blood-brain barrier (Groth et al., 1958) and has been reported to increase ACh concentration in the brain (Re 1974; Haubrich et al., 1975; Goldberg and Silbergeld, 1974). However, other investigators have been unable to confirm this deanol-induced increase in ACh (Pepeu et al., 1960; Zahniser et al., 1977).

The most rational and successful therapeutic trial of an ACh precursor has been the use of choline. Plasma choline is a precursor of ACh synthesized in the brain (Haubrich et al., 1972; Jenden et al., 1974). Choline injected intraperitoneally into rats and guinea pigs has been shown to increase brain choline and ACh (Cohen and Wurtman, 1975; Haubrich et al., 1975). In a study of four patients with tardive dyskinesias Davis et al., (1975, 1976) observed significant improvement in four of them during treatment with up to 20 g of oral choline daily. This therapeutic usefulness of choline in tardive dyskinesias has been confirmed by Growdon et al., (1977b).

Huntington's Chorea

Huntington's chorea is an autosomal dominant genetic disease in which chorea and dementia develop at an average age of 44 years. Pathological changes consist of a loss of small neurons in the striatum and additional degenerative changes in the cerebral cortex, globus pallidus and subthalamic nuclei (Bruyn, 1968).

Changes in the concentrations of neurotransmitters have been reported in the basal ganglia of patients who died with Huntington's chorea (Bird and Iversen, 1974; Stahl and Swanson, 1974; Enna et al., 1976; Perry et al., 1973). GABA and the activity of its synthetic enzyme glutamic acid decarboxylase (GAD) were consistently reduced in the caudate, putamen, globus pallidus and substantia nigra of the Huntington's chorea brain (Perry et al., 1973; Bird and Iversen, 1974; Stahl and Swanson, 1974; Bird et al., 1973). These results suggest that many of the neurons in the striatum and globus pallidus which degenerate in Huntington's chorea are GABAergic neurons. There is also degeneration of some striatal cholinergic neurons since choline acetyltransferase (CAT) was slightly reduced in the caudate nucleus in some cases and markedly reduced in the putamen (Bird and Iversen, 1974; Stahl and Swanson, 1974; McGeer et al., 1973). The nigrostriatal neurons remain intact since tyrosine hydroxylase activities and DA concentrations were normal in Huntington's chorea except for the smaller subgroup with rigidity (Westphal variant) who had significantly higher brain DA concentrations (Bird and Iversen, 1974).

Serotonin receptor binding and muscarinic receptor binding were reduced in the caudate nucleus, putamen and globus pallidus in Huntington's chorea (Wastek et al., 1976; Hiley and Bird, 1974). A significant reduction in DA receptor binding sites was found in the caudate nucleus, putamen and frontal cortex of Huntington's chorea brains (Reisine et al., 1977). However, receptor binding of GABA and β-adrenergic agents were not significantly altered (Enna et al., 1976). These findings suggest that a significant portion of muscarinic cholinergic, dopaminergic and serotoninergic synaptic receptors in the striatum are located on GABAergic and/or cholinergic neurons which degenerate in Huntington's chorea.

The abnormal movements of Huntington's chorea are improved by drugs which interfere with the action of DA in the basal ganglia such as reserpine, phenothiazines, butyrophenones and AMPT. On the other hand, L-DOPA and d-amphetamine aggravate chorea and hyperkinesia presumably by increasing DA activity within the basal ganglia (Klawans and Weiner, 1974). The results of these therapeutic trials suggest that the neurological signs in Huntington's chorea may be related to a relative or absolute hyperactivity of the nigrostriatal dopaminergic input or a supersensitivity of striatal DA receptors. The degeneration of the inhibitory GABAergic striatonigral feedback pathway in Huntington's chorea might be one mechanism which enhances striatal DA turnover and release in this disease (see Figure 1).

There are animal data to support the hypothesis that excessive striatal DA receptor stimulation can produce choreoathetoid movements. For, example, administration of L-DOPA to monkeys with bilateral caudate lesions produces choreiform movements (Sax et al., 1973). Cools (1972) produced choreoathetoid hyperkinesia in cats by unilateral injections of either L-DOPA, DA, 3-methoxy-tyramine or dextroamphetamine into the caudate nucleus.

Increased striatal DA release would be expected to reduce the discharge frequency of intrastriatal cholinergic neurons in this disease. Furthermore, the biochemical studies of the autopsied brains of patients with Huntington's chorea suggest that there is a loss of some cholinergic neurons in the striatum. For these reasons clinical trials of drugs known to raise brain ACh have been undertaken in patients with Huntington's disease. Initially, the cholinesterase inhibitor, physostigmine, was tried by several investigators and the responses have been equivocal (Klawans and Rubovits, 1972b; Tarsy et al., 1973; Aquilonius and Sjostrum, 1971). Deanol was also tried with some limited improvement (Walker et al., 1973). Another approach initiated by Davis et al., (1976) is to increase brain ACh in Huntington's chorea by administering its precursor choline. Their preliminary studies indicate that oral choline chloride significantly reduced the abnormal movements associated with Huntington's chorea in two of four patients. Growdon

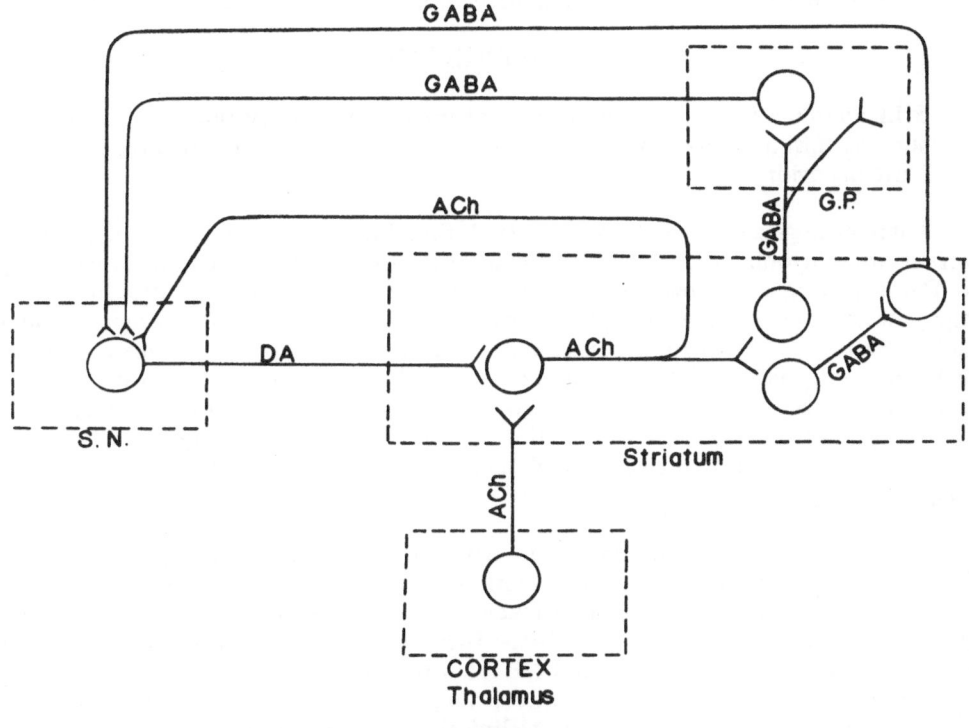

FIGURE 1

Monoamine Interactions in the Basal Ganglia. Abbreviations used: S.N. = substantia nigra, G.P. = globus pallidus, GABA = gamma-amino butyric acid, DA = dopamine, ACh = acetylcholine.

et al., (1977a) reported that oral choline produced transient improvement in speech, balance and gait in some patients with Huntington's disease but the response was not consistent or lasting. The deficiency of CAT and muscarinic receptor sites in this disease might account for the limited effectiveness of precursor therapy.

The degeneration of GABAergic neurons in Huntington's chorea suggests that therapy with drugs that enhance this neurotransmitter might afford symptomatic improvement. In general, however, administration of GABA (Barbeau, 1973), GABA-mimetics (Barbeau, 1973; Fisher *et al.*, 1974; Shoulson *et al.*, 1977; Shoulson *et al.*, 1975) and inhibitors of GABA transaminase (Shoulson *et al.*, 1975; Shoulson *et al.*, 1976) have yielded disappointing results in Huntington's chorea.

In summary, available data suggests that there is degeneration of GABA containing neurons and to a lesser extent cholinergic neurons in the striatum in Huntington's chorea. The loss of GABA inhibition of the nigrostriatal pathway would increase DA release and secondarily inhibit the remaining intrastriatal cholinergic neurons. This is the rationale for the three major pharmacological approaches to the treatment of Huntington's chorea, namely 1) DA receptor blockers, 2) cholinergic agents and 3) GABA receptor stimulants.

SCHIZOPHRENIA

Schizophrenia is a psychotic disorder of unknown etiology presenting with symptoms such as misinterpretation of reality, delusions, hallucinations, apathy, withdrawal and bizarre behavior.

Pharmacological studies have suggested that brain DA metabolism also may be aberrant in schizophrenia. All of the clinically effective antipsychotic drugs except the DA depleting agent reserpine possess DA receptor-blocking activity. In fact the antipsychotic potency of neuroleptic drugs seems to parallel their DA receptor binding affinity (Seeman et al., 1976; Creese et al., 1976). In contrast, phenothiazine compounds which lack antipsychotic efficacy do not affect the DA system (Anden et al., 1964; Roos, 1965). Carlsson et al., (1972) observed that the antipsychotic effects of neuroleptics could be potentiated by co-administration of alpha-methyl-p-tyrosine (AMPT), a drug which inhibits tyrosine hydroxylase and thereby reduces the synthesis of DA and norepinephrine (NE).

If DA receptor blocking agents are anti-schizophrenic, then dopamine agonists might be expected to have a psychomimetic effect. In fact, this is true. A large single dose of amphetamine is capable of producing the symptomatology of paranoid schizophrenia in normal subjects (Connell, 1958; Griffith et al., 1972; Angrist and Gershon, 1970). Amphetamine releases DA and NE from presynaptic nerve terminals and blocks their reuptake. Chronic administration of cocaine, another drug which blocks the neuronal reuptake of DA and NE, also produces a clinical state virtually identical to amphetamine psychosis or acute paranoid schizophrenia (Mayer-Gross, 1960). Furthermore, amphetamine and other drugs which enhance dopaminergic neurotransmission (eg. L-DOPA and methylphenidate) will exacerbate the psychotic symptomatology of schizophrenic patients. All of these observations have led to the speculation that schizophrenia is associated with a hyperactivity of dopaminergic neurons (Matthysse, 1973; Snyder et al., 1974). Thus it would appear that DA-containing neurons are not only involved in extrapyramidal function but also in mental behavior. Are we dealing with the same dopaminergic pathway? We don't know.

Both the corpus striatum and the limbic system have been discussed as possible neuroanatomical sites of the pathophysiology of schizophrenia.

Corpus Striatum

Mettler first described a disturbance of visual and auditory perception in cats produced by lesions of the striatum (Mettler, 1965; Mettler and Mettler, 1942). On the basis of these observations he proposed the hypothesis that in schizophrenia there might exist a disturbed function of the striatum.

Amphetamine-induced stereotypy in animals has been thought to be analogous to amphetamine psychosis and certain schizophrenic symptoms in man (Snyder et al., 1974). Injections of amphetamine and apomorphine produce stereotyped behavior (continuous sniffing, gnawing, licking and biting) in rats by enhancing dopaminergic activity in the neostriatum (Munkvad *et al.*, 1968; Ernst, 1967). Antipsychotic drugs, which block DA receptors in the brain (Munkvad *et al.*, 1968; van Rossum, 1966) have an antistereotypic potency which correlates with the therapeutic effects of these agents in schizophrenia (Janssen *et al.*, 1967; Munkvad *et al.*, 1968; van Rossum, 1966).

Since there is a DA-ACh interaction in the striatum, stereotypy like extrapyramidal signs also should be modified by drugs which act on the cholinergic system. As might have been anticipated, stereotyped behavior induced by amphetamine and apomorphine is potentiated by anticholinergic drugs and antagonized by cholinergic drugs such as physostigmine (Arnfred and Randrup, 1968; Scheel-Kruger, 1970). Anticholinergic drugs given alone did not produce compulsive gnawing behavior, but combined administration of anticholinergic drugs and a small ineffective dose of apomorphine produced a very high gnawing intensity. The relevance of this animal model to human schizophrenia can be seriously questioned, and recently greater emphasis has been placed on the possible involvement of the limbic system in abnormal behavior such as schizophrenia.

Limbic System

Both human and animal studies have linked schizophrenia to abnormal functioning of the limbic system. For example, schizophrenia-like symptoms are observed in cases of known limbic-system dysfunction such as can occur in temporal lobe epilepsy, encephalitis and brain tumors involving limbic structures (Torrey and Petersen, 1974). Furthermore, signs of limbic system dysfunction such as electrical abnormalities recorded from electrodes implanted in limbic structures have been reported in schizophrenic patients (Torrey and Petersen, 1974). In animals, ablation of the limbic system produces profound changes in behavior and an impairment in the animal's ability to screen out multiple visual stimuli.

Dopaminergic neurons with cell bodies dorsocranial to the interpeduncular region in the ventral mesencephalon (A10) project to the limbic system including the nucleus accumbens, the central amygdaloid nucleus and the olfactory tubercle (Anden *et al.*, 1966). Dopamine has an inhibitory action on some neurons in the limbic system. Aghajanian and Bunney (1974) have demonstrated that DA, iontophoresed on olfactory tubercle cells, inhibited their discharge frequency. Phenothiazines and butyrophenones block this effect of DA in proportion to their clinical efficacy in treating schizophrenia.

One action of DA in the limbic system is to increase locomotor activity. Direct injection of DA into the nucleus accumbens enhances locomotor activity in rats (Pijnenburg and van Rossum, 1973). This effect is antagonized by pretreatment with the DA receptor antagonist haloperidol. Psychomotor stimulant drugs like amphetamine may stimulate motor activity through a dopaminergic mechanism in the nucleus accumbens. Injection of haloperidol bilaterally into the nucleus accumbens antagonizes the stimulation of locomotor activity following intraperitoneal injection of d-amphetamine (Pijnenburg *et al.*, 1975). Thus it is apparent that amphetamine has an action on both the limbic system as well as the striatum, producing behavioral changes which are specific to each brain region.

Some investigators have explored the possibility that a comparison of the effect of neuroleptic drugs on DA metabolism in the limbic system and striatum might determine their ratio of antipsychotic to extrapyramidal potency and localize the major site of action of each drug (Anden and Stock, 1973; Carlsson, 1974). They proposed that the extrapyramidal side effects of neuroleptic drugs might be due to blockade of DA receptors in the striatum and the antipsychotic action due to DA receptor blockade in the limbic system.

Antipsychotics (eg. chlorpromazine, clozapine and haloperidol) increase the turn-over rate of DA in the caudate nucleus and nucleus accumbens resulting in a higher level of the DA metabolites homovanillic acid (HVA) and dihydroxyphenylacetic acid (DOPAC) in these nuclei (Zivkovic et al., 1975). Anden (1972) and Anden and Stock (1973) reported a greater increase of HVA content in the limbic regions compared to the striatum of rabbit brain after treatment with clozapine, an antipsychotic drug which produces little or no extrapyramidal side effects in man. In contrast, haloperidol produced an identical increase of HVA in the 2 regions. The relative increase of DA metabolites in the limbic system compared to the neostriatum after administration of clozapine, chlorpromazine and haloperidol has not been consistent in subsequent studies (Anden and Stock, 1973; Wiesel and Sedvall, 1975; Waldmeier and Maitre, 1976; Wilk et al., 1975). For example Wiesel and Sedvall (1975) observed the opposite effects in rats, i.e. a greater increase in HVA in the striatum than in the limbic system with clozapine as well as with chlorpromazine and haloperidol. It would appear that these discrepancies are related to species differences and differences in experimental protocol. Therefore it is unlikely that the antipsychotic efficacy of a drug can be determined by measuring the ratio of DA turnover in the limbic versus striatal regions. Furthermore, recent evidence strongly suggests that the propensity of a neuroleptic drug to produce extrapyramidal side effects is inversely proportional to its antimuscarinic action (Miller and Hilley, 1974). Clozapine and thioridazine which produce very few extrapyramidal side effects are potent antimuscarinic agents and have the greatest affinity for the muscarinic cholinergic receptor in the brain of any of the other neuroleptic drugs.

There is evidence for a functionally important DA-ACh interaction in the limbic system which has many similarities to that occurring in the striatum. Both the nucleus accumbens and the tuberculum olfactorum have been found to be rich in ACh and the enzymes CAT and acetylcholinesterase (AChE) (Jacobowitz and Palkovits, 1974; Palkovits et al., 1974b; Koslow et al., 1974) suggesting a dense cholinergic innervation. The numbers of cholinergic muscarinic receptors, determined by radioautographic localization of the muscarinic antagonist [3]H 3-quinuclidinyl benzilate (^{3}H QNB) was about the same or slightly higher in the nucleus accumbens compared to the striatum (Kuhar and Yamamura, 1976). Just as has been observed in the striatum, haloperidol and chlorpromazine increase ACh turnover in the nucleus accumbens (Marco et al., 1976). Therefore limbic dopaminergic neurons may inhibit the metabolism of ACh in cholinergic postsynaptic interneurons in the limbic system as well as in the striatum. This interaction of DA and ACh in the limbic system may be as relevant to the pathophysiology of schizophrenia as striatal DA-ACh balance is to extrapyramidal function. However the evidence for DA-ACh dysfunction in schizophrenia is much more circumstantial and preliminary compared to our knowledge of the extrapyramidal system.

Antimuscarinic drugs can produce a toxic confusional state characterized by disorientation, agitation, visual and auditory hallucinations, loss of short term memory, and agitation characteristic of an organic brain syndrome. Gershon (1960) believes that the anticholinergic drug N-ethyl-3-piperdyl cyclopentylphenylglycolate (Ditran) produces schizophrenic-like symptomatology and exacerbates schizophrenia in some patients. Aggravation of schizophrenia by antimuscarinic agents also has been observed by others (El-Yousef *et al.*, 1973; Singh and Kay, 1975; Singh and Smith, 1973). However, other investigators have reported that anticholinergic drugs do not reduce the antipsychotic action of phenothiazines and butyrophenones (Chien and DiMascio, 1967). On the other hand, drugs which stimulate central cholinergic neurons have been reported to improve schizophrenic symptomatology. Davis (1974) observed that methylphenidate, a potent DA releasing and re-uptake blocker, markedly worsens schizophrenic symptoms. Physostigmine, administered after the methylphenidate-induced worsening, abolished the increase in psychotic symptoms (Davis, 1974; Janowsky *et al.*, 1973). Physostigmine also blocks the increase in talkativeness, interactions and general stimulatory effect of methylphenidate-induced psychosis. Rosenthal and Bigelow (1973) reported that oral physostigmine produced marked clinical improvement in five patients with chronic schizophrenia. However, Rowntree *et al.*, (1950) did not obtain improvement in schizophrenia with an irreversible cholinesterase inhibitor diisopropylfluorophosphate (DFP). Pfeiffer and Jenny (1957) observed a brief improvement in schizophrenic patients after subcutaneous injection of the cholinomimetic drug, arecoline.

In summary, the most effective therapeutic agents for schizophrenia are the neuroleptic drugs. Their antipsychotic potency is proportional to their ability to block DA receptor sites. Preliminary investigations suggest that cholinergic stimulation in the limbic system or perhaps even in the striatum, secondary to DA receptor blockade, may also be necessary for the anti-schizophrenic action of drugs such as the phenothiazines and butyrophenones. This hypothesis does not account for the anti-psychotic potency of drugs such as clozapine and thioridazine which have significant antimuscarinic activity. At present, this proposed relationship of the DA-ACh interaction in the limbic system to schizophrenia must be considered very speculative but still worthy of further clinical and laboratory studies to determine its validity.

REFERENCES

Aghajanian, G.K., and Bunney, B.S., 1974, Central dopaminergic neurons, neurophysiological identification and responses to drugs, in *"Frontiers in Catecholamine Research"* (E. Usdin and S.H. Snyder, eds.), pp. 643-648, Pergamon, New York.

Ambani, L.M., and Van Woert, M.H., 1972, Modification of the tremorigenic activity of physostigmine, *Br. J. Pharmacol. 46:*344.

Ambani, L.M., Van Woert, M.H., and Bowers, M.B. Jr., 1973, Physostigmine effects on phenothiazine-induced extrapyramidal reactions, *Arch. Neurol. 29:*444.

Anden, N.E., 1972, Dopamine turnover in the corpus striatum and the limbic system after treatment with neuroleptic and anti-acetylcholine drugs, *J. Pharm. Pharmacol. 24:*905.

Anden, N.E., and Bedard, P., 1971, Influence of cholinergic mechanisms on the function and turnover of brain dopamine, *J. Pharm. Pharmacol. 23:*460.

Anden, N.E., and Stock, G., 1973, Effect of clozapine on the turnover of dopamine in the corpus striatum and in the limbic system, *J. Pharm. Pharmacol. 25:*346.

Anden, N.E., Roos, B.E., and Werdinius, B., 1964, Effects of chlorpromazine, haloperidol and reserpine on the levels of phenolic acids in rabbit corpus striatum, *Life Sci. 3:*149.

Anden, N.E., Dahlstrom, A., Fuxe, K., Alson, L., and Ungerstedt, U., 1966, Ascending monoamine neurons to the telencephalon and diencephalon, *Acta Physiol. Scand.* 67:313.

Anden, N.E., Carlsson, A., and Haggendal, J., 1969, Adrenergic mechanisms, *Ann. Rev. Pharmacol.* 9:119.

Angrist, B.M., and Gershon, S., 1970, The phenomenology of experimentally induced amphetamine psychosis — preliminary observations, *Biol. Psychiatry 2:*95.

Aquilonius, S.M., and Sjostrom, R., 1971, Cholinergic and dopaminergic mechanisms in Huntington's chorea, *Life Sci. 10:*405.

Arnfred, T., and Randrup, A., 1968, Cholinergic mechanism in brain inhibiting amphetamine-induced stereotyped behavior, *Acta Pharmacol. Toxicol. 26:*384.

Baker, W.W., Connor, J.D., Rossi, G.V., and Lalley, P.M., 1969, Production of tremor by intracaudate cholinergic agents and its suppression by locally administered catecholamines, in *"Progress in Neuro-Genetics"* (A. Barbeau, and J.A. Brunnette, eds.), pp. 390-403, International Congress Series No. 175, Excerpta Medica, Amsterdam.

Barbeau, A., 1961, Biochemistry of Parkinson's disease, *Excerpta Media, Amsterdam (I.C.S.) 38:*152.

Barbeau, A., 1973, G.A.B.A. and Huntington's chorea, *Lancet 2:*1499.

Barbeau, A., Mars, H., and Gillo-Joffroy, L., 1971, Adverse clinical side effects of levodopa therapy, in *"Recent Advances in Parkinson's Disease" (Contemporary Neurology Series No. 8)* (F.H. McDowell and C.H. Markham, eds.), pp. 203-237, F.A. Davis, Philadelphia.

Bird, E.D., and Iversen, L.I., 1974, Huntington's chorea: postmortem measurement of glutamic acid decarboxylase, choline acetyltransferase and dopamine in the basal ganglia, *Brain 97:*457.

Bird, E.D., MacKay, A.V.P., Rayner, C.N., and Iversen, L.L., 1973, Reduced glutamic acid-decarboxylase activity of post-mortem brain in Huntington's chorea, *Lancet 1:* 1090.

Birket-Smith, E., 1974, Abnormal involuntary movements induced by anticholinergic therapy, *Acta Neurol. Scan. 50:*801.

Birkmayer, W., and Hornykiewicz, O., 1961, Der L-3, 4-dioxyphenylalanin (-Dopa)-effect bei der Parkinson-Akinese, *Wien Klin. Wochenschr. 73:*787.

Bloom, F.E., Costa, E., and Salmoiraghi, G.C., 1965, Anesthesia and the responsiveness of individual neurons of the caudate nucleus of the cat to acetylcholine, norepinephrine and dopamine administered by microelectrophoresis, *J. Pharmacol. Exp. Ther. 150:*244.

Bowers, M.B., Jr., and Roth, R.H., 1972, Interaction of atropine-like drugs with dopamine-containing neurons in rat brain, *Br. J. Pharmacol. 44:*301.

Bruyn, G.W., 1968, Huntington's chorea: historical clinical and laboratory synopsis, in *"Vinken and Bryun Handbook of Clinical Neurology, Diseases of Basal Ganglia"*, Vol. 6, pp. 277-298, North Holland, Amsterdam.

Bunney, B.S., Aghajanian, G.K., and Roth, R.H., 1973, Comparison of effects of L-DOPA, amphetamine, and apomorphine on firing rate of rat dopaminergic neurons, *Nature (New Biol.) 245:*123.

Burt, D.R., Creese, I., and Snyder, S.H., 1977, Antischizophrenic drugs: chronic treatment elevates dopamine receptor binding in brain, *Science 196:*326.

Butcher, S.H., Butcher, L.L., and Cho, A.K., 1976, Modulation of neostriatal acetylcholine in the rat by dopamine and 5-hydroxytryptamine afferents, *Life Sci. 18:*733.

Calne, D.B., Teychenne, P.F., and Claveria, L.E., 1974, Bromocryptine in parkinsonism, *Br. Med. J. 4:*442.

Carlsson, A., 1974, Antipsychotic drugs and catecholamine synapses, *J. Psychiatr. Res. 11:*57.

Carlsson, A., Persseon, T., Roos, B.E., and Walinder, J., 1972, Potentiation of phenothiazines by alpha-methyltyrosine in the treatment of chronic schizophrenia, *J. Neural Transm. 33:*83.

Casey, D.E., and Denney, D., 1974, Dimethylaminoethanol in tardive dyskinesia, *N. Engl. J. Med. 291:*797.

Cheramy, A., Nieoullon, A., and Glowinski, J., 1977, Effects of peripheral and local administration of picrotoxin on the release of newly synthesized ^{3}H-dopamine in the caudate nucleus of the cat, *Naunyn Schmiedbergs Arch. Pharmacol. 297:*31.

Chien, C.P., and DiMascio, A., 1967, Drug-induced extrapyramidal symptoms and their relations to clinical efficacy, *Am. J. Psychiatry 123:*1490.

Cho, K., Haslett, W.L., and Jenden, D.J., 1962, The peripheral actions of oxotremorine, a metabolite of tremorine, *J. Pharmacol. Exp. Ther. 138:*249.

Clement-Cormier, Y.C., Kebabian, J.W., Petzold, G.L., and Greengard, P., 1974, Dopamine-sensitive adenylate cyclase in mammalian brain: a possible site of action of antipsychotic drugs, *Proc. Natl. Acad. Sci. 71:*1113.

Cohen, E.L., and Wurtman, R.J., 1975, Brain acetylcholine increase after systemic choline administration, *Life Sci. 16:*1095.

Connell, P.H., 1958, *"Amphetamine Psychosis",* Chapman and Hall, London.

Connor, J.D., 1970, Caudate nucleus neurons: correlation of the effects of substantia nigra stimulation with iontophoretic dopamine, *J. Physiol. London 208:*691.

Conrad, L.C.A., Leonard, C.M., and Pfaff, D.W., 1974, Connections of the median and dorsal raphe nuclei in the rat: an autoradiographic and degeneration study, *J. Comp. Neurol. 156:*79.

Consolo, S., Ladinsky, H., and Garattini, S., 1974, Effect of several dopaminergic parameters in the rat striatum, *J. Pharm. Pharmacol. 26:*275.

Cools, A.R., 1972, Athetoid and choreiform hyperkinesia produced by caudate application of dopamine in cats, *Psychopharmacologia 25:*229.

Cools, A.R., Janssen, H.J., Struyker Boudier, H.A.J., and van Rossum, J.M., 1975, Interaction between antipsychotic drugs and catecholamine receptors, in *Wenner-Gren Center, Int. Symposium Series* (G. Sedvall, B. Unvas, Y. Zotterman, eds.), pp. 73-87, Pergamon Press, Oxford.

Costall, B., and Naylor, R.J., 1975, Cholinergic modification of abnormal involuntary movements induced in the guinea pig, *J. Pharm. Pharmacol. 27:*273.

Cotzias, G.C., Van Woert, M.H., and Schiffer, L.M., 1967, Aromatic amino acids and modification of parkinsonism, *N. Engl. J. Med. 276:*374.

Creese, I., Burt, D.R., and Snyder, S.H., 1975, Dopamine receptor binding: differentiation of agonist and antagonist states with ^{3}H-dopamine and ^{3}H-haloperidol, *Life Sci. 17:*993.

Creese, I., Burt, D.R., and Snyder, S.H., 1976, Dopamine receptor binding predicts clinical and pharmacological potencies of antischizophrenic drugs, *Science 192:*481.

Creese, I., Burt, D.R., and Snyder, S.H., 1977, Dopamine receptor binding enhancement accompanies lesion-induced behavioral supersensitivity, *Science 197:*596.

Davis, J.M., 1974, A two factor theory of schizophrenia, in *"Symp. Catecholamines Enzymes Neuropathol. Schizophrenia", J. Psychiatr. Res. 11:*25.

Davis, K.L., Berger, P.A., and Hollister, L.E., 1975, Choline for tardive dyskinesia, *N. Engl. J. Med. 293:*152.

Davis, K.L., Hollister, L.E., Barchas, J.D., and Berger, P.A., 1976, Choline in tardive dyskinesia and Huntington's disease, *Life Sci. 19:*1507.

Davis, K.L., Berger, P.A., and Hollister, L.E., 1977, Deanol in tardive dyskinesia, *Am. J. Psychiatry 134:*7.

DeSilva, L., and Huang, C.Y., 1975, Deanol in tardive dyskinesia, *Br. Med. J. 3:*466.

Dray, A., Goyne, T.J., Oakley, N.R., and Tanner, T., 1976, Evidence for the existence of a raphe projection to the substantia nigra in rat, *Brain Res. 113:*45.

Duffy, M.J., Mulhall, D., and Powell, D., 1975, Subcellular distribution of substance P in bovine hypothalamus and substantia nigra, *J. Neurochem. 25:*305.

DuVigneaud, V., Chandler, J.P., Simmonds, S., Moyer, A.W., and Cohn, M., 1946, The role of dimethyl and monomethylaminoethanol in transmethylation reactions *in vivo*, *J. Biol. Chem. 164:*603.

Duvoisin, R.C., 1967, Cholinergic antagonism in parkinsonism, *Arch. Neurol. 17:*124.

Ehringer, H., and Hornykiewicz, O., 1960, Verteilung von Noradrenalin und Dopamin (3-hydroxytyramin) im Gehirn des Menschen und ihr verhalten bei Erkrankungen des extrapyramidalen Systems, *Klin Wochenschr. 39:*1236.

El-Yousef, M.K., Janowsky, D.S., Davis, J.M., and Sekerke, H.J., 1973, Reversal of anti-parkinsonian drug toxicity by physostigmine: a controlled study, *Am. J. Psychiatry 130:*141.

Enna, S.J., Bird, E.D., Bennett, J.P., Jr., Bylubd, D., Yamamura, H.L., Iversen, L.I., and Snyder, S.H., 1976, Huntington's chorea: changes in neurotransmitter receptors in the brain, *N. Engl. J. Med. 294:*1305.

Ernst, A.M., 1967, Mode of action of apomorphine and dextroamphetamine in gnawing compulsion in rats, *Psychopharmacologia 10:*316.

Escobar, J.I., and Kemp, K.F., 1975, Dimethylaminoethanol for tardive dyskinesia, *N. Engl. J. Med. 292:*317.

Fann, W.E., Lake, C.R., and McKenzie, G.M., 1975a, Adrenergic and cholinergic factors in extrapyramidal disorders, in *"Neurotransmitter Balances Regulating Behavior"* (E.F. Domino and J.M. Davis, eds.), pp. 159-174, J.M. Davis, Ann Arbor.

Fann, W.E., Sullivan, J.L. III, and Miller, R.D., 1975b, Deanol in tardive dyskinesia: a preliminary report, *Psychopharmacology 42:*135.

Feltz, P., 1971, Gamma-amino-butyric acid and a caudate-nigral inhibition, *Can. J. Physiol. Pharmacol. 49:*1113.

Fisher, R., Norris, J.W., and Gilka, L., 1974, GABA in Huntington's chorea, *Lancet 1:*506.

Fjalland, B., and Moller-Nielsen, I., 1974, Enhancement of methylphenidate induced stereotypies by repeated administration of neuroleptics, *Psychopharmacology 34:*105.

Gerlach, J., Reisby, N., and Randrup, A., 1974, Dopaminergic hypersensitivity and cholinergic hypofunction in the pathophysiology of tardive dyskinesia, *Psychopharmacologia 34:*21.

Gershon, S., 1960, Blocking effect of tetrahydroaminacrin on a new psychotomimetic agent, *Nature 186:*1072.

Giorguieff, M.F., Le Floch, M.L., Glowinski, J., and Besson, M.J., 1977, Involvement of cholinergic presynaptic receptors of nicotinic and muscarinic types in the control of spontaneous release of dopamine from striatal dopaminergic terminals in the rat, *J. Pharm. Exp. Ther. 200:*535.

Goldberg, A.M., and Silvergeld, E.K., 1974, Neurological aspects of lead induced hyperactivity, *Trans. Am. Soc. Neurochem. 5:*185.

Greengard, P., 1974, Molecular studies on the nature of the dopamine receptor in the caudate nucleus of the mammalian brain, in *"Frontiers in Neurology and Neuroscience Research 1974"* (P. Seeman and G.M. Brown eds.), pp 12-15, The University of Toronto Press, Toronto.

Griffith, J.D., Cavanaugh, J., Held, J., and Oates, J.A., 1972, Dextroamphetamine, *Arch. Gen. Psychiatry 26:*97.

Groth, D.P., Bain, J.A., and Pfeiffer, C.C., 1958, The comparative distribution of C^{14} labelled 2-dimethylaminoethanol and choline in the mouse, *J. Pharmacol. Exp. Ther. 124:*290.

Growdon, J.H., Cohen, E.L., and Wurtman, R.J., 1977a, Huntington's disease: clinical and chemical effects of choline administration, *Ann. Neurol. 1:*418.

Growdon, J.H., Hirsch, M.J., Wurtman, R.J., and Wiener, W., 1977b, Oral choline administration to patients with tardive dyskinesia, *N. Engl. J. Med. 297:*524.

Harris, L.W., Stitcher, D.L., and Heyl, W.C., 1977, Modification of striatal acetylcholine concentration by N^6, O^2-dibutyryl adenosine 3',5'monophosphate in rats injected with chlorpromazine, *Life Sci. 20:*1879.

Hattori, T., McGeer, P.L., Fibiger, H.C., and McGeer, E.G., 1973, On the source of GABA-containing terminals in the substantia nigra: electron microscopic audiographic and biochemical studies, *Brain Res. 54:*103.

Haubrich, D.R., Reid, W.D., and Gillette, J.R., 1972, Acetylcholine formation in mouse brain and effect of cholinergic drugs, *Nature (New Biol.) 238:*88.

Haubrich, D.R., Wang, P.F.L., Clody, D.E., and Wedeking, P.W., 1975, Increase in rat brain acetylcholine induced by choline or deanol, *Life Sci. 17:*975.

Hiley, C.R., and Bird, E.D., 1974, Decreased muscarinic receptor concentration in post-mortem brain in Huntington's chorea, *Brain Res. 80:*355.

Hokfelt, T., Kellerth, J.O., Nilsson, G., and Pernow, B., 1975, Substance P: localization in the central nervous system and in some primary sensory neurons, *Science 190:*889.

Holmstedt, B., and Lundgren, G., 1966, Tremorigenic agents and brain acetylcholine, in *"Mechanism and Release of Biogenic Amines"* (U.C. von Euler, S. Rosell and B. Unvas, eds.), pp. 439-468, Pergamon Press, Oxford.

Jacobowitz, D.M., and Palkovits, M., 1974, Topographic atlas of catecholamine and acetylcholinesterase-containing neurons in rat brain, *J. Comp. Neurol. 157:*13.

Janowsky, D.S., El-Yousef, M.K., Davis, J.M., and Sekerke, H.J., 1973, Antagonistic effects of physostigmine and methylphenidate in man, *Am. J. Psychiatry 130:*1370.

Janssen, P.A.J., Niemegeers, C.J.E., Schillekens, K.H.L., and Lenaerts, F.M., 1967, Is it possible to predict the clinical effects of neuroleptic drugs (major tranquilizers) from animal data?, *Arznesmettel-Forschung 17:*841.

Jenden, D.J., Choi, L., Silverman, R.W., Steinborn, J.A., Rock, M., and Booth, R.A., 1974, Acetylcholine turnover estimation in brain by gas chromatography/mass spectrometry, *Life Sci. 14:*55.

Kataoka, K., Bak, I.J., Hassler, R., Kim, J.S., and Wagner, A., 1974, L-glutamate decarboxylase and choline acetyltransferase activity in the substantia nigra and the striatum after surgical interruption of the striato-nigral fibers of the baboon, *Exp. Brain Res. 19:*217.

Kazamatsuri, H., Chien, C., and Cole, J.O., 1972, Treatment of tardive dyskinesia. I. Clinical efficacy of a dopamine-depleting agent, tetrabenazine, *Arch. Gen. Psychiatry 27:*95.

Kelley, P.H., and Miller, R., 1974, The interaction of neuroleptic and muscarinic agents with central dopaminergic systems, *Br. J. Pharmacol. 54:*115.

Kim, J.S., Bak, I.J., Hassler, R., and Okada, Y., 1971, Role of gamma-aminobutyric acid (GABA) in the extrapyramidal motor system. II. Some evidence for the existence of a type of GABA-rich striato-nigral neurons, *Exp. Brain Res. 14:*95.

Klawans, H.L., and McKendall, R.R., 1971, Observations on the effect of levodopa on tardive lingual-facial-buccal dyskinesia, *J. Neurol Sci. 14:*189.

Klawans, H.L., and Rubovits, R., 1972a, An experimental model of tardive dyskinesia, *J. Neural Transm. 33:*235.

Klawans, H.L., and Rubovits, R., 1972b, Central cholinergic-anticholinergic antagonism in Huntington's chorea, *Neurology (Minneap.) 22:*107.

Klawans, H.L., and Rubovits, R., 1974, Effect of cholinergic and anticholinergic agents on tardive dyskinesia, *J. Neurol. Neurosurg. Psychiatry 37:*941.

Klawans, H.L., and Weiner, W.J., 1974, The effect of d-amphetamine on choreiform movement disorders, *Neurology (Minneap.) 24:*312.

Klawans, H.L., Topel, J.L., and Bergen, D., 1975, Deanol in the treatment of levo-dopa-induced dyskinesia, *Neurology (Minneap.) 25:*290.

Koslow, S.H., Racagni, G., and Costa, E., 1974, Mass fragmentographic measurement of norepinephrine, dopamine, serotonin and acetylcholine in seven discrete nuclei of the rat tel-diencephalon, *Neuropharmacology 13:*1123.

Kuhar, M.H., and Yamamura, H.I., 1976, Localization of cholinergic muscarinic receptors in rat brain by light microscopic radioautography, *Brain Res. 110:*229.

Lloyd, K.G., Davidson, L., and Hornykiewicz, O., 1973, Metabolism of levodopa in the human brain, *Adv. Neurol. 3:*173.

Marco, E., Mao, C.C., Cheney, D.L., Revulta, A., and Costa, E., 1976, The effects of anti-psychotics on the turnover rate of GABA and acetylcholine in rat brain nuclei, *Nature 264:*363.

Marsden, C.D., Tarsy, D., Baldessarini, R.J., 1975, Spontaneous and drug-induced move-ment disorders in psychotic patients, in *"Psychiatric Aspects of Neurological Disease"* (D.F. Benson, D. Blumer, eds.), pp. 219-266, Grune and Stratton, New York.

Matthysse, S., 1973, Antipsychotic drug actions: a clue to the neuropathology of schizo-phrenia?, *Fed. Proc. 32:*200.

Mayer-Gross, W., Slater, E., and Roth, M., 1960, in *"Clinical Psychiatry"*, Williams and Wilkins, Baltimore, p. 377.

McGeer, P.L., and McGeer, E.G., 1971, Cholinergic enzyme systems in Parkinson's disease, *Arch. Neurol. 25:*265.

McGeer, P.L., McGeer, E.G., and Fibiger, H.C., 1973, Choline acetylase and glutamic acid decarboxylase in Huntington's chorea, *Neurology (Minneap.) 23:*912.

McGeer, E.G., McGeer, P.L., Grewaal, D.S., and Singh, V.K., 1975, Striatal cholinergic interneurons and their relation of dopaminergic nerve endings, *J. Pharmacol. 4:*143.

McLennan, H., and York, D.H., 1967, The action of dopamine on neurons of the caudate nucleus, *J. Physiol. (Lond.) 189:*393.

Mettler, F.A., 1955, Perceptual capacity, functions of the corpus striatum and schizo-phrenia, *Psychiatr. Q. 29:*89.

Mettler, F.A., and Mettler, C.C., 1942, The effects of striatal injury, *Brain 65:*242.

Miller, R.J., and Hilley, C.R., 1974, Antimuscarinic properties of neuroleptic drugs and drug-induced parkinsonism, *Nature (Lond.) 248:*596.

Mitchell, J.F., 1963, The spontaneous and evoked release of acetylcholine from the cerebral cortex, *J. Physiol. (Lond.) 165:*98.

Moore, K.E., and Thornburg, J.E., 1975, Drug-induced dopaminergic supersensitivity, *Adv. Neurol. 9:*93.

Munkvad, I., Pakkenberg, H., and Randrup, A., 1968, Aminergic systems in basal ganglia associated with stereotyped hyperactive behavior and catalepsy, *Brain Behav. Evol. 1:*89.

Nashold, B.S., 1959, Cholinergic stimulation of globus pallidus in man, *Proc. Soc. Exp. Biol. Med. 101:*68.

Ng, L.K.Y., Gelhard, R.E., Chase, T.N., and McLean, P.D., 1973, Drug-induced dyskinesia in monkeys: a pharmacological model employing 6-hydroxydopamine, *Adv. Neurol.* 1:651.

Nyback, H., and Sedvall, G., 1969, Regional accumulation of catecholamines formed from trypsine ^{14}C in the rat brain: Effect of chlorpromazine, *Eur. J. Pharmacol.* 5:245.

Nyback, H., Schubert, J., and Sedvall, G., 1970, Effect of apomorphine and pimozide on synthesis and turnover of labelled catecholamines in mouse brain, *J. Pharm. Pharmacol.* 22:622.

O'Keefe, R., Sharman, D.F., and Vogt, M., 1970, Effect of drugs used in psychosis on cerebral dopamine metabolism, *Br. J. Pharmacol.* 38:287.

Palkovits, M., Brownstein, M., and Saavedra, J.M., 1974a, Serotonin content of the brain stem nuclei in the rat, *Brain Res.* 80:237.

Palkovits, M., Saavedra, J.M., Koboyashi, P.M., and Brownstein, M., 1974b, Choline acetyltransferase content of limbic nuclei of the rat, *Brain Res.* 79:443.

Pepeu, G., Freedman, D.X., and Giarman, N.J., 1960, Biochemical and pharmacological studies on dimethylaminoethanol (Deanol), *J. Pharmacol. Exp. Ther.* 129:131.

Perry, T.L., Hansen, S., and Kloster, M., 1973, Huntington's chorea: deficiency of gamma-aminobutyric acid in brain, *N. Engl. J. Med.* 288:337.

Pfeiffer, C.C., and Jenney, J.E.H., 1957, The inhibition of the conditioned response and the counteraction of schizophrenia by muscarinic stimulation of the brain, *Ann. N.Y. Acad. Sci.* 66:953.

Pijnenburg, A.J.J., and van Rossum, J.M., 1973, Stimulation of locomotor activity following injection of dopamine into the nucleus accumbens, *J. Pharm. Pharmacol.* 25:1003.

Pijnenburg, A.J.J., Honig, W.M.M., and van Rossum, J.M., 1975, Inhibition of d-amphetamine-induced locomotor activity by injection of haloperidol into the nucleus accumbens of the rat, *Psychopharmacologia* 41:87.

Precht, W., and Yoshida, M., 1971, Blockage of caudate-evoked inhibition in the substantia nigra by picrotoxin, *Brain Res.* 32:229.

Re, O., 1974, 2-dimethylaminoethanol (Deanol): a brief review of its clinical efficacy and postulated mechanism of action, *Curr. Ther. Res. Clin. Exp.* 16:1238.

Reisine, T.D., Fields, J.Z., Stern, L.Z., Johnson, P.C., Bird, E.D., and Yamamura, H.I., 1977, Alteration in dopaminergic receptors in Huntington's disease, *Life Sci.* 21:1123.

Roos, B.E., 1965, Effects of certain tranquilizers on the level of homovanillic acid in the corpus striatum, *J. Pharm. Pharmacol.* 7:820.

Rosenthal, R., and Bigelow, L.B., 1973, The effects of physostigmine in phenothiazine resistant chronic schizophrenic patients: preliminary observations, *Compr. Psychiatry* 14:489.

Rowntree, D., Nevin, S., and Wilson, A., 1950, The effects of diisopropylfluorophosphate in schizophrenia and manic depressive psychosis, *J. Neurol. Neurosurg. Psychiatry* 13:47.

Rubovits, R., and Klawans, H.L., Jr., 1972, Implications of amphetamine-induced stereotyped behavior as a model for tardive dyskinesia, *Arch. Gen. Psychiatry* 27:502.

Salmoiraghi, G.C., Costa, E., and Bloom, F.E., 1965, Pharmacology of central synapses, *Annu. Rev. Pharmacol.* 5:213.

Sato, S., Daly, R., and Peters, H., 1971, Reserpine therapy of phenothiazine induced dyskinesia, *Dis. Nerv. Syst.* 32:680.

Sax, D.S., Butters, N., Tomlinson, E.B., and Feldman, R.G., 1973, Effects of serial caudate lesions and L-DOPA administration upon cognitive and motor behavior in monkeys, *Adv. Neurol.* 1:657.

Sayers, A.C., Burki, H.R., Ruch, W., and Asper, H., 1975, Neuroleptic-induced hypersensitivity of striatal dopamine receptors in the rat as a model of tardive dyskinesias. Effects of clozapine, haloperidol, loxapine and chlorpromazine, *Psychopharmacologia 41:*97.

Scheel-Kruger, J., 1970, Central effects of anticholinergic drugs measured by the apomorphine gnawing in mice, *Acta Pharmacol. Toxicol. (Kbh.) 28:*1.

Seeman, P., Lee, T., Chou-Wong, M., and Wong, K., 1976, Antipsychotic drug doses and neuroleptic dopamine receptors, *Nature 261:*717.

Sethy, V.H., and Van Woert, M.H., 1973a, Effect of L-DOPA on brain acetylcholine in rats, *Neuropharmacology 12:*27.

Sethy, V.H., and Van Woert, M.H., 1973b, Antimuscarinic drugs: effects on brain acetylcholine and tremors in rats, *Biochem. Pharmacol. 22:*2685.

Sethy, V.H., and Van Woert, M.H., 1974a, Modification of striatal acetylcholine concentration by dopamine receptor agonists and antagonists, *Res. Commun. Chem. Pathol. Pharmacol. 8:*13.

Sethy, V.H., and Van Woert, M.H., 1974b, Regulation of striatal acetylcholine concentration by dopamine receptors, *Nature 251:*529.

Sheppard, C., and Merlis, S., 1967, Drug-induced extrapyramidal symptoms: their incidence and treatment, *Am. J. Psychiatry 123:*886.

Shoulson, I., Chase, T.N., Roberts, E., and Van Balgooy, J.N.A., 1975, Huntington's disease: treatment with imidazole-4-acetic acid, *N. Engl. J. Med. 293:*504.

Shoulson, I., Kartzinel, R., and Chase, T.N., 1976, Huntington's disease: treatment with dipropylacetic acid and gamma-aminobutyric acid, *Neurology 26:*61.

Shoulson, I., Goldblatt, D., Charlton, M., and Joynt, R.J., 1977, Huntington's disease, treatment with Muscimol, a GABA-mimetic drug, *Ann. Neurol. (ABST.) 1:*506.

Simke, J.P., and Saelens, J.K., 1977, Evidence for a cholinergic fiber tract connecting the thalamus with the head of the striatum of the rat, *Brain Res. 126:*487.

Singh, M.M., and Kay, S.R., 1975, Therapeutic reversal with benztropine in schizophrenia, *J. Nerv. Mental Dis. 168:*258.

Singh, M.M., and Smith, J.M., 1973, Reversal of some therapeutic effects of an antipsychotic agent by an antiparkinsonian drug, *J. Nerv. Ment. Dis. 157:*50.

Snyder, S.H., Banerjie, S.P., Yamamura, H.I., and Greenberg, D., 1974, Drugs, neurotransmitters and schizophrenia, *Science 184:*1243.

Stadler, H., Lloyd, K.G., Gadea-Ciria, M., and Bartholini, G., 1973, Enhanced striatal acetylcholine release by chlorpromazine and its reversal by apomorphine, *Brain Res. 55:*476.

Stahl, W.L., and Swanson, P.D., 1974, Biochemical abnormalities in Huntington's chorea brains, *Neurology (Minneap.) 24:*813.

Tarsy, D., and Baldessarini, R.J., 1974, Behavioral supersensitivity to apomorphine following chronic treatment with drugs which interfere with the synaptic function of catecholamines, *Neuropharmacology 13:*927.

Tarsy, D., Sax, D.S., and Leopold, N., 1973, The effect of physostigmine on Huntington's chorea and L-DOPA dyskinesia, *Adv. Neurol. 1:*777.

Tarsy, D., Leopold, N., and Sax, D.S., 1974, Physostigmine in choreiform movement disorders, *Neurology (Minneap.) 24:*28.

Torrey, E.F., and Peterson, M.R., 1974, Schizophrenia and the limbic system, *Lancet 2:*942.

Trabucchi, M., Cheney, D., Racgni, G., and Costa, E., 1974, Involvement of brain cholinergic mechanisms in the action of chlorpromazine, *Nature 249:*664.

Ungerstedt, U., 1971, Postsynaptic supersensitivity after 6-hydroxydopamine induced degeneration of the nigrostriatal dopamine system, *Acta Physiol. Scand. (Suppl.) 367:*69.

van Rossum, J.M., 1966, The significance of dopamine receptor blockade for the action of neuroleptic drugs, in *"Proc. 5th Int. Congress Collegium Intern. Neuropsychopharmacologium", Int. Congress Series No. 129* (H. Brill, J.O. Cole, and P. Deniker, eds.), pp. 321-329, Excerpta Medica, Amsterdam.

Van Woert, M.H., Ambani, L.M., and Bowers, M.B., Jr., 1972, Levodopa and cholinergic hypersensitivity in Parkinson's disease, *Neurology (Minneap.) 22:*86.

Von Voigtlander, P.F., Lorenz, E.G., and Trienzenberg, H.J., 1975, Increased sensitivity to dopaminergic agents after chronic neuroleptic treatment, *J. Pharmacol. Exp. Ther. 193:*88.

Waldmeier, P.C., and Maitre, L., 1976, On the relevance of preferential increases of mesolimbic versus striatal dopamine turnover for the prediction of antipsychotic activity of psychotropic drugs, *J. Neurochem. 27:*589.

Walker, J.E., Hoehn, M., Sears, E., and Lewis, J., 1973, Dimethylaminoethanol in Huntington's chorea, *Lancet 1:*1512.

Wastek, G.J., Stern, L.Z., Johnson, P.C., and Yamamura, H.I., 1976, Huntington's disease: regional alteration in muscarinic cholinergic receptor binding in human brain, *Life Sci. 19:*1033.

Weintraub, M.I., and Van Woert, M.H., 1971, Reversal of cholinergic hypersensitivity in Parkinson's disease by levodopa, *N. Engl. J. Med. 284:*412.

Wiesel, F.A., and Sedvall, G., 1975, Effect of antipsychotic drugs on homovanillic acid levels in striatum and olfactory tubercle of the rat, *Eur. J. Pharmacol. 30:*364.

Wilk, S., Watson, E., and Stanley, M.E., 1975, Differential sensitivity of two dopaminergic structures in rat brain haloperidol and to clozapine, *J. Pharmacol. Exp. Ther. 195:*265.

Zahniser, N.R., Chou, D., and Hanin, I., 1977, Is 2-dimethylaminoethanol (Deanol) indeed a precursor of brain acetylcholine? A gas chromatographic evaluation, *J. Pharmacol. Exp. Ther. 200:*545.

Zivkovic, B., Guidotti, A., Revuelta, A., and Costa, E., 1975, Effect of thioridazine, clozapine and other antipsychotics on the kinetic state of tyrosine hydroxylase and on the turnover rate of dopamine in striatum and nucleus accumbens, *J. Pharmacol. Exp. Ther. 194:*37.

INTERACTIONS BETWEEN ACETYLCHOLINE AND DOPAMINE IN THE BASAL GANGLIA

D. Tarsy

Department of Neurology, Boston V.A. Hospital, Boston University School of Medicine, Boston, Massachusetts 02130

Division of Neurology, Department of Medicine, New England Deaconess Hospital, Harvard Medical School, Boston, Massachusetts 02115

DISTRIBUTION OF DOPAMINE AND ACETYLCHOLINE IN THE BASAL GANGLIA

Dopamine

The distribution of brain dopamine (DA) is relatively restricted to several well defined neuronal projections, the most widely studied of which are the nigrostriatal, mesolimbic, mesocortical, and tuberoinfundibular systems. The dopaminergic nigrostriatal and mesolimbic systems account for the fact that in mammalian brain approximately 80% of brain DA is located in the basal ganglia with greatest concentrations in the caudate nucleus and putamen (neostriatum), substantia nigra (SN), globus pallidus, nucleus accumbens, and amygdaloid complex (Hornykiewicz, 1973). The nigrostriatal pathway (Anden *et al.*, 1964) originates in a dense collection of DA-containing cell bodies in the pars compacta of SN which project to the neostriatum where they arborize into a network of densely packed DA-containing nerve terminals. The mesolimbic pathway originates medial to SN from DA-containing cell bodies of the ventromedial interpeduncular nucleus and projects to a group of small midline nuclei including nucleus accumbens, olfactory tubercle, and interstitial nucleus of the stria terminalis (Anden *et al.*, 1966).

Acetylcholine

Although acetylcholine (ACh) is distributed more diffusely within mammalian brain than DA, particularly high concentrations are also found in the caudate nucleus and putamen. This conclusion is based on the finding of high concentrations of ACh (Fahn and Cote, 1968; Yamamura *et al.*, 1974), choline acetylase (CAT) (Hebb and Silver, 1956), acetylcholinesterase (Burgen and Chipman, 1951; Yamamura *et al.*, 1974), and muscarinic cholinergic receptors (Yamamura *et al.*, 1974) in mammalian neostriatum and has been confirmed in studies of human brain material as well (Hebb and Silver, 1956; McGeer and McGeer, 1971; Rinne *et al.*, 1973). On the basis of similar evidence ACh is also believed to be present in large concentrations in mesolimbic nuclei in both animal (Palkovits *et al.*, 1974; Cheney *et al.*, 1975; Kuhar and Yamamura, 1976; Ben-Ari *et al.*, 1977) and human brain (McGeer and McGeer, 1976b). The neuronal localization of neostriatal ACh is well established (De Robertis *et al.*, 1963) but until recently there has been some debate concerning the distribution of afferent and efferent projections of neostriatal cholinergic neurons. Shute and Lewis (1967) identified an ascending cholinergic pathway between the SN, globus pallidus, and caudate-putamen in rat brain on the basis of lesion studies followed by histochemical staining for acetylcholinesterase activity. However, similar studies done in cat and monkey brain failed to identify an ascending cholinergic pathway and demonstrated instead a descending cholinergic projection from caudate-putamen to globus pallidus and SN (Olivier *et al.*, 1970). McGeer *et al.*, (1971) lesioned the major known afferent pathways to the neostriatum (Kemp and Powell, 1971) by placing large lesions in cortex, thalamus, globus pallidus, and ventral tegmental regions of midbrain without producing a significant drop in neostriatal CAT or ACh. On the basis of studies in other brain regions, interruption of afferent cholinergic input should produce a drop in both CAT and ACh. Thus, McGeer *et al.*, (1971) concluded that there was no significant afferent cholinergic projection to the neostriatum. With the exception of one study, (Olivier *et al.*, 1970) significant cholinergic efferent projections from the neostriatum have also not been demonstrated (McGeer *et al.*, 1969; Lynch *et al.*, 1972) leading to the conclusion that cholinergic neurons of the neostriatum are organized entirely within this nucleus and are short interneurons of the type originally demonstrated histologically by Kemp and Powell (1971). Subsequent biochemical studies (McGeer *et al.*, 1969; Lynch *et al.*, 1972) have confirmed these findings and in addition have suggested that neostriatal cholinergic interneurons have relatively short axonal and dendritic processes since small caudate lesions do not affect ACh (Butcher and Butcher, 1974) or acetylcholinesterase (Lynch *et al.*, 1972) concentration in immediately adjacent regions of caudate. Immunohistochemical studies which allow direct visualization of CAT-containing neostriatal neurons also clearly demonstrated the existence of small cholinergic cells characteristic of striatal interneurons (Hattori *et al.*, 1976; McGeer *et al.*, 1976).

NEUROPSYCHIATRIC DISORDERS

Parkinsonism

Dopamine

In idiopathic Parkinson's disease and postencephalitic parkinsonism, pathologic changes occur in the pars compacta of the SN which result in a marked reduction in concentration of DA in SN and the neostriatum to which nigrostriatal neurons project and terminate. A high correlation is found between severity of nigral cell loss and degree of striatal DA deficiency in patients with Parkinson's disease (Bernheimer *et al.*, 1973) as well as animals with experimental SN lesions (Anden *et al.*, 1964; Poirier and Sourkes, 1965). Extensive postmortem biochemical and histopathological studies have established that reduction of striatal DA concentrations is an important basis for the clinical manifestations of parkinsonism (Hornykiewicz, 1973; Bernheimer *et al.*, 1973). Since in

Parkinson's disease there is impaired dopaminergic input into a striatum containing relatively normal receptor cells, symptoms can usually be reversed following administration of L-DOPA despite the presence of relatively advanced disease of nigrostriatal neurons, (Bernheimer *et al.*, 1973; Klawans, 1973; Lloyd *et al.*, 1975a). Although direct biochemical evidence is lacking it is likely that parkinsonian features of striatonigral degeneration, hypertensive lacunar state, and olivopontocerebellar atrophy are also due to striatal DA deficiency. In these conditions, however, the effects of DA replacement are often less dramatic due to coexisting degeneration of striatal receptor cells.

The concept that parkinsonism is related to nigrostriatal DA deficiency receives support from the effect of neuroleptic (antipsychotic) drugs in animals and man. Each of the cardinal symptoms of Parkinson's disease including akinesia, rigidity, postural abnormalities, and tremor may be produced by neuroleptic drugs (Hornykiewicz, 1971; Marsden *et al.*, 1975). The fact that bradykinesia is the earliest, most common, and sometimes the sole manifestation of drug-induced parkinsonism (Marsden *et al.*, 1975; Rifkin *et al.*, 1975) is an interesting corollary of the observation that in Parkinson's disease akinesia correlates highly with striatal DA deficiency and, according to some observers (Bernheimer *et al.*, 1973) is the parkinsonian sign most sensitive to treatment with both intravenous and oral L-DOPA. Parkinsonism occurs following the use of all neuroleptic drugs including reserpine, tetrabenazine, phenothiazines, and butyrophenones. Reserpine and tetrabenazine deplete brain catecholamines by interference with presynaptic vesicular storage mechanisms. In animals reserpine produces a state of profound akinesia and rigidity which is dramatically reversed by L-DOPA (Carlsson *et al.*, 1957). Reserpine-induced parkinsonism in man is similarly reversed by treatment with L-DOPA (Hornykiewicz, 1973). Unlike reserpine, the phenothiazines and butyrophenones produce a state of functional DA deficiency by interference with DA release (Seeman and Lee, 1975) and production of receptor blockade of DA synapses (Marsden *et al.*, 1975). In laboratory animals these drugs produce states of prolonged immobility referred to as "catalepsy" and antagonize the behavioral effects of direct and indirect DA agonists such as L-DOPA, apomorphine, and amphetamine. The fact that alpha-methyl-p-tyrosine, which blocks catecholamine synthesis by inhibition of tyrosine hydroxylase, also produces parkinsonism (Chase, 1972) further supports the concept that parkinsonism results from a state of striatal DA deficiency.

Acetylcholine

There is no significant reduction in concentration of CAT or acetylcholinesterase (McGeer and McGeer, 1971, 1976b; Rinne *et al.*, 1973; Lloyd *et al.*, 1975b) in the neostriatum of patients with Parkinson's disease. It is now recognized that the vast majority of ACh containing neurons of the striatum are small interneurons which remain confined to the striatum rather than projecting to or from this structure (McGeer *et al.*, 1971; Lynch *et al.*, 1972; Butcher and Butcher, 1974; McGeer *et al.*, 1976). Since striatal neurons themselves remain normal in Parkinson's disease it is not surprising that enzymes related to ACh metabolism also remain normal. By contrast, the finding that CAT is reduced in all regions of SN in Parkinson's disease (Lloyd *et al.*, 1975b) is attributable to the degeneration of SN cell bodies characteristic of this disease.

Although ACh concentration is normal it is well recognized that a state of relative cholinergic preponderance exists in Parkinson's disease. Belladonna alkaloids with anticholinergic properties have long been used in the treatment of parkinsonism with little understanding of the mechanism their therapeutic efficacy. Subsequent recognition of the role of ACh in brain function led to the suggestion that the clinical effect of atropinic drugs might be due to a central atropine-ACh antagonism similar to that observed in experimental situations (Feldberg, 1945). The clinical efficacy of a number of anti-parkinsonian drugs including antihistamines (Gair and Ducey, 1950) and certain phenothiazines such as ethopropazine correlates highly with the anticholinergic properties of these agents *in vitro* (Ahmed and Marshall, 1962). A number of behavioral studies have suggested that pharmacologic potentiation of central cholinergic mechanisms produces behavioral responses which bear some resemblance to symptoms of clinical parkinsonism. It is known, for example, that systemic (Ahmed and Marshall, 1962; Ambani and Van Woert, 1972) or intracaudate (Connor *et al.*, 1966) injection of cholinomimetic drugs produces tremor in experimental animals which may be blocked by anticholinergic drugs. Although this high frequency tremor is an imperfect model of parkinsonian tremor, it has been useful in the secreening of new anticholinergic compounds. Intracaudate injection of cholinergic drugs in cats produces "a state of quietude" (Stevens *et al.*, 1961) while systemic administration of cholinergic drugs in rodents produces cataleptic states (Costall and Olley, 1971), although here too the relationship of these phenomena to parkinsonian akinesia is open to question. Finally, systemic administration of physostigmine, a centrally active anticholinesterase which increases brain ACh levels, produces a state of rigidity which, on neurophysiologic grounds bears close resemblance to that seen in Parkinson's disease (Arvidsson *et al.*, 1966).

The clinical observation that cholinergic drugs exacerbate parkinsonism was firmly established by Duvoisin (1967). Previous reports in small numbers of patients had suggested that physostigmine exacerbates extrapyramidal signs in postencephalitic parkinsonism. Duvoisin (1967) found that intravenous physostigmine produced obvious worsening of all parkinsonian signs in 17 of 20 patients, most of whom had idiopathic Parkinson's disease. This effect was readily reversed by immediate injection of an anticholinergic drug. Moreover, the response to physostigmine in each patient corresponded to the degree of improvement he previously had shown to anticholinergic treatment. The fact that this interaction occurred within the central nervous system was established by the lack of effect of drugs with purely peripheral cholinergic or anticholinergic properties.

DA-ACh Interaction

McGeer *et al.*, (1961) observed that anticholinergic drugs had a dramatic effect in reversing phenothiazine-induced extrapyramidal reactions and formulated the concept of a catecholamine-ACh balance which was upset by DA blocking drugs and could be restored by treatment with ACh blocking agents. Barbeau (1962) applied a more elaborate but similar concept to idiopathic Parkinson's disease by suggesting that imbalance in a see-saw like DA-ACh equilibrium results in symptoms such as rigidity and akinesia. A large number of physiologic and pharmacologic studies will be reviewed in detail below which support the concept of a reciprocal balance between DA and ACh mechanisms important for neostriatal function.

The observation that physostigmine has no extrapyramidal effect in neurologically normal subjects (Duvoisin, 1967; Ambani *et al.*, 1973) and does not produce new signs in parkinsonian patients suggests that parkinsonism is probably not due to an absolute excess of ACh but reflects instead a relative imbalance secondary to deficiency in DA neurotransmission (Duvoisin, 1967). Weintraub and Van Woert (1971) provided further support for this concept by studying the effect of physostigmine before and during L-DOPA therapy in ten patients with Parkinson's disease. As expected, all untreated patients showed an exacerbation of symptoms following physostigmine. By contrast, however, physostigmine either had no effect or produced only minimal worsening in patients receiving chronic L-DOPA therapy. Those patients on L-DOPA showing no response to physostigmine also were not benefited by the addition of anticholinergic drugs to their treatment while those with a positive physostigmine test showed further improvement with the addition of anticholinergic drugs. These results, together with similar observations in a model of parkinsonism produced in dogs (Van Woert et al., 1972), indicated that when striatal DA mechanisms are restored towards normal, cholinergic sensitivity is reduced. This confirms previous indications (McGeer and McGeer, 1971) that cholinergic sensitivity in Parkinson's disease is not a primary phenomenon but secondary to DA deficiency.

A further manifestation of cholinergic sensitivity in parkinsonism is the observation that anticholinergic drugs by themselves occasionally produce choreiform dyskinesias similar to those commonly associated with L-DOPA treatment (Fahn and David, 1973; Mano et al., 1973; Birket-Smith, 1974) while administration of anticholinergics together with L-DOPA increases the incidence of L-DOPA dyskinesias (Birket-Smith, 1975). Conversely, administration of physostigmine reduces or abolishes L-DOPA induced dyskinesias (Klawans, 1973; Tarsy et al., 1974).

It should also be mentioned that since anticholinergic drugs, particularly benztropine, block presynaptic reuptake of DA in the striatum, this mechanism has been offered as an explanation of their antiparkinsonian effect (Coyle and Snyder, 1969). Considerable doubt is cast on this theory, however, by the identification of a number of clinically effective anticholinergic drugs which are relatively weak as blockers of striatal DA uptake (Farnebo et al., 1970; Fuxe et al., 1970).

If drug-induced parkinsonism is due to functional DA deficiency then cholinergic sensitivity should be demonstrable in this condition as well. Physostigmine, in fact, has been found to exacerbate phenothiazine induced parkinsonism (Ambani et al., 1973; Rosenthal and Bigelow 1973; Gerlach et al., 1974) while anticholinergic drugs are well known to reduce the severity of drug-induced parkinsonism (Simpson, 1970). Recent studies, in fact, have found an inverse relationship between the potency of antipsychotic drugs in inducing extrapyramidal effects and their potency as anticholinergic drugs (Miller and Hiley, 1974; Snyder et al., 1974). Thus, for example, it has been suggested that thioridazine or clozapine produce little or no extrapyramidal effects because of their relatively strong anticholinergic properties. However, since the prophylactic use of anticholinergic drugs appear to reduce only the severity and not the frequency of parkinsonian symptoms (DiMascio and Demirgian, 1970; Swett et al., 1977) it seems unlikely that the anticholinergic properties of an antipsychotic drug like clozapine could alone account for its complete freedom (Ayd, 1974) from extrapyramidal effects.

Choreiform Disorders

Huntington's Disease

Clinical evidence for a reciprocal relationship between DA and ACh neurotransmission in Huntington's disease although often suggestive, has been considerably less impressive than in parkinsonism. CAT is reduced in the neostriatum of patients with Huntington's disease (McGeer *et al.*, 1973; Bird and Iversen, 1974; Stahl and Swanson, 1974), a finding which correlates with the loss of small striatal interneurons many of which are cholinergic (Bak *et al.*, 1975). The loss of CAT in the caudate nucleus and putamen is patchy, however, with some regions showing virtually absent CAT while others show normal levels (McGeer *et al.*, 1973; Bird and Iversen, 1974). Studies of DA levels in the basal ganglia of patients with Huntington's disease, on the other hand, have shown relatively mild changes. In one postmortem study of 14 patients, DA and homovanillic acid (HVA) concentrations were significantly reduced in the caudate nucleus while they were normal in the putamen, globus pallidus, and SN leading to the conclusion that in Huntington's disease the ratio of caudate DA to putamen DA is shifted in favor of the putamen (Bernheimer *et al.*, 1973). In a larger postmortem study, however, DA levels in the caudate nucleus and putamen were normal in choreic patients while DA was elevated in the putamen of rigid cases of Huntington's disease (Bird and Iversen, 1974).

Undoubtedly, the most significant biochemical disturbance identified in Huntington's disease has been the finding of reduced gamma-aminobutyric acid (GABA) and glutamic acid decarboxylase (GAD) (Perry *et al.*, 1973; McGeer *et al.*, 1973; Bird and Iversen, 1974; Stahl and Swanson, 1974), the enzyme which synthesizes GABA, in the caudate nucleus, putamen, globus pallidus, and SN which is more consistent and greater in degree than the reduction of CAT described above. As in the case of cholinergic neurons, there is evidence that the majority of GABA containing neurons in the neostriatum are small Golgi type II interneurons (McGeer and McGeer, 1975). In addition, however, there is also good evidence for striatonigral, striatopallidal, and pallidonigral efferents which are GABA-mediated. Reduced levels of GABA in the various nuclei of the basal ganglia in Huntington's disease may therefore be related to destruction of neostriatal interneurons as well as striatal efferents to globus pallidus and SN.

The point has been frequently made that Huntington's disease is in many ways the reciprocal of Parkinson's disease (Klawans and Rubovits, 1972; Klawans, 1973). In Parkinson's disease, the DA nigrostriatal pathway is destroyed while striatal neurons to which they project remain intact. The reverse is the case in Huntington's disease in which SN neurons are usually normal while there is extensive loss of small neurons of the striatum. Parkinson's disease and Huntington's disease also appear to be mirror images pharmacologically. Whereas drugs which interfere with DA mechanisms such as reserpine, tetrabenazine, or phenothiazines produce or exacerbate akinetic features of parkinsonism, they are often effective in suppressing the hyperkinetic involuntary movements of Huntington's disease. On the other hand, drugs with dopaminergic activity such as L-DOPA and amphetamine, effective as antiparkinsonian agents, produce or exacerbate chorea.

Clinical studies of manipulation of cholinergic mechanisms have provided less consistent results in Huntington's disease than in Parkinson's disease. In some studies administration of physostigmine to patients with Huntington's disease has produced mild improvement in chorea (Aquilonius and Sjostron, 1971; Klawans and Rubovits, 1972), while anticholinergic drugs have produced worsening (Klawans and Rubovits, 1972, Fahn et al., 1973). Klawans (1972, 1973) has therefore maintained that, as in Parkinson's disease, an antagonistic relationship between striatal DA and ACh is demonstrable in Huntington's disease. In other studies, however, physostigmine has either had no effect or in some cases had produced worsening in Huntington's disease (Fahn et al., 1973; Tarsy et al., 1974).

Tardive Dyskinesia

Tardive dyskinesia is a hyperkinetic, frequently permanent disorder occurring following prolonged exposure to phenothiazine or butyrophenone antipsychotic drugs. It is characterized by a variety of abnormal movements including orofacial dyskinesia, chorea, athetosis, dystonia, tics, and abnormal postures (Tarsy and Baldessarini, 1976). Although the prolonged and frequently irreversible course of this syndrome strongly suggests that permanent structural alterations are responsible, postmortem studies to date fail to demonstrate consistent neuropathologic findings (Tarsy and Baldessarini, 1976; Tarsy and Baldessarini, 1977).

As in the case of Huntington's disease, a number of clinical observations have suggested that this syndrome is associated with a state of relative DA hypersensitivity. Tardive dyskinesia closely resembles dyskinesias produced by L-DOPA in patients with Parkinson's disease, administration of L-DOPA exacerbates tardive dyskinesia (Chase, 1972; Gerlach et al., 1974), and tardive dyskinesia worsens on withdrawal and is suppressed by treatment with drugs that deplete or block the action of DA (Kazamatsuri et al., 1972).

The possibility of a reciprocal relationship between DA and ACh in tardive dyskinesia had been widely considered (Gerlach et al., 1974; Davis et al., 1977). Rubovits and Klawans (1972) have suggested that stereotyped behavior produced in animals by drugs with dopaminergic properties might serve as an animal model for tardive dyskinesia. As will be discussed below, a number of investigators have demonstrated a reciprocal relationship between DA and ACh using this model (Arnfred and Randrup, 1968; Scheel-Kruger, 1970; Klawans et al., 1972; Janowsky et al., 1972). In addition, intracaudate injection of dopamine produces stereotyped chewing behavior in guinea pigs which may be abolished by systemic administration of cholinergic drugs (Costall and Naylor, 1975). Clinically, the evidence for cholinergic hypofunction in tardive dyskinesia, although certainly suggestive, has been less consistent. Although anticholinergic drugs often worsen tardive dyskinesia (Kiloh et al., 1973; Klawans and Rubovits, 1974; Gerlach et al., 1974), some patients show either no response (Tarsy and Bralower, 1977) or improvement (Granacher et al., 1975). Similarly, attempts to produce improvement in tardive dyskinesia by administration of physostigmine have, as in the case of Huntington's disease produced mixed results. Klawans and Rubovits (1974) reported mild improvement following intravenous physostigmine but in other studies no significant changes have been observed (Tarsy et al., 1974; Gerlach et al., 1974; Grahacher et al., 1975; Tarsy and Bralower, 1977). Oral choline has produced mild improvement in tardive dyskinesia in recent studies (Davis et al., 1976; Growdon et al., 1977), presumably by elevation of brain ACh levels. The occasional occurrence of choreiform syndromes as a result of anticholinergic drug overdose in the form of tricyclic antidepressants (Burks *et al.*, 1974) or other anti-cholinergic agents (Mendelson, 1977; Klawans and Moskovitz, 1977) and their reversal with cholinergic drugs provides additional evidence that in the acute situations, cholinergic suppression can produce effects similar to those of dopaminergic stimulation.

Schizophrenia

The question of whether an important interaction between DA and ACh exists in schizophrenia is currently the subject of some debate. The widely held clinical impression that anticholinergic, antiparkinson drugs block extrapyramidal side effects of antipsychotic drugs without interfering with antipsychotic efficacy (Chien and DiMascio, 1967) is usually cited as clinical evidence against a role of cholinergic mechanisms in schizophrenia. Indeed a number of studies in which anticholinergic drugs have been discontinued in patients maintained on antipsychotic drugs have shown no indication of improvement in psychiatric status (Orlov *et al.*, 1971; Klett and Caffey, 1972; McClelland *et al.*, 1974). These studies, however, have been carried out in largely chronic populations with a primary focus of attention directed towards possible emergence of extrapyramidal rather than psychiatric symptoms. Prospective studies in recently hospitalized schizophrenics of relatively short duration with careful monitoring of psychiatric status suggest, in fact, that anticholinergic drugs may block the therapeutic efficacy of antipsychotic drugs (Singh and Kay, 1975b; 1975c). Perhaps consistent with these observations, cholinergic drugs such as arecoline and physostigmine have been reported to improve schizophrenic symptoms (Pfeiffer and Jenney, 1957) while physostigmine reversed the intensification of schizophrenic symptoms produced by methylphenidate (Janowsky *et al.*, 1973). On the other hand, the long acting anticholinesterase inhibitor diisopropylfluorophosphonate often exacerbated psychotic symptoms (Rowntree *et al.*, 1950) while physostigmine had no effect (Janowsky *et al.*, 1973).

Although the effect observed by Singh and Kay (1975a; 1975b; 1975c) was felt to be an exacerbation of the underlying psychotic disorder rather than a toxic effect of anticholinergic drugs it remains possible that the adverse effects of anticholinergic drugs on memory and attention (Safer and Allen 1971; Drachman, 1977) may have contributed to their findings. A possible peripheral mechanism for the phenomenon also worth considering is the effect of anticholinergic drugs on gastrointestinal absorption. Several studies (Rivera-Calimlim *et al.*, 1976; Gautier *et al.*, 1977) have shown that co-administration of anticholinergic drugs substantially reduces plasma levels of neuroleptic drugs. It should be noted, however, that clinical exacerbations of psychosis have not been correlated with such changes in plasma levels while Singh and Kay (1975a) found that even when given alone anticholinergic drugs seemed to worsen psychotic symptoms.

ANIMAL BEHAVIORAL STUDIES

Catalepsy

Catalepsy is a state of extreme motor passivity in which an animal is rendered immobile and unable to extract himself from externally imposed awkward postures. Neuroleptic drugs which interfere with striatal DA transmission and cholinergic drugs both produce catalepsy (Costall and Olley, 1971). In addition, neuroleptic catalepsy is enhanced or reduced by co-administration of cholinergic or anticholinergic drugs respectively (Morpurgo, 1962; Scheel-Kruger and Randrup, 1968; Zetler, 1968). Although it has usually been assumed that the interaction of DA and ACh mechanisms relevant for for drug-induced catalepsy occurs in the neostriatum, this behavioral effect may actually be relatively non-specific from both an anatomic and pharmacologic point of view (Costall and Naylor, 1973). Thus, although brain lesion and intracerebral injection studies indicate an important role for the neostriatum in neuroleptic catalepsy (Costall and Olley, 1971; Costall et al., 1972), bilateral intrastriatal injection of cholinergic drugs do not produce catalepsy while bilateral neostriatal lesions fail to prevent catalepsy following systemic administration of cholinergic drugs (Costall et al., 1972) suggesting that cholinoceptive sites important for cholinergic catalepsy may lie outside the neostriatum.

Rigidity

Neuroleptic drugs such as reserpine, chlorpromazine, or haloperidol produce rigidity in rats which is accompanied by increased alpha-motoneuron and decreased gamma-motoneuron excitability (Roos and Steg, 1964). Physostigmine produces a state of rigidity which is physiologically identical to that produced by the neuroleptics (Arvidsson et al., 1966). Treatment with L-DOPA or atropine eliminates this rigidity and reverses the reciprocal change in motor neuron excitability produced by reserpine and physostigmine respectively (Arvidsson et al., 1966). Moreover, atropine is also antagonistic to reserpine and haloperidol in this model (Arvidsson et al., 1966).

Stereotyped Behavior

Stereotyped behavior refers to a complex of repetitive, apparently purposeless motor activities produced in all animal species by direct or indirect DA agonists such as amphetamine, methylphenidate, apomorphine, and L-DOPA. In the rat, for example, such behavior consists of continuous sniffing, licking, and biting. Anticholinergic drugs also produce stereotyped behavior in rats similar to although less intense than that produced by amphetamines (Arnfred and Randrup, 1968). When anticholinergics are given in combination with amphetamines, stereotyped behavior may be produced with lower doses of amphetamines than are necessary when amphetamine is given alone (Arnfred and Randrup, 1968). On the other hand, drugs with cholinergic properties prevent the appearance of amphetamine-induced stereotyped behavior (Arnfred and Randrup, 1968). Similar results have been reported using a variety of anticholinergic, cholinergic, and dopaminergic drugs in several animal species (Scheel-Kruger, 1970; Klawans et al., 1972). The additional observation that the capacity of a neuroleptic drug to antagonize methylphenidate-induced stereotyped behavior is potentiated by cholinergic drugs and reduced by anticholinergic treatment further confirms the antagonistic effects of dopaminergic and cholinergic drugs on stereotyped behavior (Janowsky et al., 1972).

Rotational Behavior

In rodents it is well known that a relative increase in the activity of one nigrostriatal system makes the animal rotate towards the contralateral side. Thus, for example, electrical stimulation of one nigrostriatal tract, unilateral intracaudate injection of dopaminergic drugs, or unilateral destruction of one nigrostriatal system with systemic administration of drugs with dopaminergic properties all produce rotation of the animal away from the side of greater nigrostriatal activity.

Costall *et al.*, (1972) demonstrated the presence of a reciprocal balance between dopaminergic and cholinergic mechanisms in the neostriatum on the basis of intracaudate injection studies. Unilateral injection of cholinergic or neuroleptic drugs both resulted in circling behavior ipsilateral to the side of caudate injection. Conversely, intracaudate injection of anticholinergics or DA agonists (Ungerstedt *et al.*, 1969) resulted in circling contralateral to the side of injection. When atropine was injected into the same caudate nucleus as either a cholinergic or neuroleptic drug ipsilateral circling was reduced; when injected contralaterally ipsilateral circling was potentiated providing further support for a balance of neostriatal DA-ACh mechanisms in rotational behavior.

Evidence along similar lines comes from studies of systemic drug effects in animals with unilateral destruction of one nigrostriatal system. In such animals systemic administration of amphetamine produces continuous rotational behavior towards the side of the lesion due to release and inhibition of presynaptic reuptake of endogenous DA in the intact nigrostriatal tract (Ungerstedt *et al.*, 1973). Systemic anticholinergic drugs such as atropine or scopolamine given alone to such animals produces less vigorous rotation in the same direction (Ungerstedt *et al.*, 1973; Kelly and Miller, 1975; Marsden *et al.*, 1975, Pycock *et al.*, 1978). When given together with amphetamine, anticholinergic drugs potentiate (Marsden *et al.*, 1975) while cholinergic drugs antagonize amphetamine-induced rotation (Kelly and Miller, 1975; Marsden *et al.*, 1975, Pycock *et al.*, 1978).

The observation which repeatedly emerges from these animal behavioral studies is that dopaminergic and cholinergic effects are antagonistic and, as a result, dopaminergic effects are mimicked by anticholinergic drugs while antidopaminergic effects are mimicked by cholinergic drugs. Recent ontogenetic studies in rats indicate that the neuroanatomic substrate for DA-mediated behavior is present in the immediate neonatal period while functional maturity of striatal cholinergic interneurons and responses to cholinergic drugs does not appear until after the second week of life (Kelly *et al.*, 1974; Guyenet *et al.*, 1975a; Baez *et al.*, 1976). Interestingly, a reciprocal relationship between adrenergic and cholinergic effects has been described in a number of other animal behavioral models as well, including conditioned maze behavior (Schelkunov, 1967), operant shock avoidance behavior (Carlton, 1963), brain self stimulation (Wauquier *et al.*, 1975), group toxicity in mice (Morpurgo and Theobald, 1964), jumping behavior (Colpaert *et al.*, 1975) and locomotor stimulation (Thornburg and Moore, 1973) to mention only a few. Until relatively recently all that could be said regarding interactions of this sort was that an antagonistic balance accounted for the phenomenon the anatomical substrate for which was unknown.

MECHANISMS OF DA-ACH INTERACTION

Microiontophoretic Studies

In microiontophoretic studies putative neurotransmitters are administered into the immediate vicinity of individual neurons while the electrical activity of these cells is monitored extracellularly (Bloom *et al.*, 1965). Although such techniques are poorly suited for the study of interactions between putative neurotransmitters, several pertinent observations have been made for the understanding of DA and ACh interactions in the basal ganglia.

Bloom *et al.,* (1965) found that microiontophoretic application of DA onto caudate neurons usually produced depression of firing rate while facilitation occurred in only a relatively small number of cells. Following administration of ACh the opposite was observed with facilitation of spontaneous firing rate occurring more frequently than depression. Sequential application of DA and ACh onto the same neuron, carried out in only a few cases, showed that DA greatly reduced or abolished facilatory responses to ACh. Subsequent studies, all using extracellular recording techniques have confirmed the fact that, in the caudate nucleus DA depresses the firing of about 50-90% and excites about 5-15% of caudate neurons tested (McLennan and York, 1967; York, 1967; Herz and Zieglgansberger, 1968; Spehlmann, 1975; Siggins *et al.,* 1976). Investigators using intracellular recording techniques have argued that DA exerts a predominantly excitatory effect on caudate neurons and have attributed the inhibitory effect observed in extra-cellular recordings to possible DA excitation of local inhibitory neurons (Kitai *et al.,* 1976). It is possible that cells large enough to be recorded intracellularly show an excit-atory response to DA while inhibitory receptors are located on smaller caudate neurons. A possible artifactual explanation of excitatory responses in intracellular studies has also been discussed (Siggins *et al.,* 1976).

The effect of microiontophoretic ACh and other cholinomimetic substances on caudate neurons has been predominantly excitatory (Bloom *et al.,* 1965; McLennan and York, 1966; Herz and Zieglgansberger, 1968; Spehlmann, 1975) with evidence that a topographic distribution of cholinoceptive neurons may exist such that superificial caudate cells are excited while deeper cells are depressed by ACh (McLennan and York, 1966). On the basis of observations that ACh responses are blocked by previous ionto-phoretic application of atropine (McLennan and York, 1966), are mimicked by oxotrem-orine (a muscarinic agent) (Herz and Sieglgansberger, 1968), and are unaffected by drugs with nicotinic or antinicotinic properties (McLennan and York, 1966) it has been con-cluded that cholinoceptive receptors on caudate neurons are muscarinic in type. The muscarinic nature of caudate cholinergic receptors is further supported by more recent studies with radioactively labelled muscarinic antagonists which bind with high affinity to central cholinergic receptors (Hiley and Bird, 1974; Snyder *et al.,* 1974; Yamamura *et al.,* 1974).

In view of the predominantly depressant effect of DA and excitatory effect of ACh on caudate neurons it has been assumed that individual caudate cells exhibit a reciprocal response to DA and ACh. Steg (1969), studying the response of individual caudate neurons to intravenous physostigmine, atropine, L-DOPA, and reserpine, found that nearly all cells activated by physostigmine were depressed by L-DOPA and concluded that excitatory cholinergic and inhibitory monoaminergic neurons terminate on a common population of striatal cells.

Microiontophoretic studies, on the other hand, have provided little direct evidence that individual cells respond to DA and ACh in a reciprocal manner. As already men-tioned, Bloom *et al.,* (1965) found that previous application of DA onto a caudate neuron reduced or abolished the excitatory response to subsequent application of ACh. However, McLennan and York (1966), although indicating that a rigorous examination to determine whether all cholinoceptive cells were also affected by DA was not carried out, found some neurons which were depressed by both DA and ACh and others in which ACh was excitatory and DA was depressant. Connor (1970) found no correlation between

DA and ACh responses on the same unit. Cells facilitated by ACh were sometimes depressed by DA, others were facilitated by DA, and frequently a neuron responded to only one agent.

In a somewhat different approach Spehlmann (1975) has studied responses of caudate neurons to microiontophoretic application of DA or ACh in cats with unilateral nigrostriatal lesions and depletion of caudate DA. In these animals, although the proportion of neurons excited by ACh was not increased, the threshold for the excitatory effect of ACh was significantly less in lesioned than in intact animals suggesting that depletion of striatal DA may increase neuronal excitability to ACh in some undetermined way.

The origin of caudate neurons sensitive to DA and ACh in microiontophoretic studies has been the subject of extensive study (Tebecis, 1974). On the basis of stimulation, recording, and iontophoretic studies, McLennan and York (1967) originally proposed an inhibitory dopaminergic pathway from the nucleus centromedianum of the thalamus to the caudate nucleus; but subsequent neurophysiologic studies have cast doubt on such a pathway (Tebecis, 1974). Subsequently, abundant evidence had accumulated that dopaminergic terminals in the caudate nucleus originate in the SN. Electrical stimulation in the SN inhibits the firing of many caudate neurons which are also depressed by iontophoretic application of DA (Connor, 1970). On the other hand, the excitation of caudate neurons sometimes produced by stimulation of the SN may not be dopaminergic since most caudate neurons excited by nigral stimuli are either depressed or unaffected by DA (McLennan and York, 1967; Connor, 1970). The putamen also receives dopaminergic input from the SN but, unlike the caudate nucleus, iontophoretic DA and stimulation in the SN both produce excitation rather than inhibition of putamen neurons (York, 1970).

With regard to cholinoceptive caudate neurons, although it was originally proposed (McLennan and York, 1966; McLennan, 1971) that cholinergic fibers project from the ventral anterior nucleus of the thalamus to caudate, this too has been challenged (Tebecis, 1974) and receives little support from anatomic studies of cholinergic pathways (Shute and Lewis, 1967; McGeer et al., 1971).

Biochemical Studies

Dopaminergic Regulation of Cholinergic Activity

Although it has been generally assumed that an important antagonistic relationship exists between DA and ACh mechanisms in the basal ganglia, information concerning the specific nature of this relationship has become available only recently. As already discussed, microiontophoretic studies indicate that caudate neurons respond oppositely to application of dopaminergic and cholinergic substances although definite evidence that individual cells consistently do so is not available. Largely on the basis of such studies, however, it was initially suggested that there may be antagonistic DA and ACh input upon a common striatal neuron (Steg, 1969; Corrodi et al., 1972). Reduction of inhibitory dopaminergic input upon this hypothetical striatal neuron would lead to a functional preponderance of cholinergic excitatory activity thereby explaining, for example, the ameliorative effect of anticholinergic drugs in Parkinson's disease.

A major difficulty with this view is that evidence for extrastriatal cholinergic inputs onto striatal neurons has not been forthcoming. As mentioned previously, McLennan and York (1966) proposed a thalamocaudate cholinergic projection. Shute and Lewis (1967), on the basis of cholinesterase-staining techniques, identified fibers terminating in the neostriatum which arose in globus pallidus, entopenduncular nucleus, preoptic area, and brain-stem. However, doubts have been cast on the specificity of this method for identification of cholinergic neurons (Karczmar, 1969; McGeer et al., 1976) and more recently it has been shown that widespread lesions in cortex, thalamus, midbrain tegmentum, and globus pallidus produce no significant change in levels of acetylcholinesterase (Lynch et al., 1972) or CAT (McGeer et al., 1971; Lynch et al., 1972) in rat neostriatum. This data has been interpreted to indicate that cholinergic neurons in the caudate nucleus are predominantly short interneurons which originate within the striatum itself and remain confined to this structure.

An alternative view of neostriatal DA-ACh interaction suggests that cholinergic striatal neurons with excitatory properties receive a direct inhibitory dopaminergic input from the SN (Calne, 1970; Bartholini et al., 1973). This ascending dopaminergic input is believed to inhibit the activity of striatal cholinergic neurons so that reduced dopaminergic activity results in increased striatal cholinergic activity while increased dopaminergic activity results in inhibition of striatal cholinergic activity. Initial experiments supporting such a concept were carried out by means of a push-pull cannula implanted in the caudate nucleus of cats whereby release of ACh could be monitored following intravenous administration of a series of drugs (Stadler et al., 1973). Neuroleptic drugs which block striatal DA receptors such as chlorpromazine and haloperidol caused a marked increase in the output of striatal ACh, while promethazine, a phenothiazine which does not block striatal DA receptors, had no effect. Subsequent administration of apomorphine, a DA agonist, abolished this increase. This effect appeared to be specific for the striatum since ACh output in cortex and several limbic regions was unaffected by these drugs. The possibility that anticholinergic properties of some neuroleptics might in some way account for the results was excluded by the observations that atropine had no effect on ACh output and haloperidol is relatively weak in anticholinergic properties (Miller and Hiley, 1974; Snyder et al., 1974). Inhibition of acetylcholinesterase by neuroleptic drugs as an explanation for the results was also excluded (Guyenet et al., 1975c). These biochemical observations were felt to be inconsistent with a concept of balanced antagonistic DA and ACh inputs regulating the activity of a common striatal neuron but suggested instead that there is a population of striatal cholinergic neurons under the direct influence of a tonic inhibitory dopaminergic input.

A series of studies utilizing other techniques have subsequently confirmed these findings. Trabucchi et al., (1974) measuring ACh turnover rates, found that after administration of chlorpromazine or haloperidol the rate of ACh synthesis in rat striatum was increased while no change occurred in occipital cortex suggesting again the existence of a specific striatal neuronal mechanism for regulation of cholinergic activity not found in other brain regions. The opposite effect on ACh turnover rate was observed following administration of dopaminergic drugs such a L-DOPA, apomorphine, and amphetamine (Trabucchi et al., 1975). Several laboratories have shown that administration of a variety of other pre- and post-synaptic DA antagonists such a reserpine, pimozide, and clozapine leads to a decrease in striatal ACh levels (due to increased turnover and release) (Beani et al., 1966; Orzeck and Barbeau, 1970; Sethy and Van Woert, 1974; McGeer et al.,

1974; Consolo et al., 1975). In interpreting the physiological implications of these bio-chemical studies it is assumed, although not proven, that increased striatal ACh synthesis corresponds with increased activity of cholinergic neurons (Trabucchi et al., 1974) similar to the nigrostriatal system, for example, where increased rates of DA turnover correlate with increased firing rates in nigrostriatal DA neurons (Bunney et al., 1973).

Release of DA in the striatum by electrical stimulation of zona compacta of the SN produces a marked decrease of striatal ACh output similar to the effect of DA agonists (Stadler et al., 1975). However, initial studies of the effect of nigrostriatal lesions sur-prisingly failed to reproduce the effects of pharmacologic DA blockade. Thus, chemical or electrolytic destruction of nigrostriatal pathways failed to produce the decrease in neostriatal ACh concentrations expected after disinhibition of striatal cholinergic neurons, (Butcher and Butcher, 1974; Grewaal et al., 1974 Consolo et al., 1975; Guyenet et al., 1975b). Since biochemical measurements were made 1-14 days following placement of lesions, the possibility of some form of secondary adaptation by striatal cholinergic neurons to the effect of reduced nigrostriatal input was suggested (Consolo et al., 1975; Agid et al., 1975). Fibiger and Grewaal (1974) have shown that administration of apomorphine to rats with two month old unilateral SN lesions produces an increase in striatal ACh levels which is significantly greater in the neostriatum ipsilateral to the lesion than on the intact side. If this is taken as biochemical evidence that denervation can produce a form of supersensitivity in striatal cholinergic neurons (Fibiger and Grewaal, 1974) it may account for the normal rather than accelerated striatal ACh turnover observed in the chronic denervation experiments.

However, subsequent acute studies measuring striatal ACh concentration within two hours following electrolytic nigrostriatal lesions have found that striatal ACh is, in fact, significantly decreased at a time when DA release is reduced thus confirming the assumption that the nigrostriatal pathway provides a direct tonic inhibition of striatal cholinergic activity (Agid et al., 1975; Rommelspacher and Kuhar, 1975).

Direct anatomical evidence that nigrostriatal DA neurons form direct synapses with striatal cholinergic interneurons has recently come from immunohistochemical studies (Hattori et al., 1976). Administration of intraventricular 6-hydroxydopamine produces degeneration of dopaminergic nerve endings in the neostriatum which are found to make direct synaptic contact with major dendrites or dendritic spines staining positively for CAT visualized at the light and electron microscopic level. Although a definite estimate of the percentage of dopaminergic nerve endings in the striatum which innervate cholinergic neurons has not yet been made it is becoming clear that the inner-vation of cholinergic neurons by dopaminergic terminals is quite heavy (Hattori et al., 1976).

Cholinergic Regulation of Dopaminergic Activity

It has been demonstrated by numerous biochemical and physiologic techniques that the synthesis and release ("turnover") of DA in nigrostriatal neurons is increased in response to administration of neuroleptic antipsychotic drugs which interfere with synaptic transmission of DA in the neostriatum. Thus, for example, neuroleptic drugs in experimental animals produce increased conversion of radioactively labelled tyrosine to labelled DA (Bartholini and Pletscher, 1969), increased striatal release of DA (Cheramy *et al.*, 1970) increased levels of striatal homovanillic acid (Matthysse, 1973), and increased firing rates of nigrostriatal neurons (Bunney *et al.*, 1973). It is currently believed that this neuroleptic-induced acceleration of nigrostriatal activity results at least in part from a neuronally mediated feedback loop which serves to compensate for blockade of striatal dopamine receptors (Carlsson and Lindqvist, 1963). This neuronally mediated control of DA turnover is distinct from other possible mechanisms of feedback inhibition such as biochemical end-product inhibition of tyrosine hydroxylase by catecholamines (Javoy *et al.*, 1972), presynaptic receptor-mediated feedback mechanisms (Kehr *et al.*, 1972) or self-inhibitory mechanisms in DA neurons within the SN (Groves *et al.*, 1975). The anatomical substrate for this neuronal feedback loop is believed to be a recurrent striatonigral projection which modulates activity in nigrostriatal dopaminergic neurons.

A number of studies have suggested that ACh may play a major role in this neuronal feedback mechanism. Given alone, anticholinergic drugs reduce nigrostriatal DA turnover (O'Keefe *et al.*, 1970, Anden and Bedard, 1971; Bartholini and Pletscher, 1971; Corrodi *et al.*, 1972; Bowers and Roth, 1972; Westerink and Korf, 1975) while cholinergic drugs exert the opposite effect (Bartholini and Pletscher, 1971; Anden, 1974; Westerink and Korf, 1975; Javoy *et al.*, 1975; Ulus and Wurtman, 1976). When given together with neuroleptics, anticholinergic drugs block neuroleptic-induced accelerated DA turnover (O'Keefe *et al.*, 1970; Anden and Bedard, 1971; Corrodi *et al.*, 1972; Bowers and Roth, 1972; Westerink and Korf, 1975). Initially it was suggested that an excitatory cholinergic striatonigral projection which regulates the activity of nigral DA neurons could account for the turnover changes observed following anticholinergic and cholinergic drugs (Corrodi *et al.*, 1972). Thus, blockade of this facilatory mechanism by anticholinergic drugs would decrease DA turnover while potentiation with cholinergic agents would increase DA turnover. Although initially there appeared to be histochemical evidence for a striatonigral cholinergic pathway based on topographical distribution of acetylcholinesterase (Olivier *et al.*, 1970), this method may be unreliable for identification of cholinergic neurons (Karczmar, 1969; McGeer *et al.*, 1976). Moreover, surgical interruption of striatonigral pathways does not alter levels of CAT in the SN (McGeer *et al.*, 1973) while micro-iontophoretic application of ACh onto nigral neurons fails to mimic the effect of electrical stimulation of caudate neurons (Feltz, 1971).

Recent anatomical (McGeer *et al.*, 1973; Bak *et al.*, 1975), biochemical (Harris and Baldessarini, 1975; Cheramy *et al.*, 1977), physiologic (Feltz, 1971; Crossman *et al.*, 1973) and behavioral (Tarsy *et al.*, 1975; Dray *et al.*, 1975) evidence suggests, in fact, that striatonigral inhibition is mediated by GABA neurons. On the basis of the numerous studies discussed above, an alternative scheme to reconcile the data concerning the role of ACh and GABA in regulation of nigrostriatal activity is to interpose a short excitatory intrastriatal cholinergic interneuron between ascending nigrostriatal dopaminergic projections and descending GABA-mediated striatonigral or striatopallidalnigral projections (MGeer and McGeer, 1976a; Roth and Bunney, 1976; Tarsy, 1977).

There are two major difficulties with this scheme. Firstly, anticholinergic and cholinergic drugs have been shown to have no effect on firing rates of nigrostriatal neurons (Bunney and Aghajanian, 1976) thereby making it unlikely that cholinergic interneurons are directly incorporated into a recurrent neuronal loop feedback system of the sort described above. Secondly, a single excitatory cholinergic interneuron interposed between an inhibitory dopaminergic neuron and a descending monosynaptic inhibitory GABA-mediated neuron fails to fit with experimental observations. According to this scheme DA receptor blockade and cholinergic drugs should both inhibit rather than activate nigrostriatal DA turnover while anticholinergic drugs should activate rather than inhibit nigrostriatal DA turnover.

A simpler explanation of the effect of cholinergic and anticholinergic drugs on striatal DA turnover may be that these drugs act directly to affect release of DA from striatal nerve terminals. The "Burn-Rand hypothesis" (Burn and Rand, 1959), also referred to as the "cholinergic-link hypothesis" (Ferry, 1966), states that in peripheral sympathetic neurons ACh is released from adrenergic nerve terminals and acts on presynaptic nicotinic receptors to allow entry of calcium which, in turn, causes release of norepinephrine. A muscarinic mechanism whereby ACh release results in blockade of catecholamine release in peripheral adrenergic neurons has also been described (Muscholl, 1974). Recent studies in the central nervous system have shown that ACh and other cholinergic agonists stimulate the release of DA both *in vitro* in rat striatal slices and *in vivo* in the cat caudate nucleus (Giorguieff *et al.*, 1976; Giorguieff *et al.*, 1977). It is currently uncertain whether this is a purely pharmacologic phenomenon or does have physiologic importance for regulation of DA release. In view of the large number of small striatal ACh interneurons which exist however, local ACh-mediated regulation of DA release is an intriguing possibility which should be clarified by future study.

In addition to DA-ACh interaction within the striatum, there may also be cholinergic regulation of nigrostriatal DA activity at the level of the SN. The observation that injection of atropine just rostral and dorsal to the SN increases striatal DA turnover (Bartholini and Pletscher, 1971; Bartholini *et al.*, 1971) suggested the possibility of an inhibitory cholinergic influence on nigrostriatal DA neurons. The observations of Javoy *et al.*, (1974) that short infusions of carbachol, a cholinomimetic agent, into the SN inhibit neostriatal DA utilization while infusion of atropine activates DA synthesis and utilization provide additional evidence for ACh-mediated inhibition of nigrostriatal DA activity. Microiontophoretic studies have indicated, however, that DA neurons in zona compacta of SN are insensitive to ACh while zona reticulata neurons are excited by ACh (Aghajanian and Bunney, 1974). It is therefore speculated that there may be a cholinergic projection of unknown origin onto inhibitory interneurons of zona reticulata which in turn project to DA neurons in zona compacta of SN (Roth and Bunney, 1976). The finding that DA neurons in the SN contain acetylcholinesterase, speculatively to inactivate ACh released from cholinergic fibers afferent to DA neurons (Butcher and Bilezikjian, 1975), must be regarded as of uncertain significance in view of the fact that concentrations of ACh and CAT in animal (Cheney *et al.*, 1975) and human (Lloyd *et al.*, 1975b; McGeer and McGeer, 1976b) SN are relatively small.

Unfortunately, behavioral studies to date have produced conflicting results which are not entirely consistent with cholinergic inhibition of nigrostriatal DA neurons in the SN. Reports that intranigral arecoline produces ipsilateral rotation (Costall *et al.*, 1972) while intranigral atropine produces an assymetrical posture with rotation towards the contralateral side (Javoy *et al.*, 1974) are consistent with the notion of cholinergic inhibition of nigrostriatal DA activity. On the other hand, results of other behavioral studies are more consistent with cholinergic facilitation than inhibition of nigral DA mechanisms. Thus, intranigral injection of a series of cholinergic drugs in rats has been found to produce contralateral postural deviation or circling while intranigral injection of anticholinergic drugs has produced ipsilateral postural deviation or circling (C.D. Marsden, personal communication). Further observations that intranigral injection of physostigmine produces stereotyped behavior in rats (Smelik and Ernst, 1966) while bilateral intranigral injection of ACh, methacholine, or neostigmine all produce stereotyped behavior and increased locomotor activity in rabbits (Wolfarth et al., 1974) would also support a facilatory effect of ACh on nigral DA neurons.

The results of the behavioral studies cited above are obviously conflicting and for the present should not be taken as evidence for or against cholinergic regulation of nigrostriatal DA activity at the level of the SN, whether inhibitory or facilatory. Most studies of this type have been done without simultaneous biochemical measurement of nigrostriatal DA activity, have not been replicated in more than one laboratory, have utilized different animal species, and are dealing with injections into a relatively small brain region leaving open the question of whether effects are mediated in zona compacta, zona reticulata, or some other immediately adjacent brain region with cholinoceptive sensitivity.

DA-ACH INTERACTION IN THE LIMBIC SYSTEM

Largely because of methodologic considerations mechanisms of DA-ACh interaction have been far more extensively studied in the nigrostriatal than mesolimbic or mesocortical DA systems. However, in addition to containing high concentrations of DA, various limbic nuclei including nucleus accumbens and amygdaloid nucleus have also been shown to be rich in ACh (Cheney et al., 1975), CAT (Palkovits et al., 1974; Cheney et al., 1975), and muscarinic receptors (Kuhar and Yamamura, 1976). In the case of nucleus accumbens concentrations of ACh, CAT, and muscarinic receptors are as high as in caudate nucleus (Cheney et al., 1975; Kuhar and Yamamura, 1976).

The observation that DA receptor blockade with neuroleptic drugs increases ACh turnover in the neostriatum appears to be specific for this region and has not been observed in limbic nuclei or other brain regions. Chlorpromazine or haloperidol did not increase release of ACh collected by a push-pull cannula technique from the nucleus accumbens of cats despite increased release of DA in this region (Bartholini et al., 1974; Stadler et al., 1975). On the other hand, data concerning cholinergic regulation of DA activity have been contradictory. In two studies administration of the anticholinergic drug trihexyphendyl has been found to suppress neuroleptic-induced increases in DA turnover in neostriatum but less so or not at all in pooled limbic structures (Anden, 1974; Bartholini et al., 1975). However, microdissection studies of individual limbic nuclei have shown that trihexyphendyl does suppress neuroleptic-induced increases in DA turnover here as well as in the neostriatum (Westerink and Korf, 1975). Moreover, administration of cholinergic drugs oxotremorine or physostigmine increases DA turnover at least as much if not more so in mesolimbic nuclei than in neostriatum (Anden, 1974; Bartholini et al., 1975; Westerink and Korf, 1975).

Thus, on the basis of a limited number of studies, limbic nuclei appear to resemble the neostriatum with regard to cholinergic regulation of dopaminergic function but differ in the absence of dopaminergic inhibition of cholinergic activity. In view of a close proximity of the heavily cholinergic nucleus interpeduncularis to cell bodies of midbrain area A-10 from which dopaminergic mesolimbic neurons originate, it has been suggested that the habenula-interpeduncular system may play a role in feedback regulation of the mesolimbic system (Cheney *et al.*, 1975). On the other hand, it is possible that more recently studied mechanisms of cholinergic regulation of striatal DA release (Giorguieff *et al.*, 1977) may play a role in limbic DA turnover as well.

CONCLUSIONS

The experimental studies discussed above provide evidence for DA-ACh interaction at several levels in the basal ganglia. Evidence for dopaminergic inhibition of striatal cholinergic activity, cholinergic regulation of nigral dopaminergic activity, and ACh-mediated release of DA within the striatum have all been described. Whether any or all of these mechanisms adequately explain the numerous animal behavioral and clinical examples of a reciprocal interaction between DA and ACh in the basal ganglia remains open to debate.

A major role of the dopaminergic nigrostriatal system, at least in its projection to the caudate nucleus, appears to be inhibition of striatal cholinergic neurons. By means of this relationship, the inhibitory effect of a DA agonist on striatal cholinergic activity should be mimicked or potentiated by an anticholinergic drug. Conversely, the effect of a DA antagonist in disinhibiting and thereby facilitating activity in striatal cholinergic neurons should be mimicked by administration of a cholinergic drug. Similarly, the effect of a DA antagonist should be blocked by an anticholinergic drug. As already discussed, animal behavioral and clinical studies in patients with extrapyramidal disorders appear to support this reciprocal relationship.

The role of the large number of intrastriatal cholinergic neurons which receive this inhibitory dopaminergic innervation is presently unknown. In the past it was suggested that striatonigral and striatopallidal efferent projections are cholinergic (Poirier, 1971). If so, nigrostriatal dopaminergic neurons might be expected to play a role in inhibiting this large efferent system which is obviously important in the control and regulation of motor behavior. As reviewed above, however, the weight of evidence indicates that the vast majority of striatal cholinergic neurons remain exclusively intrastriatal while the bulk of striatal efferents to globus pallidus and SN are instead GABA-mediated.

Although mechanisms for cholinergic facilitation of dopaminergic activity have also been described it currently appears doubtful that they play a significant role in the animal behavioral and clinical effects of systemically administered cholinergic and anticholinergic drugs. The possibility that striatal cholinergic interneurons play a role in feedback regulation of nigrostriatal activity has been discussed. This could be either as part of a polysynaptic ACh- and GABA-mediated system or by exerting direct presynaptic effects on DA release. However, the capacity of cholinergic and anticholinergic drugs to stimulate DA release and interfere with DA turnover respectively are the results of relatively large doses (Javoy, 1975) and are actually the opposite of what would be expected on the basis of their animal behavioral and clinical effects. On the other hand, if a mechanism also exists at the level of the SN for cholinergic inhibition of nigrostriatal DA activity (Javoy *et al.*, 1974, 1975), systemic anticholinergic drugs in relatively low, clinically relevant doses acting at both striatal and nigral levels may produce opposite and cancelling effects on DA turnover (Javoy *et al.*, 1975). It is thus possible that these apparently antagonistic cholinergic influences on DA activity bear little or no relationship to the effects of these drugs used clinically (Javoy *et al.*, 1975).

It should be emphasized that in both animals and man the effects of DA agonists are considerably more powerful than those of anticholinergic drugs. Thus, the effect of DA-mediated inhibition of cholinergic neurons is mimicked by an anticholinergic drug qualitatively but not necessarily in a quantitative manner. The most obvious explanation is the fact that nigrostriatal DA neurons also project to non-cholinergic striatal neurons (Hattori et al., 1976). Although the chemical neurotransmission of these neurons has not yet been identified it seems likely that at least some will turn out to be GABA-mediated.

To what extent can clinical observations be explained by what we know at this time about DA-ACh interactions? In Parkinson's disease it is well known that anticholinergic drugs tend to be more effective early than later in the course of the disease while L-DOPA treatment can be effective at any time. If parkinsonian symptoms occur exclusively because of loss of DA inhibition of striatal neurons, then anticholinergic drugs should maintain their therapeutic effectiveness. One explanation offered for the limited useful-ness of anticholinergic drugs is that anticholinergic therapy restores DA-ACh equilibrium at a level of DA activity well below normal while L-DOPA, in normalizing striatal DA levels, results in equilibrium at closer to physiologic levels (Hornykiewicz, 1971).

Another possible explanation is that, although initially DA depletion produces disinhibition of striatal cholinergic activity, with time an adaptive change occurs such that striatal cholinergic activity returns to normal levels thereby reducing the efficacy of cholinergic suppression by pharmacologic means. We have already seen that in the experimental animal disinhibition of striatal cholinergic activity can only be observed within the first two hours following a nigrostriatal lesion and is no longer evident 1-14 days later. Precisely because of this relatively transient effect of nigrostriatal destruction on striatal ACh turnover it has been suggested that loss of inhibitory DA input on striatal cholinergic neurons cannot by itself explain cholinergic sensitivity in Parkinson's disease (Spehlmann and Stahl, 1976). An alternative hypothesis suggests that death of nigro-striatal DA neurons results in sprouting of axons of striatal cholinergic interneurons which innervate vacated postsynaptic terminals thereby resulting in a great increase in striatal cholinergic activity (Spehlmann and Stahl, 1976).

Observations concerning the extrapyramidal effect of neuroleptic drugs are also relevant. Firstly, acute dyskinesias which appear following exposure to small doses of neuroleptic drugs are exquisitely sensitive to anticholinergic treatment (Marsden et al., 1975). By contrast, neuroleptic-induced parkinsonism responds less dramatically and, in fact, is unaffected by intravenous administration of anticholinergic drugs (Simpson, 1970). Could this phenomenon be explained by an adaptation of cholinergic neurons to the effect of DA blockade? Further evidence that some form of adaptation may occur is the observation that tolerance to extrapyramidal effects appears to occur in the first three months of exposure of neuroleptic drugs (DiMascio and Demirgian, 1970; Orlov et al., 1971; Klett and Caffey, 1972; McClelland et al., 1974). Similar tolerance to the neuroleptic effects of chronically administered antipsychotic drugs has been demonstrated in laboratory animals (Asper et al., 1973). The fact that in idiopathic Parkinson's disease anticholinergic drugs become increasingly ineffective, while in drug-induced parkinsonism they become unnecessary in most patients after three months of exposure undoubtedly relates to the fact that in Parkinson's disease there is progressive degeneration of nigro-striatal neurons while DA "deficiency" in drug-induced parkinsonism is produced by pharmacological blockade of DA receptors for which some degree of tolerance appears possible.

In chronic choreiform syndromes in man there is less convincing clinical evidence for a reciprocal balance between DA-ACh mechanisms. In animal models of hyperkinetic motor activity such as sterotyped behavior, on the other hand, it has been relatively easy to demonstrate a reciprocal relationship (Rubovits and Klawans, 1972). The most obvious difference in the two situations is that pharmacological experiments in animals involve study of drug interactions in a normal brain. In the case of Huntington's disease, damage in some striatal cholinergic interneurons may be compensated for by blocking DA inhibition of remaining cholinergic neurons (McGeer *et al.*, 1976). However, coexistant and more extensive pathologic changes in striatal GABA interneurons may confound the effect of cholinergic drugs in this condition. Since physostigmine, an anticholinesterase, depends for its cholinergic activity on the presence of endogenous ACh neurons, its variable effect in Huntington's chorea may also be due to the patchy loss of striatal cholinergic neurons which is known to occur in this disease (McGeer *et al.*, 1973; Bird and Iversen, 1974). The fact that the number of striatal cholinergic receptors, many of which are likely to be on GABA neurons, are also reduced in Huntington's disease (Hiley and Bird, 1974) makes it even less likely that cholinergic drugs such as choline will have beneficial effects in this condition (Davis *et al.*, 1976; Aquilonius and Eckernas, 1977).

Less can be said about the situation in tardive dyskinesia in which neuropathological changes have been inconsistent and neurochemical changes have not yet been studied. Although anticholinergic drugs sometimes worsen this condition it has been difficult to show a consistent beneficial effect by administration of physostigmine. Recent attempts to raise brain levels of ACh by administration of oral choline to patients with tardive dyskinesia (Davis *et al.*, 1976; Growdon *et al.*, 1977) have shown some promising results however and will be watched with interest in the future.

As discussed in previous sections the role of DA-ACh interaction in the limbic system has been less extensively studied than in the nigrostriatal system. The observation that anticholinergic drugs may interfere with the therapeutic effect of antipsychotic drugs (Singh and Kay, 1975a; 1975b; 1975c) is intriguing but requires further clinical confirmation. Importantly, however, if such an effect does exist, it need not be necessarily due to a direct interaction between DA and ACh neurons within individual limbic nuclei as discussed in connection with extrapyramidal disorders but may be related to effects on other limbic cholinergic projections (Singh and Kay, 1975a) or even adverse effects of anticholinergic drugs on memory and attention (Safer and Allen, 1971; Drachman, 1977).

In conclusion, a reciprocal relationship between DA and ACh mechanisms is demonstrable in a number of models of animal motor activity, in parkinsonism, and to a somewhat lesser extent in choreiform syndromes. It is possible that clinical demonstration of cholinergic responsiveness has been limited simply by the relatively small number of practical or safe cholinergic drugs which exist, especially those which might be effective in the presence of damage to cholinergic neurons or cholinergic receptors. New approaches to the treatment of extrapyramidal disorders by manipulation of cholinergic mechanisms have begun to appear and will undoubtedly continue to be forthcoming in the near future.

REFERENCES

Aghajanian, G.K., and Bunney, B.S., 1974, Central dopaminergic neurons: neurophysio-logical identification and responses to drugs, *Biochem. Pharmacol. (Suppl.) 23:*523.

Agid, Y., Guyenet, P., Glowinski, J., Beajouan, J.C., and Javoy, F., 1975, Inhibitory influence of the nigrostriatal dopamine system on the striatal cholinergic neurons in the rat, *Brain Res. 86:*488.

Ahmed, A., and Marshall, P.B., 1962, Relationship between anti-acetylcholine and anti-tremor activity in anti-parkinsonian and related drugs, *Br. J. Pharmacol. 18:*274.

Ambani, L.H., and Van Woert, M., 1972, Modification of the tremorigenic activity of physostigmine, *Br. J. Pharmacol. 46:*344.

Ambani, L.H., and Van Woert, M., and Bowers, M.B., Jr., 1973, Physostigmine effects on phenothiazine-induced extrapyramidal reactions, *Arch. Neurol. 29:*444.

Anden, N.E., 1974, Effects of oxotremorine and physostigmine on the turnover of dopamine in the corpus striatum and the limbic system, *J. Pharm. Pharmacol. 26:*738.

Anden, N.E., and Bedard, P., 1971, Influences of cholinergic mechanisms on the function and turnover of brain dopamine, *J. Pharm. Pharmacol. 23:*460.

Anden, N.E., Carlsson, A., Dahlstrom, A., Fuxe, K., Hillarp, N.A., and Larsson, K., 1964, Demonstration and mapping out of nigro-neostriatal dopamine neurons, *Life Sci. 3:* 523.

Anden, N.E., Dahlstrom, A., Fuxe, K., Larsson, K., Olson, L., and Ungerstedt, U., 1966, Ascending monoamine neurons to the telencephalon and diencephalon, *Acta Physiol. Scan. 67:*313.

Aquilonius, S., and Eckernas, S., 1977, Choline therapy in Huntington's chorea, *Neurology 27:*887.

Aquilonius, S.M., and Sjostrom, R., 1971, Cholinergic and dopaminergic mechanisms in Huntington's chorea, *Life Sci. 10:*405.

Arnfred, T., and Randrup, A., 1968, Cholinergic mechanisms in brain inhibiting amphet-amine induced stereotyped behavior, *Acta Pharmacol. Toxicol. 26:*384.

Arvidsson, J., Roos, B.E., and Steg, G., 1966, Reciprocal effects on a- and γ-motoneurons of drugs influencing monoaminergic and cholinergic transmission, *Acta Physiol. Scan. 67:*398.

Asper, H., Baggliolini, M., Burki, H.R., Lauener, H., Ruch, W., and Stille, G., 1973, Tolerance phenomena with neuroleptics, *Eur. J. Pharmacol. 22:*287.

Ayd, F.J., Jr., 1964, Clozapine – a unique new neuroleptic, *Int. Drug Ther. Newsletter 9:*5.

Baez, L.A., Eskridge, N.K., and Schein, R., 1976, Postnatal development of dopaminergic and cholinergic catalepsy in the rat, *Eur. J. Pharmacol. 36:*155.

Bak, I.J., Choi, W.B., Hassler, R., Usunoff, K.G., and Wagner, A., 1975, Fine structural synaptic organization of the corpus striatum and substantia nigra in rat and cat, *Adv. Neurol. 9:*25.

Barbeau, A., 1962, The pathogenesis of Parkinson's disease: A new hypothesis, *Can. Med. Assoc. J. 87:*802.

Bartholini, G., and Pletscher, A., 1969, Enhancement of tyrosine hydroxylation within the brain by chlorpromazine, *Experientia 25:*919.

Bartholini, G., and Pletscher, A., 1971, Atropine-induced changes of cerebral dopamine turnover, *Experientia 27:*1302.

Bartholini, G., Stadler, H., and Lloyd, K.G., 1973, Cholinergic-dopaminergic interactions in the extrapyramidal system, *Adv. Neurol. 3:*233.

Bartholini, G., Stadler, H., and Lloyd, K.G., 1974, Cholinergic-dopaminergic relation in different brain structures, *Biochem. Pharmacol. (Suppl.) 23:*610.

Bartholini, G., Keller, H.H., and Pletscher, A., 1975, Drug-induced changes of dopamine turnover in striatum and limbic system of the rat, *J. Pharm. Pharmacol. 27:*439.

Beani, L., Ledda, F., Bianchi, C., and Baldi, V., 1966, Reversal by 3, 4-dihydroxyphenyl-alanine of reserpine-induced regional changes in acetylcholine content in guinea-pig brain, *Biochem. Pharmacol. 15:*779.

Ben-Ari, Y., Zigmond, R.E., Shute, C.C.D., and Lewis, P.R., 1977, Regional distribution of choline acetyltransferase and acetylcholinesterase within the amygaloid complex and stria terminalis system, *Brain Res. 120:*435.

Bernheimer, H., Birkmayer, W., Hornykiewicz, O., Jellinger, K., and Seitelberger, F., 1973, Brain dopamine and the syndromes of Parkinson and Huntington's, *J. Neurol. Sci. 20:*415.

Bird, E.D., and Iversen, L.L., 1974, Huntington's chorea: post mortem measurement of glutamic acid decarboxylase, choline acetyltransferase and dopamine in the basal ganglia, *Brain 97:*457.

Birket-Smith, E., 1974, Abnormal involuntary movements induced by anticholinergic therapy, *Acta Neurol. Scand. 50:*801.

Birket-Smith, E., 1975, Abnormal involuntary movements in relation to anticholinergics and levodopa therapy, *Acta Neurol. Scand. 52:*158.

Bloom, F.E., Costa, E., and Salmoiraghi, G.C., 1965, Anesthesia and the responsiveness of individual neurons of the caudate nucleus of the cat to acetylcholine, norepinephrine and dopamine administered by microelectrophoresis, *J. Pharm. Exp. Ther. 150:*244.

Bowers, M.B., Jr., and Roth, R.H., 1972, Interaction of atropine-like drugs with dopamine containing neurons in rat brain, *Br. J. Pharmacol. 44:*301.

Bunney, B.S., and Aghajanian, G.K., 1976, The effect of antipsychotic drugs on the firing of dopaminergic neurons: A reappraisal, in *"Antipsychotic Drugs, Pharmacodynamics and Pharmacokinetics"* (G. Sedvall, B. Unvass, and Y. Zotterman, eds.), pp. 305-318, Pergamon Press, New York.

Bunney, B.S., Walters, J.R., Roth, R.H., and Aghajanian, G.K., 1973, Dopaminergic neurons: effect of antipsychotic drugs and amphetamine on single cell activity, *J. Pharm. Exp. Ther. 185:*560.

Burgen, A.S.V., and Chipman, L.M., 1951, Cholinesterase and succinic dehydrogenase in the central nervous system of the dog, *J. Physiol. 114:*296.

Burks, J.S., Walker, J.E., Rumack, B.H., and Ott, J.E., 1974, Tricyclic antidepressant poisoning, *JAMA 230:*1405.

Burn, J.H., and Rand, M.J., 1959, Sympathetic postganglionic mechanism, *Nature 184:*163.

Butcher, L., and Bilezikjian, L., 1975, Acetylcholinesterase-containing neurons in the neostriatum and substantia nigra revealed after punctate intracerebral injection of diisopropylfluorophosphate, *Eur. J. Pharmacol. 34:*115.

Butcher, S.G., and Butcher, L.L., 1974, Origin and modulation of acetylcholine activity in the neostriatum, *Brain Res. 71:*167.

Calne, D.B., 1970, *"Parkinsonism: Physiology, Pharmacology, and Treatment,"* pp. 66-67, Edward Arnold Ltd., London.

Carlsson, A., and Lindqvist, M., 1963, Effect of chlorpromazine or haloperidol on formation of 3-methoxytyramine and normetanephrine in mouse brain, *Acta Pharmacol. Toxicol. 20:*140.

Carlsson, A., Lindqvist, M., and Magnusson, T., 1957, 3, 4-dihydroxyphenylalanine and 5-hydroxytryptophan as reserpine antagonists, *Nature 180:*1200.

Carlton, P.L., 1963, Cholinergic mechanisms in the control of behavior by the brain, *Psychol. Rev. 70:*19.

Chase, T.N., 1972, Drug-induced extrapyramidal disorders, *Res. Publ. Assoc. Res. Nerv. Ment. Dis. 50:*448.

Cheramy, A., Besson, J.J., and Glowinski, J., 1970, Increased release of dopamine from striatal dopaminergic terminals in the rat after treatment with a neuroleptic: thioproperazine, *Eur. J. Pharmacol. 10:*206.

Cheramy, A., Nieoullon, A., and Glowinski, J., 1977, Effects of peripheral and local administration of picrotoxin on the release of newly synthesized ^{3}H-dopamine in the caudate nucleus of the cat, *Naunyn Schmiedebergs Arch. Pharmacol. 297:*31.

Cheney, D.L., LeFevre, H.F., and Racagni, G., 1975, Choline acetyltransferase activity and mass fragmentographic measurement of acetylcholine in specific nuclei and tracts of rat brain, *Neuropharmacology 14:*801.

Chien, C.P., and DiMascio, A., 1967, Drug-induced extrapyramidal symptoms and their relations to clinical efficacy, *Am. J. Psychiatry 123:*1490.

Colpaert, F.C., Wauquier, A., Niemegeers, C., and Lal, H., 1975, Reversal by a central antiacetylcholine drug of pimozide-induced inhibition of mouse-jumping in amphetamine-dopa treated mice, *J. Pharm. Pharmacol. 27:*536.

Connor, J.D., 1970, Caudate nucleus neurons: correlation of the effects of substantia nigra stimulation with iontophoretic dopamine, *J. Physiol. 208:*691-703.

Connor, J.D., Rossi, G.V., and Baker, W.W., 1966, Analysis of the tremor induced by injection of cholinergic agents into the caudate nucleus, *Int. J. Neuropharmacol. 5:*207.

Consolo, S., Ladinsky, H., and Bianchi, S., 1975, Decrease in rat striatal acetylcholine levels by some direct and indirect-acting dopaminergic antagonists, *Eur. J. Pharmacol. 33:*345.

Corrodi, H., Fuxe, K., and Lidbrink, P., 1972, Interaction between cholinergic and catecholaminergic neurons in rat brain, *Brain Res. 43:*397.

Costall, B., and Naylor, R.J., 1973, Neuroleptic and non-neuroleptic catalepsy? *Arzneim Forsch. 23:*674.

Costall, B., and Naylor, R.J., 1975, Cholinergic modification of abnormal involuntary movements induced in the guniea pig by intrastriatal dopamine, *J. Pharm. Pharmacol. 27:*273.

Costall, B., and Olley, J.E., 1971, Cholinergic and neuroleptic induced catalepsy: modification by lesions in the caudate-putamen, *Neuropharmacology 10:*297.

Costall, B., Naylor, R.J., and Olley, J.E., 1972, Catalepsy and circling behavior after intracerebral injections of neuroleptic, cholinergic and anticholinergic agents into the caudate-putamen, globus pallidus, and substantia nigra of rat brain, *Neuropharmacology 11:*645.

Coyle, J.T., and Snyder, S.H., 1969, Antiparkinsonian drugs: inhibition of dopamine uptake in the corpus striatum as a possible mechanism of action, *Science 166:*899.

Crossman, A.R., Walker, R.J., and Woodruff, G.N., 1973, Picrotoxin antagonism of gamma-aminobutyric acid inhibiting responses and synaptic inhibition in the rat substantia nigra, *Br. J. Pharmacol. 49:*696.

Davis, K.L., Hollister, L.E., Barchas, J.D., and Berger, P.A., 1976, Choline in tardive dyskinesia and Huntington's disease, *Life Sci. 19:*1507.

Davis, K.L., Berger, P.A., and Hollister, L.E., 1977, Cholinergic mechanisms in tardive dyskinesia and Huntington's chorea, in *"Neurotransmitter Function: Basic and Clinical Aspects"* (W.S. Fields, ed.), pp. 247-262, Stratton Intercontinental, New York.

DeRobertis, E., Rodriguez de Lores Arnaiz, G., Salganicoff, L., Peregrino de Iraldi, A., and Zieher, L.M., 1963, Isolation of synaptic vesicles and structural organization of the acetylcholine system within brain nerve endings, *J. Neurochem. 10:*225.

DiMascio, A., and Demirgian, E., 1970, Antiparkinson drug overuse, *Psychosomatics 11:* 596.

Drachman, D.A., 1977, Memory and cognitive function in man: Does the cholinergic system have a specific role? *Neurology 27:*783.

Dray, A., Oakley, N.R., and Simmonds, M.A., 1975, Rotational behavior following inhibition of GABA metabolism unilaterally in the rat substantia nigra, *J. Pharm. Pharmacol. 27:*627.

Duvoisin, R.C., 1967, Cholinergic-anticholinergic antagonism in parkinsonism, *Arch. Neurol. 17:*124.

Fahn, S., and Cote, L.J., 1968, Regional distribution of choline acetylase in the brain of the rhesus monkey, *Brain Res. 7:*323.

Fahn, S., and David, E., 1973, Oral-facial-lingual dyskinesia due to anticholinergic medication, *Trans. Am. Neurol. Assoc. 97:*277.

Fahn, S., Mishkin, M.M., and Hoffman, R.R., 1973, Pharmacologic and radiologic investigations in Huntington's chorea, *Adv. Neurol. 1:*581.

Farnebo, L.O., Fuxe, K., Hamberger, B., and Ljundahl, H., 1970, Effects of some antiparkinson drugs on catecholamine neurons, *J. Pharm. Pharmacol. 22:*733.

Feldberg, W., 1945, Present views on the mode of action of acetylcholine in the central nervous system, *Physiol. Rev. 25:*596.

Feltz, P., 1971, Gamma-amino butyric acid and a caudate-nigral inhibition, *Can. J. Physiol. Pharmacol. 49:*1113.

Ferry, C.B., 1966, Cholinergic link hypothesis in adrenergic neuroeffector transmission, *Physiol. Rev. 46:*420.

Fibiger, H.C., and Grewaal, D.S., 1974, Neurochemical evidence for denervation supersensitivity: The effect of unilateral substantia nigra lesions on apomorphine-induced increases in neostriatal acetylcholine levels, *Life Sci. 15:*57.

Fuxe, K., Goldstein, M., and Ljungdahl, A., 1970, Antiparkinsonian drugs and central dopamine neurons, *Life Sci. 9:*811.

Gair, D.S., and Ducey, J., 1950, Chemical structure of substances effective in treatment of parkinsonism, *Arch. Intern. Med. 85:*284.

Gautier, J., Jus, A., Villeneuve, A., Jus, K., Pires, P., and Villeneuve, R., 1977, Influence of the antiparkinsonian drugs on the plasma level of neuroleptics, *Biol. Psychiatry 12:*389.

Gerlach, J., Reisby, N., and Randrup, A., 1974, Dopaminergic hypersensitivity and cholinergic hypofunction in the pathophysiology of tardive dyskinesia, *Psychopharmacologia 34:*21.

Giorguieff, M.F., LeFloc'h, M.L., Westfall, T.C., Glowinski, J., and Besson, M.J., 1976, Nicotinic effect of acetylcholine on the release of newly synthesized ^{3}H-dopamine in rat striatal slices and cat caudate nucleus, *Brain Res. 106:*117.

Giorguieff, M.F., LeFloc'h, M.L., Glowinski, J., and Besson, M.J., 1977, Involvement of cholinergic presynaptic receptors of nicotinic and muscarinic types in the control of the spontaneous release of dopamine from striatal dopaminergic terminals in the rat, *J. Pharmacol. Exp. Ther. 200:*535.

Granacher, R.P., Baldessarini, R.J., and Cole, J.O., 1975, The pharmacologic evaluation of tardive dyskinesia, *N. Engl. J. Med. 292:*326.

Grewaal, D.S., Fibiger, H.C., and McGeer, E.G., 1974, 6-hydroxydopamine and striatal acetylcholine levels, *Brain Res. 73:*372.

Groves, P.M., Wilson, C.J., Young, S.J., and Rebec, G.V., 1975, Self-inhibition by dopaminergic neurons, *Science 190:*522.

Growdon, J.H., Hirsch, M.J., Wurtman, R.J., and Weiner, W., 1977, Oral choline administration to patients with tardive dyskinesia, *N. Engl. J. Med. 297:*524.

Guyenet, P.G., Beaujouan, J.C., and Glowinski, J., 1975a, Ontogenesis of neostriatal cholinergic neurones in the rat and development of their sensitivity to neurologic drugs, *Naunyn Schmiedebergs Arch. Pharmacol. 288:*329.

Guyenet, P.G., Javoy, F., Agid, Y., Beaujouan, J.C., and Glowinski, J., 1975b, Dopamine receptors and cholinergic neurons in the rat neostriatum, *Adv. Neurol. 9:*43.

Guyenet, P.G., Agid, Y., Javoy, F., Beaujouan, J.C., Rossier, J., and Glowinski, J., 1975c, Effects of dopaminergic receptor agonists and antagonists on the activity of the neo-striatal cholinergic system, *Brain Res. 84:*227.

Harris, J.E., and Baldessarini, R.J., 1975, Amphetamine-induced inhibition of tyrosine hydroxylation in homogenates of rat corpus striatum, *Neuropharmacology 14:*457.

Hattori, T., Singh, V.K., McGeer, E.G., and McGeer, P.L., 1976, Immunohistochemical localization of choline acetyltransferase containing neostriatal neurons and their relationship with dopaminergic synapses, *Brain Res. 102:*164.

Hebb, C.O., and Silver, A., 1956, Choline acetylase in the central nervous system of man and some other animals, *J. Physiol. 134:*718.

Herz, A., and Zieglgansberger, W., 1968, The influence of microelectrophoretically applied biogenic amines, cholinomimetics and procaine on synaptic excitation in the corpus striatum, *Int. J. Neuropharmacol. 7:*221.

Hiley, R., and Bird, E.D., 1974, Decreased muscarinic receptor concentration in post-mortem brain in Huntington's chorea, *Brain Res. 80:*355.

Hornykiewicz, O., 1971, Neurochemical pathology of Parkinson's disease, in *"Recent Advances in Parkinson's Disease"* (F.H. McDowell and C.H. Markham, eds.), pp. 33-65, F.A. Davis, Philadelphia.

Hornykiewicz, O., 1973, Dopamine in the basal ganglia, *Br. Med. Bull. 29:*172.

Janowsky, D.S., El-Yousef, M.K., Davis, J.M., and Sekerke, H.J., 1972, Cholinergic antagonism of methylphenidate-induced stereotyped behavior, *Psychopharmacologia 27:*295.

Janowsky, D.S., El-Yousef, M.K., Davis, J.M., and Sekerke, H.J., 1973, Antagonistic effects of physostigmine and methylphenidate in man, *Am. J. Psychiatry 130:*1370.

Javoy, F., Agid, Y., Bouvet, D., and Glowinski, J., 1972, Feedback control of dopamine synthesis in dopaminergic terminals of the cat striatum, *J. Pharm. Exp. Ther. 182:*454.

Javoy, F., Agid, Y., Bouvet, D., and Glowinski, J., 1974, Changes in neostriatal DA metabolism after carbachol or atropine microinjections into the substantia nigra, *Brain Res. 68:*253.

Javoy, F., Agid, Y., and Glowinski, J., 1975, Oxotremorine and atropine-induced changes of dopamine metabolism in the rat striatum, *J. Pharm. Pharmacol. 27:*677.

Karczmar, A.G., 1969, Is the central cholinergic nervous system over-exploited? *Fed. Proc. 28:*147.

Kazamatsuri, H., Chien, C.P., and Cole, J.O., 1972, Therapeutic approaches to tardive dyskinesia, *Arch. Gen. Psychiatry 27:*491.

Kehr, W., Carlsson, A., Lindqvist, M., Magnusson, T., and Atack, C.B., 1972, Evidence for a receptor-mediated feedback control of striatal tyrosine hydroxylase activity, *J. Pharm. Pharmacol. 24:*744.

Kelly, P.H., and Miller, R.J., 1975, The interaction of neuroleptic and muscarinic agents with central dopaminergic systems, *Br. J. Pharmacol. 54:*115.

Kelley, P.H., Miller, R.J., and Sahakian, B., 1974, Interaction of neuroleptic and cholinergic drugs with central dopaminergic mechanisms, *Br. J. Pharmacol. 52:*430P.

Kemp, J., and Powell, T.P.S., 1971, The connections of the striatum and globus pallidus: synthesis and speculation, *Philos. Trans. R. Soc. Lond. (BIOL) 262:*441.

Klawans, H.L., Jr., 1973, *"The Pharmacology of Extrapyramidal Movement Disorders,"* Karger, Basel.

Klawans, H.L., Jr., and Moskovitz, C., 1977, Cyclizine-induced chorea, *J. Neurol. Sci. 31:*237.

Klawans, H.L., Jr., and Rubovits, R., 1972, Central cholinergic-anticholinergic antagonism in Huntington's chorea, *Neurology 22:*107.

Klawans, H.L., Jr., and Rubovits, R., 1974, Effect of cholinergic and anticholinergic agents in tardive dyskinesia, *J. Neurol. Neurosurg. Psychiatry 27:*941.

Klawans, H.L., Jr., Rubovits, R., Patel, B.C., and Weiner, W.J., 1972, Cholinergic and anticholinergic influences on amphetamine-induced stereotyped behavior, *J. Neurol. Sci. 17:*303.

Klett, C.J., and Caffey, E., Jr., 1972, Evaluating the long-term need for antiparkinson drugs by chronic schizophrenics, *Arch. Gen. Psychiatry 26:*374.

Kiloh, L.G., Smith, S.J., and Williams, S.E., 1973, Antiparkinson drugs as casual agents in tardive dyskinesia, *Med. J. Aust. 2:*591.

Kitai, S.T., Sugimori, M., and Kocsis, J.D., 1976, Excitatory nature of dopamine in the nigro-caudate pathway, *Exp. Brain Res. 24:*351.

Kuhar, M.J., and Yamamura, H.I., 1976, Localization of cholinergic muscarinic receptors in rat brain by light microscopic radioautography, *Brain Res. 110:*229.

Lloyd, K.G., Davidson, L., and Hornykiewicz, O., 1975a, The neurochemistry of Parkinson's disease: effect of L-DOPA therapy, *J. Pharmacol. Exp. Ther. 195:*453.

Lloyd, K.G., Mohler, H., Heitz, Ph., and Bartholini, G., 1975b, Distribution of choline acetyltransferase and glutamate decarboxylase within the substantia nigra and in other brain regions from control and parkinsonian patients, *J. Neurochem. 25:*789.

Lynch, G.S., Lucas, P.A., and Deadwyler, S.A., 1972, The demonstration of acetylcholinesterase containing neurons within the caudate nucleus of the rat, *Brain Res. 45:*617.

Mano, T., Sobue, I., Hirose, K., Takagi, S., Watanabe, H., and Okamoto, S., 1973, Dyskinesias induced by anticholinergic drugs: an electrophysiological analysis, *Excer. Med. Int. Contr. Ser. (10th Int. Cong. Neurol.) 296:*44.

Marsden, C.D., Tarsy, D., and Baldessarini, R.J., 1975, Spontaneous and drug-induced movement disorders in psychotic patients, in *"Psychiatric Aspects of Neurologic Disease"* (D.F. Benson and D. Blumer, eds.), pp. 219-266, Grune and Stratton, New York.

Marsden, C.D., Milson, J., Parkes, J.D., Pycock, C., and Tarsy, D., 1975, The effect of cholinergic and anticholinergic drugs on rotational behavior in mice with destruction of one nigrostriatal pathway, *J. Physiol. 249:*64P.

Matthysse, S., 1973, Antipsychotic drug actions: Clue to the neuropathology of schizophrenia? *Fed. Proc. 32:*200.

McClelland, H.A., Blessed, G., Bhate, S., Ali, N., and Clarke, P.A., 1974, The abrupt withdrawal of antiparkinsonian drugs in schizophrenic patients, *Br. J. Psychiatry 124:* 151.

McGeer, E.G., Wada, J.A., Terao, A., and Jung, E., 1969, Amine synthesis in various brain regions with caudate or septal lesions, *Exp. Neurol. 24:*277.

McGeer, E.G., Fibiger, H.C., McGeer, P.L., and Brooke, S., 1973, Temporal changes in amine synthesizing enzymes of rat extrapyramidal structures after hemitransections or 6-hydroxydopamine administration, *Brain Res. 52:*289.

McGeer, P.L., and McGeer, E.G., 1971, Cholinergic enzyme systems in Parkinson's disease, *Arch. Neurol. 25:*265.

McGeer, P.L., and McGeer, E.G., 1975, Evidence for glutamic acid decarboxylase-containing interneurons in the neostriatum, *Brain Res. 91:*331.

McGeer, P.L., and McGeer, E.G., 1976a, The GABA system and function of the basal ganglia: Huntington's disease, in *"GABA in Nervous System Function"* (E. Roberts, T.N. Chase, D.B. Tower, eds.), pp. 487-495, Raven Press, New York.

McGeer, P.L., and McGeer, E.G., 1976b, Enzymes associated with the metabolism of catecholamines, acetylcholine and GABA in human controls and patients with Parkinson's disease and Huntington's chorea, *J. Neurochem. 26:*65.

McGeer, P.L., Boulding, J.E., Gibson, W.C., and Foulkes, R.G., 1961, Drug-induced extrapyramidal reactions, *JAMA 177:*665.

McGeer, P.L., McGeer, E.G., Fibiger, H.C., and Wickson, V., 1971, Neostriatal choline acetylase and cholinesterase following selective brain lesions, *Brain Res. 35:*308.

McGeer, P.L., McGeer, E.G., and Fibiger, H.C., 1973, Choline acetylase and glutamic acid decarboxylase in Huntington's chorea, *Neurology 23:*912.

McGeer, P.L., Grewaal, D.S., and McGeer, E.G., 1974, Influence of noncholinergic drugs on rat striatal acetylcholine levels, *Brain Res. 80:*211.

McGeer, P.L., Hattori, T., Singh, V.K., and McGeer, E.G., 1976, Cholinergic systems in extrapyramidal function, in *"The Basal Ganglia"* (M. Yahr, ed.), pp. 213-222, Raven Press, New York.

McLennan, H., 1971, Possible chemical mediators of synaptic action in certain basal ganglial pathways, in *"Recent Advances in Parkinson's Disease"* (F.H. McDowell and C.H. Markham, eds.), pp. 67-82, F.A. Davis, Philadelphia.

McLennan, H., and York, D.H., 1966, Cholinergic mechanisms in the caudate nucleus, *J. Physiol. 187:*163.

McLennan, H., and York, D.H., 1967, The action of dopamine on neurons of the caudate nucleus, *J. Physiol. 189:*393.

Mendelson, G., 1977, Pheniramine aminosalicylate overdosage, *Arch. Neurol. 34:*313.

Miller, R.J., and Hiley, C.R., 1974, Antimuscarinic properties of neuroleptics and drug-induced parkinsonism, *Nature 248:*596.

Morpurgo, C., 1962, Effects of antiparkinson drugs on a phenothiazine-induced catatonic reaction, *Arch. Int. Pharmacodyn. Ther. 137:*84.

Morpurgo, C., and Theobald, W., 1964, Influence of antiparkinson drugs and amphetamine on some pharmacological effects of phenothiazine derivitives used as neuroleptics, *Psychopharmacologia 6:*178.

Muscholl, E., 1974, Regulation of catecholamine release. The muscarinic inhibitory mechanism, *Biochem. Pharmacol. (Suppl.) 23:*430.

O'Keefe, R., Sharman, D.F., and Vogt, M., 1970, Effect of drugs used in psychoses on cerebral dopamine metabolism, *Br. J. Pharmacol. 38:*287.

Olivier, A., Parent, A., Simard, H., and Poirier, L.J., 1970, Cholinesterase striatopallidal and striatonigral efferents in the cat and the monkey, *Brain Res. 18:*273.

Orlov, P., Kasparian, G., DiMascio, A., and Cole, J.O., 1971, Withdrawal of antiparkinson drugs, *Arch. Gen. Psychiatry 25:*410.

Orzeck, A., and Barbeau, A., 1970, Interrelationship among dopamine, serotonin, and acetylcholine, in *"L-DOPA and Parkinsonism"* (A. Barbeau and F.H. McDowell, eds.), pp. 88-94, F.A. Davis, Philadelphia.

Palkovits, M., Saavedra, J.M., Kobayashi, R.M., and Brownstein, M., 1974, Choline acetyltransferase content of limbic nuclei of the rat, *Brain Res. 79:*443.

Perry, T.L., Hansen, S., and Kloster, M., 1973, Huntington's chorea: deficiency of γ-aminobutyric acid in brain, *N. Engl. J. Med. 288:*337.

Pfeiffer, C.C., and Jenney, E.H., 1957, The inhibition of the conditioned response and the counteraction of schizophrenia by muscarinic stimulation of the brain, *Ann. NY Acad. Sci. 66:*753.

Poirier, L.J., 1971, The development of animal models for studies in Parkinson's disease, in *"Recent Advances in Parkinson's Disease"* (F.H. McDowell and C.H. Markham, eds.), pp. 83-117, F.A. Davis, Philadelphia.

Poirier, L.J., and Sourkes, T.L., 1965, Influence of the substantia nigra on the catecholamine content of the striatum, *Brain 88:*181.

Pycock, C., Milsen, J., Tarsy, D., and Marsden, C.D., 1978, The effect of manipulations of cholinergic mechanisms on turning behavior in mice with unilateral destruction of the nigro- neostriatal dopaminergic system, *Neuropharmacology 17:*175.

Rifkin, A., Quitkin, F., and Klein, D.F., 1975, Akinesia: a poorly recognized drug-induced extrapyramidal behavioral disorder, *Arch. Gen. Psychiatry 32:*672.

Rinne, U.K., Riekkinen, P., Sonninen, V., and Laaksonen, H., 1973, Brain acetylcholinesterase in Parkinson's disease, *Acta Neurol. Scand. 49:*215.

Rivera-Calimlim, L., Nasrallah, H., Strauss, J., and Lasagna, L., 1976, Clinical response and plasma levels: effect of dose, dosage schedules, and drug interactions on plasma chlorpromazine levels, *Am. J. Psychiatry 133:*646.

Rommelspacher, H., and Kuhar, M.J., 1975, Effects of dopaminergic drugs and acute medial forebrain bundle lesions on striatal acetylcholine levels, *Life Sci. 16:*65.

Roos, B.E., and Steg, G., 1964, The effect of L-3, 4-dihydroxyphenylalanine and DL-5-hydroxytryptophan on rigidity and tremor induced by reserpine, chlorpromazine, and phenoxybenzamine, *Life Sci. 3:*351.

Rosenthal, R., and Bigelow, L.B., 1973, The effects of physostigmine in phenothiazine resistant chronic schizophrenic patients: preliminary observation, *Compr. Psychiatry 14:*489.

Roth, R.H., and Bunney, B.S., 1976, Interaction of cholinergic neurons with other chemically defined neuronal systems in the CNS, in *"Biology of Cholinergic Function"* (I. Hanin and A. Goldberg, eds.), pp. 379-395, Raven Press, New York.

Rowntree, D.W., Nevin, S., and Wilson, A., 1950, The effect of diisopropylfluorophosphonate in schizophrenia and manic depressive psychosis, *J. Neurol. Neurosurg. Psychiatry 13:*47.

Rubovits, R., and Klawans, H.L., Jr., 1972, Implications of amphetamine-induced stereotyped behavior as a model for tardive dyskinesia, *Arch. Gen. Psychiatry 27:*502.

Safer, D.J., and Allen, R.P., 1971, The central effects of scopolamine in man, *Biol. Psychiatry 3:*347.

Scheel Kruger, J., 1970, Central effects of anticholinergic drugs measured by the apomorphine gnawing test in mice, *Acta Pharmacol. Toxicol. 28:*1.

Scheel Kruger, J., and Randrup, A., 1968, Pharmacological evidence for a cholinergic mechanism in brain involved in a special stereotyped behavior of reserpinized rats, *Br. J. Pharmacol. 34:*217P.

Schelkunov, E.L., 1967, Integrated effect of psychotropic drugs on the balance of cholino-, adreno-, and serotoninergic processes in the brain as a basis of their gross behavioral and therapeutic actions, *Activ. Ner. Sup. 9:*207.

Seeman, P., and Lee, T., 1975, Antipsychotic drugs: direct correlation between clinical potency and presynaptic action on dopamine neurons, *Science 188:*1217.

Sethy, V.H., and Van Woert, M.H., 1974, Modification of striatal acetylcholine concentration by dopamine receptor agonists and antagonists, *Res. Commun. Chem. Pathol. Pharmacol. 8:*13.

Shute, C.C.D., and Lewis, P.R., 1967, The ascending cholinergic reticular system: neocortical, olfactory, and subcortical projections, *Brain 90:*497.

Siggins, G.R., Hoffer, B.J., Bloom, F.E., and Ungerstedt, U., 1976, Cytochemical and electrophysiological studies of dopamine in the caudate nucleus, in *"The Basal Ganglia"* (M.D. Yahr, ed.), pp. 227-247, Raven Press, New York.

Simpson, G.M., 1970, Controlled studies of antiparkinsonism agents in the treatment of drug-induced extrapyramidal symptoms, *Acta Psychiatry Scand. (Suppl.) 212:*44.

Singh, M.M., and Kay, S.R., 1975a, Therapeutic reversal with benztropine in schizophrenics, *J. Nerv. Ment. Dis. 160:*258.

Singh, M.M., and Kay, S.R., 1975b, A comparitive study of haloperidol and chlorpromazine in terms of clinical effects and therapeutic reversal with benztropine in schizophrenia. Theoretical implications for potency differences among neuroleptics, *Psychopharmacologia 43:*103.

Singh, M.M., and Kay, S.R., 1975c, A longitudinal comparison between two protypic neuroleptics (haloperidol and chlorpromazine) in matched groups of schizophrenics. Nontherapeutic interactions with trihexyphenidyl. Theoretical implications for potency differences, *Psychopharmacologia 43:*115.

Smelik, P.G., and Ernst, A.M., 1966, Role of the nigrostriatal dopaminergic fibers in compulsive gnawing behavior in rats, *Life Sci. 5:*1485.

Snyder, S., Greenberg, D., and Yamamura, H.I., 1974, Antischizophrenic drugs and brain cholinergic receptors, *Arch. Gen. Psychiatry 31:*58.

Spehlmann, R., 1975, The effects of acetylcholine and dopamine on the caudate nucleus depleted of biogenic amines, *Brain 98:*219.

Spehlmann, R., and Stahl, S.M., 1976, Dopamine acetylcholine imbalance in Parkinson's disease, *Lancet 1:*724.

Stadler, H., Lloyd, K.G., Gadea-Ciria, M., and Bartholini, G., 1973, Enhanced striatal acetylcholine release by chlorpromazine and its reversal by apomorphine, *Brain Res. 55:*476.

Stadler, H., Gadea-Ciria, M., and Bartholini, G., 1975, *"In vivo"* release of endogenous neurotransmitters in cat limbic regions: effect of chlorpromazine and of electrical stimulation, *Naunyn Schmiedebergs Arch. Pharmacol. 288:*1.

Stahl, W.L., and Swanson, P.D., 1974, Biochemical abnormalities in Huntington's chorea, *Neurology 24:*813.

Steg, G., 1969, Striatal cell activity during systemic administration of monoaminergic and cholinergic drugs, in *"Third Symposium on Parkinson's Disease"* (F.J. Gillingham and I.M.L. Donaldson, eds.), pp. 26-29, E.S. Livingstone, Edinburgh.

Stevens, J.R., Kim, C., and MacLean, P., 1961, Stimulation of caudate nucleus, *Arch. Neurol. 4:*47.

Swett, C., Cole, J.O., and Shapiro, S., 1977, Extrapyramidal side effects in chlorpromazine recipients, *Arch. Gen. Psychiatry 34:*942.

Tarsy, D., 1977, Dopamine-acetylcholine interaction in the basal ganglia, in *"Neuro-transmitter Function: Basic and Clinical Aspects"* (W.S. Fields, ed.), pp. 213-246, Stratton Intercontinental, New York.

Tarsy, D., and Baldessarini, R.J., 1976, The tardive dyskinesia syndrome, in *"Clinical Neuropharmacology, Vol. 1"* (H.L. Klawans, ed.), pp. 29-61, Raven Press, New York.

Tarsy, D., and Baldessarini, R.J., 1977, The pathophysiologic basis of tardive dyskinesia, *Biol. Psychiatry 12:*431.

Tarsy, D., and Bralower, M., 1977, Deanol acetamidobenzoate treatment in choreiform movement disorders, *Arch. Neurol. 34:*756.

Tarsy, D., Leopold, N., and Sax, D.S., 1974, Physostigmine in choreiform movement disorders, *Neurology 24:*28.

Tarsy, D., Pycock, C., Meldrum, B., and Marsden, C.D., 1975, Rotational behavior induced in rats by intranigral picrotoxin, *Brain Res. 89:*160.

Tebecis, A.K., 1974, *"Transmitters and Identified Neurons in the Mammalian Central Nervous System,"* pp. 168-185, Scientechnica, Bristol.

Thornburg, J.E., and Moore, K.E., 1973, Inhibition of anticholinergic drug-induced locomotor stimulation in mice by a-methyltyrosine, *Neuropharmacology 12:*1179.

Trabucchi, M., Cheney, D., Racagni, G., and Costa, E., 1974, Involvement of brain cholinergic mechanisms in the action of chlorpromazine, *Nature 249:*664.

Trabucchi, M., Cheney, D.L., Racagni, G., and Costa, E., 1975, *In vivo* inhibition of striatal acetylcholine turnover by L-DOPA, apomorphine, and (+)-amphetamine, *Brain Res. 85:*130.

Ulus, I.H., and Wurtman, R.J., 1976, Choline administration: activation of tyrosine hydroxylase by dopaminergic neurons of rat brain, *Science 194:*1060.

Ungerstedt, U., Avemo, A., Avemo, E., Ljungberg, T., and Ranje, C., 1973, Animal models of parkinsonism, *Adv. Neurol. 3:*257.

Ungerstedt, U., Butcher, L., Butcher, S.G., Anden, N.E., and Fuxe, K., 1969, Direct chemical stimulation of dopaminergic mechanisms in the neostriatum of the rat, *Brain Res. 14:*461.

Van Woert, M.H., Ambani, L., and Bowers, M.B., Jr., 1972, Levodopa and cholinergic hypersensitivity in Parkinson's disease, *Neurology (Suppl.) 22:*86.

Wauquier, A., Niemegeers, C.J., and Lal, H., 1975, Differential antagonism by the anticholinergic dexetimide of inhibitory effects of haloperidol and fentanyl on brain self-stimulation, *Psychopharmacologia 41:*229.

Weintraub, M.I., and Van Woert, M., 1971, Reversal by levodopa of cholinergic hypersensitivity in Parkinson's disease, *N. Engl. J. Med. 284:*412.

Westerink, B.H.C., and Korf, J., 1975, Influence of drugs on striatal and limbic homovanillic acid concentration in the rat brain, *Eur. J. Pharmacol. 33:*31.

Wolfarth, S., Dulska, E., and Lacki, M., 1974, Comparison of the effects of the intranigral injection of cholinomimetics with systemic injections of the dopamine receptor stimulating and blocking agents in the rabbit, *Neuropharmacology 13:*867.

Yamamura, H.I., Kuhar, M.J., Greenberg, D., and Snyder, S., 1974, Muscarinic cholinergic receptor binding: regional distribution in monkey brain, *Brain Res. 66:*541.

York, D.H., 1967, The inhibitory action of dopamine on neurons of the caudate nucleus, *Brain Res. 5:*263.

York, D.H., 1970, Possible dopaminergic pathway from substantia nigra to putamen, *Brain Res. 20:*233.

Zetler, G., 1968, Cataleptic state and hypothermia in mice, caused by central cholinergic stimulation and antagonized by anticholinergic and antidepressant drugs, *Int. J. Neuropharmacol. 7:*325.

EVIDENCE FOR THE EXISTENCE OF TWO STRIATAL DOPAMINE RECEPTORS

H. L. Klawans, A. Hitri, P. A. Nausieda and W. J. Weiner

Department of Neurological Sciences, Rush Presbyterian St. Luke's Medical Center, 1725 West Harrison Street, Chicago, Illinois 60612

INTRODUCTION

Striatal dopaminergic mechanisms have been implicated in two separate human neurologic syndromes. The first of these is parkinsonism; a syndrome consisting of rigidity, akinesia, resting tremor and loss of postural reflexes which is felt to be related to decreased activity of dopamine (DA) at striatal DA receptors (Hornykiewicz, 1966; Klawans, 1973). The second is chorea which is felt to reflect increased dopaminergic activity at at least some striatal DA receptors (Klawans, 1971; Klawans, 1973).

A detailed review of the data which supports the role of decreased DA effect in the pathogenesis of parkinsonian signs and symptoms is beyond the scope of this chapter but can be briefly summarized as follows:

1. Both idiopathic and post encephalitic parkinsonism are associated by degeneration of the nigrostriatal neurons (Greenfield and Bosanquet, 1953) with subsequent loss of ipsilateral striatal DA (Hornykiewicz, 1966).

2. Neuroleptic-induced parkinsonism is due to the ability of neuroleptics to block striatal DA receptors (Klawans, 1968).

3. Reserpine-induced parkinsonism is due to the ability of reserpine to deplete striatal DA stores (Klawans, 1968).

The role of DA in chorea is not as widely understood as its role in parkinsonism and since the role of DA in one choreatic disorder is cogent to the discussion of the possible existence of two separate striatal DA receptors, the pathophysiology of chorea and especially Huntington's chorea will be reviewed in detail.

The term chorea is used to describe an entire class of abnormal involuntary movements, each of which is a rapid, uncoordinated jerk. The simultaneous or successive occurrence of two or more such isolated movements results in complex movement patterns, while the superimposition of these movements on normal movements can cause a dance-like gait. Chorea is a manifestation of malfunction of the striatum and not a specific disease state. The physiological basis of these movements has been best studied in Huntington's chorea.

Huntington's chorea is a progressive degenerative disease of the brain which is inherited as a dominant autosomal gene with complete penetrance. It is usually manifested by progressive extrapyramidal and mental symptoms. Chorea is the most frequent extra-pyramidal manifestation. In a small percentage of patients, rigidity and akinesia dominate the clinical picture. Dementia is the most common mental symptom, although organic psychosis or even schizophrenic reactions may be the primary mental manifestation.

The essential pathologic alteration in Huntington's chorea is a loss of neurons in the caudate and putamen. Two different types of neurons are normally found in the striatum. The smaller neurons are characteristically more involved in Huntington's chorea than the larger striatal ones (Doon *et al.*, 1973). In most instances there is a marked loss of the small ganglion cells associated with an equal proliferation of astrocytes. The latter may be so great as to give an impression of increased cellularity to the atrophied caudate and putamen. There is also diffuse cerebral cortical atrophy. It is generally accepted that the abnormal movements are related to changes in the striatum, whereas the mental symptoms are usually attributed to the pathologic alterations of the cerebral cortex.

Bruyn has pointed out that Huntington's chorea seems in certain respects to be the opposite of Parkinson's disease (Bruyn, 1968). This is particularly true in relation to the dopaminergic nigrostriatal neuronal system. In parkinsonism there is degeneration of the DA-rich cells of the substantia nigra, while the neurons of the striatum are intact. In Huntington's chorea the dopaminergic cells of the substantia nigra are not involved, but the neurons of the striatum that normally receive the DA input are markedly altered. In parkinsonism the DA input to the normal striatum is decreased. In Huntington's chorea the DA input is intact, and the striatal cells are abnormal. Although the lack of DA input apparently results in parkinsonism, it is not as clear what relationship DA has to chorea. It has been proposed that abnormal sensitivity of some striatal receptors to a normal input of DA underlies the disorder (Klawans, 1973; Klawans *et al.*, 1972; Klawans and Weiner, 1975).

If increased responsiveness to DA produces chorea, then drugs that decrease the effect of DA at striatal receptor sites should improve chorea. The classes of drugs that decrease the effect of DA at DA receptors include reserpine and neuroleptic compounds such as chlorpromazine and haloperidol. All of these agents produce parkinsonism in man with some degree of regularity, and all of them have been used to treat chorea with some degree of success. It has been suggested that the suppressive effect of reserpine on chorea is secondary to the production of parkinsonism in choreic individuals. The amelioration of chorea however appears to be due to a biochemical or physiologic alteration which is similar to the alteration that produces parkinsonism and is not secondary to the induction of parkinsonism. Both the production of parkinsonism and improvement in chorea may be related to a similar mechanism without the presence of a cause-and-effect relationship. In fact the appearance of drug-induced parkinsonism is not a prerequisite for drug-induced improvement of chorea.

Reserpine and neuroleptic agents decrease the activity of DA at DA receptors and improve chorea, functions suggesting that DA is of primary importance in initiating the movement. Blocking the action of DA at the striatal receptors improves chorea despite the fact that the striatal DA content is normal. This observation supports the hypothesis that the defect producing chorea involves an abnormal cellular or receptor response to normal amounts of DA and not abnormal synthesis turnover or release of DA.

The significance of DA in chorea is also supported by observations involving a number of amino acids. a-Methyl-paratyrosine (AMPT) is an inhibitor of tyrosine hydroxylase that greatly decreases levels of catecholamines in the brain stem and striatum but does not affect the level of serotonin. AMPT improves choreatic restlessness (Birkmayer, 1969). Since L-DOPA increases striatal DA levels, it may increase the amount of DA reaching the receptors and thereby intensify the symptoms. It is fairly clear that long-term oral administration of L-DOPA usually increases hyperkinesia in Huntington's chorea.

Patients with Huntington's chorea may manifest rigidity and akinesia, two of the cardinal manifestations of parkinsonism. As mentioned above, akinesia and rigidity are at times seen late in the course of Huntington's chorea. In other patients, the initial motor manifestation is slowness in motor activity. These patients manifest increasing akinesia as the disease progresses and often have no chorea. It is generally felt that in parkinsonism rigidity and akinesia are related to loss of DA influence on the striatal neurons. If the pathogenesis of rigidity and akinesia in Huntington's chorea is also due to a decreased dopaminergic influence on striatal neurons, then L-DOPA might also improve rigidity in these patients. Barbeau (1969), Bird and Paulson (1970) have both·given long-term oral L-DOPA to young patients with the rigid form of Huntington's chorea and have both observed some improvement in the rigidity. This is consistent with the suggestion that decreased DA activity may be related to the rigidity in Huntington's chorea. Since DA levels are normal in this disease (Bernheimer and Hornykiewicz, 1973) the decreased DA influence would have to be related to decreased response to the normal levels of DA. Since the striatal neurons are primarily altered in this disease, it is not unreasonable to assume that their response to putative neurotransmitters is altered. It is proposed here that rigidity is related to an overall decreased response of effect of DA on certain striatal neurons, while chorea is related to a hypersensitivity to DA.

This at first seems contradictory. The paradox of having striatal receptors which are hypersensitive to DA at the same time that other striatal receptors are hyposensitive to the same amine is resolved by several considerations. The neurons of the striatum are not all involved in the disease process to the same degree at any one point in time. Some could easily be hypersensitive even though overall the response to DA is decreased. If this is true, then patients receiving L-DOPA for Huntington's chorea with rigidity could have improved rigidity but worsened chorea. This appears to be the case. In fact, treatment of rigidity can bring out previously undetected chorea (Barbeau, 1969). The cell population of the normal striatum is not at all uniform. There is not only a noticeable histologic difference among the cells, there is also a difference in the apparent effect of DA on such cells. While most cells are inhibited by DA, some are facilitated. It is possible that chorea may be related to cells which are normally facilitated, rigidity to those which are normally inhibited. While this is clearly speculative, the cell population is diverse, and the normal striatal cells can react in different ways to DA.

Initial studies on the striatum emphasized that DA has an inhibitory action on striatal neurons. Recent work has shown that a significant percentage of the DA-responsive caudate neurons are facilitated by DA. York (1970) actually found that following ionto-phoretic dopamine, 53 putamen neurons showed facilitation, while 37 putamen neurons showed inhibition. Two separate striatal nerve cell populations are suggested by these observations: a DA-facilitated nerve cell population, which possesses predominantly or exclusively facilitory DA membrane receptors, and DA-inhibitory DA membrane receptors. It is suggested that in Huntington's chorea the predominant defect occurs at this facilitory neuron. In contrast to normal facilitory neurons which fire in an orderly manner, the altered neurons fire abnormally and perhaps hypersynchronously in response to DA stimulation. This could result in choreiform movements. Although altered striatal neurons responsible for chorea may be derived from either the DA-inhibited or the DA-facilitated striatal neurons, it would appear that they are primarily derived from the DA-facilitated nerve cells.

It is of major interest that the pathology of the rigid-akinetic form of Huntington's chorea is not identical to the pathology of the usual choreic form. Bruyn (1968) notes that, although the small neurons of the striatum usually bear the brunt of the pathological process, the large striatal neurons are often involved, being shrunken and showing evidence of degenerative changes. This involvement of the large neurons is particularly marked in the hypokinetic rigid cases. This pathologic difference between classic hyperkinetic Huntington patients and the less frequently seen hypokinetic patients is consistent with the hypothesis that the DA-facilitated and DA-inhibited striatal cell populations are impaired to different degrees in the two forms of Huntington's chorea.

The evidence reviewed above suggests that the small cells are DA-facilitated and that their involvement in Huntington's chorea is directly related to the production of chorea. The larger striatal neurons would be DA-inhibited, and involvement of these cells in Huntington's chorea is manifested by hypokinesia and rigidity. As discussed before, the course of chorea in most patients also suggests that the small cells are related to these movements.

Parkinsonism may be analogous to Huntington's chorea in the simultaneous occurrence of different DA responses. It has been proposed that failure of L-DOPA in parkinsonism is related to decreased receptor responsiveness to DA, while the L-DOPA-induced dyskinesia is related to receptor site hypersensitivity. L-DOPA can induce chorea in patients with parkinsonism (Klawans, 1973). Chorea can be induced in such patients without relief of parkinsonian akinesia or rigidity. This suggests that while both of these clinical states are related in some way to striatal DA receptors, they are not mutually exclusive. The production of chorea without the relief of rigidity suggests that an abnormal (hypersensitive) response can be elicited without restoring normal function. This supports the concept that the dopaminergic mechanisms of chorea and rigidity, although related, are not identical. The production of parkinsonism is not a prerequisite for drug-induced improvement in chorea, and similarly, improvement in parkinsonism is not a prerequisite for L-DOPA-induced chorea.

These observations then suggest the possible existence of two separate striatal dopaminergic mechanisms and possibly two separate types of striatal DA receptors. The question of course is how to demonstrate the existence of two different DA receptors.

The investigation of the binding of biologically active substances to membranous preparations from nervous tissue is well established as a direct biochemical method for the evaluation of specific receptor sites. In our recent work we have studied DA receptor binding characteristics in the caudate-putamen of guinea pig brain. In this study a tritiated form of the naturally occurring agonist DA was used to estimate membrane binding. Since DA as well is the other biogenic amines are able to bind *in vitro* as well as *in vivo* to membrane structures other than the receptor site, various criteria must be fulfilled to identify the specific receptor binding. The receptor binding should be of high affinity, saturable, reversible, stereospecific and the affinity of agents to displace DA from the receptors should parallel their pharmacological potencies. In a recent attempt to characterize the DA receptor sites many investigators have studied the DA receptors by labelling them with various neuroleptics, which are known to interfere with the action of endogenous DA at its receptor sites (Creese *et al.*, 1975; Seeman *et al.*, 1975; Seeman *et al.*, 1976; Tittler *et al.*, 1977; Fields *et al.*, 1978). Haloperidol is most widely used neuroleptic in such DA receptor binding studies. However, haloperidol is not only a DA antagonist; it also has activity at norepinephrine (Ohta, 1976) and muscarinic (Snyder *et al.*, 1974) receptor sites, and it is possible that haloperidol or neuroleptic receptor sites may also exist (Leysen *et al.*, 1978). Because of these considerations, haloperidol binding should not be expected to be identical to or necessarily representative of DA binding at its receptor site. In our opinion the binding of naturally occurring agonist DA may better reflect the characteristic of the DA receptor site, than an artifical agonist or antagonist.

METHODS

The binding studies were carried out as follows: white male outbred guinea pigs weighing 250-350 g were housed six to a cage in environmentally controlled quarters lighted between 0600-1800 hours. Animals were allowed free access to food and water. A group of six guinea pigs was decapitated every three weeks. The brains were quickly removed and frozen on dry ice. The corpus striata were dissected in a cold room (4°C) from the serially sectioned brains.

For the binding studies the striatal tissue from six animals was pooled and homogenized in 40 volumes of ice cold 0.05M tris HCl buffer pH7.4 containing 120 mM NaCl, 5m M KCl, 2 mM CaCl$_2$ and 1mM MgCl$_2$ according to the method of (Creese *et al.*, 1975). The homogenate was centrifuged at 50,000 x g for 10 min. The supernatant fluid was discarded and the pellet was rehomogenized in 100 volumes of the same buffer. One ml aliquots corresponding to 10 mg of original tissue wet weight were incubated with various concentrations 0.1-20nM of H^3 dopamine, in the same buffer as previously described for the tissue preparation with the addition of 0.1% ascorbic acid. The incubation was carried out at 4°C. After equilibration the samples were rapidly filtered under vacuum through Whatman GF/B filters. Each filter was rinsed with a single 5 ml ice cold buffer. The filters were counted by liquid scintillation spectrometry. Specific binding of H^3 dopamine was measured as the excess over blank tubes containing 200 nM apomorphine, whereas the stereospecific binding was determined as the excess over blank tubes containing 1 μM (+) Butaclamol as previously described by Creese *et al.*, (1975).

Since all of the methods for the determination of the kinetic parameters of binding are based on the first order mass action law and most of these require equilibrium or steady state conditions, the first step was to determine the equilibrium of the binding under experimental conditions.

The equilibrium was reached after 20 min incubation (Hitri, 1978). In all subsequent studies where the amount of bound radioactive DA to the striatal membranes was monitored as a function of ^{3}H-DA concentration, the incubation time was 20 min in order to assure equilibrium.

RESULTS

Figure 1 illustrates the saturation curves of total, specific and stereospecific ^{3}H-DA binding to guinea pig striatal membranes. The specific binding was calculated by subtracting the nonspecific binding obtained in the presence of 200 nM apomorphine from the total binding, while the stereospecific binding was determined as the excess over blank tubes containing 1 μM (+) Butaclamol, the clinically effective enantiomere of this new antipsychotic drug. The stereospecific binding obtained was 10-15% of the total binding in the concentration range of 0.2-10 nM H^3-DA. In order to determine the number of binding sites and the affinity constants, the data were analyzed according to the method of Scatchard.

Figure 2A represents the Scatchard plot of ^{3}H-DA stereospecific binding to striatal membranes of young guinea pigs weighing 250-300 g. The slope on the Scatchard plot represents the binding site affinity while the intercept on the abscissa represents the receptor sites concentration. As can be seen there is only one regression line present in the membranes derived from such young animals (6 weeks old). This line demonstrates a receptor site concentration of 65 pmoles/g with the affinity constant of 4×10^7M.

Figure 2B demonstrates the ^{3}H-DA binding to guinea pig striatal membranes in 11 week old animals. The statistical evaluation of the data revealed one binding site characterized by the receptor site concentration of 67 pmoles/g and an affinity constant (Ka) equal to 9×10^7M. However there is a suggestion for the appearance of the second higher affinity binding site.

Figure 2C illustrates the ^{3}H-DA stereospecific binding to the striatal membranes of 15 week old guinea pigs. The Scatchard analysis revealed two distinct binding sites. One regression line is described by the slope of 1×10^9M representing the association constant and receptor site concentration of 22 pmoles/g. The low affinity binding site is characterized by an association constant of 7×10^7M and receptor site concentration of 55 pmoles/g.

DISCUSSION

The data demonstrates the development of two different populations of DA receptors in the striatum of normal guinea pigs. The existence of separate classes of receptors with different biochemical characteristics could of course have profound clinical implication if such receptors have different functions and different affinities for agents other than DA itself. The clinical data suggesting that there are at least two classes of striatal DA receptors was reviewed above. The concept that the two biochemically distinct receptors might subserve different functions is seductive but unproven. If this is true

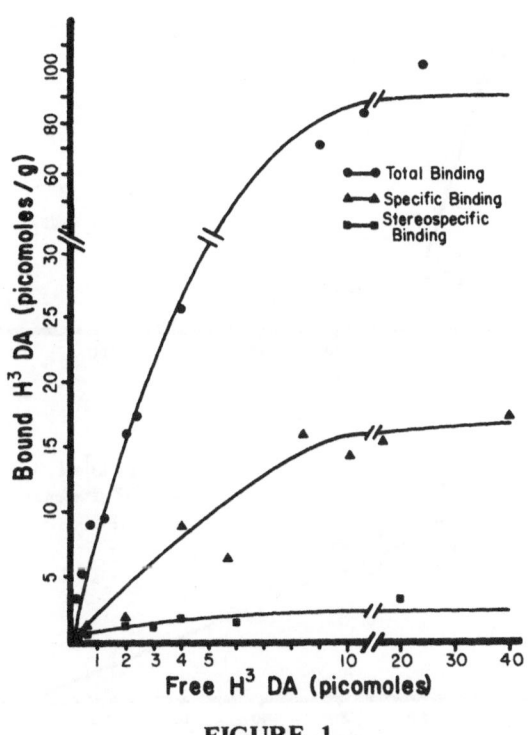

FIGURE 1

Saturation curves of ^{3}H-dopamine binding to the guinea pig striatal membranes. The specific binding was obtained as the excess over blank tubes containing 200 M apomorphine. The stereospecific binding was determined as the excess over blank tubes containing 1 μM (+) Butaclamol.

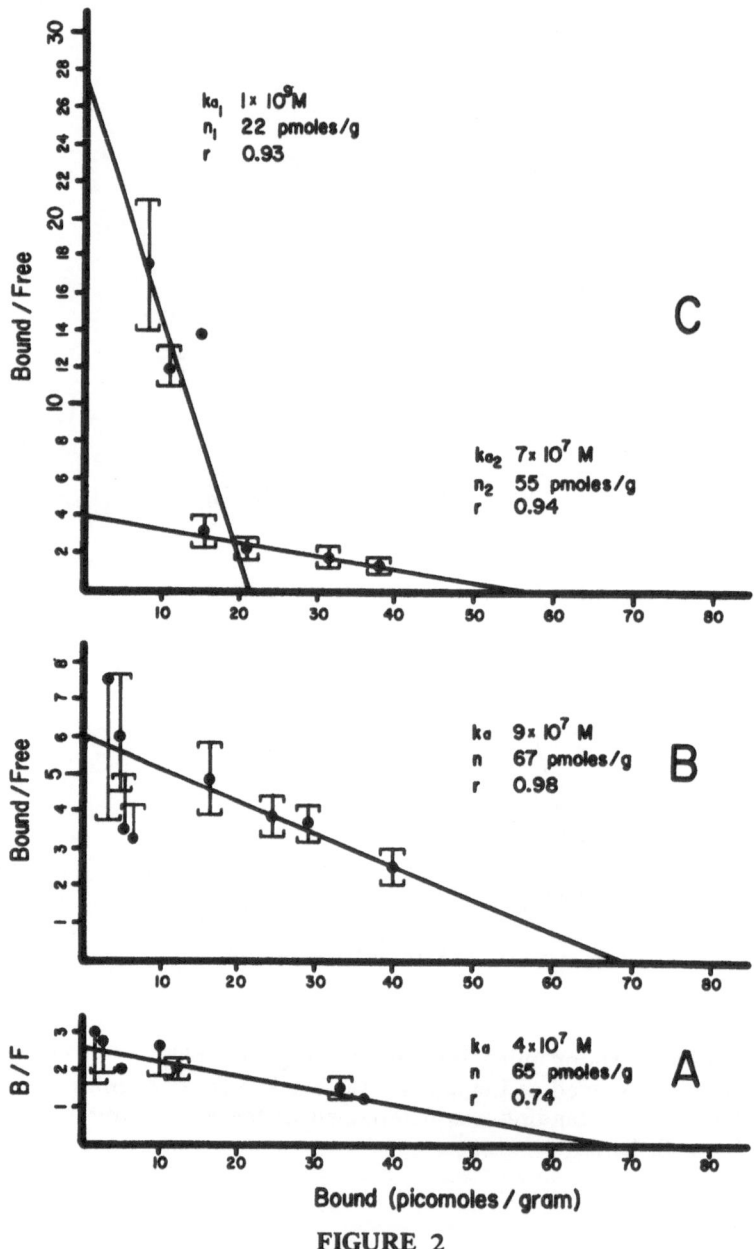

FIGURE 2

Scatchard plots of ^{3}H-dopamine stereospecific binding to guinea pig striatal membranes. The slopes of the regression lines denote the affinity of the receptor binding, whereas the receptor density is represented by the intercept on the abscissa. A — 6-week-old guinea pigs; B — 11-week-old guinea pigs; C — 15-week-old guinea pigs.

and drugs can be found with differential affinity for the two receptors, numerous therapeutic advantages can be hypothesized including improvement of parkinsonism without eliciting chorea, improvement of schizophrenia without eliciting extrapyramidal side effects, and total amelioration of chorea without any parkinsonism.

Recent studies with the DA agonist bromocriptine are consistent with the concept of two functionally and biochemically different classes of receptors with differential affinity for a specific agent. High doses of bromocriptine (Kartzinel *et al.*, 1976) worsen chorea while low doses improve chorea (Frattola *et al.*, in press). This suggests that there is one set of receptors for which bromocriptine has high affinity which when occupied by DA or a DA agonist improve chorea, and another lower affinity type which when occupied worsens chorea. Whether the high affinity site for bromocriptine is presynaptic and the low affinity site is post-synaptic (Trabucchi *et al.*, in press) is solely conjectural.

The differential affinity with differential functional effect appears however to be true. The fact that this is only a qualitative difference in affinity will probably limit the long-term clinical efficacy of bromocriptine in chorea but the observation of differential effect makes the search of agents which will act at only one DA receptor more attractive. Only time will tell if such agents can be found and, if found, if they will be of any clinical value.

ACKNOWLEDGEMENTS

This work was supported by grants from the United Parkinson Foundation and Boothroyd Foundation Chicago, Illinois.

REFERENCES

Barbeau, A., 1969, L-DOPA and juvenile Huntington's disease, *Lancet:* 1066.

Bernheimer, H., and Hornykiewicz, O., 1973, Brain amines in Huntington's chorea, *Adv. Neurol. 1:*525.

Bird, M.T., and Paulson, G.W., 1970, Early onset rigid Huntington's chorea, *Neurology 20:*400.

Birkmayer, W., 1969, The a-methyl-p-tryrosine effect in extrapyramidal disorders, *Wien Klin Wochenschr 81:*10.

Bruyn, G.W., 1968, Huntington's chorea, in *"Handbook of Clinical Neurology"* (P.J. Vinken, and C.W. Bruyn, eds.), pp. 298.

Creese, J., Burt, D.R., and Snyder, S.H., 1975, Dopamine receptor binding: differentiation of agonist and antagonist states with H^3-dopamine and H^3-haloperidol, *Life Sci. 17:*993.

Doon, R., Baro, F., and Brucher, J.M., 1973, A cytemetric study of the putamen in different types of Huntington's chorea in *"Huntington's Chorea, 1872-1972"* (A. Barbeau, T.N. Chase, and G.W. Paulson, eds.), *Adv. Neurol 1:*369.

Fields, J.Z., Reisine, T.D., and Yamamura, H.I., 1977, Biochemical demonstration of dopaminergic receptors in rat and human brain using ^{3}H-spiroperidol, *Brain Res. 136:*578.

Frattola, L., Albizzati, M., Spano, P., and Trabucchi, M., 1977, The treatment of Huntington's chorea and bromocriptine, *Acta Neurol. Scand. 56(1):*37.

Greenfield, J.G., and Bosanquet, F.D., 1953, The brain stem lesions in parkinsonism, *J. Neurol. Neurosurg. Psychiat. 16:*213.

Hitri, A., Weiner, W.J., Borison, R.L., Diamond, B.I., Nausieda, P.A., and Klawans, H.L., 1978, Dopamine binding following prolonged haloperidol pretreatment, *Ann. Neurology 3:*134.

Hornykiewicz, O., 1966, Dopamine (3-hydroxytyramine) and brain function, *Pharmacol. Rev. 18:*925.

Kartzinel, R., Hunt, R.D., and Calne, D.B., 1976, Bromocriptine in Huntington's chorea, *Archives Neurol 33:*517.

Klawans, H.L., 1968, The pharmacology of parkinsonism, *Dis. Nerv. Syst. 29:*805.

Klawans, H.L., 1973, *"The Pharmacology of Extrapyramidal Movement Disorders,"* Karger, Basel.

Klawans, H.L., and W.J., Weiner, 1975, The pharmacology of choreatic movement disorders, in *"Progress in Neurobiology,"* (G.A. Kerkut, and J.W. Phillis, eds.), pp. 1-32, Oxford Pergamon Press.

Klawans, H.L., Ilahi, M.M., and Rengel, S.P., 1971, Toward an understanding of the pathophysiology of Huntington's chorea, *Conf. Neural. 33:*297.

Klawans, H.L., Paulson, G.W., Ringel, S.P., and Barbeau, A., 1972, The use of L-DOPA in the detection of presymptomatic Huntington's chorea, *N. Engl. J. Med. 286:*1332.

Leysen, J.E., Gommeren, W., and Laduron, P.M., 1978, Spiperone: a ligand of choice for neuroleptic receptors I. Kinetics and characteristics of *in vitro* binding, *Biochem. Pharm. 27:*307.

Ohta, M., 1976, Haloperidol blocks an alpha adrenergic receptor in the reticulo cortical inhibitory input, *Physiol. Behav. 16:*505.

Seeman, P., Chau-Wong, M., Tedesco, J., and Wong, K., 1975, Brain receptors for antipsychotic drugs and dopamine: direct binding assays, *Proc. Natl. Acad. Sci. USA 72:* 4376.

Seeman, P., Lee, T., Chau-Wong, M., Tedesco, J., and Wong, K., 1976, Dopamine receptors in human calf brains, using H^3-apomorphine and an antipsychotic drug, *Proc. Natl. Acad. Sci. USA 73:*4354.

Snyder, S.H., Greenberg, D., and Yamamura, H., 1974, Antischizophrenic drugs and brain cholinergic receptors, *Arch Gen. Psychiatry 31:*58.

Tittler, M., Weinreich, P., and Seeman, P., 1977, New detection of brain dopamine receptors with H^3-dihydroergocryptine, *Proc. Natl. Acad. Sci. USA 74(9):*3750.

Trabucchi, M., Andreoli, V.M., Frattola, L., *et al.,* 1977, Pre- and post-synaptic actions of bromocriptine: its pharmacological effects on schizophrenia and neurological diseases, *Adv. Biochem. Psychopharmacol. 16:*661.

York, D.H., 1970, Possible dopaminergic pathway from substantia nigra to putamen, *Brain Res. 20:*233.

PHYSOSTIGMINE RELATED CHANGES IN CEREBROSPINAL FLUID NEUROTRANSMITTER METABOLITES IN MAN

K. L. Davis[1,2], K. F. Faull[2], L. E. Hollister[1,2], J. D. Barchas[2] and P. A. Berger[1,2]

[1]Veterans Administration Hospital, 3801 Miranda Avenue, Palo Alto, California 94304

[2]Department of Psychiatry and Behavioral Sciences, Stanford University School of Medicine, Stanford, California 94305

INTRODUCTION

Administration of the acetylcholinesterase inhibitor physostigmine to man produces a range of behavioral changes that can be of therapeutic benefit to some patients with Huntington's disease, tardive dyskinesia, mania and memory deficits (Aquilonius and Sjostrom, 1971; Janowsky et al., 1973; Klawans and Rubovits, 1974; Davis et al., 1976; 1978a; 1978b). The scope and complexity of the actions of physostigmine suggest that the neurochemical basis of these effects might extend beyond the ability of the drug to increase cholinergic activity. It is possible that some of the behavioral consequences of physostigmine result from the action of increased central cholinergic activity on other neurotransmitters.

Animal studies indicate there is an interaction in the substantia nigra and corpus striatum between acetylcholine and dopamine (Laverty and Sharman, 1965; Corrodi et al., 1967; O'Keefe et al., 1970; Perez-Cruet et al., 1971; Anden and Bedard, 1971; Bowers and Roth, 1972; Corrodi et al., 1972; Bhatnagar, 1973; Bartholini et al., 1973; Anden, 1974; Nose and Takemoto, 1974; Javoy et al., 1974; 1975; Westernick and Korf, 1975; Giorguieff et al., 1976). However, the nature of this interaction is extremely complex. Muscarinic and nicotinic stimulation may have opposite effects on dopamine release (Giorguieff et al., 1976).

Furthermore, cholinergic regulation of dopamine activity at the nigral level is the opposite of striatal regulation (Laverty and Sharman, 1965; Corrodi et al., 1967; Perez-Cruet et al., 1971; Bhatnagar, 1973; Bartholini et al., 1973; Anden, 1974; Nose and Takemoto, 1974; Javoy et al., 1974; 1975; Westernick and Korf, 1975).

A series of investigators have demonstrated that administration of a central cholino-mimetic elevates brain concentrations of homovanillic acid (HVA). However, such eleva-tions can be seen following increased or decreased dopamine release (Carlsson *et al.,* 1972; Roth *et al.,* 1978). Thus, these data do not clarify the effect of increased central cholinergic activity upon dopaminergic activity, although there can be little question that increasing central cholinergic activity can affect dopaminergic activity.

One approach to this problem is to study cerebrospinal fluid concentrations of HVA and dihydroxyphenylacetic acid (DOPAC) following the administration of physo-stigmine to man. Cerebrospinal fluid HVA largely derives from the third and fourth ventricles, and has been regarded as reflecting dopamine metabolism in the striatum (Portig and Vost, 1969; Papeschi *et al.,* 1971). The spinal cord contributes little HVA to the CSF pool (Post *et al.,* 1973; Kessler *et al.,* 1976). Although CSF concentrations of 3,4-dihydroxyphenylacetic acid (DOPAC) are far less than CSF concentrations of HVA, CSF DOPAC is also believed to largely derive from dopamine metabolism in the striatum. HVA can be the result of either intraneuronal or extraneuronal dopamine metabolism (Roffler-Tarlov *et al.,* 1971). DOPAC formation only occurs intraneuronally, although it may reflect the breakdown of dopamine taken back into the neuron from the synaptic cleft. By simultaneously measuring DOPAC and HVA in lumbar CSF after the infusion of physostigmine, some inferences concerning the effect of increased cholinergic activity upon dopaminergic activity in the basal ganglia of man are possible. Whatever change increased striatal cholinergic activity produced on dopaminergic activity must be consis-tent with the ameliorative effects of physostigmine on the abnormal movements of patients with tardive dyskinesia and on the movements of some patients with Huntington's disease.

METHODS

Subjects

Eight male subjects between the ages of 22 and 50 without a history of psychiatric illness gave their informed consent to participate in this investigation. Subjects received an infusion of 2 mg of physostigmine dissolved in 200 cc of normal saline, and an infusion of 200 cc of normal saline. The order of infusions was randomized, and seven days intervened between infusions.

Beginning at 8:00 p.m. on the day before the infusion, subjects were given 100 mg/kg of probenecid in five divided doses over the next 16 hr. At 9:30 a.m. on the infusion days, subjects were given 0.5 mg of methscopolamine bromide subcutaneously. By 10:00 a.m., when the subjects' pulse rates were at least 100 beats per minute, the infusions were begun. The infusions proceeded at a constant rate, concluding in 60 min. At 2:00 p.m. subjects underwent a lumbar puncture. 24 cc of spinal fluid were with-drawn. None of the lumbar punctures were traumatic. The measurement of concentra-tions was always performed on the fifth through tenth cc of CSF for DOPAC, HVA and probenecid according to the gas chromatographic/mass spectrometric methods of Karoum and Swahn (Karoum *et al.,* 1975; Swahn *et al.,* 1976).

RESULTS

Table 1 summarizes the HVA, DOPAC and probenecid values after physostigmine and placebo infusions. Total HVA and DOPAC concentrations were calculated. A paired t-test was used to determine if total HVA, total DOPAC, total HVA/probenecid and total DOPAC/probenecid concentrations were significantly higher following the physostigmine infusion than following the saline infusion. After physostigmine, subjects had significantly elevated levels of total DOPAC/probenecid ($p \leq .01$, one tailed) and total HVA/probenecid ($p \leq .025$, one tailed) than after receiving saline infusions. The ratios for saline and physostigmine conditions are shown in Table 2. No significant differences were found between the saline and physostigmine conditions in probenecid, total HVA or total DOPAC.

TABLE 1

Cerebrospinal Fluid Values of DOPAC, HVA and Probenecid

Subject	Saline			Physostigmine		
	DOPAC ng/ml	HVA ng/ml	Probenecid μg/ml	DOPAC ng/ml	HVA ng/ml	Probenecid μg/ml
H.T.	2.0	117.2	11.1	2.6	168.2	14.0
F.F.	2.0	134.0	13.8	1.5	93.0	7.3
D.B.	2.3	114.9	10.4	1.8	104.1	7.0
S.B.	8.4	204.9	25.0	5.9	159.0	13.6
W.C.	2.2	110.0	11.2	2.6	115.2	11.7
M.B.	11.1	370.5	23.8	10.7	353.7	19.8
R.H.	5.5	222.9	18.3	5.2	196.2	18.8
M.R.	4.9	165.4	12.7	6.0	216.1	12.7
$\bar{X}$	4.8	180.0	15.8	4.5	175.7	13.1
σ	3.4	88.0	5.9	3.1	84.3	4.7

TABLE 2

Ratios of DOPAC/Probenecid and HVA/Probenecid

	Saline		Physostigmine	
Subject	DOPAC/Probenecid ng/μg	HVA/Probenecid ng/μg	DOPAC/Probenecid ng/μg	HVA/Probenecid ng/μg
H.T.	0.18	10.56	0.19	12.01
F.F.	0.15	9.71	0.21	12.74
D.B.	0.22	11.05	0.26	14.87
S.B.	0.34	8.20	0.43	11.69
W.C.	0.20	9.82	0.22	9.85
M.B.	0.47	15.57	0.54	17.86
R.H.	0.30	12.18	0.28	10.44
M.R.	0.39	13.02	0.47	17.02
$\bar{X} \pm \sigma$	0.28 ± 0.11	11.26 ± 2.29	0.33 ± 0.13	13.33 ± 2.95

$$t_{(DOPAC/Probenecid)} = 3.02$$

$$p \leqslant .01 \text{ (one tailed)}$$

$$t_{(HVA/Probenecid)} = 2.86$$

$$p \leqslant .025 \text{ (one tailed)}$$

DISCUSSION

These results confirm and extend our previous findings that physostigmine elevated CSF HVA (Davis et al., 1977). Administration of physostigmine significantly elevated CSF concentrations of DOPAC/μg probenecid and HVA/μg probenecid. Probenecid blocks the outflow of both HVA and DOPAC from the CSF. Our data indicate that a significant positive correlation exists between CSF HVA and DOPAC concentrations, and the CSF probenecid concentrations obtained after administration of 100 mg/kg of probenecid (Berger et al., in press). Consequently, the ratio of CSF DOPAC and HVA to probenecid partially corrects for the differences in CSF probenecid concentrations, and the variable degree of transport blockade produced by these unequal concentrations of probenecid. This ratio facilitates comparisons between subjects and experimental conditions. The significant differences between DOPAC/μg probenecid and HVA/μg probenecid indicates that dopamine turnover was higher when subjects received physostigmine than after the same subjects received saline. CSF HVA and DOPAC are mostly derived from the third and fourth ventricles. Thus, physostigmine elevated the turnover of striatal dopamine (Portig and Vost, 1969; Papeschi et al., 1971). As pointed out, these data should be integrated with the favorable clinical effects of increased central cholinergic activity in patients with tardive dyskinesia and in some patients with Huntington's disease. Preclinical and clinical data can be made consistent if increased cholinergic activity would inhibit dopaminergic impulse flow. This has been proposed to occur and be mediated by a GABA neuron (Groves et al., 1975). There is evidence to support an inhibitory striato-nigral GABA tract. Striatal stimulation inhibits the activity of nigral cells (Voneida, 1960; Szabo, 1962; Nauta and Mehler, 1966; Niimi et al., 1970; Szabo, 1970; Precht and Yoshida, 1971; Yoshida et al., 1971; Yoshida and Precht, 1971; McNair et al., 1972; Szabo, 1972; McGeer et al., 1974). In addition, these inhibitory neurons have been shown to contain GABA, and the application of GABA by iontophoresis onto the substantia nigra also inhibits the activity of nigral neurons (Feltz, 1971; Aghajanian and Bunney, 1973; Anden and Stock, 1973; Okada and Hassler, 1973; Crossman et al., 1974).

If cholinergic stimulation inhibits dopaminergic impulse flow via an inhibitory striato-nigral pathway, there are a predictable series of effects on dopamine synthesis. It has been shown that diminished dopaminergic impulse flow is associated with increased dopamine synthesis (Walters, 1972; Roth et al., 1973; Murrin and Roth, 1976). Ultimately, this would be reflected in elevated concentrations of DOPAC and HVA, as neuronal storage granules overflow. This is consistent with the results of this study.

This interpretation can also explain the ameliorative effect of physostigmine on the frequency of abnormal involuntary movements in some patients with Huntington's disease and tardive dyskinesia. Diminished dopaminergic activity, which has been produced by a number of drugs, decreases the frequency and severity of the abnormal involuntary movements of patients with tardive dyskinesia and Huntington's disease (Klawans, 1970; Baldessarini and Tarsy, 1976). Consequently, if increased cholinergic activity in the striatum diminishes dopaminergic activity in the nigra, improvement in patients with these movement disorders would be anticipated.

Investigations of the effects of cholinomimetics on apomorphine- and amphetamine-induced stereotypy are consistent with an inhibitory action of striatal cholinergic neurons on nigral dopaminergic activity. Physostigmine, oxotremorine and choline chloride have all been reported to suppress methylphenidate- or apomorphine-induced stereotypy (Anfred and Randrup, 1968; Janowsky et al., 1972; Davis et al., 1978c; 1978d). Furthermore, intranigral injections of arecoline produces ipsilateral rotation, while intranigral atropine yields contralateral rotation. These data also suggest an inhibitory role for striatal acetylcholine upon nigral dopaminergic activity (Roth et al., 1973; 1976).

Other explanations for elevated dopamine turnover following cholinomimetic administration, and the ability of these drugs to inhibit stereotypy and diminish the abnormal involuntary movements of patients with tardive dyskinesia and Huntington's disease are possible. For example, if there are two dopamine receptors, one inhibitory and the other excitatory, it is conceivable that cholinomimetics could increase dopamine impulse flow only on neurons that synapse onto inhibitory dopamine receptors. In fact, there is some evidence to suggest two dopamine receptors in the striatum (Cools et al.,

1976; Cools, 1977). Furthermore, others have concluded that cholinomimetics stimulate the release of dopamine from nigral dopaminergic neurons (Bartholini *et al.*, 1975). This possibility deserves further study. If, on the other hand, centrally acting cholinomimetics inhibit nigral dopaminergic impulse flow, there are important implications for the long-term use of cholinomimetics in the treatment of tardive dyskinesia. A chronic diminution of nigral dopaminergic activity could supersensitize post-synaptic dopaminergic neurons. Consequently, cholinomimetics would not be a viable chronic treatment for patients with tardive dyskinesia. Additional studies are underway to investigate this possibility.

ACKNOWLEDGEMENTS

This research was supported by the Medical Research Service of the Veterans Administration, the NIMH Specialized Research Center Grant MH-30854, U.S. Public Health Service Grant MH-03030, NIMH Grant MH-24161 and the Kate Pande Memorial Research Fund.

REFERENCES

Aghajanian, G.K., and Bunney, B.S., 1973, Central dopaminergic neurons: Neurophysiological identification and response to drugs, in *"Frontiers in Catecholamine Research"* (E. Usdin, and S. Snyder, eds.), pp. 643-648, Pergamon Press, New York.

Anden, N.E., 1974, Effect of oxotremorine and physostigmine on the turnover of dopamine in the corpus striatum and limbic system, *J. Pharm. Pharmacol. 26:*738.

Anden, N.E., and Bedard, P., 1971, Influences of cholinergic mechanisms on the function and turnover of brain dopamine, *J. Pharm. Pharmacol. 23:*460.

Anden, N.E., and Stock, G., 1973, Effect of clozapine on the turnover of dopamine in the corpus striatum and in the limbic system, *J. Pharm. Pharmacol. 25:*346.

Anfred, T., and Randrup, A., 1968, Cholinergic mechanisms in brain inhibiting amphetamine-induced stereotyped behavior, *Acta Pharmacol. Toxicol. 26:*384.

Aquilonius, S.M., and Sjostrom, R., 1971, Cholinergic and dopaminergic mechanisms in Huntington's chorea, *Life Sci. 10:*405.

Baldessarini, R.J., and Tarsy, D., 1976, Mechanisms underlying tardive dyskinesia, in *"The Basal Ganglia"* (M.D. Yahr, ed.), pp. 433-446, Raven Press, New York.

Bartholini, G., Stadler, H., and Lloyd, F.G., 1973, Cholinergic-dopaminergic interactions in the extrapyramidal system, *Adv. Neurol. 3:*233.

Bartholini, G., Keller, H.H., and Pletscher, A., 1975, Drug-induced changes of dopamine turnover in striatum and limbic system of the rat, *J. Pharm. Pharmacol. 27:*439.

Berger, P.A., Faull, K., Davis, K.L., and Barchas, J.L., in press, Amine metabolites in CSF in psychiatric disorders, in *"Fourth International Catecholamine Symposium"* (E. Usdin, ed.), Pergamon Press, New York.

Bhatnagar, S.P., 1973, Studies related to the cholinergic influence on the accumulation and disappearance of monoamines in the rat brain, *Can. J. Physiol. Pharmacol. 51:*893.

Bowers, M.B., and Roth, R.H., 1972, Interactions of atropine-like drugs with dopamine-containing neurones in rat brain, *Br. J. Pharmacol. 44:*301.

Carlsson, A., Kehr, W., Lindquist, M., Magnusson, T., and Atack, C.U., 1972, Regulation of monoamine metabolism in the central nervous system, *Pharmacol. Rev. 24:*371.

Cools, A.R., 1977, Two functionally and pharmacologically distinct dopamine receptors in the rat brain, in *"Advances in Biochemical Psychopharmacology, Vol. 16"* (E. Costa, and G.L. Gessa, eds.), pp. 215-225, Raven Press, New York.

Cools, A.R., Honig, W.M.M., Pijnenburg, A.J.J., and van Rossom, J.M., 1976, The nucleus accumbens of rats and dopaminergic mechanisms regulating locomotor behavior, *Neurosci. Lett. 3:*335.

Corrodi, H., Fuxe, K., Hammer, W., *et al.,* 1967, Oxotremorine and central monoamine neurones, *Life Sci. 6:*2557.

Corrodi, H., Fuxe, K., and Lidbrink, P., 1972, Interaction between cholinergic and catecholaminergic neurones in rat brain, *Brain Res. 43:*397.

Crossman, A.R., Walker, R.J., and Woodruff, G.N., 1974, Proceedings: Pharmacological studies on single neurones in the substantia nigra, *Br. J. Pharmacol. 51:*137P.

Davis, K.L., Hollister, L.E., Barchas, J.D., and Berger, P.A., 1976, Choline in tardive dyskinesia and Huntington's disease, *Life Sci. 19:*1507.

Davis, K.L., Hollister, L.E., Goodwin, F.K., and Gordon, E.K., 1977, Neurotransmitter metabolites in the cerebrospinal fluid of man following physostigmine, *Life Sci. 21:* 933.

Davis, K.L., Berger, P.A., Hollister, L.E., and DeFraites, E.G., 1978a, Physostigmine in mania, *Arch. Gen. Psychiatry 35(1):*119.

Davis, K.L., Mohs, R., Tinklenberg, J.R., Pfefferbaum, A., Hollister, L.E., and Kopell, B.S., 1978b, Physostigmine: improvement of long-term memory processes in normal humans, *Science 201:*4352.

Davis, K.L., Hollister, L.E., and Tepper, J., 1978c, Cholinergic inhibition of methylphenidate induced stereotypy: oxotremorine, *Psychopharmacology 56:*1.

Davis, K.L., Hollister, L.E., Vento, A.L., and Simonton, S., 1978d, Choline chloride in methylphenidate- and apomorphine-induced stereotypy, *Life Sci. 22:*2171.

Feltz, P., 1971, Gamma-aminobutyric acid and a caudato-nigral inhibition, *Can. J. Physiol. Pharmacol. 49:*1113.

Giorguieff, M.F., Lefloch, M.L., Westfall, T.C., Glowinski, J., and Besson, M.J., 1976, Nicotinic effect of acetylcholine on the release of newly synthesized ^{3}H dopamine in rat striatal slices and cat caudate nucleus, *Brain Res. 106:*117.

Groves, P.M., Wilson, C.J., Young, S.J., and Rebec, G.V., 1975, Self-inhibition by dopaminergic neurons: an alternative to the "Normal Feedback Loop" hypothesis for the mode of action of certain psychotropic drugs, *Science 190:*522.

Janowsky, D.S., El-Yousef, M.K., Davis, J.M., and Sekerke, H.J., 1972, Cholinergic antagonism of methylphenidate-induced stereotyped behavior, *Psychopharmacologia 27:*295.

Janowsky, D.S., El-Yousef, J.K., and Davis, J.M., 1973, Parasympathetic suppression of manic-symptoms by physostigmine, *Arch. Gen. Psychiatry 28:*542.

Javoy, F., Agid, Y., Bouvet, D., *et al.,* 1974, Changes in neostriatal dopamine metabolism after carbachol or atropine microinjections into the substantia nigra, *Brain Res. 68:* 253.

Javoy, F., Agid, Y., and Glowinski, J., 1975, Oxotremorine and atropine-induced changes of dopamine metabolism in the rat brain, *J. Pharm. Pharmacol. 27:*677.

Karoum, F., Gillin, J.C., Wyatt, R.J., and Costa, E., 1975, Mass fragmentography of nanogram quantities of biogenic amine metabolites in human cerebrospinal fluid and whole rat brain, *Biomed. Mass. Spectrom. 2:*183.

Kessler, J.A., Gordon, E.K., Reid, J.L., and Kopin, I.J., 1976, Homovanillic acid and 3-methoxy, 4-hydroxyphenylethyleneglycol production by the monkey spinal cord, *J. Neurochem. 26:*1057.

Klawans, H.L., 1970, A pharmacologic analysis of Huntington's chorea, *Eur. Neurol. 4:* 148.

Klawans, H.L., and Rubovits, R., 1974, Effect of cholinergic and anticholinergic agents on tardive dyskinesia, *J. Neurol. Neurosurg. Psychiatry 37:*941.

Laverty, R., and Sharman, D.F., 1965, Modification by drugs of the metabolism of 3, 4-dihydroxyphenylethylamine, noradrenaline, and 5-hydroxytryptamine in the brain, *Br. J. Pharmacol. 24:*759.

McGeer, P.A., Fibiger, H.C., Haltoris, T., Singh, V.K., McGeer, E.G., and Maler, L., 1974, Biochemical neuroanatomy of the basal ganglia, *Adv. Behav. Biol. 10:*27.

McNair, J.L., Sutin, J., and Tsubokawa, T., 1972, Suppression of cell firing in the substantia nigra by caudate nucleus stimulation, *Exp. Neurol. 37:*395.

Murrin, L.C., and Roth, R.H., 1976, Dopaminergic neurons: reversal of effects elicited by gamma-butyrolactone by stimulation of the nigra-neostriatal pathway, *Naunyn Schmiedebergs Arch. Pharmacol. 295:*15.

Nauta, W.J.H., and Mehler, W.R., 1966, Projections of the lentiform nucleus in the monkey, *Brain Res. 1:*3.

Niimi, K., Ikeda, T., Kawamura, S., and Inoshita, H., 1970, Efferent projections of the head of the caudate nucleus in the cat, *Brain Res. 21:*327.

Nose, T., and Takemoto, H., 1974, Effect of oxotremorine on homovanillic acid concentration in striatum of the rat, *Eur. J. Pharmacol. 25:*51.

Okada, V., and Hassler, R., 1973, Uptake and release of γ-aminobutyric acid (GABA) in slices of substantia nigra of rat, *Brain Res. 49:*214.

O'Keefe, R., Shapman, D.R., and Vogt, M., 1970, Effect of drugs used in psychoses on cerebral dopamine metabolism, *Br. J. Pharmacol. 38:*287.

Papeschi, R., Sourkes, T.L., Piorier, L.J., and Boucher, R.L., 1971, On the intracerebral origin of homovanillic acid of the cerebrospinal fluid of experimental animals, *Brain Res. 28:*527.

Perez-Cruet, J., Gessa, G.L., Taliamonte, A., *et al.*, 1971, Evidence for a balance in the basal ganglia between cholinergic and dopaminergic activity, *Fed. Proc. 30:*216.

Portig, P.J., and Vost, M., 1969, Release into the cerebral ventricles of substances with possible transmitter function in the caudate nucleus, *J. Physiol. (Lond) 204:*687.

Post, R.M., Goodwin, R.K., Gordon, E., and Watkin, D., 1973, Amine metabolites in human cerebrospinal fluid: effects of cord transection and spinal fluid block, *Science 179:*897.

Precht, W., and Yoshida, M., 1971, Blockage of caudate-evoked inhibition of neurons in the substantia nigra by picrotoxin, *Brain Res. 32:*229.

Roffler-Tarlov, S., Sharman, D.F., and Tegerdine, P., 1971, 3-4-dihydroxyphenylacetic acid in the mouse striatum: a reflection of intra- and extra-neuronal metabolism of dopamine? *Br. J. Pharmacol. 42:*343.

Roth, R.H., Walters, J.R., and Aghajanian, G.K., 1973, Effect of impulse flow on the release and synthesis of dopamine in the rat striatum, in *"Frontiers in Catecholamine Research"* (E. Usdin, and S.H. Snyder, eds.), pp. 567-574, Pergamon Press, New York.

Roth, R.H., Murrin, L.C., and Walter, J.R., 1976, Central dopaminergic neurons: effects of alterations in impulse flow on the accumulation of dihydroxyphenylacetic acid, *Eur. J. Pharmacol. 36:*163.

Roth, R.H., Salzman, P.M., and Nowycky, M.C., 1978, Impulse flow and short-term regulation of transmitter biosynthesis in central catecholaminergic neurons, in *"Psychopharmacology: A Generation of Progress"* (M.A. Lipton, A. Dimascio, and K.F. Killam, eds.), pp. 185-198, Raven Press, New York.

Swahn, C.G., Sandgarde, B., Wiesel, F.A., and Sedvall, G., 1976, Simultaneous determination of the three major monoamine metabolites in brain tissue and body fluids by a mass fragmentographic method, *Psychopharmacology 48:*147.

Szabo, J., 1962, Topical distribution of the striatal efferents in the monkey, *Exp. Neurol.* *5:*21.

Szabo, J., 1970, Projections from the body of the caudate nucleus in the rhesus monkey, *Exp. Neurol.* *27:*1.

Szabo, J., 1972, The course and distribution of efferents from the tail of the caudate nucleus in the monkey, *Exp. Neurol.* *37:*562.

Voneida, T.J., 1960, An experimental study in the course and destination of fibers arising in the head of caudate nucleus in the cat and monkey, *J. Comp. Neurol.* *115:* 75.

Walters, J.R., 1972, Effect of gamma hydroxybutyrate on dopamine and dopamine metabolites in the rat striatum, *Biochem. Pharmacol.* *21:*2111.

Westernick, B.H.C., and Korf, J., 1975, Influence of drugs on striatal and limbic homovanillic acid concentration in the rat brain, *Eur. J. Pharmacol.* *33:*31.

Yoshida, M., and Precht, W., 1971, Monosynaptic inhibition of neurons of the substantia nigra by caudato-nigral fibers, *Brain Res.* *32:*275.

Yoshida, M., Rabin, A., and Anderson, M., 1971, Two types of monosynaptic inhibition of pallidal neurons produced by stimulation of the diencephalon and substantia nigra, *Brain Res.* *30:*235.

ACETYLCHOLINE AND ANTERIOR PITUITARY HORMONE SECRETION

B. M. Davis and K. L. Davis

Department of Psychiatry, Veterans Administration Hospital,
3801 Miranda Avenue, Palo Alto, California 94304

INTRODUCTION

This chapter deals with the effects of acetylcholine (ACh) on anterior pituitary hormone secretion. The literature is reviewed. In general, previous investigations of the effects of cholinergic stimuli indicate stimulation of the hypothalamo-hypophyseal-adrenal and gonadal axes. Cholinergic stimulation seems to inhibit prolaction secretion. Little information is available on growth hormone.

A study is reported in which physostigmine, an acetylcholinesterase inhibitor was administered in order to increase cholinergic transmission. Cortisol, prolactin, growth hormone and luteinizing hormone (LH) were measured in peripheral blood. No significant changes were seen at low doses of physostigmine and higher doses produced a stress response in which cortisol, prolactin and growth hormone were all elevated. The results are discussed.

ACTH AND CORTICOSTEROIDS

Cholinergic agents can stimulate the hypothalamo-hypophyseal-adrenal (H-P-A) axis. Evidence from *in vivo* and *in vitro* investigations indicates that cholinomimetic and anticholinergic drugs can have profound effects upon basal corticosteroid secretion, the diurnal rise, the stress response, and on feedback inhibition.

Basal cortisol or corticosterone production have been found to be increased by cholinergic agonists. One experimental approach demonstrating this effect has been the implantation of carbachol, an agonist with mixed nicotinic and muscarinic properties, and physostigmine, into the hypothalamus. In rats, guinea pigs and cats, hypothalamic implantation of these drugs has increased adrenal secretion (Naumenko, 1968; Krieger and Krieger, 1970; Endroczi *et al.*, 1963). Control implantation of inert material had no effect, ruling out the possibility that physical stimulation of the hypothalamus caused adrenocorticotrophic hormone (ACTH) release. The site of action of carbachol and

445

physostigmine in these studies was the hypothalamus itself. This was established by the lack of response when these agents were implanted into other parts of the brain or given intravenously (Krieger and Krieger, 1970).

In a second approach, large doses of centrally-acting cholinomimetics were administered intravenously. Nicotinic agonists and mixed cholinergic agonists stimulated basal cortisol secretion in dogs (Suzuki *et al.,* 1964; Otsuka, 1966). However, hypophysectomized animals, or animals with lesions of the anterior median eminence did not demonstrate an augmentation in basal cortisol levels following the intravenous administration of pilocarpine, a mixed cholinergic agonist (Suzuki *et al.,* 1975a). This suggests that an intact pituitary and hypothalamus are necessary for cholinergic stimulation of the adrenal, and is consistent with the studies indicating a hypothalamic involvement in the augmentation of basal cortisol levels.

A third approach to the investigation of a possible cholinergic regulation of serum cortisol has been to study the effect of cholinomimetics on cortisol levels in man. Nicotine administration by inhalation was associated with a dose dependent increase in serum cortisol (Hill and Wynder, 1974). That the effect of cholinomimetics upon cortisol levels in man is central and not peripheral is suggested by a study of galanthamine and neostigmine, both acetylcholinesterase inhibitors. Galanthamine, which crosses the blood brain barrier, produced significantly higher serum cortisol concentrations than neostigmine, which acts only peripherally (Cozanitis, 1974).

Although these studies indicate that there is cholinergic stimulation of the H-P-A axis, they do not establish specific cholinergic activation of a corticotrophin releasing factor (CRF) or of ACTH. In the studies cited above, after the administration of a cholinomimetic, animals are often reported to exhibit autonomic and behavioral changes such as stertorous respiration, salivation, defecation, sham rage and electroencephalographic changes (Suzuki *et al.,* 1964; Otsuka, 1966; Naumenko, 1967; Naumenko, 1968; Krieger and Krieger, 1970; Endroczi *et al.,* 1963). Thus cholinergic agonists may be inducing a nonspecific stress response.

The induction of stress would elevate ACTH. Measurement of the other stress-induced hormones, such as growth hormone and prolactin, would help to differentiate between specific cholinergic stimulation of only ACTH release and nonspecific stress resulting in ACTH and growth hormone or prolactin secretion.

On the other hand, *in vitro* studies offer some evidence for acetylcholine as a specific activator of the H-P-A axis. Hypothalamic CRF release has been stimulated by ACh. Incubation of excised whole rat hypothalami in a medium containing 10^{-14} to 10^{-15} M ACh resulted in the production of a substance with CRF-like properties (Bradbury *et al.,* 1974). This effect was abolished by atropine, although dose-dependence was not demonstrated in the range tested. A dose-dependent decrease was produced by hexamethonium, a nicotinic blocker, while bethanechol, a muscarinic agonist, was without effect. These data point to a predominately nicotinic mechanism of action (Hillhouse *et al.,* 1975).

Further support for cholinergic release of a CRF-like material comes from studies of isolated synaptosomes from sheep hypothalami. This preparation, when incubated with 10^{-9} to 10^{-11}M ACh also produced a substance capable of releasing ACTH from an *in vitro* pituitary preparation (Edwardson and Bennett, 1974).

Cholinergic mechanisms have been implicated in the diurnal variations of serum cortisol. Blockage of the diurnal cortisol rise has been observed in cats receiving a dose of atropine specific for inhibition of muscarinic receptor stimulation (Krieger and Krieger, 1967; Krieger *et al.*, 1968).

The diurnal rise in cortisol in man has also been prevented by anticholinergic agents. During a "critical period" from 4 p.m. to midnight, administration of 30 mg of "Pervagal," a methantheline derivative with antimuscarinic and ganglionic blocking properties abolished the expected early morning plasma cortisol rise and markedly reduced 24 hr urinary 17-hydroxycorticosteroids (Ferrari *et al.*, 1977).

There are a number of studies suggesting that the stress induced secretion of cortisol has a cholinergic basis. Inhibition of the stress response follows an intraventricular infusion of 50 mg/ml atropine solution (Porter *et al.*, 1970), or the hypothalamic implantation of atropine pellets (Hedge and Smelik, 1968; Hedge and deWied, 1971; Kaplanski and Smelik, 1973). However, the local concentrations of drug achieved by this method are extremely high and cast doubt on the specificity of atropine's action as a pure muscarinic antagonist. Atropine, in doses exceeding 1.4 mg/kg, inhibits responses to histamine, serotonin and norepinephrine and has local anesthetic activity (Innes and Nickerson, 1970; Makara and Stark, 1976).

Additional studies using a dose of atropine that is specific for blockade of muscarinic receptors (0.4 mg/kg) did not show diminution of cortisol secretion in response to insulin hypoglycemia, bacterial pyrogen, or lysine vasopressin (Krieger *et al.*, 1968). In fact, when atropine was administered systemically to conscious dogs in a dose of 1 mg/kg (Suzuki *et al.*, 1964; Otsuka, 1966), they became extremely agitated and showed a rise in 17-hydroxycorticosteroid production. Thus, in this investigation, atropine induced the behavioral concomitants of the stress response without abolishing cortisol secretion. This result is not consistent with the participation of muscarinic cholinergic synapses in the cortisol component of the stress response. On the other hand, nicotine administration to rats raised plasma corticosterone to the levels seen in pole-sitting stress; administration to stressed rats produced no further increase, but delayed the return to baseline (Balfour *et al.*, 1975).

Feedback inhibition of cortisol secretion may be mediated by central cholinergic transmission. Suppression of cortisol by dexamethasone has been overcome by intra-hypothalamic implants of carbachol. Physostigmine administration may also override dexamethasone suppression of cortisol secretion in man (Carroll, B., personal communication). Further investigation into this relationship will be of great interest in light of the abnormalities in dexamethasone suppressibility and cholinergic transmission that have been alleged in patients with depression (Janowsky *et al.*, 1972; 1973; Davis *et al.*, 1975; Carroll *et al.*, 1976; Davis *et al.*, 1978).

PROLACTIN

The effect of cholinergic function on prolactin secretion in rats has been evaluated in various physiological and pharmacological states. Cholinergic mixed agonists in general reduce prolactin secretion, but nicotinic and muscarinic effects appear to account for suppression under different biological conditions.

Basal prolactin secretion has been investigated in two conditions in which it is somewhat elevated: in the proestrus and the estrogen-treated rat. In the proestrus animal, ACh injected into the lateral ventricle produced a significant decrease in serum prolactin levels (Grandison *et al.*, 1974). The nicotinic blocking agent mecamylamine increases prolactin levels in a dose dependent fashion in the estrogen-treated rat. However, the time course of the prolactin increase following mecamylamine is not consistent with the long-acting nicotinic blocking properties of the drug, but rather with a short-lived stress response possibly due to sudden ganglionic blockade. There is no convincing data that nicotinic blockade increases prolactin levels, nor is there evidence that alterations in muscarinic activity affect prolactin levels. Neither atropine nor arecoline, a muscarinic agonist, influenced prolactin levels in the estrogen-treated rat (Lawson and Gala, 1975). It is significant that atropine and arecoline produced behavioral effects, indicating CNS activity. Thus, muscarinic agents which are clearly active in the brain did not affect basal prolactin secretion.

Prolactin surges which occur in various hyperestrogenic states in the rat are inhibited by muscarinic, nicotinic and mixed cholinergic agonists (Blake *et al.*, 1973; Grandison and Meites 1976a; Subramanian and Gala, 1976). Atropine alone in extremely high doses (350-700 mg/kg) which are not specific for blockade of the muscarinic receptor (see above), is uniformly reported to block prolactin surges (Libertun and McCann, 1973; Donoso and Bacha, 1975a; McLean and Nikitovitch-Winer, 1975). However, physostigmine has been reported to prevent high dose atropine inhibition of prolactin secretion (McLean and Nikitovitch-Winer, 1975). This data does not permit a conclusion about the importance of a muscarinic mechanism in the mediation of prolactin surges.

Prolactin secretion during pregnancy and lactation has been markedly reduced by treatment with nicotine in the rat. Pup size at birth was decreased and pups died of starvation because of failure of milk production by nicotine-treated mothers (Terkel *et al.*, 1973). Thus, in the rat, nicotinic stimulation may decrease serum prolactin during pregnancy and lactation.

Mixed cholinergic agonists appear to inhibit stress-induced prolactin secretion (Blake and Sawyer, 1972). Injection of pilocarpine or physostigmine prevents the prolactin increase that follows stress due to control injections of saline (Grandison *et al.*, 1974; Grandison and Meites, 1976a). Nicotine alone does not prevent prolactin release in response to either stress (Grandison and Meites, 1976b). Thus it appears that cholino-mimetic agents can prevent stress-induced secretion of prolactin, and that the mechanism may be predominately muscarinic. However, cholinergic influences on prolactin release are probably mediated by dopaminergic mechanisms. When dopaminergic transmission is impaired by 6-hydroxydopamine, reserpine, or neuroleptic treatment; cholinergic agents do not alter prolactin levels (Grandison and Meites, 1976a; Kato *et al.*, 1974; Donoso and Bacha, 1975b).

GROWTH HORMONE

Little information is available on the effects of ACh on growth hormone (GH) secretion. A preliminary report indicates inhibition of the sleep-related growth hormone rise by methscopolamine, a peripheral muscarinic blocking agent (Mendelson and Gillin, personal communication).

A different relationship has been proposed in patients with tardive dyskinesia. A positive correlation between basal growth hormone levels and dose of anticholinergic medication has been reported in these patients (Burnett *et al.*, 1978). It has been shown that nicotine administration suppresses chlorpromazine-induced elevations of growth hormone in the rat (Kato *et al.*, 1974). Since dopamine blocking agents suppress growth hormone secretion in the human, the relevance to human physiology of growth hormone studies performed in the rat is questionable.

LUTEINIZING HORMONE

In vitro and *in vivo* studies in animals indicate that LH secretion is increased by ACh and decreased by nicotine. Basal LH secretion in intact adult male rats was markedly increased by injection of 10 μg ACh into the third ventricle. This was abolished by atropine (Justo *et al.*, 1975). In ovariectomized, estrogen-primed rats, subcutaneous administration of pilocarpine and physostigmine was followed by an immediate small decrease and then a marked increase in LH levels. Both effects were blunted by atropine (Libertun and McCann, 1974).

That endogenous ACh is involved in the control of gonadotropin secretion was also shown by the effects of anticholinergic drugs. The copulation-ovulation reflex in the rabbit is blocked if methantheline, a blocking agent with antimuscarinic and anti-nicotinic potency, is injected intravenously a few seconds post-coitum (Sawyer *et al.*, 1951). Atropine implantations into the hypothalamus have been found to inhibit the increased LH secretion that occurs after castration (Libertun and McCann, 1976).

Further evidence for anticholinergic inhibition of LH secretion comes from the report that an intrahypothalamic implant of atropine blocks compensatory ovarian hypertrophy after unilateral castration (Monti *et al.*, 1970).

In vitro evidence corroborates the conclusions drawn from animal studies that cholinomimetics and blocking agents do affect the control of LH secretion at the level of the hypothalamus. When incubated with rat anterior pituitaries and hypothalamic fragments, ACh produced a dose-dependent increase in LH release. Prostigmine, an AChE inhibitor yielded the same result in this system, implying the presence of endogenous ACh. No drug directly affected the pituitary release of LH, as all the drugs required the presence of hypothalamic fragments for their effect on LH. The addition of atropine to the pituitary-hypothalamic preparation with ACh reduced LH secretion to a fraction of baseline, in a manner dependent on the dose of atropine (Fiorindo and Martini, 1975). This reduction below baseline could be understood if the effect of muscarinic blockade on cholinergic agonism were to unmask nicotinic stimulation. There is considerable evidence that nicotine administration inhibits LH secretion. In ovariectomized rats, LH levels are decreased by nicotine (Blake, 1974). This effect is seen even in rats with deaf-ferentation of the medial basal hypothalamus. The ovulatory LH surge in rats is delayed by subcutaneous nicotine injections given on the afternoon of proestrous (Blake *et al.*, 1972). When this surge is artifically advanced by progesterone, nicotine can suppress ovulation (Kanematsu and Sawyer, 1973).

Cholinergic effects upon LH secretion seem to occur at the level of the hypothalamus. Pretreatment with nicotine or atropine does not influence the action of luteinizing-hormone releasing factor (LRH) on the release of LH by the pituitary (Blake, 1974; Blake *et al.*, 1974; Libertun and McCann, 1974). Therefore, cholinergic regulation of LH secretion is probably mediated via LRH.

EFFECTS OF PHYSOSTIGMINE ON ANTERIOR PITUITARY HORMONE SECRETION

We investigated the effect of intravenous administration of physostigmine on levels of cortisol, LH, growth hormone and prolactin in the human.

The subjects were 17 normal female and male, paid volunteers, aged 18-35, who gave their informed consent to participate in the study. Each underwent two identical infusion procedures on nonconsecutive days (Figure 1). After an overnight fast, subjects reported to the Palo Alto VA Hospital at 8:30 AM. An intravenous infusion of normal saline was begun, followed by administration of 0.5-0.75 mg methscopolamine subcutaneously. Methscopolamine is an anticholinergic agent which does not cross the blood brain barrier and is necessary to counteract the cardiovascular effects of physostigmine. When cholinergic blockade was achieved, as evidenced by a pulse rate of 100, 200 ml normal saline or saline with 1.0, 1.5 or 2.0 mg physostigmine sulfate was infused at a constant rate over one hour. Drug and control infusions occurred in random order. Patients were blind to the contents of the infusion, however some patients experienced nausea and vomiting on the physostigmine day. No patient became ill on the control day. Blood was sampled in the basal state, on reaching a pulse of 100, and at the end of control and physostigmine infusions. Hormone determinations were performed by radioimmunoassay by Smith Kline & French Laboratories in San Francisco.

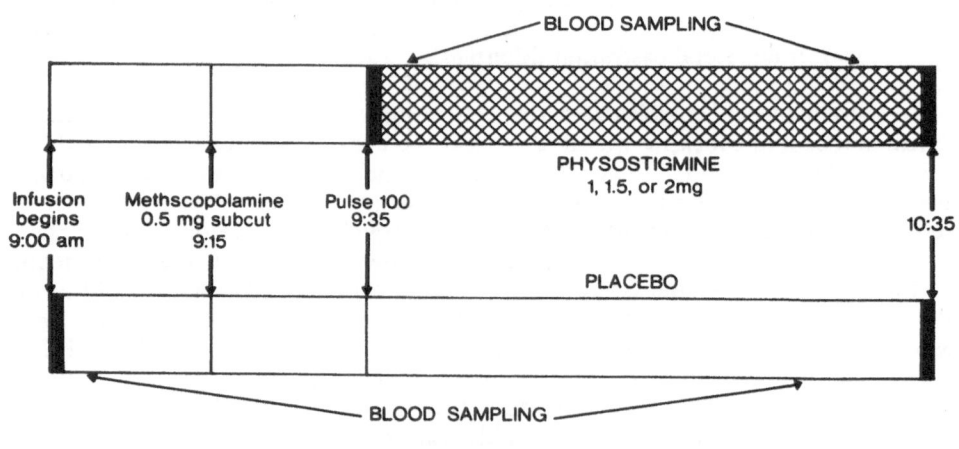

FIGURE 1

Infusion Design

RESULTS

Hormone levels 15 or 75 minutes after administration of methscopolamine were not significantly different from baseline (Figure 2).

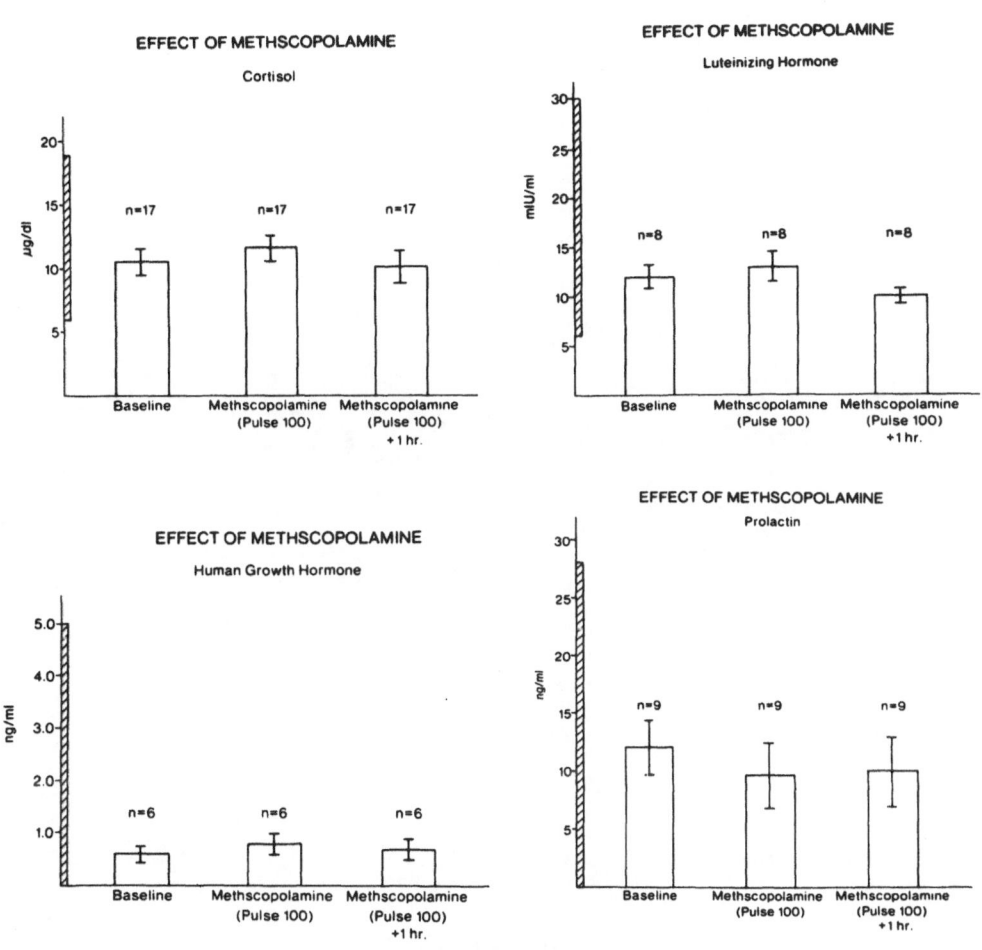

FIGURE 2

Effect of Methscopolamine

Data from those subjects receiving 1 mg physostigmine who did not become nauseated are presented in Figure 3. There was no significant difference between values obtained at the end of physostigmine or control infusions, nor between those levels and baseline.

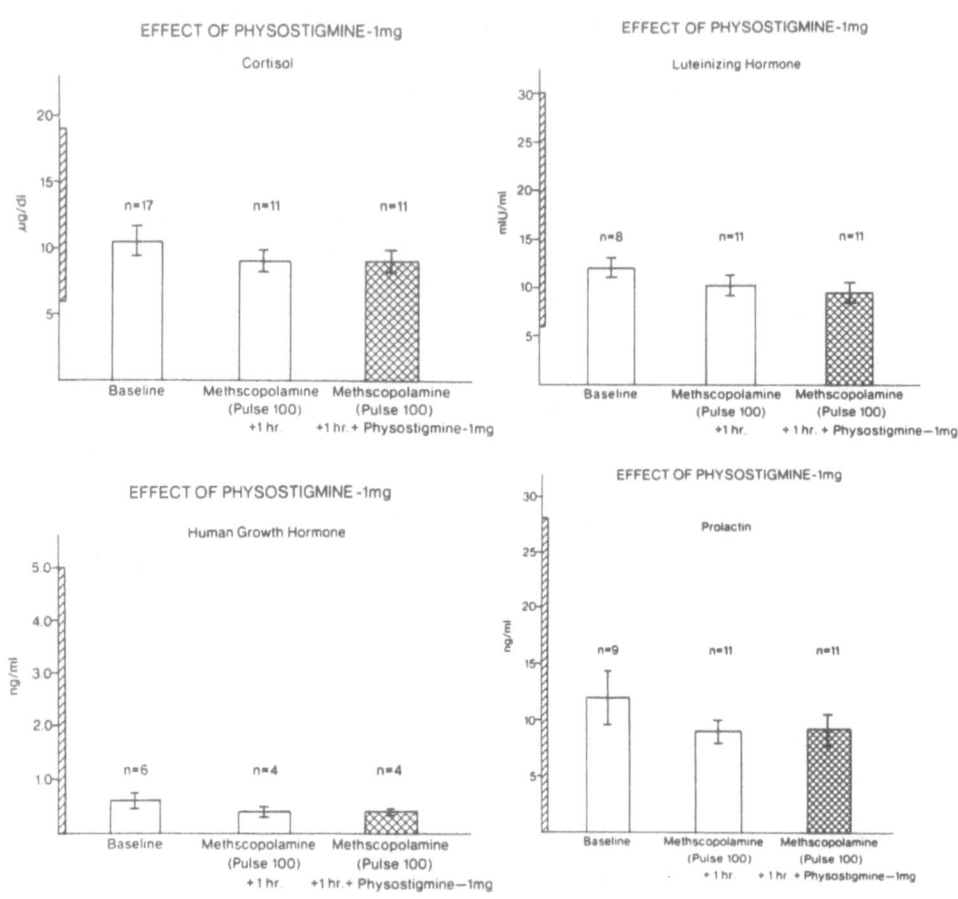

FIGURE 3

Effect of Physostigmine — 1 mg

A marked rise of cortisol, growth hormone and prolactin was seen in those patients with nausea or vomiting (Figure 4). This appeared to be an "all-or-none" response, as the degree of elevation appeared to be independent of the dose of physostigmine (Figure 5).

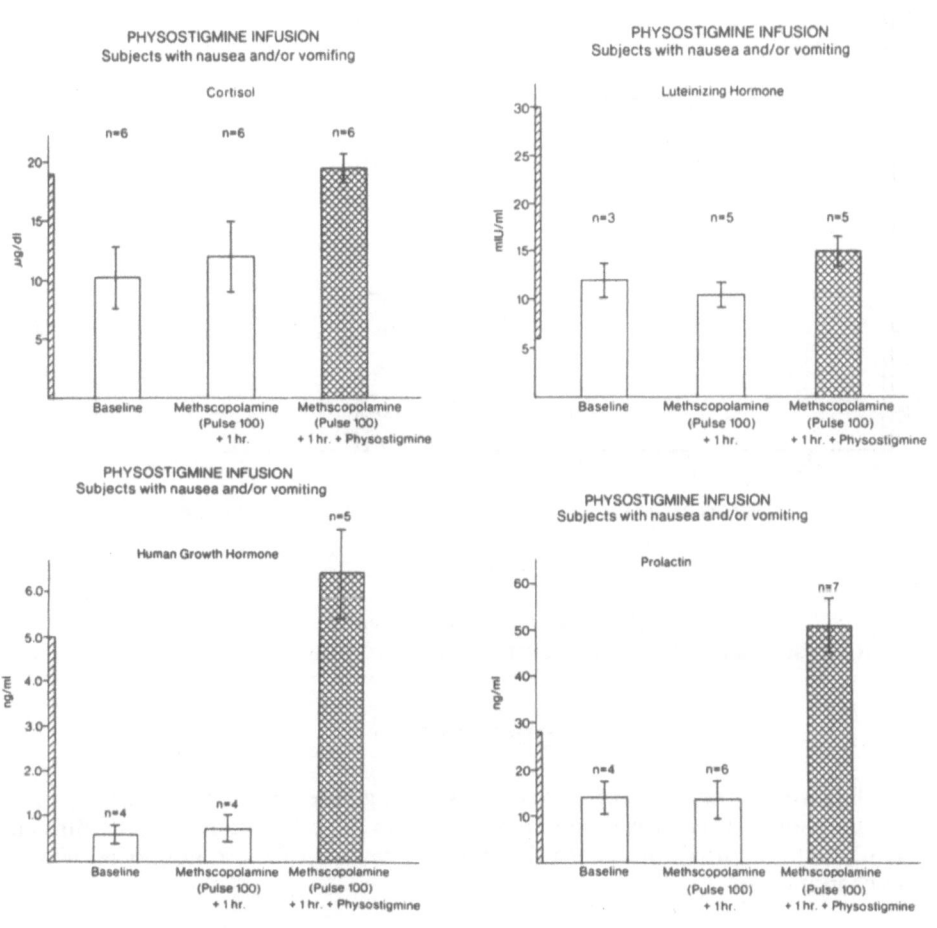

FIGURE 4

Physostigmine Infusion
Subjects with Nausea and/or Vomiting

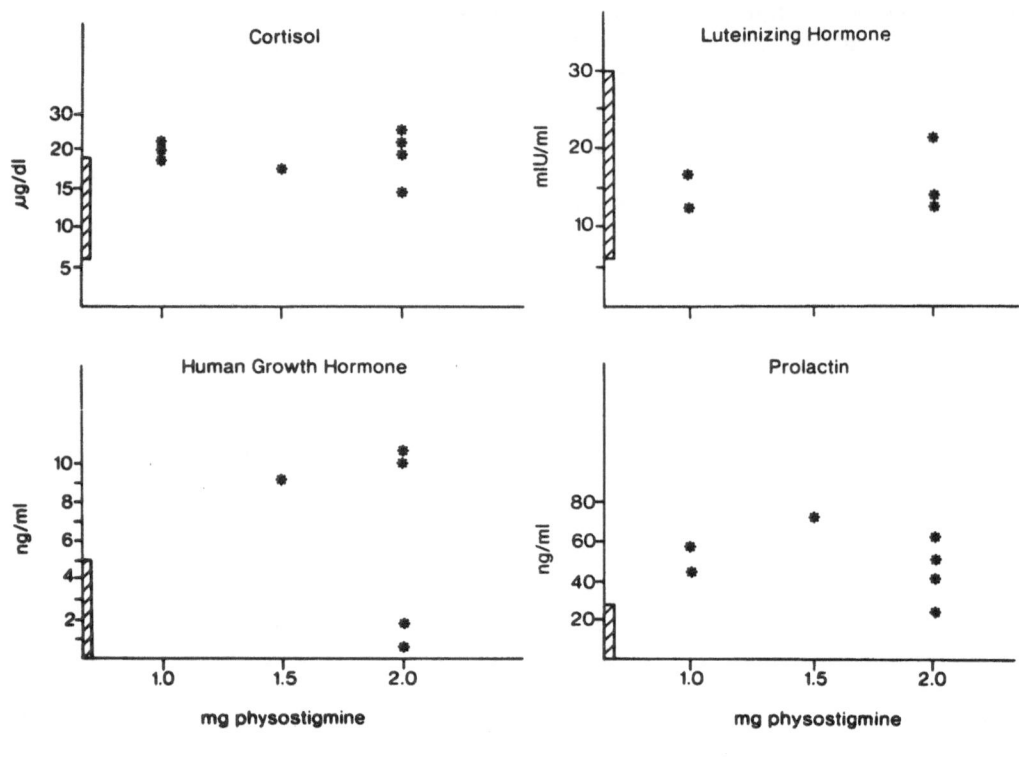

FIGURE 5

Lack of Effect of Physostigmine Dose
Post Physostigmine Hormone Levels in Subjects with Nausea and/or Vomiting

DISCUSSION

In this study, infusion of 1 mg of physostigmine produced no change in basal
levels of cortisol, LH, growth hormone or prolactin. The literature suggests that cholinergic manipulations should influence the levels of several of these hormones. Why, then,
were no changes seen?

The relative dose of physostigmine used here was much lower than in investigations
in animals. In a study of cortisol levels in dogs, a physostigmine dose (0.05 mg/kg) roughly
comparable to that used in these infusions, no changes were demonstrated (Harwood and
Mason, 1956). It would seem of interest to know the endocrine effects of a larger dose of
physostigmine in humans. However, all subjects receiving greater than 1 mg reported
nausea and some vomited. This situation was reflected by an endocrine stress response:
simultaneous elevations of cortisol, growth hormone and prolactin. Thus, it was not
possible to evaluate the influence of greater cholinergic agonist activity on basal individual
hormone secretion. The increases in growth hormone and prolactin seen here question
the specificity of studies in which only corticosteroids or ACTH were measured, and were

elevated by larger doses of cholinomimetics. No subject in this study demonstrated behavioral or endocrine evidence of stress on the control day. Yet a stress response was unavoidable in humans receiving larger doses of physostigmine and may account for parts of the data currently in the literature (see introduction). Parenthetically, these data do not rule out the possibility that physostigmine mediated or influenced the expression of the stress response.

It is not likely that the use of methscopolamine prior to physostigmine infusion accounted for the lack of change in hormone levels. Since methscopolamine does not cross the blood-brain barrier, its effect should be apparent only on the pituitary. *In vitro* studies, those involving hypothalamic lesions and drugs with peripheral and central actions, and releasing factor administration, indicate that the pituitary itself is not the site of action of cholinergic agonists or blocking agents (Cozanitis, 1974; Bradbury *et al.*, 1974; Libertun and McCann, 1974; Blake, 1974; Blake *et al.*, 1974; Suzuki *et al.*, 1975a; 1975b; McLean and Mikitovitch-Winer, 1975; Fiorindo and Martini, 1975; Grandison and Meites, 1976a).

A more specific analysis of the results must take into account the normal secretory patterns and control mechanisms of hormone secretion.

Animal studies indicate that cholinergic stimulation lowers prolactin. Our subjects were drug-free normals, predominantly male, whose prolactin levels were therefore at the low end of the physiologic range. Even if ACh is in part responsible for maintenance of these low levels, it may not have been possible to observe a further decrease. It will be of interest to investigate the effect of physostigmine on prolactin secretion in the various physiologic and pharmacologic states in which it is elevated.

The experimental conditions were more appropriate for evaluation of a possible stimulatory effect on LH secretion. The subjects were intact young normals with relatively low levels of gonadotropins, and hypothalamic-pituitary axes presumably capable of responding to appropriate stimulation. Yet no significant increase in LH was shown. If augmentation of gonadotropin secretion by cholinomimetics is to be demonstrated in the human, it may be necessary to begin with conditions of greater potential secretion, such as pre-ovulatory, castrated, or short-term estrogen primed individuals.

Basal secretion of growth hormone did not appear to be influenced by physostigmine. This does not rule out the possibility that other aspects of growth hormone secretion can be modified by cholinergic agents.

In summary, intravenous infusion of 1 mg of physostigmine in the morning into normal young subjects did not change basal levels of cortisol, LH, growth hormone or prolactin. It is not clear whether physostigmine influenced the induction of the stress response. The participation of cholinergic synapses in the other physiologic and pharmacologic states of anterior pituitary hormone secretion is not refuted by these data.

ACKNOWLEDGEMENTS

This research was supported by the National Institute of Mental Health Specialized Research Center Grant MH-30854, the Medical Research Service of the Veterans Administration, Nichols Institute for Endocrinology, and the Kate Pande Memorial Research Fund.

REFERENCES

Balfour, D.J.K., Khyllar, A.K., and Longden, A., 1975, Effects of nicotine on plasma corticosterone and brain amines in stressed and unstressed rats, *Pharmacol. Biochem. Behav. 3:*179.

Blake, C.A., 1974, Parallelism and divergence in luteinizing hormone and follicle-stimulating hormone release in nicotine-treated rats (37881), *Proc. Soc. Exp. Biol. Med. 145:*716.

Blake, C.A., and Sawyer, C.H., 1972, Nicotine blocks the suckling-induced rise in circulating prolactin in lactating rats, *Science 177:*619.

Blake, C.A., Scaramuzzi, R.J., Norman, R.L., Kanematsu, S., and Sawyer, C.H., 1972, Nicotine delays the ovulatory surge of luteinizing hormone in the rat (36922), *Proc. Soc. Exp. Biol. Med. 141:*1014.

Blake, C.A., Norman, R.L., Scaramuzzi, R.J., and Sawyer, C.H., 1973, Inhibition of the proestrous surge of prolactin in the rat by nicotine, *Endocrinology 92(5):*1334.

Blake, C.A., Norman, R.L., and Sawyer, C.H., 1974, Localization of the inhibitory actions of estrogen and nicotine on release of luteinizing hormone in rats, *Neuroendocrinology 16:*22.

Bradbury, M.W.B., Burden, J., Hillhouse, E.W., and Jones, M.T., 1974, Stimulation electrically and by acetylcholine of the rat hypothalamus *in vitro, J. Physiol. (Lond) 239:*269.

Burnett, G.R., Prange, A.J., Wilson, E.C., and Snyder, S.H., 1978, Neuroendocrine-drug relations in tardive dyskinesia. Abstract NR21 for the Annual Meeting of the American Psychiatric Association, Atlanta, Georgia.

Carroll, B.J., Curtis, G.C., and Mendels, I., 1976, Neuroendocrine regulation in depression. II. Discrimination in depressed from nondepressed patients, *Arch. Gen. Psychiatry 33(9):*1051.

Cozanitis, D.A., 1974, Galanthamine hydrobromide versus neostigmine, *Anesthesia 29:* 163.

Davis, K.L., Hollister, L.E., Berger, P.A., and Barchas, J.D., 1975, Cholinergic imbalance hypotheses of psychoses and movement disorders: Strategies for evaluation, *Psychopharmacol. Comm. 1(5):*533.

Davis, K.L., Berger, P.A., Hollister, L.E., and De Fraites, E.G., 1978, Physostigmine in mania, *Arch. Gen. Psychiatry 35(1):*119.

Donoso, A.O., and Bacha, J.C., 1975a, Role of the blood-brain barrier in the anticholinergic differential effects on LH and prolactin release in proestrous rats, *J. Neural. Transm. 37:*155.

Donoso, A.O., and Bacha, J.C., 1975b, Acetylcholine induced responses of plasma LH and prolactin in normal and 6-hydroxydopamine treated rats, *J. Neural. Transm. 37:* 269.

Edwardson, J.A., and Bennett, G.W., 1974, Modulation of corticotrophin-releasing factor release from hypothalamic synaptosomes, *Nature 251:*425.

Endroczi, E., Schreiberg, G., and Lissak, K., 1963, The role of central nervous activating and inhibitory structures in the control of pituitary-adrenocortical function. Effects of intracerebral cholinergic and adrenergic stimulation, *Acta Physiol. Acad. Hung. 24:* 211.

Ferrari, E., Bossolo, P.A., Vailati, A., Martinelli, I., Rea, A., and Nosari, I., 1977, Variations circadiennes des effets d'une substance vagolytique sur le systeme ACTH-secretant chez l'homme, *Ann. Endocrinol. (Paris) 38:*203.

Fiorindo, R.P., and Martini, L., 1975, Evidence for a cholinergic component in the neuro-endocrine control of luteinizing hormone (LH) secretion, *Neuroendocrinology 18:*322.

Grandison, L., and Meites, J., 1976a, Evidence for adrenergic mediation of cholinergic inhibition of prolactin release, *Endocrinology 99(3):*775.

Grandison, L., and Meites, J., 1976b, Inhibition of pseudopregnancy and stress induced by prolactin release in rats by pilocarpine, *Fed. Proc. 35:*306.

Grandison, L., Gelato, M., and Meites, J., 1974, Inhibition of prolactin secretion by cholinergic drugs (37988), *Proc. Soc. Biol. Med. 145:*1236.

Harwood, C.T., and Mason, I.W., 1956, Effects of intravenous infusion of autonomic agents in peripheral blood 17-hydroxycorticosteroid levels in the dog, *Am. J. Physiol. 186:*445.

Hedge, G.A., and de Wied, D., 1971, Corticotropin and vasopressin secretion after hypo-thalamic implantation of atropine, *Endocrinology 88:*1257.

Hedge, G.A., and Smelik, P.G., 1968, Corticotropin release: Inhibition by intrahypo-thalamic implantation of atropine, *Science 159:*891.

Hill, P., and Wynder, E.L., 1974, Smoking and cardiovascular disease, *Am. Heart J. 87(4):*491.

Hillhouse, E.W., Burden, J., and Jones, M.T., 1975, The effect of various putative neuro-transmitters on the release of corticotrophin releasing hormone from the hypothalamus of the rat *in vitro*. I. The effect of acetylcholine and noradrenaline, *Neuroendocrinology 17:*1.

Innes, I.R., and Nickerson, M., 1970, Drugs inhibiting the action of acetylcholine on structures innervated by postganglionic parasympathetic nerves (antimuscarinic or atropinic drugs), in *"The Pharmacological Basis of Therapeutics"* (L.S. Goodman and A. Gilman, eds.), pp. 528-548, MacMillan Company, New York.

Janowsky, D.S., El-Yousef, M.K., Davis, J.M., and Sekerke, H.J., 1972, A cholinergic adrenergic hypothesis of mania and depression, *Lancet 2:*632.

Janowsky, D.S., El-Yousef, J.K., and Davis, J.M., 1973, Parasympathetic suppression of manic symptoms by physostigmine, *Arch. Gen. Psychiatry 28:*542.

Justo, G., Motta, M., and Martin, L., 1975, *In vivo* effects of acetylcholine on LH secre-tion, *Experientia 31(5):*598.

Kanematsu, S., and Sawyer, C.H., 1973, Inhibition of the progesterone-advanced LH surge at proestrus by nicotine (37497), *Proc. Soc. Exp. Biol. Med. 143:*1183.

Kaplanski, J., and Smelik, P.G., 1973, Analysis of the inhibition of the ACTH release by hypothalamic implants of atropine, *Acta Endocrinol. (Kbh) 73:*651.

Kato, Y., Chihara, K., Ohgo, S., and Imura, H., 1974, Effect of nicotine on the secretion of growth hormone and prolactin in rats, *Neuroendocrinology 16:*237.

Krieger, D.T., and Krieger, H.P., 1967, Circadian pattern of plasma 17-hydroxycorti-costeroid. Alteration by anticholinergic agents, *Science 155:*1421.

Krieger, H.P., and Krieger, D.T., 1970, Chemical stimulation of the brain: Effect on adrenal corticoid release, *Am. J. Physiol. 218:*1632.

Krieger, D.T., Silverberg, A.I., Rizzo, F., and Krieger, H.P., 1968, Abolition of circadian periodicity of plasma 17-OHCS levels in the cat, *Am. J. Physiol. 215(4):*959.

Lawson, D.M., and Gala, R.R., 1975, The influence of adrenergic, dopaminergic, cholin-ergic and serotoninergic drugs on plasma prolactin levels in ovariectomized, estrogen-treated rats, *Endocrinology 96(1):*313.

Libertun, C., and McCann, S.M., 1973, Blockade of the release of gonadotropins and prolactin by subcutaneous or intraventricular injection of atropine in male and female rats, *Endocrinology 92(6):*1714.

Libertun, C., and McCann, S.M., 1974, Further evidence for cholinergic control of gonadotropin and prolactin secretion (38374), *Proc. Soc. Exp. Biol. Med. 147:*498.

Libertun, C., and McCann, S.M., 1976, Blockade of the postorchidectomy increase gonadotropins by implants ʻof atropine into the hypothalamus (39347), *Proc. Soc. Exp. Biol. Med. 152:*143.

Makara, G.B., and Stark, E., 1976, The effects of cholinomimetic drugs and atropine on ACTH release, *Neuroendocrinology 21:*31.

McLean, B.K., and Nikitovitch-Winer, M.B., 1975, Cholinergic control of the nocturnal prolactin surge in the pseudopregnant rat, *Endocrinology 97(4):*763.

Monti, J.M., Sala, M.A., Otegui, J.T., and Benedeth, W.L., 1970, Inhibition of ovarian compensatory hypertrophy by implants of atropine in the hypothalamus, *Experientia 26(11):*1263.

Naumenko, E.V., 1967, Role of adrenergic and cholinergic structures in the control of the pituitary-adrenal system, *Endocrinology 80:*69.

Naumenko, E.V., 1968, Hypothalamic chemoreactive structures and the regulation of pituitary-adrenal function. Effects of local injections of norepinephrine, carbachol and serotonin into the brain of guinea pigs with intact brains after mesencephalic transection, *Brain Res. 11:*1.

Otsuka, K., 1966, Effects of atropine, eserine and tetramethylammonium on the adrenal 17-hydroxycorticosteroid secretion in anesthetized dogs, *Tohoku J. Exp. Med. 88:* 165.

Porter, J.C., Goldman, B.D., and Wilber, J.F., 1970, Hypophysiotropic hormones in portal vessel blood, in *"Hypophysiotrophic Hormones of the Hypothalamus"* (J. Meites, ed.), pp. 282-293, Williams and Wilkins, Baltimore.

Sawyer, C.H., Markee, J.E., and Everett, J.W., 1951, Blockade of neurogenic stimulation of the rabbit adenohypophysis by banthine, *Am. J. Physiol. 166:*223.

Subramanian, M.G., and Gala, R.R., 1976, The influence of cholinergic, adrenergic, serotonergic drugs on the afternoon surge of plasma prolactin in ovariectomized, estrogen-treated rats, *Endocrinology 98(4):*842.

Suzuki, T., Hirai, K., Yoshio, H., Kurouji, K.I., and Hirose, T., 1964, Effect of eserine and atropine on adrenocortical hormone secretion in unanaesthetized dogs, *Endocrinology 31:*81.

Suzuki, T., Abe, K., and Hirose, T., 1975a, Adrenal cortical secretion in response to pilocarpine in dogs with hypothalamic lesions, *Neuroendocrinology 17:*75.

Suzuki, T., Hirose, T., Abe, K., and Matsumoto, I., 1975b, Dissociation of adrenocortical secretory responses to cyanide and pilocarpine in dogs with hypothalamic lesions, *Neuroendocrinology 19:*269.

Terkel, J., Blake, C.A., Hoover, V., and Sawyer, C.H., 1973, Pup survival and prolactin levels in nicotine-treated lactating rats (37485), *Proc. Soc. Exp. Biol. Med. 143:*1131.

BIOCHEMICAL AND PHARMACOLOGICAL ASPECTS OF CHOLINERGIC TREATMENT STRATEGIES

DIETARY CONTROL OF CENTRAL CHOLINERGIC ACTIVITY

R. J. Wurtman and J. H. Growdon*

Laboratory of Neuroendocrine Regulation, Department of
Nutrition and Food Science, Massachusetts Institute of
Technology, Cambridge, Massachusetts 02139

*Department of Neurology, Tufts University Medical School,
Boston, Massachusetts 02111

INTRODUCTION

This chapter describes the relationship between choline — administered as choline chloride or as phosphatidylcholine (lecithin), by injection or via the diet — and tissue acetylcholine (ACh) levels, and shows that choline administration, by raising blood and brain choline levels, can be a major determinant of the rate of ACh synthesis and, probably, of the amount of the neurotransmitter released when cholinergic neurons are depolarized.

It is surprising, to say the least, that the availability of a circulating precursor should have any effect whatsoever on the synthesis of a ubiquitous neurotransmitter. We may speculate as to why the evolutionary process "allowed" the formation of ACh to be "open-loop," and not simply coupled to the maintenance of those ACh levels needed to sustain cholinergic neurotransmission. At the present time, we are not aware of any really compelling hypothesis which might explain this precursor dependence; however, it is possible that cholinergic neurons, like those which release serotonin (a transmitter whose rate of synthesis varies with plasma amino acid levels [Fernstrom and Wurtman, 1972, 1974; Wurtman and Fernstrom, 1976]), may function as "sensors" that inform other brain neurons about the general metabolic state of the organism, as reflected in its plasma choline concentrations. The particular physiological circumstances which cholinergic neurons might "sense" remain to be characterized. Even though we are unable to explain why cholinergic neurons should be "open-loop," we can, just the same, take advantage of this precursor dependence in order to modify their functional activities, and thereby explore the physiological consequences of enhanced cholinergic tone, and treat disease states associated with inadequate release of ACh into synapses.

ACETYLCHOLINE AS A TYPE I NEUROTRANSMITTER

At the present time, perhaps twenty to thirty compounds are thought to function as neurotransmitters within synapses of the mammalian central nervous system. These

461

compounds fall into three main classes, based on the mechanisms that control their synthesis (Table 1) (Wurtman and Scally, 1977).

TABLE 1

Classification of Neurotransmitters by Mode of Synthesis

TYPE I: Synthesized by *enzymes* from a *circulating precursor* which the brain cannot make.

Transmitter	Precursor	Enzyme
Acetylcholine (ACh)	Choline	Choline Acetyltransferase (CAT)
Dopamine, Nor-epinephrine	Tyrosine	Tyrosine Hydroxylase (TH)
Serotonin (5HT)	Tryptophan	Tryptophan Hydroxylase
Histamine	Histidine	Histidine Decarboxylase

TYPE II: Synthesized by *polyribosomes* (i.e., *peptides*).

Type IIa: Polysomal synthesis generates the active transmitter.

Type IIb: Compound synthesized on the polysome is subsequently activated by *enzymes* (for example, by cleavage of a "propeptide," amidation, ring closure [to form pyroglutamate]).

TYPE III: Non-essential amino acids.

Type IIIa: Synthesis catalyzed by an *enzyme* specifically localized within the neurons that make that transmitter (for example, glutamic acid decarboxylase for GABA; serine hydroxymethyl transferase for glycine).

Type IIIb: Synthesis may not involve a neuron-specific enzyme (aspartate and glutamate).

The first group (Type I) includes all of the best-characterized transmitters: water-soluble amines of low molecular weight, carrying an ionic charge at physiological pH, that are synthesized by enzymes from specific precursors that the brain cannot make, but must obtain from the circulation. These precursors — tyrosine (or phenylalanine), tryptophan, choline, histidine — have little or no intrinsic activity at synapses; rather, metabolic transformations catalyzed by one or more neuronal enzymes are required to convert them to the transmitters that are recognized by synaptic receptors. In some cases (e.g., tryptophan), the diet is the sole source of the circulating precursor; in others (e.g., tyrosine, choline), the precursor may be derived either from dietary sources or form hepatic synthesis.

The Type II neurotransmitters include the peptides. The initial steps in the synthesis of these compounds are probably mediated not by enzymes but by polyribosomes. The precursors of the peptides are amino acids, some of which must be obtained from the circulation (e.g., tryptophan, the branched-chain amino acids) and some of which can be made by neurons from glucose or other metabolic substrates. The peptide moiety that acts on synaptic receptors might be the same compound as that produced on the poly-ribosomes (Type IIa). Alternatively, its activation might require one or more enzymes that, for example, cleave it from a "propeptide," couple it to a non-peptide constituent (perhaps analogous to the glyco-moiety that forms a part of the pituitary hormones FSH, LH, and TSH), amidate a terminal carboxyl group, or convert a terminal glutamate to pyroglutamate (Type IIb).

The Type III compounds include three non-essential amino acids (glutamate, aspartate, glycine) and gamma aminobutyrate (GABA), which is formed from a non-essential amino acid (glutamate). Neurons synthesize these neurotransmitters at rates that are largely independent of plasma levels of their precursors. Some of these com-pounds (Type IIIa) are synthesized by specific enzymes that are highly localized within the neurons containing the particular transmitter (glutamic acid decarboxylase for GABA; serine hydroxymethyltransferase for glycine). Too little is now known about the synthesis of the particular glutamate or aspartate molecules that function as neurotransmitters to allow any conclusions as to the specificity of the enzymatic pathways responsible for their production; hence, they are, for the present, categorized in another subgroup (Type IIIb).

While the above grouping must be regarded as highly tentative, it may be of value in predicting the behaviors of synapses that utilize transmitters from a particular group. For example, Type I transmitters should be expected to be influenced by plasma amino acid levels (and, consequently, by the diet or by hormones affecting amino acid metabo-lism), while Type II neurotransmitters should not. In order to show that amino acid availability materially affects the synthesis of brain peptides, it would be necessary to show that processes that modify brain amino acid uptake (e.g., food consumption; time of day; amino acid administration) cause parallel changes in (a) the saturation (or charging) of the tRNA's to which the amino acids must bind prior to their incorpo-ration into peptide chains, and (b) the proportion of the cell's ribosomal RNA that is aggregated with strands of messenger RNA to form the polyribosomes (or polysomes), which actually carry out the synthesis of the peptides. Neither relationship probably occurs *in vivo* except under grossly abnormal conditions (e.g., in immature rats given 1 g/kg of phenylalanine [Aoki and Siegel, 1970]).

It is likely that the synthesis of Type III transmitters also proceeds at rates that are independent of food consumption. Even though the brain's uptake of glucose, their major precursor, does seem to vary with plasma glucose concentrations, the utilization of glucose by the brain apparently does not (Pardridge and Oldendorf, 1977); moreover, plasma glucose concentrations tend to be well buffered, and to change relatively little after food consumption.

CONTROL OF THE SYNTHESIS OF TYPE I TRANSMITTERS
BY PRECURSOR AVAILABILITY

Five types of evidence are needed in order to prove that the concentration of a neurotransmitter's precursor in the plasma normally influences the rate at which the transmitter is synthesized in brain neurons. It must be shown that:

1. The level of the precursor in the blood (or, in the case of tryptophan or tyrosine, its concentration relative to the concentrations of other blood constituents that compete with it for uptake into the brain [Fernstrom and Wurtman, 1972; Gibson and Wurtman, 1977]) normally fluctuates. This may occur, for example, in response to eating particular foods, or to fasting.

2. The brain cannot synthesize the precursor from glucose, monocarboxylic acids, or other amino acids, and thus is totally dependent on the blood stream for its supply of the precursor. (There is some evidence that tyrosine hydroxylase in brain neurons can convert phenylalanine to L-DOPA [Ikeda *et al.*, 1965]); in that case, phenylalanine, and not tyrosine, becomes the "essential" circulating precursor. Similarly, brain tissue may be able to liberate free choline from lecithin (Freeman and Jenden, 1976), just as it can liberate tryptophan, tyrosine and other amino acids by breaking down its own proteins. If the choline thus formed is capable of reutilization for neurotransmitter synthesis, and if circulating lecithin is actively transported into the brain, then both this compound and choline itself may serve as circulating precursors for brain ACh.

3. The rate at which the precursor is taken up into the brain changes as a function of its plasma concentration, or the ratio of that concentration to the effective net concentration of its competitors; that is, the blood-brain-barrier uptake mechanism for that precursor located within the endothelial cells of cerebral capillaries (Pardridge, 1977) is unsaturated when the precursor's plasma concentration is within its normal range. Moreover, this uptake mechanism must specifically determine the precursor's concentration within those particular neurons that convert it to the neurotransmitter.

4. The enzyme that limits the rate at which the precursor is transformed to the synaptically-active transmitter also is unsaturated when the precursor's brain concentration is within its normal range (i.e., the true *in vivo* K_m of the enzyme for the precursor-substrate is near to, or greater than, the precursor's *in vivo* concentration). As a corollary, substrate concentrations measured in homogenates of whole brain are equal to, or at least proportionate to, the concentrations present in the vicinity of the neurotransmitter-forming enzymes. This is shown by observations that the rates at which tryptophan (Carlsson *et al.*, 1972; Colmenares *et al.*, 1975) and tyrosine (Gibson and Wurtman, 1977) are hydroxylated within those few brain cells that can convert them to serotonin (5HT) and the catecholamines are proportional to whole-brain tryptophan and tyrosine levels.

5. The enzyme that controls the synthesis of the transmitter should not be encumbered by a feedback loop that decreases its activity after transmitter levels have been increased (e.g., after administration of the precursor), nor should its activity be more limited by the concentration of some scarce cofactor than by concentrations of the substrate itself. Apparently, no such feedback loops operate within cholinergic or sero-

toninergic neurons; hence, the rates at which these neurons synthesize ACh or 5HT can — and do — vary in proportion to plasma choline or amino acid concentrations. End-product inhibition of tyrosine hydroxylase, the catecholamine-synthesizing enzyme, is demonstrable after catecholamine levels have been raised pharmacologically; however, it is not certain that this mechanism also operates in normal, drug-free animals. Moreover, whether or not tyrosine hydroxylase happens to be in its active or inactive form influences the extent to which neurotransmitter synthesis in catecholaminergic neurons is limited by precursor availability. Treatments that accelerate the firing rate of the neurons activate the enzyme, thus enhancing its relatively poor affinity for its tetrahydrobiopterin cofactor, and amplifying its dependence on tyrosine levels (Scally and Wurtman, 1977).

CHOLINE AND THE BIOSYNTHESIS OF ACETYLCHOLINE

The following discussion summarizes the evidence currently available that plasma choline levels — which normally reflect the consumption of the compound — can control the synthesis of ACh in brain neurons.

The synthesis of ACh, a Type I neurotransmitter, from choline and acetyl-coenzyme A (acetyl-CoA) is catalyzed by the enzyme choline acetyltransferase (CAT) (Figure 1). Although a few reports suggest that the brain can synthesize choline (Kewitz and Pleul, 1976), most investigators agree that, unlike the liver, the brain cannot carry out the stepwise methylation of enthanolamine (Ansell and Spanner, 1967; Bremer and Greenberg, 1961), and thus cannot form choline *de novo*. (The choline that appears, in some experiments, to be formed by the brain probably represents material liberated by the hydrolysis of lecithins present in cell membranes or provided by the circulation [Browning and Schulman, 1968]). The major immediate source of brain choline is thus "free" choline, taken up from the bloodstream at the blood-brain barrier (Pardridge and Oldendorf, 1977).

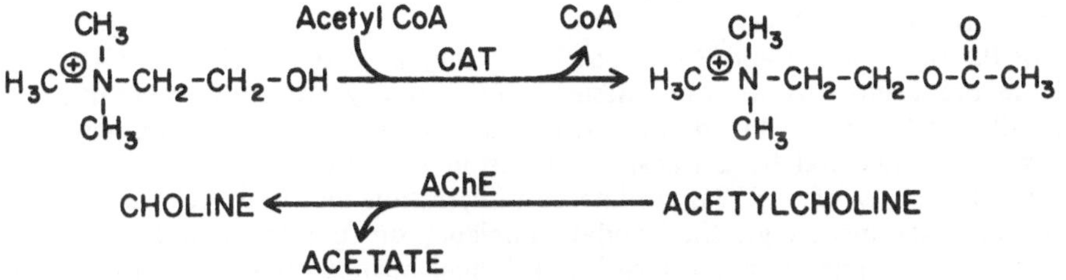

FIGURE 1

Acetylcholine (ACh) biosynthesis: the enzyme choline acetyltransferase (CAT) catalyzes the acetylation of choline, using acetyl-CoA as the acetate donor.

Choline levels in serum and plasma do vary widely, depending on the quantities of choline and lecithin consumed in the diet; this relationship has been demonstrated both in human samples (Growdon *et al.*, 1977a; Wurtman *et al.*, 1977) and in samples from rats (Cohen and Wurtman, 1976) (Figure 2). The transport of choline into the intact brain is mediated by a low-affinity system similar to that described for the neutral amino acids

(Pardridge, 1977; Pardridge and Oldendorf, 1977). Deanol (dimethylaminoethanol), a synthetic choline analog, acts competitively at this locus (Millington *et al.*, unpublished observations), as may circulating polyamines. A high-affinity choline uptake system (K_m = 1.5 μM) has also been observed in synaptosomes prepared from cholinergic nerve terminals (Haga and Noda, 1973; Yamamura and Snyder, 1973); this carrier is sodium-dependent, and is blocked by hemicholinium and related drugs. The high-affinity system may affect the distribution of choline within the brain by preferentially shunting it to loci of ACh synthesis (Figure 3); it also may serve to allow neurons to reutilize choline formed from the hydrolysis of ACh released into synapses.

The K_m of the system that transports choline into the intact brain is 0.22 mM (Pardridge and Oldendorf, 1977). Since plasma choline levels normally fall below this concentration (Cohen and Wurtman, 1976; Schuberth and Jenden, 1975), the uptake system is highly unsaturated; hence, any significant variation in plasma choline levels should generate corresponding changes in brain choline uptake, and ultimately, in brain choline levels. This has been shown to be the case: brain choline levels normally bear a linear relationship to plasma choline concentrations throughout their dynamic range (Cohen and Wurtman, 1976).

The K_m's of CAT for choline (0.4 mM) and acetyl-CoA (18 μM) are both well above the normal brain concentrations of these substances (30-50 μM and 7-11 μM, respectively). Therefore, changes in the brain levels of either of the precursors for ACh might be expected to modify the rate at which the neurotransmitter is synthesized. Several years ago, Cohen and Wurtman began to examine the effects on ACh synthesis of treatments that changed plasma choline levels. Our interest in exploring the relationship between the choline precursor and its neurotransmitter product arose from prior studies on 5HT synthesis (Fernstrom and Wurtman, 1974), that had demonstrated that brain 5HT levels vary inversely with the protein content of each meal (which changes the extent to which the 5HT-forming enzyme, tryptophan hydroxylase, is saturated with its amino acid precursor [Figure 4]). We soon found that the administration of choline by injection (Cohen and Wurtman, 1975), stomach tube (Hirsch *et al.*, 1977; Ulus *et al.*, 1977a) or the diet (Cohen and Wurtman, 1976) increased the levels of choline, and then of ACh, in brain and various other tissues. Concurrently and independently, Haubrich and his collaborators (1974) were drawing similar conclusions from experiments in which choline was administered by intracarotid infusion or intraventricular injection. In our laboratory (Hirsch *et al.*, 1977), choline administration elevated ACh levels within all brain regions examined, e.g., the caudate nucleus, the cortex, and the hippocampus (which contains cholinergic nerve terminals). It had been shown some years earlier that when weanling rats consumed a choline-free diet for five days, brain ACh levels decreased by 35% (Nagler *et al.*, 1968). We observed that when adult rats consumed 0, 20, or 129 mg of choline/day for 11 days (Cohen and Wurtman, 1976), or even for 3 days, dose-related differences were generated in caudate ACh levels. Since the predominant source of choline in the diet normally is phosphatidylcholine (lecithin), we compared the effect of consuming a given amount of choline as the chloride salt or as lecithin on plasma choline and neuronal ACh levels. Choline ingested as lecithin was far more effective than choline chloride in elevating plasma choline levels in humans (Wurtman *et al.*, 1977) (Figure 5), and brain and adrenal ACh levels in rats (Hirsch and Wurtman, unpublished observations) (Table 2).

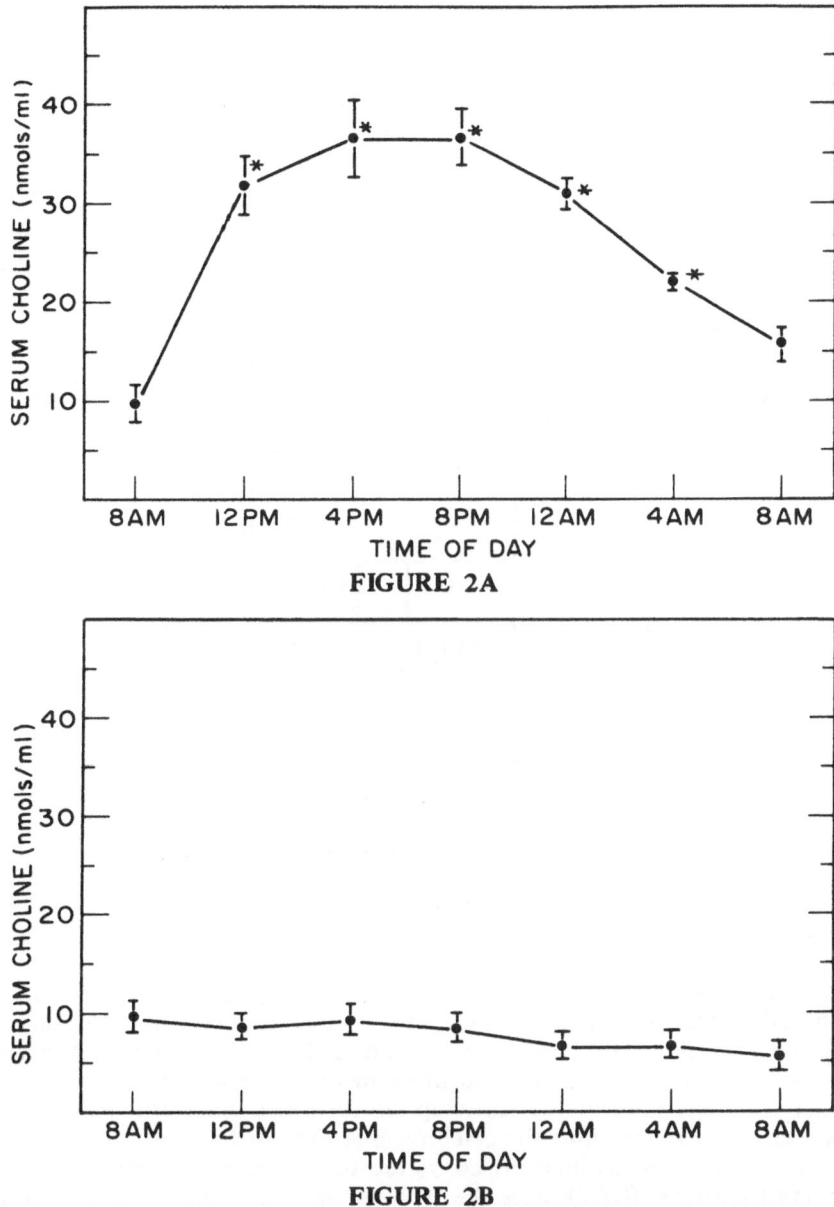

FIGURE 2A

FIGURE 2B

Serum choline levels during consumption of a high choline (A) and a low choline (B) diet by 6 normal human subjects for 2 days. The high choline diet provided 5 g choline (largely as lecithin)/day, or about 67 mg/kg; the low choline diet contained 50 mg/day, or about 0.67 mg/kg. Meals were eaten starting at 8:30 a.m., 12 noon, and 5:00 p.m. Blood samples were obtained at 8:00 a.m. on the second day, and at 4 hr intervals thereafter for 24 hr. Each point represents the mean ± S.D. Data were analyzed by 2-way ANOVA and paired t-test. *P < .01. (Reproduced with permission from Hirsch, M.J., Growdon, J.H., and Wurtman, R.J., (in press), Relations between dietary choline or lecithin intake, serum choline levels, and various metabolic indices, *Metabolism*).

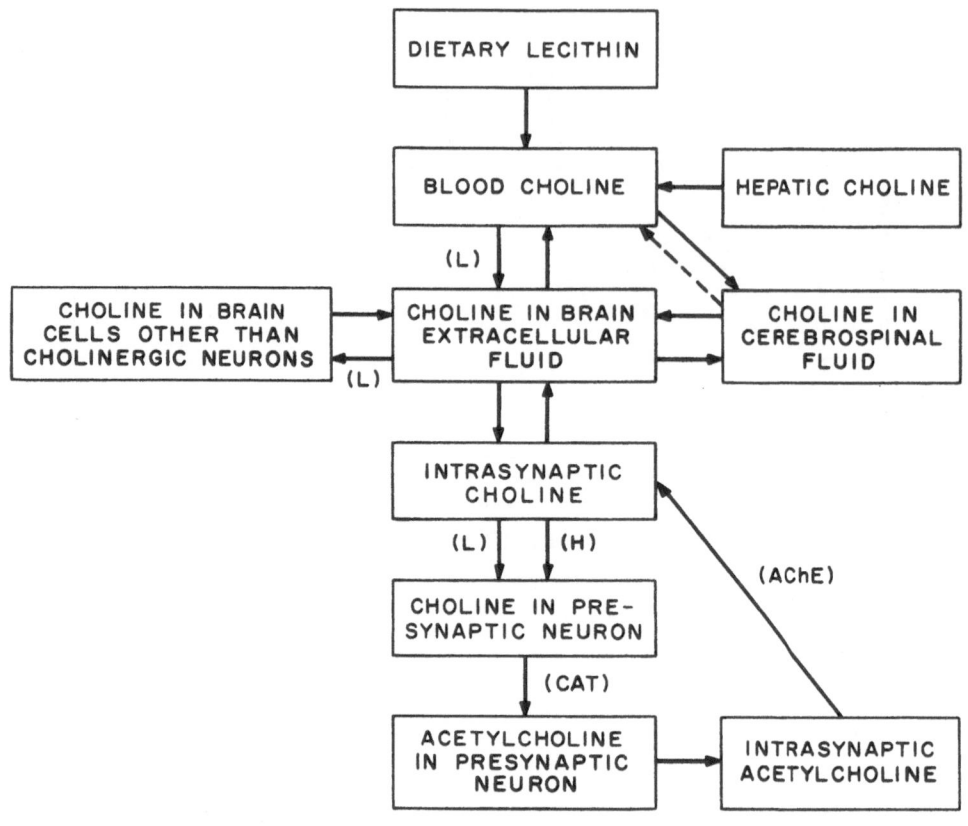

FIGURE 3

Model illustrating sources of choline for brain acetylcholine synthesis. Choline enters the blood either from dietary sources (primarily lecithin) or hepatic synthesis. It is transported into the brain's extracellular fluid by a low-affinity transport system (L) localized within the capillary endothelium of the blood-brain barrier. It then can be (1) taken up within terminals of cholinergic neurons. This might be mediated by a high-affinity (H) or a low-affinity (L) transport system; (2) taken up within other brain cells by a low-affinity mechanism (L); or (3) pass into the cerebrospinal fluid or back into the blood stream. The choline within nerve terminals is converted to acetylcholine through the action of choline acetyltransferase (CAT); once the transmitter is released into the synaptic cleft, it is hydrolyzed to choline by the enzyme acetylcholinesterase (AChE), after which the choline may again enter the presynaptic neuron via the high-affinity uptake system. Moreover, a part of the choline taken up within cholinergic terminals may be utilized for functions other than acetylcholine synthesis (e.g., production of lecithin for incorporation into membranes).

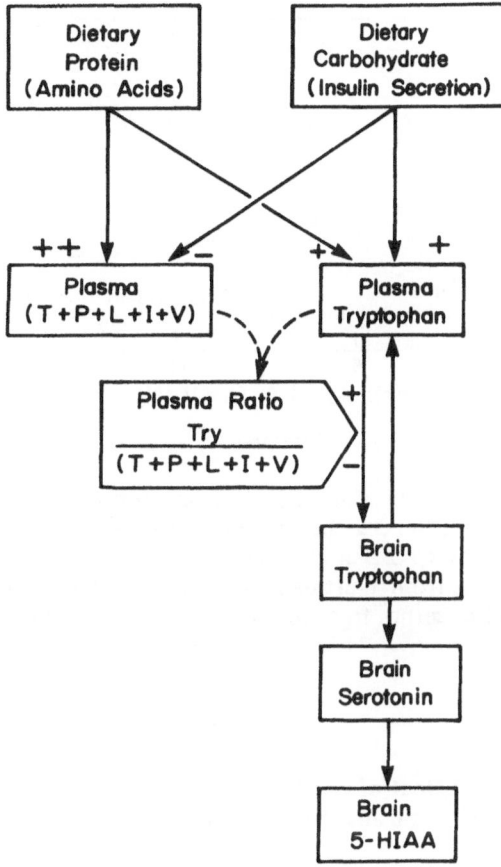

FIGURE 4

Proposed model describing diet-induced changes in brain serotonin (5HT) levels in rats. Consumption of a meal containing carbohydrate but lacking protein (upper right box) elicits insulin secretion, causing major depressions in the plasma concentrations of tyrosine (T), phenylalanine (P), leucine (L), isoleucine (I), and valine (V) — all neutral amino acids which compete with tryptophan for uptake into the brain — without lowering plasma tryptophan levels. Hence, the ratio of tryptophan to its competitors rises, causing more tryptophan to enter the brain, thereby enhancing the substrate saturation of tryptophan hydroxylase, accelerating 5HT synthesis, and ultimately raising the brain levels of 5HT and its principal metabolite, 5-hydroxyindoleacetic acid (5-HIAA). If the meal contains large amounts of protein (upper left box), the direct contribution of this protein to plasma neutral amino acid levels has the opposite effect on the tryptophan: competitor ratio, because tryptophan is scarce in all natural proteins while its competitors are abundant. Thus, 5HT-containing neurons, by coupling transmitter synthesis to the tryptophan: competitor ratio, are able to "sense" the protein content of each meal. (Reprinted with permission from Fernstrom, J.D., and Wurtman, R.J., 1972, Brain serotonin content: physiological regulation by plasma amino acids, *Science 178*:414).

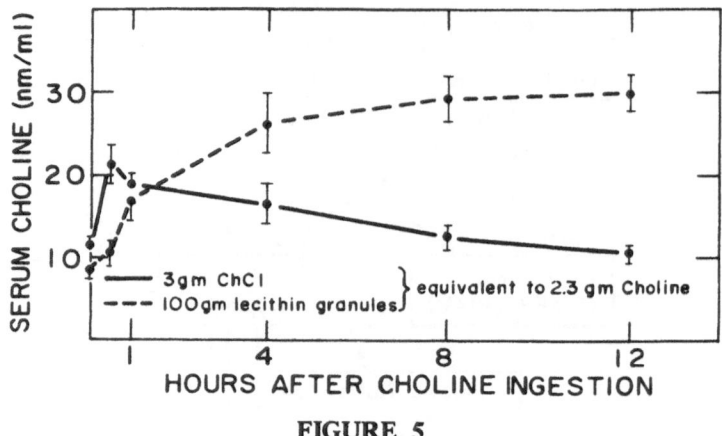

Effects of consuming choline chloride or lecithin on serum choline concentrations. Ten healthy subjects consumed either 3 g choline chloride or 100 g lecithin granules in a single meal; both were equivalent to 2.3 g choline. Subjects fasted for the following 12 hr. (Reprinted with permission from Wurtman, R.J., Hirsch, M.J., and Growdon, J.H., 1977, Lecithin consumption raises serum free choline levels, *Lancet* 2:68).

TABLE 2

**Effect of Lecithin Consumption on
Brain Choline and Acetylcholine Levels in the Rat**

Hours After Food Presented	Choline		Acetylcholine	n
	Blood nmole/ml	Brain nmole/g	Brain nmole/g	
0	12.4 ± 0.8	35.2 ± 2.3	19.6 ± 0.8	13
10	35.5 ± 2.5*	53.9 ± 5.6**	24.7 ± 1.1*	13

Adult rats were fasted overnight and then allowed access for 2 hr to a diet containing 50% lecithin granules. Each rat consumed an amount of lecithin equivalent to about 0.28 g/kg choline base.

*$P < .001$ compared with 0 hr controls
**$P < .01$ compared with 0 hr controls

(Hirsch, M.J., and Wurtman, R.J., unpublished data)

The finding that choline administration rapidly elevates neuronal ACh levels provided us with an opportunity to determine whether or not the activity of CAT is subject to significant feedback regulation *in vivo*. Previous studies by Kaita and Goldberg (1969) showed that ACh failed to inhibit CAT significantly, except at very high concentrations, which were probably unattainable *in vivo*. We reasoned that if feedback control exists at all, it would operate either allosterically, by end-product inhibition of CAT in the presence of elevated ACh concentrations, or, over a longer interval, by slowing the synthesis (or accelerating the degradation) of the enzyme protein. Neither mode of control could be demonstrated; enzyme activity was not depressed acutely in the presence of high ACh levels (i.e., in tissues from animals pretreated with choline), nor did it decline among rats given repeated doses of choline sufficient to cause prolonged elevations in ACh levels (Hirsch and Wurtman, unpublished observations) (Table 3). This lack of feedback control makes us optimistic that choline administration will retain its clinical utility (Growdon et al., 1977b) in those patients capable of responding, even after repeated use.

TABLE 3

Effect of Choline Administration on
Choline Acetyltransferase (CAT) Activity in the Rat Caudate Nucleus

Hours After Choline	CAT Activity	Choline Level	Acetylcholine Level
8	127 ± 5*	332 ± 20*	148 ± 12*
24	128 ± 6*	118 ± 10	85 ± 7
48	100 ± 6	108 ± 7	92 ± 5

Rats were killed at the intervals listed after receiving choline chloride (2.8 g/kg) by stomach tube. Each experimental group contained 8-12 animals. Data are given as percents of control. Control CAT activity was 7.2 ± 2.7 nmole ACh formed per hr per mg tissue; control caudate choline and ACh contents were 42.4 ± 13.9 and 27.9 ± 9.3 nmole/g, respectively.

*$P < .001$ differs from control values

(Hirsch, M.J., and Wurtman, R.J., unpublished observations)

In order to determine whether increased tissue ACh levels induced by choline administration result from increased *de novo* synthesis, we gave rats an acetylcholinesterase (AChE) inhibitor, physostigmine, in conjunction with choline. The resulting increase in brain ACh was equal to the sum of the effects of either agent alone, a finding compatible with the hypothesis that choline acts by affecting ACh synthesis and not by slowing its degradation (Cohen and Wurtman, 1976). The presence of very high choline levels, or of a high choline-ACh ratio, may also inhibit AChE activity; the K_i for choline's inhibition of AChE is 1.2 mM. However, AChE is present in the brain in such excess that only major inhibition of this enzyme would be expected to have any effect on ACh hydrolysis *in vivo*.

CHOLINE AND CHOLINERGIC FUNCTION

The increase in neuronal ACh levels caused by choline administration to animals might lead to increased ACh release; on the other hand, increased levels don't necessarily change the quantities of the transmitter released into synapses following each nerve impulse, or per unit time. It was equally possible, for example, that the choline-induced increase occurred within a metabolic "pool," or compartment, which was not accessible for release. In such a situation, the number of ACh molecules liberated following each neuronal depolarization could be relatively constant, from animal to animal and time to time, and independent of presynaptic ACh levels. To examine the relationship between precursor-induced increases in ACh levels and the amounts of the transmitter released into synapses, we have utilized indirect experimental approaches, which involve measuring biochemical changes in cells that are postsynaptic to the cholinergic neurons.* Two such cells are the dopaminergic neurons that terminate in the caudate nucleus and the chromaffin cells of the adrenal medulla (Figure 6). Both contain the enzyme tyrosine hydroxylase (TH), and presumably lack the enzyme CAT, which is needed to acetylate choline. Tyrosine hydroxylase in the caudate nucleus is known to undergo a rapid and short-lived activation when the neuron containing it is depolarized (Murrin *et al.*, 1976); the enzyme in chromaffin cells apparently does not exhibit short-term activation, but is induced 24-48 hr after the cells are subjected to prolonged cholinergic stimulation (Thoenen, 1974).

Choline administration (60 mg/kg, i.p.) increased striatal TH activity by approximately 25% within 2 hr of injection; this effect was dose-related, and was blocked by pretreatment with atropine, a cholinergic muscarinic antagonist (Table 4) (Ulus and Wurtman, 1976). Choline administration also caused a parallel acceleration in the accumulation of L-DOPA, the product of this enzyme, in animals treated with an inhibitor of dopa decarboxylase.

When a large dose of choline (20 mmoles/kg) was given to animals by stomach tube, the levels of choline and ACh in the adrenal medulla rose markedly (Ulus *et al.*, 1977a); ACh levels returned to normal 16 hr after intubation. Tyrosine hydroxylase activity did not change significantly for the initial 12 to 16 hr, but increased by about 30% 24 hr after intubation. When this dose of choline was administered daily by stomach tube for 4 days, adrenal TH activity increased by 50% (Ulus *et al.*, 1977a). This increase was not simply a nonspecific response to stress, since it did not occur in animals intubated with saline or ammonium chloride; it was blocked by pretreatment with cycloheximide, an inhibitor of protein synthesis, or by prior adrenal denervation (Figure 7) (Ulus *et al.*, 1977a). Choline administration similarly elevated urinary epinephrine levels in intact

---

*This approach denies the investigator the opportunity to make direct, quantitative estimates of the numbers of molecules released; however, the information it provides may be even more likely to reflect physiological changes than methods based on assaying directly the ACh liberated into a test medium. The phenomena it records — biochemical changes in post-synaptic cells — require three sets of events in order to occur: (1) release of more transmitter molecules; (2) occupancy by the transmitter of additional cholinergic receptors on post-synaptic cells; (3) biochemical responses to this enhanced receptor occupancy on the part of the post-synaptic cell. In the absence of any of these events (for example, if there are no unoccupied receptors to combine with the transmitter), post-synaptic responses to choline will not occur.

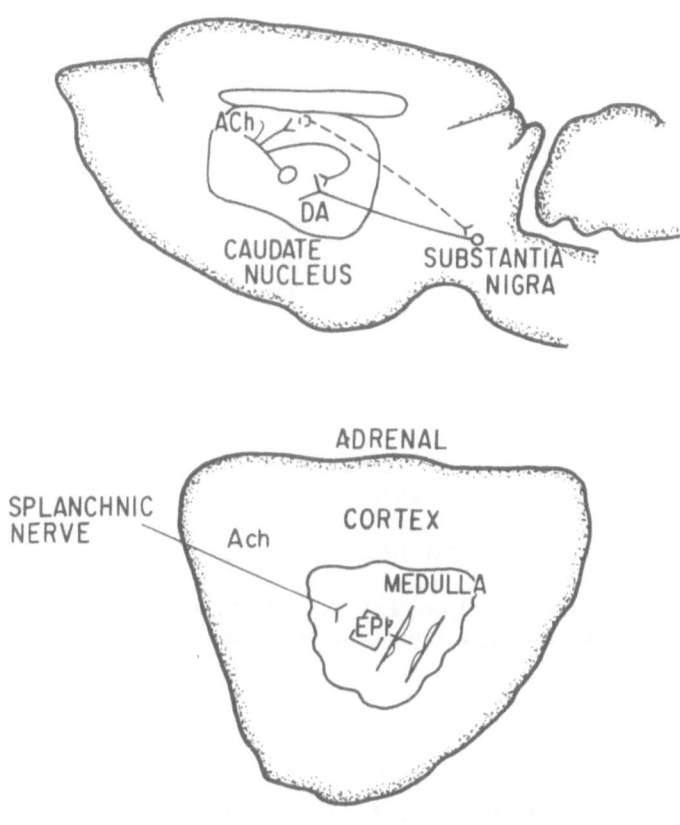

FIGURE 6

Preparations used in experiments to examine the effects of choline administration on TH activity in post-synaptic cells. The top diagram shows dopaminergic neurons running from the substantia nigra to the caudate nucleus (which contains the TH activated following choline administration), where their axons make inhibitory synapses with cholinergic neurons. These latter neurons take up exogenous choline and convert it to ACh. The transmitter may be released directly onto the terminals of the dopaminergic neurons, via axo-axonal synapses; alternatively (dotted line), its effect on the nigro-neostriatal neurona may be mediated by a multisynaptic pathway. The bottom diagram shows the adrenal cortex and medulla, which is innervated by a cholinergic nerve, the splanchnic nerve. Choline administration causes the terminals of this nerve to synthesize, and probably to release, more ACh; the transmitter then causes the medullary chromaffin cells to a) release epinephrine into the circulation, and b) produce more TH — this process becomes apparent after 24 hr.

TABLE 4

Effect of Atropine on the Choline-Induced Increase
in Striatal Tyrosine Hydroxylase (TH) Activity

Treatment	TH Activity (nmole/hr/mg)	(nmole/hr/mg)
Control	2.23 ± 0.09	(8)
Choline Chloride	2.68 ± 0.10*	(9)
Atropine Sulfate	2.29 ± 0.08	(8)
Atropine Sulfate and Choline Chloride	2.36 ± 0.05	(7)

Animals received choline chloride (60 mg/kg) and atropine sulfate (40 mg/kg) intraperitoneally 2 hr before they were killed. Values are expressed as mean ± S.E.M. The number of samples is indicated in parentheses. Data were analyzed by analysis of variance.

(P < .05 differs from control groups or from atropine-treated groups.

(Reprinted with permission from Ulus, I.H., and Wurtman, R.J., 1976, Choline administration: activation of tyrosine hydroxylase in dopaminergic neurons of rat brain, *Science* *194:*1060.

animals (Figure 8), but not in rats subjected previously to bilateral adrenal denervation (Scally, Ulus, and Wurtman, unpublished observations). These observations are all compatible with the view that choline is taken up within the presynaptic terminals of cholinergic neurons and converted to ACh, causing more of the transmitter to be released per unit of time. However, they do not, in themselves, allow one to dissociate an effect of choline on the frequency of splanchnic nerve impulses (perhaps mediated centrally) from an effect on the quantity of transmitter released per impulse.

To distinguish between these two possible actions, we again utilized the two adrenomedullary responses to ACh: induction of TH and secretion of epinephrine. In these experiments, groups of rats received two treatments: choline, which presumably acts by increasing presynaptic ACh levels, and an additional treatment designed to accelerate the firing rate of the cholinergic splanchnic nerve to the adrenals. These treatments included hypotension induced by reserpine (Table 5) (Ulus *et al.*, 1977b), systemic 6-hydroxydopamine (Table 6), and phenoxybenzamine, doses of insulin sufficient to produce severe hypoglycemia (Table 7), or prolonged exposure to a cold environment (Ulus *et al.*, in press). In all cases, administration of both choline and the other treatment had significantly greater effects on adrenomedullary function than the sum of the effects produced by either alone. These observations support the view that choline acts primarily by increasing the amount of ACh released per nerve firing, and not by changing the rate of firing.

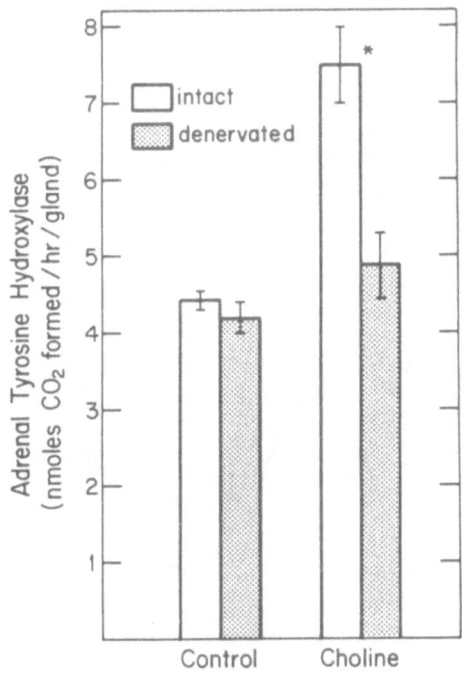

FIGURE 7

The effect of prior denervation on the response of adrenal TH activity to choline administration. The left adrenal was denervated 4 days before animals received the first of 4
daily injections of choline chloride (20 mmole/kg/day by stomach tube). Animals were
killed 24 hr after the final injection. Each point represents the mean ± S.D. of 5-7 animals.
*P < .01 when compared with enzyme activities in denervated glands or in innervated
adrenals from animals receiving water. (Reprinted with permission from Ulus, I.H.,
Hirsch, M.J., and Wurtman, R.J., 1977, Trans-synaptic induction of adrenomedullary
tyrosine hydroxylase activity by choline: evidence that choline administration increases
cholinergic transmission, *Proc. Natl. Acad. Sci. USA 74:*798).

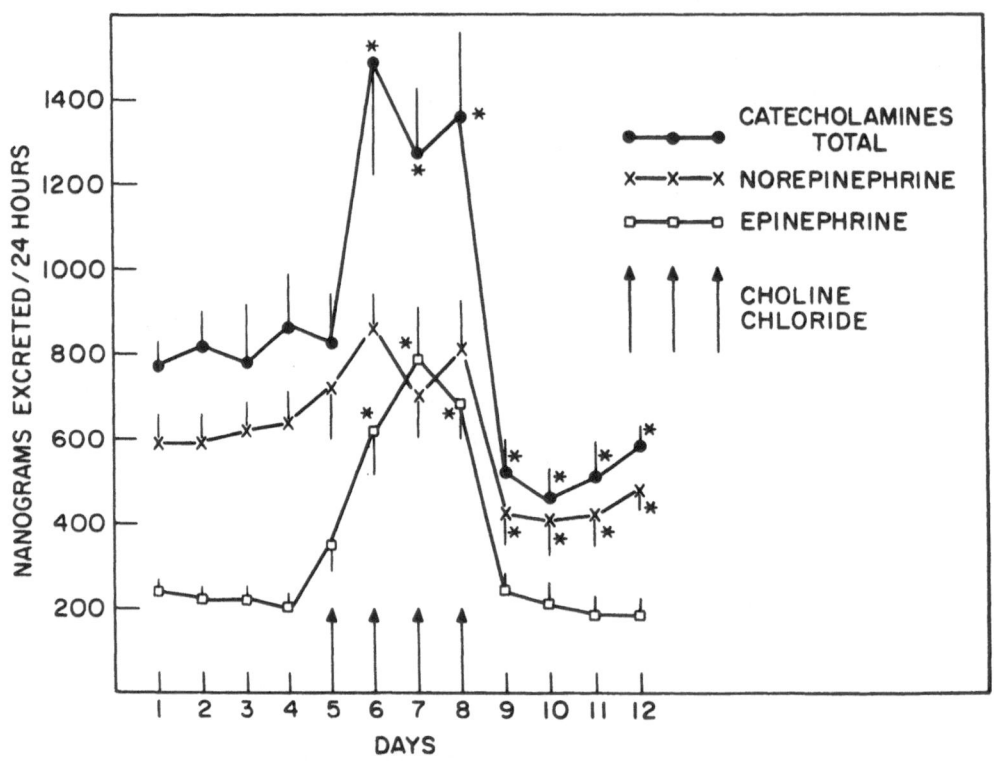

FIGURE 8

Daily urinary catecholamine excretion by rats treated with choline. On days 1-4 and 9-12, rats received water by stomach tube; on days 5-8 (indicated by arrows), they received choline (20 mmole/kg/day). Each point represents the mean of data for 6 animals; the vertical bars represent the S.D. *P < .01 compared with the mean of days 1-4. (Scally, M.C., Ulus, I.H., and Wurtman, R.J., unpublished observations).

TABLE 5

Effect of Choline and Reserpine on the Activity of Tyrosine Hydroxylase (TH) and Choline Acetyltransferase (CAT) in Rat Adrenals

Treatment	TH (nmole $^{14}CO_2$ formed per adrenal per hr)	Δ (Difference from Control)	CAT (nmole ^{14}ACh formed per adrenal per hr)	Δ (Difference from Control)
Control	3.3 ± 0.3	−	4.0 ± 0.2	−
Choline	5.5 ± 0.3*	+2.2	4.5 ± 0.4	+0.5
Reserpine	5.7 ± 0.4*	+2.4	5.8 ± 0.4*	+1.8
Reserpine and Choline	9.9 ± 0.6**	+6.6	5.6 ± 0.4*	+1.6

Animals received choline chloride (20 mmole/kg/day, by stomach tube, for 4 days), or both agents (daily for 4 days), reserpine (4 μmole/kg/day, intraperitoneally, for 4 days), and were killed 24 hr after the last treatment. Data are shown as means ± S.E.M., and analyzed by one-way analysis of variance. Both choline and reserpine caused significant increases in TH; their effects on this enzyme were more than additive. Reserpine, but not choline, also produced a significant elevation in CAT activity; this effect — which was not modified by the concurrent administration of choline — probably reflects the increased frequency of firing of the nerve (the splanchnic nerve) that contains the CAT.

*P < .01 differs from control group
**P < .01 differs from adrenals of rats receiving choline or reserpine alone

(Reprinted with permission from Ulus, I.H., Scally, M.C., and Wurtman, R.J., 1977, Choline potentiates the trans-synaptic induction of adrenal tyrosine hydroxylase by reserpine, probably by enhancing the release of acetylcholine, *Life Sci. 21:*145).

TABLE 6

Effect of Choline on Adrenal Tyrosine Hydroxylase (TH) Activity in Control or 6-Hydroxydopamine-Treated Rats

Treatment	(TH) (nmole/$^{14}CO_2$ formed/hr/gland)	Difference
Control	7.48 ± 0.36	-
Choline	9.95 ± 0.31*	+2.47
6-Hydroxydopamine	13.44 ± 0.31*	+5.96
6-Hydroxydopamine and Choline	24.64 ± 1.22**	+17.16

Rats (200-g males) received 6-hydroxydopamine hydrobromide (200 mg/kg, intravenously) twice, at 48-hr intervals; rats were killed 48 hr after the second injection. Choline chloride (1.4 g/kg, by stomach tube) was given at the same time as the first 6-hydroxydopamine dose, and at 12-hr intervals thereafter, until 24 hrs before the rats were killed. Data, shown as means ± S.E.M. of 4-6 determinations, were analyzed by one-way analysis of variance.

*$P < .05$ differs from control
**$P < .01$ differs from adrenals of rats receiving choline or 6-hydroxydopamine alone

(Reprinted with permission from Ulus, I.H., Scally, M.C., and Wurtman, R.J., (in press), Potentiation by choline of the induction of adrenal tyrosine hydroxylase by phenoxybenzamine, 6-hydroxydopamine, insulin, or exposure to cold, *J. Pharmacol. Exp. Ther.*).

TABLE 7

Effect of Choline on Adrenal Tyrosine Hydroxylase (TH) Activity in Control or Insulin-Treated Rats

Treatment	TH (nmole/$^{14}CO_2$ formed/hr/gland)	Difference
Control	4.86 ± 0.38	–
Choline	6.53 ± 0.53*	+1.67
Insulin	6.35 ± 0.28*	+1.49
Insulin and Choline	11.88 ± 0.72**	+7.02

Rats (220-g males) received insulin (2 units/rat, intraperitoneally) and choline chloride (2.8 g/kg, by stomach tube) daily for 4 days; rats were killed 24 hr after the last treatment. Data, shown as means ± S.E.M. of 6-8 determinations, were analyzed by one-way analysis of variance.

*P < .02 compared with control
**P < .001 compared with control; P < .01 differs with adrenals of rats receiving choline or insulin alone

(Reprinted with permission from Ulus, I.H., Scally, M.C., and Wurtman, R.J., (in press), Potentiation by choline of the induction of adrenal tyrosine hydroxylase by phenoxybenzamine, 6-hydroxydopamine, insulin, or exposure to cold, *J. Pharmacol. Exp. Ther.*).

Cholinergic transmission occurs at a variety of synapses, including nicotinic synapses at skeletal muscle and in ganglia, muscarinic synapses on peripheral smooth muscle and secretory cells, and muscarinic and possibly nicotinic synapses in the central nervous system. It is possible that choline administration enhances cholinergic neurotransmission at all of these loci; however, this cannot be assumed. Experiments must be performed to test the effects of choline on ACh release and on post-synaptic responses at all of these loci. It might be found, for example, that the number or orientation of cholinergic receptors at a particular synapse is such that precursor-induced increases in the quantities of ACh released into the synapse are not associated with enhanced receptor occupancy, and thus fail to produce changes in post-synaptic function. It might also be found that some types of cholinergic neurons fail to synthesize and store more ACh in response to exogenous choline, perhaps because they lack the requisite low-affinity uptake system for choline, because they contain a low-K_m variant of CAT, or because they are unable to store additional ACh. It seems safe to prophesize that such studies will be done, and that we will soon know the scope of choline's effects on cholinergic functions, when the choline is provided as a normal dietary component or taken in larger quantities as a drug. Meanwhile, we already know enough to be grateful to nature — which is not generally regarded as excessively generous to scientists and physicians — for giving us the extraordinary "window" of precursor control through which to study and manipulate cholinergic function.

ACKNOWLEDGEMENTS

These studies were supported in part by grants from ADAMHA (MH-28783), the National Aeronautics and Space Administration (NGR-22-009-627), and the Ford Foundation.

REFERENCES

Ansell, G.B., and Spanner, S., 1967, The metabolism of labeled ethanolamine in the brain of the rat *in vivo*, *J. Neurochem. 14:*873.

Aoki, K., and Siegel, F.L., 1970, Hyperphenylalanemia: disaggregation of brain polyribosomes in young rats, *Science 168:*129.

Bremer, J., and Greenberg, D.M., 1961, Methyl transferring enzyme system in the biosynthesis of lecithin (phosphatidylcholine), *Biochim. Biophys. Acta 46:*205.

Browning, E.T., and Schulman, M.P., 1968, (^{14}C) acetylcholine synthesis by cortex slices of rat brain, *J. Neurochem. 15:*1391.

Carlsson, A., Kehr, W., Lindquist, M., Magnusson, T., and Atack, C.V., 1972, Regulation of monoamine metabolism in the central nervous system, *Pharmac. Rev. 24:*371.

Cohen, E.L., and Wurtman, R.J., 1975, Brain acetylcholine: increase after systemic choline administration, *Life Sci. 16:*1095.

Cohen, E.L., and Wurtman, R.J., 1976, Brain acetylcholine: control by dietary choline, *Science 191:*561.

Colmenares, J.L., Wurtman, R.J., and Fernstrom, J.D., 1975, Effect of ingesting a carbohydrate-fat meal on the levels and synthesis of 5-hydroxyindoles in various regions of the rat central nervous system, *J. Neurochem. 25:*825.

Fernstrom, J.D., and Wurtman, R.J., 1972, Brain serotonin content: physiological regulation by plasma amino acids, *Science 178:*414.

Fernstrom, J.D., and Wurtman, R.J., 1974, Nutrition and the brain, *Sci. Am. 230:*84.

Freeman, J.J., and Jenden, D.J., 1976, The source of choline for acetylcholine synthesis in brain, *Life Sci. 19:*949.

Gibson, C.J., and Wurtman, R.J., 1977, Physiological control of brain catecholamine synthesis by brain tyrosine concentration, *Biochem. Pharmacol. 26:*1137.

Growdon, J.H., Cohen, E.L., and Wurtman, R.J., 1977a, Effects of oral choline administration on serum and CSF choline levels in patients with Huntington's Disease, *J. Neurochem. 28:*229.

Growdon, J.H., Hirsch, M.J., Wurtman, R.J., and Wiener, W., 1977b, Oral choline administration to patients with tardive dyskinesia, *N. Engl. J. Med. 297:*524.

Haga, T., and Noda, H., 1973, Choline uptake systems of rat brain synaptosomes, *Biochim. Biophys. Acta 291:*564.

Haubrich, D.R., Wang, P.F.L., and Wedeking, P., 1974, Role of choline in biosynthesis of acetylcholine, *Fed. Proc. 33:*477.

Hirsch, M.J., Growdon, J.H., and Wurtman, R.J., 1977, Increase in hippocampal acetylcholine after choline administration, *Brain Res. 332:*383.

Ikeda, M., Levitt, M., and Udenfriend, S., 1965, Hydroxylation of phenylalanine by purified preparations of adrenal and brain tyrosine hydroxylase, *Biochem. Biophys. Res. Commun. 18:*482.

Kaita, A.A., and Goldberg, A.M., 1969, Control of acetylcholine synthesis: inhibition of choline acetyltransferase by acetylcholine, *J. Neurochem. 16:*1185.

Kewitz, H., and Pleul, O., 1976, Synthesis of choline from ethanolamine in rat brain, *Proc. Natl. Acad. Sci. USA 73(7):*2181.

Murrin, C.L., Morgenroth, V.H., and Roth, R.H., 1976, Dopaminergic neurons: effects of electrical stimulation on tyrosine hydroxylase, *Mol. Pharmacol. 12:*1070.

Nagler, A.L., Dettbarn, W.D., Seifter, E., and Levenson, S.M., 1968, Tissue levels of acetylcholine and acetylcholinesterase in weanling rats subjected to acute choline deficiency, *J. Nutr. 94:*13.

Pardridge, W.M., 1977, Regulation of amino acid availability to the brain, in *"Nutrition and the Brain"* (R.J. Wurtman and J.J. Wurtman, eds.), Vol. 1 pp. 141-204, Raven Press, New York.

Pardridge, W.M., and Oldendorf, W.H., 1977, Transport of metabolic substrates through the blood-brain barrier, *J. Neurochem. 28:*5.

Scally, M.C., and Wurtman, R.J., 1977, Brain tyrosine level controls striatal dopamine synthesis in haloperidol-treated rats, *J. Neural Transm. 41:*1.

Schuberth, J., and Jenden, D.J., 1975, Transport of choline from plasma to cerebrospinal fluid in the rabbit, with reference to the origin of choline and acetylcholine metabolism in the brain, *Brain Res. 84:*245.

Thoenen, H., 1974, Trans-synaptic enzyme induction, *Life Sci. 14:*223.

Ulus, I.H., and Wurtman, R.J., 1976, Choline administration: activation of tyrosine hydroxylase in dopaminergic neurons of rat brain, *Science 194:*1060.

Ulus, I.H., Hirsch, M.J., and Wurtman, R.J., 1977a, Trans-synaptic induction of adrenomedullary tyrosine hydroxylase activity by choline: evidence that choline administration increases cholinergic transmission, *Proc. Natl. Acad. Sci. USA 74:*798.

Ulus, I.H., Scally, M.C., and Wurtman, R.J., 1977b, Choline potentiates the trans-synaptic induction of adrenal tyrosine hydroxylase by reserpine, probably by enhancing the release of acetylcholine, *Life Sci. 21:*145.

Ulus, I.H., Scally, M.C., and Wurtman, R.J., (in press), Potentiation by choline of the induction of adrenal tyrosine hydroxylase by phenoxybenzamine, 6-hydroxydopamine, insulin, or exposure to cold, *J. Pharmacol. Exp. Ther.*

Wurtman, R.J., and Fernstrom, J.D., 1976, Control of brain neurotransmitter synthesis by precursor availability and nutritional state, *Biochem. Pharmacol. 25:*1691.

Wurtman, R.J., and Scally, M.C., 1977, Precursor control of neurotransmitter synthesis, in *"Biochemistry and Function of Monoamine Enzymes"* (E. Usdin, ed.), pp. 231-261, Marcel Dekker, New York.

Wurtman, R.J., Hirsch, M.J., and Growdon, J.H., 1977, Lecithin consumption raises serum free choline levels, *Lancet 2:*68.

Yamamura, H.I., and Snyder, S.H., 1973, High affinity transport of choline into synaptosomes of rat brain, *J. Neurochem. 21:*1355.

THE NEUROCHEMICAL BASIS OF ACETYLCHOLINE PRECURSOR LOADING AS A THERAPEUTIC STRATEGY

D. J. Jenden

Department of Pharmacology, School of Medicine and The Brain Research Institute, University of California, Los Angeles, California 90024

INTRODUCTION

With the recognition that deficits in central cholinergic function may play a role in several pathological states (Davis *et al.*, 1975b; Van Woert, 1976; Weiss *et al.*, 1976; Aquilonius, 1977; Davis *et al.*, 1977a; Drachman, 1977; Eckernas, 1977; Jenden, 1977a; Barbeau, 1978; Davis and Berger, 1978; Davis *et al.*, 1978b), increasing attention has been directed to the possibility that administration of metabolic precursors of acetylcholine (ACh) may promote its synthesis, availability and utilization. This therapeutic strategy is certainly effective in the treatment of disorders characterized by deficits in the synthesis and metabolism of other neurotransmitters, particularly dopamine (Barbeau, 1976; Growdon *et al.*, 1977a). At present there is suggestive although not compelling evidence of causative associations between cholinergic deficits and several clinical illnesses. There is very little information regarding the possible mechanisms by which administration of ACh precursors favors the synthesis and utilization of ACh, and whether other less direct mechanisms underlie the therapeutic successes which have been reported. In this chapter the origins of the choline (Ch) and acetyl moieties will be reviewed, with particular reference to ACh synthesis in the brain and its regulation. The experimental, clinical and laboratory evidence of the impact of precursor loading will be examined and some of the more promising directions for future research in this area will be identified.

PRECURSORS OF ACh

ACh is formed from Ch and acetyl-coenzyme A (AcCoA) in a reaction catalyzed by choline acetyltransferase (CAT) which is generally present in great excess relative to the maximum rate at which ACh is normally formed. For example, in the mouse brain the CAT activity in various regions is linearly related to ACh content, and is sufficient to catalyze the synthesis of the ACh they contain in about 30 sec (Nordberg and Sundwall, 1975). The excess of CAT is even greater in most regions of the rat brain, particularly those with an abundant population of cholinergic cells (Cheney *et al.*, 1976). It is unlikely that the activity of CAT can limit the rate of ACh synthesis in most structures, although an opposite view has recently been proposed (Rossier and Benda, 1977). Inhibitors of CAT have little effect on cholinergic function (Krell and Goldberg, 1975; Carson et al., 1976), confirming that CAT is not rate limiting. It follows that the rate of synthesis of ACh is limited by the availability of its precursors at the site of its synthesis, where the concentration of ACh is likely to be approximated by the equilibrium between Ch, ACh, coenzyme A (CoA) and AcCoA (Glover and Potter, 1971).

CAT is a cytoplasmic enzyme (Fonnum, 1970). Both of the substrates of the forward reaction appear to be formed elsewhere, and admitted to the cytoplasm by processes which under some circumstances appear to be rate limiting and potentially subject to regulation. It has been proposed that at least part of the transport mechanism which admits Ch to cholinergic terminals is directly coupled with CAT in the sense that transport and acetylation of Ch are stoichiometrically equivalent (Barker and Mittag, 1975). CAT is also present in other parts of cholinergic neurons where access to it may not be well regulated.

Choline and Its Precursors

There is abundant evidence that ACh synthesis in nerve terminals selectively utilizes Ch which is admitted into the terminals by a sodium-dependent, high affinity transport system (Haga and Noda, 1973; Yamamura and Snyder, 1973). This is primarily localized in cholinergic nerve terminals (Kuhar et al., 1973; Kuhar and Murrin, 1978). The ACh formed in synaptosomal preparations is a remarkably consistent fraction of the Ch which is taken up by the high affinity transport system (approximately 1:2: Haga and Noda, 1973; Barker, 1976; Simon et al., 1976; Jope et al., in press) unless circumstances are established in which the availability of AcCoA is reduced. In this case, acetylation almost stops while transport is relatively unaffected (Jope and Jenden, 1977; Jope et al., in press). The dissociation constant of the high affinity carrier on the extracellular side is approximately 1 μM (Yamamura and Snyder, 1973), which is below the concentration of free Ch in plasma, CSF or whole brain (Bligh, 1952; Stavinoha et al., 1974; Schuberth and Jenden, 1975; see also Table 3). The carrier therefore appears to be essentially saturated under normal circumstances, unless the extracellular Ch concentration is very much lower in the microenvironment of the cholinergic terminal. These considerations raise the possibility that the high affinity carrier may function not only as a mechanism to ensure that sufficient Ch is available in the terminal for ACh synthesis, but as a gate with a regulatory function through which the admission of Ch and synthesis of ACh are controlled (Jenden et al., 1976; Simon et al., 1976).

This interpretation appears more plausible in view of the existence of a net efflux of Ch from the brain, which has been demonstrated both in vitro (Bhatnagar and MacIntosh, 1967; Browning, 1971) and in vivo (Dross and Kewitz, 1972; Freeman and Jenden, 1976) in several species including man (Aquilonius et al., 1975). Mammalian brain is apparently not capable of de novo synthesis of Ch (Freeman and Jenden, 1976; Ansell and Spanner, 1977) at least in significant amounts (L'Hermite and Levy, 1975), although there are reports to the contrary (Kewitz and Pleul, 1976). Ch must therefore be transported to the brain in a bound form. Lecithin was proposed by Ansell and Spanner (1970) as the carrier molecule; plasma lysolecithin was shown to be a precursor of brain Ch in the squirrel monkey (Illingsworth and Portman, 1972) and appears to provide a major source of Ch for ACh synthesis in rats (Jope and Jenden, unpublished observations).

Free Ch has been shown unequivocally to enter the brain from the bloodstream, and to be converted there to ACh (Schuberth *et al.*, 1969, 1970; Diamond, 1971); a transport mechanism with a K_t of 220 μM has been described which facilitates its transfer (Oldendorf and Braun, 1976). Pardridge and Oldendorf (1977) have argued that this transport system is the limiting factor in determining the influx of circulating Ch into the brain, since under normal conditions the rate of transport through it is less than the calculated rate of high affinity transport. Since the high affinity system is specifically associated with ACh synthesis in cholinergic endings (v.s.) it follows that most of the Ch derived from plasma is not utilized for ACh synthesis. The relative importance for ACh metabolism of Ch generated in brain and Ch transported from plasma appears to vary from species to species (Schuberth and Jenden, 1975) and may also depend on other variables such as age, diet, functional state and pathology which have not yet been extensively studied. The available evidence supports the view that the normal mammalian brain is amply supplied with Ch from both sources. It is nevertheless quite possible that pathological or functional states exist in which a temporary or extended deficiency may develop in the supply of Ch for ACh synthesis.

The sources and metabolic pathways from which Ch can be derived have been reviewed (Freeman and Jenden, 1976; Ansell and Spanner, 1977). There are basically two sources of Ch:

1. Ch and phosphatidylcholine (lecithin) in the diet.

2. Methylation of phosphatidylethanolamine (PEA) in the liver to form lecithin. This requires a source of methyl groups to provide the cofactor of PEA methyltransferase, S-adenosylmethionine.

Precursors of Ch have been considered as alternatives to Ch itself to promote its availability for ACh synthesis. Their status at the present time has not been established, and further work is needed both on the metabolic transformations required for normal utilization of Ch in the brain and pathological abnormalities which may possibly disrupt them.

Deanol (2-dimethylaminoethanol) was originally introduced (Pfeiffer *et al.*, 1957; Pfeiffer, 1959) with the expectation that it would enter the brain freely (which it does) and be converted there to Ch and ACh, which does not occur (Ansell and Spanner, 1971; Freeman and Jenden, 1976; Ansell and Spanner, 1977). Deanol is, however, incorporated into N,N-dimethyl-PEA in the liver, where it is methylated to form lecithin. Deanol was shown many years ago to provide a source of methyl groups and to prevent some of the effects of Ch deficiency (Du Vigneaud *et al.*, 1946). In these respects it must be regarded as a Ch precursor, although not in the direct sense originally conceived (Pfeiffer *et al.*, 1957; Pfeiffer, 1969).

AcetylCoA and Its Precursors

The origin of the acetyl group of ACh has also been recently reviewed (Quastel, 1977). There seems no doubt that AcCoA used in the synthesis of ACh by the mammalian brain is derived from pyruvate by the multi-enzyme complex pyruvate dehydrogenase (PDH), and thence from glucose via the Embden-Meyerhof pathway, the major route of cerebral glucose metabolism (DiPietro and Weinhouse, 1959). The only other substrates which appear to make a significant — but smaller — contribution are acetoacetate and β-hydroxybutyrate, while acetate and citrate are much less effective (Tucek and Cheng, 1974). The absence of significant acetate reutilization after release and hydrolysis of ACh from brain preparations simplifies the interpretation of experiments utilizing an isotopic label at this site, in contrast to the substantial reuptake and utilization of Ch which occurs. It is important to recognize however that utilization of acetate for ACh synthesis occurs in some species, e.g. lobster (Cheng and Nakamura, 1970) and Torpedo (Israel and Tucek, 1974; Morel, 1975), and in some mammalian tissues (Fitzgerald and Cooper, 1971; Dreyfus, 1975), including a cholinergic neuroblastoma clone (Kato et al., 1977).

Surprisingly little attention seems to have been directed to the possibility that ACh synthesis may in some circumstances be limited by the availability of AcCoA. Total pyruvate oxidation is highly correlated with the rate of synthesis of ACh in brain minces and synaptosomes (Gibson et al., 1975; Gibson and Blass, 1976b). The distribution of PDH parallels that of CAT in brain (Reynolds, 1974), but AcCoA, like Ch, shows no specific association with cholinergic neurons (Shea and Aprison, 1977). PDH is a thiamine-dependent enzyme and thiamine deficiency might therefore be expected to reduce AcCoA production. Experimental studies of thiamine deficiency have given conflicting results on brain ACh levels (Hosein et al., 1966; Cheney et al., 1969; Speeg et al., 1970; Heinrich et al., 1973; Reynolds and Blass, 1975); a recent study using modern methods of sacrifice and analysis yielded evidence of reduced ACh utilization in some brain areas without alteration of ACh levels (Vorhees et al., 1977). A similar reduction of ACh synthesis rate proportional to brain glucose level has been observed following a large dose of insulin (Gibson and Blass, 1976b). Jope (Jope, 1977; Jope and Jenden, 1977; Jope et al., in press) has recently shown that transport and acetylation of Ch in rat brain synaptosomes may be functionally uncoupled by glucose deprivation or PDH inhibition, both of which impair AcCoA availability. Perhaps most importantly, a number of clinical disorders may involve cholinergic malfunction due to hypoxia or disorders of carbohydrate catabolism (Blass and Gibson, 1977), both of which could lead to impairment of AcCoA utilization for ACh synthesis.

PRECURSOR LOADING: THE EXPERIMENTAL EVIDENCE

Choline

Although it had been known for some time that precursor availability may limit ACh synthesis and cholinergic function in vitro (Quastel et al., 1936; Kahlson and Mac-Intosh, 1939; Birks and MacIntosh, 1961), it was not until 1968 that Kuntscherova and Vlk reported that ACh levels in brain, intestine and atria were depleted after a 24 hr fast, and could be restored by the administration of Ch (1.4 mmole/kg) and glucose (2.8 mmole/kg) or by a single feeding. Ch (1.4 mmole/kg s.c.) was found to elevate ACh levels in these tissues significantly in continuously fed animals, although a greater effect was seen in fasted animals. No further change was obtained from the additional administration of glucose (2.8 mmole/kg) in continuously fed animals (Kuntscherova, 1971, 1972).

Several investigators have since reported that administration of Ch parenterally, by gastric tube or in the diet may result in an elevation of ACh levels in at least some regions of brain, although the disagreement in the literature suggests that not all the relevant factors have been identified. The effect appears to differ in different areas of the brain and may not be detectable in whole brain (Tables 1 and 2). There seems to be no doubt that ACh levels in several peripheral tissues show larger and more reproducible changes than does the brain (Nagler et al., 1968; Haubrich et al., 1974b; Haubrich et al., 1976; Ulus et al., 1977a) in response to alterations in the availability of Ch.

An increased ACh level does not in itself prove increased function, and considerable attention has been directed to the question of whether the rates of synthesis, release and turnover are affected. Cohen and Wurtman (1976) reported that the increase in caudate ACh level following the addition of Ch to drinking water (0.1 mM for 7 days) was additive with the rise produced by physostigmine (1 mg/kg i.p.), and concluded that Ch accelerated the synthesis rate of ACh. However, this argument does not distinguish between a direct effect of Ch on synthesis rate and indirect effects, such as might occur as a result of an increase in synaptic activity in response to some effect of Ch at a remote site. Wurtman and his colleagues have attempted to demonstrate increased synaptic utilization of ACh by showing that changes occur following Ch which are attributable to increased activity of post-synaptic cells at cholinergic synapses. For example, Ch has been shown to cause increased urinary catecholamine levels (Scally et al., in press) and to antagonize the hot-plate response to morphine (Botticelli et al., 1977). Another series of experiments used the trans-synaptic induction of tyrosine hydroxylase (TH) as an endpoint. TH is known to be activated in the caudate nucleus (Murrin et al., 1976) when the cells containing it are depolarized, and is induced in the adrenal medulla 12-24 hr after prolonged cholinergic stimulation (Thoenen, 1974). TH activity was shown to be increased in the corpus striatum (Ulus and Wurtman, 1976) after administration of Ch (0.43-0.86 mmole/kg), an effect which was blocked by atropine. Although it is possible that multineuronal mechanisms could be involved in this effect, induction of TH was also demonstrated in the adrenal medulla (Ulus et al., 1977a). However, in this case the dose of Ch was so high (20 mmole/kg p.o.) that the specificity of the effect is open to question. Stress has also been reported to cause induction of TH in the adrenal (Kvetnansky et al., 1970). The induction was found to be prevented by denervation, showing that it is not postsynaptically induced (Patrick and Kirshner, 1971). It could not be duplicated by an equal dose of ammonium chloride (Ulus et al., 1977) indicating that it is not a response to non-specific osmotic stress, but ammonium chloride lacks the pharmacological actions of Ch which could be responsible. The effect was not believed to be a centrally mediated action of Ch because adrenal CAT was not induced, in contrast to reserpine, which induces adrenal CAT as a result of the prolonged increase in preganglionic neuronal activity which it causes (Oesch, 1974). However, unlike reserpine, the effect of Ch is relatively brief, and may be too short for significant induction of CAT to occur.

Wurtman and his colleagues have argued on the basis of indirect evidence that Ch increases the amount of ACh released per impulse, although no direct investigation of this question has been reported. The indirect evidence cited consists mainly of nonlinear interactions which have been found between Ch and other experimental manipulations which are designed to increase neuronal firing rates. For example, increased sympathetic impulse flow is believed to be responsible for the induction of TH which occurred after reserpine (2.5 mg/kg i.p.), phenoxybenzamine (20 mg/kg i.p.), insulin (2 U/rat i.p. x 4 days), or 6-hydroxydopamine (200 mg/kg iv x 2) or a cold environment (Ulus et al., 1977c; Ulus et al., in press). When these treatments were given after 4 days of treatment

TABLE 1

Published Data on the Effect of Choline Administration on Acetylcholine Levels in Brain

Species	Choline Dose µmole/kg	Route[a]	Duration	Structure	Changed[d] ACh Levels	Time After Dose (min)	Method of Sacrifice[b]	Assay[c]	Comments	Ref.
Rat	1430	SC	Single	Whole brain	+	60	DC	BIO	Rats were fasted for 24 hr. A further increase was seen after glucose	1
Rat	1430	SC	Single	Whole brain	+	80-100	DC	BIO	Rats were fasted for 24 hr; plasma Ch was normal by the time brain ACh was significantly raised	2
Guinea pig	200	IV	Single	Whole brain	=	2	NS	RE	Pentobarbital anesthesia	3
Guinea pig	150	IA	15 min	Whole brain	+	0	NS	RE		4
Rat	1430	IP	Single	C. striatum	+	40	MW	RE		5
Rat	150	IV	6 min	C. striatum Occip. cortex	+	0	MW	GCMS		6
Rat	430	IP	Single	Whole brain	+	40	MW	RE		7

TABLE 1 (CONTINUED)

Published Data on the Effect of Choline Administration on Acetylcholine Levels in Brain

Species	Choline Dose µmole/kg	Route[a]	Duration	Structure	Changed[d] ACh Levels	Time After Dose (min)	Method of Sacrifice[b]	Assay[c]	Comments	Ref.
Rat	1-256	IV	1 min	Whole brain	=	0	DC	GCMS		8
Rat	225	IA	15 min	C. striatum	+	0	MW	RE		9
Rat	0.5	IVT	Single	C. striatum	+	15	DC	RE		10
Rat	2.5	IVT	Single	C. striatum Hippocampus	+	15	DC	RE		11
Rat	430	IP	Single	Hippocampus Caudate n.	+	20,40	MW	RE	Rats were on Ch-deficient diet	12
Rat	270	IV	18 min	Cortex C. striatum	= / +	0	MW	RE	No change in ACh turnover	13
Rat	10,000-20,000	IG	Single	Cortex Caudate n.	+ / +	300	MW	RE		14
Mouse	1000	IP	Single	Whole brain	+	40	MW	GCMS		15

TABLE 1 (CONTINUED)

Published Data on the Effect of Choline Administration on Acetylcholine Levels in Brain

Species	Choline Dose μmole/kg	Route[a]	Duration	Structure	Changed[d] ACh Levels	Time After Dose (min)	Method of Sacrifice[b]	Assay[c]	Comments	Ref.
Rat	430	IP	Single	C. striatum Hippocampus Hypothalamus Cortex	=	15-90	MW	P/GC	Ch blocked atropine-induced depletion of ACh in cortex and hippocampus	16
Rat	430	IP	Single	Hippocampus C. striatum	=	-	MW	P/GC	Ch potentiated paraoxon-induced rise in ACh in C. striatum	17

[a]SC: subcutaneous; IV: intravenous; IA: intracarotid; IP: intraperitoneal; IVT: intracerebroventricular; IG: intragastric

[b]DC: decapitation; MW; microwave fixation; NS: not stated

[c]BIO: bioassay; RE: radioenzymatic; P/GC: pyrolysis/gas chromatography; GCMS: gas chromatography/mass spectrometry

[d] +: increase; =: no change

References: (1) Kuntscherova and Vlk, 1968; (2) Kuntscherova, 1972; (3) Haubrich et al., 1974b; (4) Haubrich et al., 1974a; (5) Haubrich et al., 1975; (6) Racagni et al., 1975; (7) Cohen and Wurtman, 1975; (8) Freeman et al., 1975; (9) Haubrich et al., 1975; (10) Haubrich et al., 1975; (11) Haubrich and Chippendale, 1977; (12) Hirsch et al., 1977a; (13) Eckernas et al., 1977; (14) Ulus et al., 1977c; (15) Jenden; unpublished observation; (16) Wecker et al., 1978; (17) Wecker and Dettbarn, 1978.

TABLE 2

Summary of Published Data on Effects of Dietary Manipulation on Brain Acetylcholine Levels in the Rat

Dietary Regimen	Duration	Structure	Effect	Method of Sacrifice	Assay	Comments	Ref.
Ch-deficient ± 11 μM Ch in drinking water	6 days	Whole brain	Decrease in Ch-deficient animals	ether anes.	Bio	Brain AChE unchanged	1
Fast	24 hr	Whole brain	Decrease	DC	RE	Brain ACh restored by Ch + glucose or by meal	2
Ch-free + 0.01, 0.14 or 0.93 μmole/day	7 or 11 days	Caudate n., Brain stem	Increase with Ch supplement	MW	RE	Increase additive with that produced by physostigmine	3
Ch-deficient or normal diet	1,5 or 11 days; 21 weeks from birth	Whole brain	No change	DC or MW	RE	Brain Ch levels also normal, but rate of physostigmine increase small in Ch-deficient animals	4
Overnight fast, then lecithin (≡ 2 mmole/kg Ch)	—	Whole brain	Increase 10 hr after lecithin	MW	RE		5

Bio: bioassay; DC: decapitation; MW: microwave fixation; RE: radioenzymatic

References: (1) Nagler et al., 1968; (2) Kuntscherova and Vlk, 1968; Kuntscherova, 1972; (3) Cohen and Wurtman, 1976; (4) Haubrich et al., 1976; (5) Hirsch and Wurtman, 1978.

with Ch (20 mmole/kg/day by stomach tube) the change in TH was found to be greater than the sum of the changes produced by Ch and the treatments alone (Ulus *et al.*, 1977c; Ulus *et al.*, 1977b; Ulus *et al.*, in press). However, increased presynaptic release of ACh is not the only possible explanation of an enhanced trans-synaptic induction of TH after Ch. In this connection it is of interest that hepatic microsomal enzyme induction by phenobarbital is Ch-dependent (Cooper and Feuer, 1973). Another possibility which requires investigation is an increased number of nicotinic receptors following Ch which could enhance the postsynaptic response to an unchanged release of ACh. Morley *et al.*, (1977) have recently reported increased a-bungarotoxin binding in brain following Ch. Finally, nonlinear summation of effects is commonplace in pharmacology, since dose/response curves are generally nonlinear. Potentiation is not established unless the nature of the dose-response curve is documented and taken into account when interpreting the interaction.

Although there is no direct evidence currently available on the effect of Ch on ACh release, Eckernas *et al.*, (1977) have studied the effect of a Ch load on brain ACh turnover in rats. Using the infusion of a tracer dose of ^{3}H-Ch (47 nmole/kg/min) to estimate ACh turnover in the corpus striatum and cortex, no significant change in turnover was found in either region when unlabelled Ch was infused at a rate (15 μmole/kg/min) sufficient to elevate the plasma Ch level almost 10-fold, although a small but significant increase in striatal ACh levels was found. They concluded (Eckernas *et al.*, 1977) that a direct agonist action of Ch, like that of oxotremorine (Choi *et al.*, 1973; Nordberg, 1977), may be responsible for both the increased striatal level and small (insignificant) decrease in turnover.

Choline Loading and the Regulation of ACh Synthesis

It is difficult to reconcile the hypothesis of increased ACh synthesis after Ch with the evidence that uptake of Ch by high affinity Ch transport is rate limiting (Jenden *et al.*, 1976; Simon *et al.*, 1976; Kuhar and Murrin, 1978). The normal level of Ch in the plasma and CSF exceeds the K_m of the high affinity transport system, which therefore appears to be close to saturation under normal conditions. One possibility which has been suggested (Jenden, 1977b) is that elevations in extracellular Ch level promote synthesis of ACh at sites where only the low affinity transport system is operating. Suszkiw *et al.*, (1976; Suszkiw and Pilar, 1976) have provided evidence that in cholinergic somata in the ciliary body, Ch is taken up by the low affinity transport system and acetylated. This would explain a selective effect of Ch in the corpus striatum which is rich in cholinergic cell bodies, while in regions such as the hippocampus in which the high affinity transport system and most of the CAT are associated with cholinergic terminals (Kuhar *et al.*, 1973), the effect is less reproducible (Table 1). Wecker and colleagues have recently reported no change in striatal, hippocampal or cortical ACh levels after Ch premedication (Wecker and Dettbarn, 1978; Wecker *et al.*, 1978), which nevertheless prevented the depletion of ACh produced by atropine in the cerebral cortex and hippocampus (Wecker *et al.*, 1978) and markedly potentiated the rise induced by paraoxon in the corpus striatum. These findings were interpreted as suggesting that action of Ch is dependent on the dynamics of the system (Wecker and Dettbarn, 1978).

The apparent incompatibility of a Ch induced increase in ACh synthesis rate with our present knowledge of the high affinity transport system warrants a closer examination.

Barker and Mittag (1975) proposed two models of the coupling between the high affinity transport system and CAT: a) direct coupling, in which the two systems are directly linked and Ch transport is stoichiometrically related to acetylation (Fonnum, 1973); and b) a "free pool" or kinetic model, in which a cytoplasmic pool of Ch is balanced by influx from the high affinity transport system and efflux by acetylation. Suszkiw and and Pilar (1976) presented data on the cholinergic terminals in the avian iris which supported the kinetic coupling model, and suggested the existence of a cytoplasmic Ch pool with a concentration of $\sim$500 μM. This exceeds the plasma concentration by 100-fold, and would require a Na^+- coupled transport system to maintain it (cf Schultz and Curran, 1973). In the kinetic coupling model, the cytoplasmic Ch concentration is determined by the relative rates of transport and acetylation. An increased rate of acetylation (resulting, perhaps, from release-induced depletion of ACh) would tend to deplete cytoplasmic Ch and hence increase the inward gradient of Ch, so that net influx would increase (Jenden et al., 1976). An increased net influx might also result from increased extracellular Ch concentration, depending on the cytoplasmic Ch concentration, membrane potential (Blaustein and Goldring, 1975), Na^+ distribution and capacity of the high affinity transport system. Whether this in turn would increase the rate of ACh synthesis depends on the change in Ch concentration in the cytoplasmic pool relative to the K_m of CAT (400 μM: White and Wu, 1973) and the equilibrium constant of the acetylation reaction (Pieklik and Guynn, 1975).

The kinetic coupling model may be regarded as a generalized hypothesis from which two special cases may be identified. When the capacity for acetylation greatly exceeds the rate of transport, all the Ch transported is acetylated and the system appears to be directly coupled. On the other hand, if the rate of the whole sequence is limited by the rate at which AcCoA becomes available, both the transport and acetylation processes may be close to equilibrium (Glover and Potter, 1971; Weiler et al., in press), and a relatively constant ratio of acetylation/transport is achieved which depends on the AcCoA/CoA ratio in the cytoplasm. This could be referred to as a quasi equilibrium model. Although the direct coupling model appears incompatible with a major influence of extracellular Ch on ACh synthesis in terminals, the quasi equilibrium model predicts that the extracellular Ch and intracellular ACh levels should always be directly related to each other if the AcCoA supply remains unchanged, since cytoplasmic concentrations of Ch, ACh, CoA and AcCoA will approximate an equilibrium:

$$\frac{[ACh]}{[Ch]} \frac{[CoA]}{[AcCoA]} \simeq 12 \quad \text{(Pieklik and Guynn, 1975)}$$

If the availability of AcCoA is rate limiting (Polak et al., 1977; Weiler et al., in press), the distribution of Ch across the cell membrane may also be close to equilibrium, with a

$$\frac{[Ch] \text{in}}{[Ch] \text{out}} \quad \text{ratio of} \sim 10 \quad \text{(Jenden et al., 1976)}$$

given a membrane potential of 25 mV (Blaustein and Goldring, 1975) or a considerably larger ratio if the only transport for Ch at cholinergic endings is sodium-coupled. It is worth pointing out that the Michaelis constants of the transport system and of CAT do not affect the relationship, provided only that the transport and acetylation capacities substantially exceed the synthesis rate. There is a great deal of evidence that CAT activity is greatly in excess of the normal ACh synthesis rate in cholinergic nerve terminals from mammalian brain (see above), but it is difficult to make a similar comparison for the capacity of the high affinity transport system because of losses in preparation of synaptosomes. A considerable reserve appears to exist in the superior cervical ganglion (Collier and MacIntosh, 1969) relative to the resting rate of synthesis of ACh. The quasi equilibrium model therefore provides a satisfactory reconciliation of the effects of Ch loading and the properties of the high affinity Ch transport system.

Deanol

The available evidence does not support the rationale originally proposed (Pfeiffer *et al.*, 1957; Pfeiffer, 1959) for the clinical use of deanol. Although deanol is rapidly taken up into the brain after systemic administration (Groth *et al.*, 1958), it is generally agreed that the brain lacks the metabolic potential for methylation of deanol (Ansell and Spanner, 1971; Freeman and Jenden, 1976; Ansell and Spanner, 1977) although Kewitz and his colleagues have maintained that methylation does occur in the brain (Kewitz and Pleul, 1976). Regardless of this question, it is certain that deanol can serve as a Ch precursor in a more general sense (Du Vigneaud *et al.*, 1946), and its chemical similarity to Ch suggests that it could influence Ch and ACh metabolism in a number of ways, some of which may be therapeutically useful.

Goldberg and Silbergeld have reported (1974) that whole brain ACh levels were elevated in the mouse after deanol (300 mg/kg), and both Ch and ACh are reported to increase in the rat corpus striatum (Haubrich *et al.*, 1975). These studies employed radioenzymatic assays which are claimed to be immune from interference by deanol. The elevation in striatal ACh was confirmed by Zahniser *et al.*, (1977) using a gas chromatographic method, although a massive dose of deanol was required (900 mg/kg). Earlier work using bioassay methods had given conflicting results (Pepeu *et al.*, 1960; Danysz *et al.*, 1967).

The observation that deanol antagonizes some of the behavioral effects of intraventricular hemicholinium (Jenden *et al.*, 1977) prompted a reinvestigation (Jope and Jenden, 1978; Jope and Jenden, unpublished observation) of the influence of deanol on Ch and ACh metabolism using rigorous gas chromatography/mass spectrometry (GCMS) methods and deuterium labelling (Jenden, in press). No evidence was found for the formation of Ch from deanol in brain tissue *in vitro* or *in vivo*, although administration of ^{2}H-labelled deanol to rats for several days led to the appearance of Ch and ACh containing the label. Neither single nor repeated administration of deanol altered the concentration of ACh in corpus striatum, hippocampus or cortex, in agreement with the results of Pepeu *et al.*, (1960) and Zahniser *et al.*, (1977). Deanol did increase the concentration of Ch in the plasma and brain after both single and repeated doses of deanol, as others have also found (Dahlberg and Schuberth, 1977; Schuberth, 1977; Zahniser, 1977). The mechanism of this effect remains to be investigated. If it occurs in human subjects after therapeutic doses of deanol, it may provide the basis for a therapeutic effect; on the other hand, deanol inhibits the transport of Ch by the high affinity system (Jope and Jenden, 1978; Jope and Jenden, unpublished observation) and the uptake of Ch into the brain (Cornford *et al.*, 1978), which may interfere with its utilization. Since deanol alters the phospholipid composition of brain (Dormard *et al.*, 1975; Yavin, 1977), there is some reason for caution in its use for long periods or in high doses. The synthesis of acetyldeanol and its release as a false transmitter had been suggested as a possible mechanism of its antagonism of hemicholinium (Osuide, 1968; Jenden *et al.*, 1977), since deanol has been shown to be a substrate of CAT *in vitro* (Korey *et al.*, 1951; Berman *et al.*, 1953) and acetyldeanol is a weak muscarinic agonist (Cho *et al.*, 1972). However, acetyldeanol was not detected *in vivo* under any conditions (Jope and Jenden, 1978; Jope and Jenden, unpublished observation).

Summary

In summary, the experimental evidence indicates that a sufficiently large dose of Ch can increase ACh levels in some areas of the brain and in other structures. This increase may occur primarily in cholinergic cell bodies. While Ch appears not to have any direct effect on the spontaneous turnover rate of ACh, there is evidence that it may have an enabling effect on ACh synthesis, allowing synthesis to keep pace with utilization under circumstances of increased demand which normally have a depleting effect. The increased synthesis of ACh may occur primarily in areas remote from the nerve terminal following uptake of Ch through the low affinity transport system. Mechanisms have been reviewed under which increased ACh levels might be brought about at cholinergic nerve terminals following an increased extracellular Ch concentration, taking into account the known properties of the high affinity transport system. Deanol is a remote precursor of Ch, large doses of which cause an increase in plasma and brain Ch levels but not of ACh levels.

PRECURSOR LOADING: THE CLINICAL EVIDENCE

Choline

Although the early studies of Kuntscherova (Kuntscherova and Vlk, 1968; Kuntscherova, 1972) aroused little interest, the reports by Haubrich, Wurtman and their colleagues (Haubrich *et al.*, 1974a; Haubrich *et al.*, 1974b; Cohen and Wurtman, 1975; Haubrich *et al.*, 1975) on Ch loading led to an immediate investigation (Aquilonius and Eckernas, 1975; Davis *et al.*, 1975) of the possible efficacy of Ch in several clinical disorders in which a cholinergic deficit was believed to exist, particularly tardive dyskinesia and Huntington's chorea. These studies have been reviewed (Barbeau, 1978; Davis and Berger, 1978), and are summarized in Table 3.

As early as 1975 Aquilonius and Eckernas showed (1975, 1976a) that Ch administered orally in doses of 3-9 g/day to human subjects resulted in a prompt and long-lasting elevation of plasma Ch levels, and in the same year Davis *et al.*, (1975a) reported improvement in a case of tardive dyskinesia who was given Ch (16 g/day). Subsequent studies have shown that most patients with tardive dyskinesia respond favorably to Ch (Davis *et al.*, 1976; Growdon *et al.*, 1977d; Hirsch *et al.*, 1977b; Tamminga *et al.*, 1977; Barbeau, 1978) and most reports have also described some improvement in Huntington's disease, although this is inconsistent (Aquilonius and Eckernas, 1975, 1977; Davis *et al.*, 1976, 1977a, 1977b; Davis and Berger, 1978; Growdon *et al.*, 1977b; Barbeau, 1978), perhaps because the neuronal defect in Huntington's chorea prevents the effective utilization of Ch (McGeer *et al.*, 1973; Bird and Iversen, 1974; Stahl and Swanson, 1974) or because the muscarinic receptors upon which the neurotransmitter acts have degenerated (Enna

TABLE 3

Summary of Clinical Data on Response to Choline Administration

Subjects	Diagnosis[c]	Daily Dose of Choline (g)	Plasma Ch			CSF Ch			Comments	Ref.
			Before (µM)	After (µM)	Time After Dose (hr)	Before (µM)	After (µM)	Time After Dose (hr)		
2	HC	3-9							Oral Ch causes dose dependent increase in plasma Ch level	1
4	HC	12-20							Significant improvement in 2 patients; same patients responded to physostigmine	2
4	TD	6							Improvement in 2; onset of depression required discontinuation of Ch in 2 patients	3
20	TD	150-200 mg/kg	12.4±1.0	33.5±2.5	1				9 improved, 10 unchanged, 1 worse; no relation between Ch level and response or side effects	4 5
10	HC	8-20	13.6±1.7	39.7±2.7[a]	1	1.8±0.1	3.1±0.3	1	No consistent or lasting improvement in any patient; minor improvement in some; physostigmine also ineffective in 5 patients tested	6

TABLE 3 (CONTINUED)

Summary of Clinical Data on Response to Choline Administration

Subjects	Diagnosis[c]	Daily Dose of Choline (g)	Plasma Ch			CSF Ch			Comments	Ref.
			Before (μM)	After (μM)	Time After Dose (hr)	Before (μM)	After (μM)	Time After Dose (hr)		
23	NS	meal	10.6±0.4	11.5±0.3	1				Plasma concentration not related to age, except newborn infants	7
4	TD	12-20							Significant improvement in all patients; physostigmine also effective in all patients	8
5	HC	3-15	9.0	28.1	1				Minor improvement in 2 patients	9
7	AD	10							Minor improvement; all patients were severely demented but became more manageable[b]	10
10	NS	2.3[d]	~9	~30	12				Plasma Ch rose slowly to peak at ≥ 12 hr	11
4	HC	10							Improvement in 2[b]	12

TABLE 3 (CONTINUED)

Summary of Clinical Data on Response to Choline Administration

Subjects	Diagnosis[c]	Daily Dose of Choline (g)	Plasma Ch			CSF Ch			Comments	Ref.
			Before (µM)	After (µM)	Time After Dose (hr)	Before (µM)	After (µM)	Time After Dose (hr)		
2	TD	10							Improvement in 1[b]	12
3	GT	10							Improvement in 1[b]	12
6	FA	10							Improvement in all[b]	12
6	HC								Significant improvement in 3 patients	
4	TD	20	11.1±3.8	23.7±3.9[e,f]		2.5±1.0	3.9±1.4[e]		Significant improvement in all patients	13
1	Mania								Improvement in BPRS, Petterson score	14
6	SCH								Dramatic improvement in 1 patient; minor (spontaneous?) improvement in 3 patients	

TABLE 3 (CONTINUED)

NOTES:

[a]25.8±1.7 during treatment at 8 g/day

[b]Preliminary data

[c]AD: Alzheimer's disease; FA: Friedreich's ataxia; GT: Gilles de la Torrette syndrome; HC: Huntington's disease; TD: tardive dyskinesia; NS: normal subjects; SCH: schizophrenia

[d]Single dose of lecithin equivalent to 2.3 g Ch

[e]Not all patients were included in analytical data

[f]Peak plasma level after a single 5 g dose was 20.2±6.5 μM at 2 hr, compared to 10.5±4.0 at 0 hr in 10 subjects

REFERENCES:

1   Aquilonius and Eckernas, 1975

2   Davis *et al.*, 1976

3   Tamminga *et al.*, 1976, 1977

4   Growdon *et al.*, 1977d

5   Hirsch *et al.*, 1977b

6   Growdon *et al.*, 1977c

7   Eckernas and Aquilonius, 1977

8   Davis *et al.*, 1976

9   Aquilonius and Eckernas, 1977

10   Boyd *et al.*, 1977

11   Wurtman *et al.*, 1977

12   Barbeau, 1978

13   Davis *et al.*, 1977b

14   Davis and Berger, 1978

et al., 1976; Yamamura *et al.*, 1977). There is evidence that patients who respond to Ch can be predicted on the basis of their response to intravenous physostigmine (Davis *et al.*, 1976, 1977a, 1977b), which is not suitable for treatment because of its short duration of action. Ch, on the other hand, has a duration of action greatly exceeding the elevation of plasma Ch levels (Davis *et al.*, 1976). This suggests that its effects depend in part on its conversion to a lipid-bound form for transportation and utilization by the brain. No information has been published on the relative utilization of free and lipid-bound Ch in man, and laboratory animals show considerable species dependence in this regard (Schuberth and Jenden, 1975). That elevations in plasma may lead to corresponding changes in the brain is indicated by a report of dose-dependent increases of CSF Ch levels (Growdon 1977c), although this is apparently inconsistent (Davis and Berger, 1978) and does not necessarily imply that Ch gains entry to the central nervous system primarily in the free form. It would be of interest to determine whether the elevation of CSF Ch, like the symptomatic improvement, outlasts the rise in Ch plasma levels.

Very large doses of Ch have been given with few serious side effects. The most common is certainly the fishy odor which is due to the secretion of trimethylamine in the sweat; trimethylamine is formed from Ch by bacteria in the gastrointestinal tract which apparently metabolize most of the administered dose (de la Huerga and Popper, 1951; Higgins *et al.*, 1972). This effect of Ch makes a true double blind study very difficult and may be less prominent when Ch is given in the form of lecithin. Several other side effects of Ch confirm its cholinergic action, including nausea, vomiting, salivation, sweating and anorexia. These effects are dose-dependent and can be treated effectively with a quaternary antimuscarinic agent such as propantheline without reducing the therapeutic effect. The cognitive impairment associated with physostigmine is not seen during treatment with Ch (Davis *et al.*, 1975a, 1975b). The most serious effect associated with Ch is depression (Tamminga *et al.*, 1976, 1977), which is also dose-dependent and reversible. This effect, seen also with physostigmine, has been interpreted as the result of an altered cholinergic/dopaminergic balance (Davis and Berger, 1978; Janowsky *et al.*, 1972), and suggests a possible therapeutic use of Ch in affective disorders; a therapeutic response to physostigmine in mania has been reported (Janowsky *et al.*, 1973; Davis *et al.*, 1977b; 1978).

Deanol

Deanol was proposed many years ago (Pfeiffer *et al.*, 1957; Pfeiffer, 1959) as a means of promoting ACh synthesis and utilization in the brain. Although its proposed rationale as a Ch precursor in the brain is not supported by recent work (see above), a number of clinical studies have reported success with deanol in the treatment of Huntington's disease, tardive dyskinesia, L-DOPA induced dyskinesia and minimal brain dysfunction. Not all studies have been positive and no double-blind crossover study appears to have been completed with deanol in any movement disorder. In view of the lack of side effects associated with this drug and the low doses in which it has been used, a controlled trial of deanol in larger doses seems indicated. Although the original rationale for its use appears incorrect, it can suppress some of the effects of Ch deficiency (DuVigneaud *et al.*, 1946) and is converted to Ch after incorporation into the phospholipid pathway in the liver (Jope and Jenden, 1978; Jope and Jenden, unpublished observation). Ch levels in the plasma and brain are elevated in experimental studies after large doses of deanol, perhaps as a result of competition with Ch for a metabolic or excretory mechanism. There is at present no evidence as to whether the clinical effects of deanol which have been reported are the result of an elevation of Ch levels or whether some more complex mechanism may be involved. No clinical studies have been published on the metabolism of deanol and its impact on Ch metabolism. In view of the resurgence of interest in this drug, such studies are clearly needed.

Lecithin

A recent study on human volunteers (Wurtman *et al.*, 1977) suggests that lecithin may provide a more efficient source of Ch than the oral administration of Ch itself. This report awaits confirmation using pure lecithin rather than a crude phospholipid fraction.* Only fragmentary information is available on the metabolism of lecithin and other phospholipids in the gastrointestinal tract before and during absorption. In view of the potential importance of this finding, studies are urgently required to determine to what extent Ch is absorbed from the gut in esterified form and whether lecithin or some other phospholipid may be transported and utilized by the brain as a Ch source without hydrolysis and resynthesis in the liver. The only other form of esterified Ch which seems to have been used therapeutically is cytidinediphosphorylcholine, the immediate source of Ch for lecithin synthesis in brain and liver. Paradoxically, its rationale and possible therapeutic effects appear to be unrelated to those of Ch (Manaka *et al.*, 1974; Ogashiwa *et al.*, 1975; Salvadorini *et al.*, 1975).

LABORATORY ASSESSMENT OF CHOLINERGIC FUNCTION

Despite the substantial advances which have been made in the last decade in analytical methodology for the study of cholinergic function (Hanin, 1974; Jenden, 1977c), there has been little progress in devising ways of using analyses of clinically accessible samples for the evaluation of cholinergic function in the central nervous system. This is due in large measure to three features of ACh metabolism:

1. The enzymes catalyzing its synthesis and destruction are normally present in such large amounts that these processes can occur in time intervals of the order of seconds or less, making it difficult to measure the kinetics in experimental studies and virtually impossible clinically.

2. Neither of the precursors of ACh is unique to ACh metabolism but turn over in relatively large amounts in all cells.

3. Ch is both a precursor and a metabolite of ACh, which complicates the interpretation of its concentration in body fluids. This contrasts to most neurotransmitter pathways in which analyses of a discrete precursor and/or product facilitate a kinetic assessment of the system.

Plasma Ch levels are clearly of value in monitoring precursor loading therapy and ensuing compliance, although no definite correlation has been established between plasma Ch level and therapeutic response. The plasma Ch level is normally within a narrow range (Bligh, 1952, 1953), but response to dietary status or exogenously adminstered Ch has

*The "lecithin" granules used in this study were apparently only 10-20% lecithin in view of the stated equivalence of 100 g "lecithin" to 3 g of Ch chloride; analytical data were not provided.

been clearly established (Table 3). Pathological conditions may also influence plasma Ch (Rennick *et al.*, 1976), but only fragmentary data are so far available. Since brain Ch is derived at least in part from an esterified Ch source present in blood, plasma concentrations of lecithin, lysolecithin, Ch plasmalogen and other Ch-containing compounds may prove to be of value.

There is some indication that erythrocyte Ch levels may be of clinical interest (Hanin *et al.*, 1977; Jope *et al.*, unpublished data). Ch is transported by erythrocytes (Martin, 1972), although their characteristics appear to be quite different to those of the high affinity transport system associated with synaptosomes. Hanin (Hanin *et al.*, 1977) has reported elevated erythrocyte Ch levels in two unipolar depressed patients being treated with tricyclic antidepressants, and Jope *et al.*, (unpublished data) have shown that in patients undergoing treatment with lithium, the erythrocyte Ch level rises 10-fold (424 μM compared to a normal value of 40 μM), while the plasma level remains in the normal range. Although Martin (1974) has reported inhibition of Ch influx in red blood cells from patients treated with lithium, it appears that inhibition of efflux of Ch may be of greater significance.

It seems likely that erythrocyte Ch levels will prove to be of diagnostic importance and perhaps provide clues regarding alterations in Ch transport and metabolism in mental disease. Further data on erythrocyte Ch levels are urgently needed both in normal subjects and in naive and drug-treated patients to establish the significance of these preliminary findings.

Early studies on Ch levels in CSF (Jonsson and Schuberth, 1969; Aquilonius *et al.*, 1970) suggested that this might be a useful marker for the release of ACh in the central nervous system. Subsequent work in the rabbit using ^{2}H-labelled Ch as a tracer (Schuberth and Jenden, 1975) led to the conclusion that CSF Ch was derived principally from plasma Ch, while only a small fraction arises from ACh. Nevertheless, Aquilonius *et al.*, (1972) reported that patients with Huntington's chorea had a significantly lower concentration of Ch (1.9 ± 0.12 μM) in the lumbar CSF than a control group (2.5 ± 0.09 μM). Two subsequent studies (Welsh *et al.*, 1976; Consolo *et al.*, 1977) also found a lower concentration in Huntington's disease, although in neither was the difference significant. If it is significant for the population as a whole, the difference is small and unlikely to be of value for purposes of diagnosis or assessment. No significant differences were found between controls and patients with Parkinson's disease (Aquilonius *et al.*, 1972; Welsh *et al.*, 1976) nor did drug treatment yield a significant effect (Aquilonius *et al.*, 1972; Consolo *et al.*, 1977). Interpretation of lumbar CSF Ch concentration is further complicated by the fact that it increases as the volume withdrawn increases (Welsh *et al.*, 1976). This was interpreted to reflect a gradient from the ventricles because of efficient removal of Ch during the ventriculocysternal passage (Aquilonius and Winbladh, 1971) since the ventricular concentration is considerably higher (Aquilonius *et al.*, 1972). As in the case of plasma, measurement of esterified forms of Ch in CSF may be more informative. There is so far little information available, but the concentration of Ch phospholipids is apparently larger than that of Ch (Sastry and Stancer, 1968).

Significant ACh levels have been reported in CSF (Schain, 1960; Duvoisin and Dettbarn, 1967; Welsh *et al.*, 1976; Davis *et al.*, 1977b), plasma (Okonek and Kilbinger, 1974; Hanin *et al.*, 1977), erythrocytes (Hanin *et al.*, 1977), platelets (Green *et al.*, 1972) and whole blood (Stavinoha and Modak, 1976; Hanin *et al.*, 1977). Although some early reports might be questioned on the basis of the specificity of the bioassay used, the basic findings have now been reproduced by GCMS (Stavinoha and Modak, 1976; Welsh *et al.*, 1976; Hanin *et al.*, 1977; Davis *et al.*, 1977b). This must be considered a reliable identification, although it is difficult to exclude the possibility that the ACh was introduced accidentally as a result of an artefact in the sample workup or derivatization procedures used. In view of the very high concentration of acetylcholinesterase in blood* it is unlikely that ACh would survive unless the enzyme is inhibited (Okonek and Kilbinger, 1974) or the ACh is bound in some inaccessible form. Survival of ACh in CSF for long enough to reach the lumbar region seems less improbable** since it disappears only slowly on standing at room temperature (Duvoisin and Dettbarn, 1967) and is not significantly more stable when the sample is treated with an anticholinesterase (Welsh *et al.*, 1976). Although the early literature suggests that trauma (Tower and McEachern, 1949a) and epilepsy (Tower and McEachern, 1949b) may be associated with elevated CSF ACh levels, recent data provide little basis for optimism for the clinical utility of this difficult measurement (Aquilonius *et al.*, 1972; Welsh *et al.*, 1976; Consolo *et al.*, 1977), although more data are clearly needed (Davis *et al.*, 1977b).

Cholinesterase (Duvoisin and Dettbarn, 1967; Consolo *et al.*, 1977) and CAT (Johnson and Domino, 1971; Aquilonius and Eckernas, 1976b) have both been reported in CSF, but have not been extensively studied. Measurements of CAT are complicated by non-enzymatic catalysis of the reaction between AcCoA and Ch (Burt and Silver, 1973; Aquilonius and Eckernas, 1976b); the residual activity attributable to CAT is extremely small in relation to the CAT present in brain (Aquilonius and Eckernas, 1976b).

More information is needed about the dynamics of the system which provides the brain with Ch for ACh synthesis. This is an area in which isotopic tracers will be required, and deuterium-labelled Ch has proven to be valuable in experimental studies of this kind (Hanin and Schuberth, 1974; Choi *et al.*, 1975; Freeman *et al.*, 1975; Schuberth and Jenden, 1975). Hazards from the clinical use of stable isotopes are minimal (Knapp and Gaffney, 1972; Jenden, 1978), although the use of ^{13}C instead of ^2H might be a wise precaution to eliminate the possibility of significant isotope effects. Following experimental designs which have already been established in laboratory animals, this could yield information about the kinetics of formation, transport and utilization of free and esterified forms of Ch, which is badly needed in the human subject. This may well provide the insight necessary to understand the neurochemical changes accompanying some kinds of cholinergic dysfunction in man and its more rational management.

ACKNOWLEDGEMENTS

I would like to thank Kevin Haynes for his expert bibliographic assistance and Flo Comes for her excellent editorial work and final preparation of the manuscript. The unpublished research reported herein was supported by USPHS grant MH-17691.

*Assuming a cholinesterase activity of 5 mmole/1/min and a Michaelis constant of 2×10^{-4} mole/1, the time constant for hydrolysis of ACh in high dilution would be 2.4 s.

**Assuming a cholinesterase activity of 60 μmole/1/min (Duvoisin and Dettbarn, 1967) and a Michaelis constant of 2×10^{-4} mole/1, the time constant for hydrolysis of ACh at high dilution would be approximately 3 min.

REFERENCES

Ansell, G.B., and Spanner, S., 1970, The origin and turnover of choline in the brain, in *"Drugs and Cholinergic Mechanisms in the CNS"* (E. Heilbronn, and A. Winter, eds.), pp. 143-162, Res. Inst. Natl. Defence, Stockholm.

Ansell, G.B., and Spanner, S., 1971, Studies on the origin of choline in the brain of the rat, *Biochem. J. 122:*741.

Ansell, G.B., and Spanner, S., 1977, The source of choline for acetylcholine synthesis, in *"Cholinergic Mechanisms and Psychopharmacology"* (D.J. Jenden, ed.), pp. 431-445, Plenum Press, New York.

Aquilonius, S.M., 1977, Role of acetylcholine in the central nervous system, in *"Metabolic and Deficiency Diseases of the Nervous System Part III"* (H.L. Klawans, ed.), pp. 435-458, North-Holland Publishing Company, New York.

Aquilonius, S.M., and Eckernas, S.A., 1975, Plasma concentration of free choline in patients with Huntington's chorea on high doses of choline chloride, *N. Engl. J. Med. 293:*1105.

Aquilonius, S.M., and Eckernas, S.A., 1976a, Free choline (Ch) in plasma from healthy volunteers and patients on high oral doses of Ch, *Acta Physiol. Scand. (Suppl) 440:*114.

Aquilonius, S.M., and Eckernas, S.A., 1976b, Choline acetyltransferase in human cerebrospinal fluid: non-enzymatically and enzymatically catalyzed acetylcholine synthesis, *J. Neurochem. 27:*317.

Aquilonius, S.M., and Eckernas, S.A., 1977, Choline therapy in Huntington's chorea, *Neurology 27:*887.

Aquilonius, S.M., and Winbladh, B., 1971, Cerebrospinal fluid clearance of choline, *Acta Pharmacol. Toxicol. (Kbh.) 29:*64.

Aquilonius, S.M., Schuberth, J., and Sundwall, A., 1970, Choline in the cerebrospinal fluid as a marker for the release of acetylcholine, in *"Drugs and Cholinergic Mechanisms in the CNS"* (E. Heilbronn, and A. Winter, eds.), pp. 399-407, Res. Inst. Natl. Defence, Stockholm.

Aquilonius, S.M., Nystrom, B., Schuberth, J., and Sundwall, A., 1972, Cerebrospinal fluid choline in extrapyramidal disorders, *J. Neurol. Neurosurg. Psychiatry 35:*720.

Aquilonius, S.M., Ceder, G., Lying-Tunnell, U., Malmlund, H.O. and Schuberth, J., 1975, The arteriovenous difference of choline across the brain of man, *Brain Res. 99:*430.

Barbeau, A., 1976, Six years of high level levodopa therapy in severely akinetic Parkinsonian patients, *Arch. Neurol. 33:*333.

Barbeau, A., 1978, Emerging treatments: replacement therapy with choline or lecithin in neurological diseases, *Can. J. Neurol. Sci. 5:*157.

Barker, L.A., 1976, Modulation of synaptosomal high affinity choline transport, *Life Sci. 18:*725.

Barker, L.A., and Mittag, T.W., 1975, Comparative studies of substrates and inhibitors of choline transport and choline acetyltransferase, *J. Pharmacol. Exp. Ther. 192:*86.

Berman, R., Wilson, I.B., and Nachmansohn, D., 1953, Choline acetylase specificity in relation to biological function, *Biochim. Biophys. Acta 12:*315.

Bhatnagar, S.P., and MacIntosh, F.C., 1967, Effects of quaternary bases and inorganic cations on acetylcholine synthesis in nervous tissue, *Can. J. Physiol. Pharmacol. 45:*249.

Bird, E.D., and Iversen, L.L., 1974, Huntington's chorea: postmortem measurement of glutonic acid decarboxylase, choline acetyltransferase and dopamine in basal ganglia, *Brain 97:*457.

Birks, R., and MacIntosh, F.C., 1961, Acetylcholine metabolism of a sympathetic ganglion, *Can. J. Biochem. Physiol. 39:*787.

Blass, J.P., and Gibson, G.E., 1977, Cholinergic systems and disorders of carbohydrate catabolism, in *"Cholinergic Mechanisms and Psychopharmacology"* (D.J. Jenden, ed.), pp. 791-803, Plenum Press, New York.

Blaustein, M.P., and Goldring, J.M., 1975, Membrane potentials in pinched-off presynaptic nerve terminals monitored with a fluorescent probe: evidence that synaptosomes have potassium diffusion potentials, *J. Physiol. (Lond.) 247:*589.

Bligh, J., 1952, The level of free choline in plasma, *J. Physiol. (Lond.) 117:*234.

Bligh, J., 1953, The role of the liver and the kidneys in the maintenance of the level of free choline in plasma, *J. Physiol. (Lond.) 120:*53.

Botticelli, L.J., Lytle, L.D., and Wurtman, R.J., 1977, Choline induced attenuation of morphine analgesia in the rat, *Commun. Psychopharmacol. 1:*519.

Boyd, W.D., Graham-White, J., Blackwood, G., Glen, I., and McQueen, J., 1977, Clinical effects of choline in Alzheimer senile dementia, *Lancet 2:*711.

Browning, E.T., 1971, Free choline formation by cerebral cortical slices from rat brain, *Biochem. Biophys. Res. Commun. 45:*1586.

Burt, A.M., and Silver, A., 1973, Non-enzymatic imidazole-catalyzed acetyl transfer reaction and acetylcholine synthesis, *Nature (New Biol.) 243:*157.

Carson, V.G., Jenden, D.J., Cho, A.K., and Green, R., 1976, Effects of the choline acetyltransferase inhibitor 3'chloro-4-stilbazole, *Biochem. Pharmacol. 25:*195.

Cheney, D.L., Gubler, C.J., and Jaussi, A.W., 1969, Production of acetylcholine in rat brain following thiamine deprivation and treatment with thiamine antagonists, *J. Neurochem. 16:*1283.

Cheney, D.L., Racagni, G., and Costa, E., 1976, Appendix II: Distribution of acetylcholine and choline acetyltransferase in specific nuclei and tracts of rat brain, in *"Biology of Cholinergic Function"* (A.M. Goldberg, and I. Hanin, eds.), pp. 655-659, Raven Press, New York.

Cheng, S.C., and Nakamura, R., 1970, A study on the tricarboxylic acid cycle and the synthesis of acetylcholine in the lobster nerve, *Biochem. J. 118:*451.

Cho, A.K., Jenden, D.J., and Lamb, S.I., 1972, Rates of alkaline hydrolysis and muscarinic activity of some amino acids and their quaternary ammonium analogs, *J. Med. Chem. 15:*391.

Choi, R.L., Roch, M., and Jenden, D.J., 1973, A regional study of acetylcholine turnover in rat brain and the effect of oxotremorine, *Proc. West. Pharmacol. Soc. 16:*188.

Choi, R.L., Freeman, J.J., and Jenden, D.J., 1975, Kinetics of plasma choline in relation to turnover of brain choline and formation of acetylcholine, *J. Neurochem. 24:*735.

Cohen, E.L., and Wurtman, R.J., 1975, Brain acetylcholine: increase after systemic choline administration, *Life Sci. 16:*1095.

Cohen, E.L., and Wurtman, R.J., 1976, Brain acetylcholine: control by dietary choline, *Science 191:*561.

Collier, B., and MacIntosh, F.C., 1969, The source of choline for acetylcholine synthesis in a sympathetic ganglion, *Can. J. Physiol. Pharmacol. 47:*127.

Consolo, S., Ladinsky, H., Bianchi, S., and Caraceni, T., 1977, The cerebrospinal fluid choline levels in patients with Huntington's chorea, *Arch. Psychiatr. Nervenkr. 223:* 265.

Cooper, S.D., and Feuer, G., 1973, Effects of drugs or hepatotoxins on the relation between drug-metabolizing activity and phospholipids in hepatic microsomes during choline deficiency, *Toxicol. Appl. Pharmacol. 25:*7.

Cornford, E.M., Braun, L.D., and Oldendorf, W.H., 1978, Carrier mediated blood-brain barrier transport of choline and certain choline analogs, *J. Neurochem. 30:*299.

Dahlberg, L., and Schuberth, J., 1977, Regulation of plasma choline by base exchange, *J. Neurochem. 29:*933.

Danysz, A., Kocmierska-Grodzka, D., Kostro, B., Polocki, B., and Kruszcuska, J., 1967, Pharmacological properties of 2-dimethylaminoethanol (bimanol-DMAE) Part II. An analysis of the pharmacological action of DMAE upon the CNS, *Diss. Pharm. Pharmacol. 19:*469.

Davis, K.L., and Berger, P.A., 1978, Pharmacological investigations of the cholinergic imbalance hypotheses of movement disorders and psychosis, *Biol. Psychiatry 13:*23.

Davis, K.L., Berger, P.A., and Hollister, L.E., 1975a, Choline for tardive dyskinesia, *N. Engl. J. Med. 293:*152.

Davis, K.L., Hollister, L.E., Berger, P.A., and Barchas, J.D., 1975b, Cholinergic imbalance hypotheses of psychoses and movement disorders: strategies for evaluation, *Psychopharmacol. Commun. 1:*533.

Davis, K.L., Hollister, L.E., Barchas, J.D., and Berger, P.A., 1976, Choline in tardive dyskinesia and Huntington's disease, *Life Sci. 19:*1507.

Davis, K.L., Berger, P.A., and Hollister, L.E., 1977a, Cholinergic mechanisms in tardive dyskinesia and Huntington's chorea, in *"Neurotransmitter Function"* (W.S. Fields, ed.), pp. 247-262, Symposia Specialists Medical Books, New York.

Davis, K.L., Berger, P.A., Hollister, L.E., DoAmaral, J.R., and Barchas, J.D., 1977b, Cholinergic dysfunction in mania and movement disorders, in *"Cholinergic Mechanisms and Psychopharmacology"* (D.J. Jenden, ed.) pp. 755-779, Plenum Press, New York.

Davis, K.L., Berger, P.A., Hollister, L.E., and Defraites, E., 1978, Physostigmine in mania, *Arch. Gen. Psychiatry 35:*119.

Davis, K.L., Berger, P.A., Hollister, L.E., and Barchas, J.D., (in press), Cholinergic involvement in mental disorders, *Life Sci.*

de la Huerga, J., and Popper, H., 1951, Urinary excretion of choline metabolites following choline administration in normals and patients with hepatobiliary diseases, *J. Clin. Invest. 30:*463.

Diamond, I., 1971, Choline metabolism in brain: the role of choline transport and the effects of phenobarbital, *Arch. Neurol. 24:*333.

Di Pietro, D., and Weinhouse, S., 1959, Glucose oxidation in rat brain slices and homogenates, *Arch. Biochem. Biophys. 80:*268.

Dormard, Y., Levron, J.C., and LeFur, J.M., 1975, Pharmacokinetic study of maleate acid of 2-(N,N-dimethylaminoethanol-$^{14}C_1$)-cyclohexylpropionate (cyprodenate) and of N,N-dimethylaminoethanol-$^{14}C_1$ in annals II. Study and identification of the metabolites of ^{14}C-cyproclinate and ^{14}C-dimethylaminoethanol in animals. *Arzneim. Forsch. 25:*201.

Drachman, D.A., 1977, Memory and cognitive function in man: does the cholinergic system have a specific role? *Neurology 27:*783.

Dreyfus, P., 1975, Identification de l'acetate comme precurseur du rocidal acetate de l'acetylcholine des junctions neuromusculaires du rat, *Cr. Acad. Sci. Paris Ser. D 280:*1893.

Dross, K., and Kewitz, H., 1972, Concentration and origin of choline in the rat brain, *Naunyn Schmiedebergs Arch. Pharmacol. 274:*91.

DuVigneaud, V., Chandler, J.P., Simmonds, S., Moyer, A.W., and Cohen, M., 1946, The role of dimethyl- and monoethylaminoethanol in transmethylating reactions *in vivo*, *J. Biochem. 164:*603.

Duvoisin, R.C., and Dettbarn, W.D., 1967, Cerebrospinal fluid acetylcholine in man, *Neurology 17:*1077.

Eckernas, S.A., 1977, Plasma choline and cholinergic mechanisms in the brain: methods, function and role in Huntington's chorea, *Acta Physiol. Scand. (Suppl) 449:*1.

Eckernas, S.A., and Aquilonius, S.M., 1977, Free choline in human plasma analyzed by simple radio-enzymatic procedure: age distribution and effect of a meal, *Scand. J. Clin. Lab. Invest. 37:*183.

Eckernas, S.A., Sahlstrom, L., and Aquilonius, S.M., 1977, *In vivo* turnover rate of acetylcholine in rat brain parts at elevated steady-state concentration of plasma choline, *Acta Physiol. Scand. 101:*404.

Enna, S.J., Bird, E.D., Bennett, J.P., Bylund, D.B., Yamamura, H.I., Iversen, L.L., and Synder, S.H., 1976, Huntington's chorea: changes in neurotransmitter receptors in the brain, *N. Engl. J. Med. 94:*1305.

Fitzgerald, G.G., and Cooper, J.R., 1971, Acetylcholine as a possible sensory mediator in rabbit corneal epithelium, *Biochem. Pharmacol. 20:*2741.

Fonnum, F., 1970, Subcellular localization of choline acetyltransferase, in *"Drugs and Cholinergic Mechanisms in the CNS"* (E. Heilbronn, and A. Winter, eds.), pp. 83-95, Res. Inst. Natl. Defence, Stockholm.

Fonnum, F., 1973, Recent developments in biochemical investigations of cholinergic transmission, *Brain Res. 62:*497.

Freeman, J.J., and Jenden, D.J., 1976, Minireview: the source of choline for acetylcholine synthesis in brain, *Life Sci. 19:*949.

Freeman, J.J., Choi, R.L., and Jenden, D.J., 1975, Plasma choline: its turnover and exchange with brain choline, *J. Neurochem. 24:*729.

Gibson, G.E., and Blass, J.P., 1976a, Inhibition of acetylcholine synthesis and of carbohydrate utilization by maple-syrup urine disease metabolites, *J. Neurochem. 26:*1073.

Gibson, G.E., and Blass, J.P., 1976b, Impaired synthesis of acetylcholine in brain accompanying mild hypoxia and hypoglycemia, *J. Neurochem. 27:*37.

Gibson, G.E., Jope, R., and Blass, J.P., 1975, Decreased synthesis of acetylcholine accompanying impaired oxidation of pyruvic acid in rat brain minces, *Biochem. J. 148:*17.

Glover, V.A.S., and Potter, L.T., 1971, Purification and properties of choline acetyltransferase from ox brain striate nuclei, *J. Neurochem. 18:*571.

Goldberg, A.M., and Silbergeld, E.K., 1974, Neurochemical aspects of lead-induced hyperactivity, *Trans. Am. Soc. Neurochem. 5:*185.

Green, A.R., Boullin, D.J., Massarelli, R., and Hanin, I., 1972, Can the human blood platelet be used as a model for the cholinergic nerve endings? *Life Sci. 11:*1049.

Groth, D.P., Bain, J.A., and Pfeiffer, C.C., 1958, The comparative distribution of C^{14}-labelled 2-dimethylaminoethanol and choline in the mouse, *J. Pharmacol. Exp. Ther. 124:*290.

Growdon, J.H., Cohen, E.L., and Wurtman, R.J., 1977a, Treatment of brain disease with dietary precursors of neurotransmitters, *Ann. Int. Med. 86:*337.

Growdon, J.H., Cohen, E.L., and Wurtman, R.J., 1977b, Huntington's disease: clinical and chemical effects of choline administration, *Ann. Neurol. 1:*418.

Growdon, J.H., Cohen, E.L., and Wurtman, R.J., 1977c, Effects of oral choline administration on serum and CSF choline levels in patients with Huntington's disease, *J. Neurochem. 28:*229.

Growdon, J.H., Hirsch, M.J., Wurtman, R.J., and Wiener, W., 1977d, Oral choline administration to patients with tardive dyskinesia, *N. Engl. J. Med. 297:*524.

Haga, T., and Noda, H., 1973, Choline uptake systems of rat brain synaptosomes, *Biochim. Biophys. Acta 291:*564.

Hanin, I., 1974, *"Choline and Acetylcholine: Handbook of Chemical Assay Methods"* Raven Press, New York.

Hanin, I., and Schuberth, J., 1974, Labeling of acetylcholine in the brain of mice fed on a diet containing deuterium labeled choline: studies utilizing gas chromatography mass spectrometry, *J. Neurochem. 23:*819.

Hanin, I., Kopp, U., Zahniser, N.H., Shih, T.M., Spiker, D.G., Merikangas, J.R., Kupfer, D.J., and Foster, F.G., 1977, Acetylcholine and choline in human plasma and red blood cells: a gas chromatograph mass spectrometric evaluation, in *"Cholinergic Mechanisms and Psychopharmacology"* (D.J. Jenden, ed.), pp. 181-195, Plenum Press, New York.

Haubrich, D.R., and Chippendale, T.J., 1977, Minireview: regulation of acetylcholine synthesis in nervous tissue, *Life Sci. 20:*1465.

Haubrich, D.R., Wang, P.F.L., and Wedeking, P., 1974a, Role of choline in biosynthesis of acetylcholine, *Fed. Proc. 33:*477.

Haubrich, D.R., Wedeking, P.W., and Wang, P.F.L., 1974b, Increase in tissue concentration of acetylcholine in guinea pigs *in vivo* induced by administration of choline, *Life Sci. 14:*921.

Haubrich, D.R., Wang, P.F.L., Clody, D.E., and Wedeking, P.W., 1975, Increase in rat brain acetylcholine induced by choline or deanol, *Life Sci. 17:*975.

Haubrich, D.R., Wang, P.F.L., Chippendale, T., and Procter, E., 1976, Choline and acetylcholine in rats: effect of dietary choline, *J. Neurochem. 27:*1305.

Heinrich, C.P., Stadler, H., and Weiser, H., 1973, The effect of thiamine deficiency on the acetylcoenzymeA and acetylcholine levels in the rat brain, *J. Neurochem. 21:*1273.

Higgins, T., Chaykin, S., Hammond, K.B., and Humbert, J.R., 1972, Trimethylamine N-oxide synthesis: a human variant, *Biochem. Med. 6:*392.

Hirsch, M.J., and Wurtman, R.J., 1978, Acute lecithin consumption elevates brain acetylcholine content, *Fed. Proc. 37:*3164.

Hirsch, M.J., Growdon, J.H., and Wurtman, R.J., 1977a, Increase in hippocampal acetylcholine after choline administration, *Brain Res. 125:*383.

Hirsch, M.J., Growdon, J.H., and Wurtman, R.J., 1977b, Oral choline administration to patients with tardive dyskinesia, *Neurology 27:*391.

Hosein, E.A., Chabrol, J.G., and Freedman, G., 1966, The effect of thiamine deficiency in rats and pigeons on the content of materials with acetylcholine-like activity in brain, heart and skeletal muscle, *Rev. Can. Biol. 25:*129.

Illingsworth, D.R., and Portman, O.W., 1972, The uptake and metabolism of plasma lysophosphatidylcholine *in vivo* by the brain of squirrel monkeys, *Biochem. J. 130:*557.

Israel, M., and Tucek, S., 1974, Utilization of acetate and pyruvate for the synthesis of "total," "bound," and "free" acetylcholine in the electric organ of Torpedo, *J. Neurochem. 22:*487.

Janowsky, D.S., El-Yousef, M.K., Davis, J.M., and Sekerke, M.J., 1972, A cholinergic-adrenergic hypothesis of mania and depression, *Lancet 2:*632.

Janowsky, D.S., El-Yousef, M.K., Davis, J.M., and Sekerke, H.J., 1973, Parasympathetic suppression of manic symptoms by physostigmine, *Arch. Gen. Psychiatry 28:*542.

Jenden, D.J., 1977a, *"Cholinergic Mechanisms and Psychopharmacology"* (D.J. Jenden, ed.), Plenum Press, New York.

Jenden, D.J., 1977b, Some recent developments in the biochemical pharmacology of cholinergic systems, in *"Neuroregulators and Psychiatric Disorders"* (E. Usdin, D.A. Hamburg, and J.D. Barchas, eds.), pp. 425-433, Oxford University Press, New York.

Jenden, D.J., 1977c, Estimation of acetylcholine and the dynamics of its metabolism, in *"Cholinergic Mechanisms and Psychopharmacology"* (D.J. Jenden, ed.), pp. 139-162, Plenum Press, New York.

Jenden, D.J., 1978, Applications of gas chromatography mass spectrometry in psychopharmacology, in *"Psychopharmacology: A Generation of Progress"* (M.A. Lipton, A. Di Mascio, and K.F. Killam, eds.), pp. 879-886, Raven Press, New York.

Jenden, D.J., Jope, R.S., and Weiler, M.H., 1976, Regulation of acetylcholine synthesis: does cytoplasmic acetylcholine control high affinity choline uptake, *Science 194:*635.

Jenden, D.J., Macri, J., Roch, M., and Russell, R.W., 1977, Antagonism by deanol of some behavioral effects of hemicholinium, *Commun. Psychopharmacol. 1:*575.

Jenden, D.J., Roch, M., and Fainman, F., (in press), Estimation of deanol and choline by gas chromatography mass spectrometry, *Life Sci.*

Johnson, S., and Domino, E.F., 1971, Cholinergic enzymatic activity of cerebrospinal fluid of patients with various neurologic diseases, *Clin. Chim. Acta 35:*421.

Jonsson, L.E., and Schuberth, J., 1969, Amphetamine effect on the choline concentration of human cerebrospinal fluid, *Life Sci. 8:*977.

Jope, R.S., 1977, Pyruvate utilization choline uptake and acetylcholine synthesis, in *"Cholinergic Mechanisms and Psychopharmacology"* (D.J. Jenden, ed.), pp. 497-509, Plenum Press, New York.

Jope, R.S., and Jenden, D.J., 1977, Synaptosomal transport and acetylation of choline, *Life Sci. 20:*1389.

Jope, R.S., and Jenden, D.J., 1978, Deanol utilization by rat brain, *Fed. Proc. 37:*3164.

Jope, R.S., Weiler, M.H., and Jenden, D.J., (in press), Regulation of acetylcholine synthesis: control of choline transport and acetylation in synaptosomes, *J. Neurochem.*

Kahlson, G., and MacIntosh, F.C., 1939, Acetylcholine synthesis in a sympathetic ganglion, *J. Physiol. 96:*277.

Kato, A.C., Lefresne, P., Berwald-Netter, Y., Beaujouan, J.C., Glowinski, J., and Gros, F., 1977, Choline stimulates the synthesis and accumulation of acetate in a cholinergic neuroblastoma clone, *Biochem. Biophys. Res. Commun. 78:*350.

Kewitz, H., and Pleul, O., 1976, Synthesis of choline from ethanolamine in rat brain, *Proc. Natl. Acad. Sci. USA 73:*2181.

Knapp, D.R., and Gaffney, T.E., 1972, Use of stable isotopes in pharmacology — clinical pharmacology, *Clin. Pharmacol. Ther. 13:*307.

Korey, S.R., de Braganza, B., and Nachmansohn, D., 1951, Choline acetylase: V. esterification and transacetylations, *J. Biol. Chem. 189:*705.

Krell, R.D., and Goldberg, A.M., 1975, Effect of choline acetyltransferase inhibitors on mouse and guinea pig brain choline and acetylcholine, *Biochem. Pharmacol. 24:*391.

Kuhar, M.J., and Murrin, L.C., 1978, Sodium-dependent high affinity choline uptake, *J. Neurochem. 30:*15.

Kuhar, M.J., Sethy, V.H., Roth, R.H., and Aghajanian, G.K., 1973, Choline: selective accumulation by central cholinergic neurons, *J. Neurochem. 20:*581.

Kuntscherova, J., 1971, Vliv kratkodobeho bladoveni na hladinu volneho cholinu v krevni plasme bilych krys, *Plzen. Lek. Sborn. 36:*17.

Kuntscherova, J., 1972, Effect of short-term starvation and choline on the acetylcholine content of organs of albino rats, *Physiol. Bohemoslov. 21:*655.

Kuntscherova, J., and Vlk, J., 1968, Uber die bedeutung der cholin und glukosezufuhr fur die normalisierung der durch hungern herabgesetzten acetylcholinvorrate in der geweben, *Plzen. Lek. Sborn. 31:*5.

Kvetnansky, R., Weise, V.K., and Kopin, I.J., 1970, Elevation of adrenal tyrosine hydroxylase and phenylethanolamine-N-methyl transferase by repeated immobilization of rats, *Endocrinology 87:*744.

L'Hermite, P., and Levy, J.C., 1975, Contingency of the action of the dimethylamino-ethanol and of its esters as precursors of the choline during the synthesis of acetyl-choline, *Ann. Pharm. Fr. 33:*137.

Manaka, S., Sano, K., Fuchinoue, T., and Sekino, H., 1974, Mechanism of action of CDP-choline in Parkinsonism. *Experientia 30:*179.

Martin, K., 1972, Extracellular cations and the movement of choline across the erythrocyte membrane, *J. Physiol. 224:*207.

Martin, K., 1974, Effects of lithium on choline transport in synaptosomes and human erythrocytes, in *"Drugs and Transport Processes"* (B.A. Callingham, ed.), pp. 347-361, University Park Press, Baltimore.

McGeer, P.L., McGeer, E.G., and Fibiger, H.C., 1973, Choline acetylase and glutanic acid decarboxylase in Huntington's chorea, *Neurology 23:*912.

Morel, M.N., 1975, Incorporation d'acetate dons l'acetylcholine de l'organe electrique de torpille: effets des concentrations d'acetate et de choline, *Cr. Acad. Sci. Paris Ser. D. 250:*999.

Morley, B.J., Robinson, G.R., Brown, G.B., Kemp, G.E., and Bradley, R.J., 1977, Effects of dietary choline on nicotinic acetylcholine receptors in brain, *Nature 266:*848.

Murrin, L.C., Morgenroth III, V.H., and Roth, R.H., 1976, Dopaminergic neurons: effects of electrical stimulation on tyrosine hydroxylase. *Mol. Pharmacol. 12:*1070.

Nagler, A.L., Dettbarn, W.D., Seifter, E., and Levenson, S.M., 1968, Tissue levels of acetylcholine and acetylcholinesterase in weanling rats subjected to acute choline deficiency. *J. Nutr. 94:*13.

Nordberg, A., 1977, Apparent regional turnover of acetylcholine in mouse brain, *Acta Physiol. Scand. S455:*1.

Nordberg, A., and Sundwall, A., 1975, Effect of pentobarbital on endogenous acetyl-choline and biotransformation of radioactive choline in different brain regions, in *"Cholinergic Mechanisms"* (P.G. Waser, ed.), pp. 229-239, Raven Press, New York.

Oesch, F., 1974, Trans-synaptic induction of choline acetyltransferase in the preganglionic neuron of the peripheral sympathetic nervous system. *J. Pharmacol. Exp. Ther. 188:*439.

Ogashiwa, M., Takeuchi, K., Hara, M., Tanaka, Y., and Okada, J., 1975, Studies on the intrathecal pharmacotherapy Part I: CDP-choline. *Int. J. Clin. Pharmacol. 12:*327.

Okonek, S., and Kilbinger, H., 1974, Determination of acetylcholine, nitrostigmine and acetylcholinesterase activity in four patients with severe nitrostigmine (E605 forte) intoxication. *Arch. Toxicol. 32:*97.

Oldendorf, W.H., and Braun, L.D., 1976, [^{3}H]-Tryptoamine and ^{3}H-water as diffusible internal standards for measuring brain extraction of radiolabelled substances following carotid injection. *Brain Res. 113:*219.

Osuide, G., 1968, Dimethylaminoethanol and neuromuscular transmission. *W. Afr. J. Biol. Appl. Chem. 11:*66.

Pardridge, W.M., and Oldendorf, W.H., 1977, Transport of metabolic substrates through the blood brain barrier. *J. Neurochem. 28:*5.

Patrick, R.L., and Kirshner, N., 1971, Effect of stimulation on the levels of tryrosine hydroxylase, dopamine β-hydroxylase and catecholamines in intact and denervated rat adrenal glands. *Mol. Pharmacol. 7:*87.

Pepeu, G., Freedman, D.X., and Giarman, N.J., 1960, Biochemical and pharmacological studies of dimethylaminoethanol (deanol), *J. Pharmacol. Exp. Ther. 129:*291.

Pfeiffer, C.C., 1959, Parasympathetic neurohumors; possible precursors and effect on behavior, *Int. Rev. Neurobiol. 1:*195.

Pfeiffer, C.C., Jenney, E.H., and Gallagher, W., 1957, Stimulant effect of 2-dimethylaminoethanol — possible precursor of brain acetylcholine, *Science 126:*610.

Pieklik, J.R., and Guynn, R.W., 1975, Equilibrium constants of the reactions of choline acetyltransferase, carnitine acetyltransferase and acetylcholinesterase under physiological conditions, *J. Biol. Chem. 250:*4445.

Polak, R.L., Molenaar, P.C., and Braggaar-Schaap, P., 1977, Regulation of acetylcholine synthesis in rat brain, in *"Cholinergic Mechanisms and Psychopharmacology"* (D.J. Jenden, ed.), pp. 511-524, Plenum Press, New York.

Quastel, J.H., 1977, Source of the acetyl group in acetylcholine, in *"Cholinergic Mechanisms and Psychopharmacology"* (D.J. Jenden, ed.), pp. 411-430, Plenum Press, New York.

Quastel, J.H., Tennenbaum, M., and Wheatley, A.H.M., 1936, Choline ester formation in, and choline esterase activities of, tissues *in vitro*, *Biochem. J. 30:*1668.

Racagni, G., Trabucchi, M., and Cheney, D.L., 1975, Steady-state concentrations of choline and acetylcholine in rat brain parts during a constant rate infusion of deuterated choline, *Naunyn Schmiedebergs Arch. Pharmacol. 290:*99.

Rennick, B., Acara, M., Hysert, P., and Mookerjee, B., 1976, Choline loss during hemodialysis: homeostatic control of plasma choline concentrations, *Kidney Int. 10:*329.

Reynolds, S.F., 1974, The distribution of pyruvate dehydrogenase in the cat central nervous system in relation to normal and abnormal neural function, Ph.D. dissertation, University of California Los Angeles.

Reynolds, S.F., and Blass, J.P., 1975, Normal levels of acetyl coenzyme A and of acetylcholine in the brains of thiamine-dependent rats, *J. Neurochem. 24:*185.

Rossier, J., and Benda, P., 1977, Activation of choline acetyltransferase by chloride: a possible regulatory mechanism, in *"Cholinergic Functions and Psychopharmacology"* (D.J. Jenden, ed.), pp. 207-221, Plenum Press, New York.

Salvadorini, F., Galeone, F., Nicotera, M., Ombrato, M., and Saba, P., 1975, Clinical evaluation of CDP-choline (Nicholin[R]): efficacy as antidepressant treatment, *Curr. Ther. Res. 18:*513.

Sastry, P.S., and Stancer, H.C., 1968, Quantitative analysis and fatty acid composition of phospholipid constituents in cerebrospinal fluid of various age groups, *Clin. Chim. Acta 22:*301.

Scally, M.C., Ulus, I.H., and Wurtman, R.J., (in press), Choline administration to the rat increases urinary catecholamines, *Naunyn Schmiedebergs Arch. Pharmacol.*

Schain, R.J., 1960, Neurohumors and other pharmacologically active substances in cerebrospinal fluid: a review of the literature, *Yale J. Biol. Med. 33:*15.

Schuberth, J., 1977, Central cholinergic dysfunction in man: clinical manifestations and approaches to diagnosis and treatment, in *"Cholinergic Mechanisms and Psychopharmacology"* (D.J. Jenden, ed.), pp. 733-745, Plenum Press, New York.

Schuberth, J., and Jenden, D.J., 1975, Transport of choline from plasma CSF in the rabbit with reference to the origin of choline and to acetylcholine metabolism in the brain, *Brain Res. 84:*245.

Schuberth, J., Sparf, B., and Sundwall, A., 1969, A technique for the study of acetylcholine turnover in mouse brain *in vivo*, *J. Neurochem. 16:*695.

Schuberth, J., Sparf, B., and Sundwall, A., 1970, On the turnover of acetylcholine in nerve endings of mouse brain *in vivo*, *J. Neurochem. 17:*461.

Schultz, S.G., and Curran, P.F., 1973, Coupled transport of sodium and organic solutes, *Physiol. Rev. 50:*637.

Shea, P.A., and Aprison, M.H., 1977, Distribution of acetyl-CoA in specific areas of the CNS of the rat as measured by a modification of a radio-enzymatic assay for acetylcholine and choline, *J. Neurochem. 28:*51.

Simon, J.R., Atweh, S., and Kuhar, M.J., 1976, Sodium-dependent high affinity choline uptake: a regulatory step in the synthesis of acetylcholine, *J. Neurochem. 26:*909.

Speeg, K.V., Chen, D., McCandless, D.W., and Schenker, S., 1970, Cerebral acetylcholine in thiamine deficiency, *Proc. Soc. Exp. Biol. Med. 134:*1005.

Stahl, W.L., and Swanson, P.D., 1974, Biochemical abnormalities in Huntington's chorea brains, *Neurology 24:*813.

Stavinoha, W.B., and Modak, A.T., 1976, Identification and quantitation of acetylcholine (ACh) in mouse blood, *Trans. Am. Soc. Neurochem. 7:*132.

Stavinoha, W.B., Weintraub, S.T., and Modak, A.T., 1974, Regional concentrations of choline and acetylcholine in the rat brain. *J. Neurochem. 23:*885.

Suszkiw, J.B., and Pilar, G., 1976, Selective localization of a high affinity choline uptake system and its role in ACh formation in cholinergic nerve terminals, *J. Neurochem. 26:*1133.

Suszkiw, J.B., Beach, R.C., and Pilar, G., 1976, Choline uptake by cholinergic neuron cell somas, *J. Neurochem. 26:*1123.

Tamminga, C., Smith, R.C., Chang, S., Haraszti, J.S., and Davis, J.M., 1976, Depression associated with oral choline, *Lancet 2:*905.

Tamminga, C.A., Smith, R.C., Ericksen, S.E., Chang, S., and Davis, J.M., 1977, Cholinergic influences in tardive dyskinesia. *Am. J. Psychiatry 134:*769.

Thoenen, H., 1974, Minireview: trans-synaptic enzyme induction, *Life Sci. 14:*223.

Tower, D.B., and McEachern, D., 1949a, Acetylcholine and neuronal activity I. cholinesterase patterns and acetylcholine in the cerebrospinal fluid of patients with craniocerebral trauma, *Can. J. Biochem. 27:*105.

Tower, D.B., and McEachern, D., 1949b, Acetylcholine and neuronal activity II. acetylcholine and cholinesterase activity in the cerebrospinal fluids of patients with epilepsy, *Can. J. Biochem. 27:*120.

Tucek, S., and Cheng, S.C., 1974, Provenance of the acetyl group of acetylcholine and compartmentation of acetyl-CoA and Krebs cycle intermediates in the brain *in vivo*, *J. Neurochem. 22:*893.

Ulus, I.H., and Wurtman, R.J., 1976, Choline administration: activation of tyrosine hydroxylase in dopaminergic neurons of rat brain, *Science 194:*1060.

Ulus, I.H., Hirsch, M.J., and Wurtman, R.J., 1977a, Trans-synaptic induction of adrenomedullary tyrosine hydroxylase activity by choline: evidence that choline administration can increase cholinergic transmission, *Proc. Natl. Acad. Sci. USA 74:*798.

Ulus, I.H., Scally, M.C., and Wurtman, R.J., 1977b, Choline potentiates the trans-synaptic induction of adrenal tyrosine hydroxylase by reserpine, probably by enhancing the release of acetylcholine, *Life Sci. 21:*145.

Ulus, I.H., Wurtman, R.J., Scally, M.C., and Hirsch, M.J., 1977c, Effect of choline on cholinergic function, in *"Cholinergic Mechanisms and Psychopharmacology"* (D.J. Jenden, ed.), pp. 525-528, Plenum Press, New York.

Ulus, I.H., Scally, M.C., and Wurtman, R.J., (in press), Potentiation by choline of the induction of adrenal tyrosine hydroxylase by phenoxybenzamine, 6-hydroxydopamine, insulin or exposure to cold, *J. Pharmacol. Exp. Ther.*

Van Woert, M.H., 1976, Parkinson's disease, tardive dyskinesia and Huntington's chorea, in *"Biology of Cholinergic Function"* (A. M. Goldberg, and I. Hanin, eds.), pp. 583-601, Raven Press, New York.

Vorhees, C.V., Schmidt, D.E., Barrett, R.J., and Schenker, S., 1977, Effects of thiamine deficiency on acetylcholine levels and utilization *in vivo* in rat brain, *J. Nutr. 107:* 1902.

Wecker, L., and Dettbarn, W.D., 1978, Differential control of acetylcholine levels in striatal and hippocampal areas of rat brain, *Fed. Proc. 37:*820.

Wecker, L., Dettbarn, W.D., and Schmidt, D.E., 1978, Choline administration: modification of the central actions of atropine, *Science 199:*86.

Weiler, M.H., Jope, R.S., and Jenden, D.J., (in press), Effect of pretreatment under various cationic conditions on acetylcholine content and choline transport in rat whole brain synaptosomes, *J. Neurochem.*

Weiss, B.L., Foster, F.G., and Kupfer, D.J., 1976, Cholinergic involvement in neuropsychiatric syndromes, in *"Biology of Cholinergic Function"* (A.M. Goldberg, and I. Hanin, eds.), pp. 603-617, Raven Press, New York.

Welsh, M.J., Markham, C.H., and Jenden, D.J., 1976, Acetylcholine and choline in cerebrospinal fluid of patients with Parkinson's disease and Huntington's chorea, *J. Neurol. Neurosurg. Psychiatry 39:*367.

White, H.L., and Wu, J.C., 1973, Kinetics of choline acetyltransferase (EC 2.3.1.6) from human and other mammalian control and peripheral nervous tissues, *J. Neurochem. 20:*297.

Wurtman, R.J., Hirsch, M.J., and Growdon, J.H., 1977, Lecithin consumption raises serum free choline levels, *Lancet 2:*68.

Yamamura, H.T., and Snyder, S.H., 1973, High affinity transport of choline into synaptosomes of rat brain, *J. Neurochem. 21:*1355.

Yamamura, H.I., Wastek, G.J., Johnson, P.C., and Stern, L.Z., 1977, Biochemical characterization of muscarinic cholinergic receptors in Huntington's disease, in *"Cholinergic Mechanisms and Psychopharmacology"* (D.J. Jenden, ed.), pp. 35-47, Plenum Press, New York.

Yavin, E., 1977, Base stimulation of phospholipid metabolism in neuroblastoma cells II. Estimates of rates of synthesis and degradation of phosphoglycerides by base manipulations, *Biochim. Biophys. Acta 489:*290.

Zahniser, N.R., 1977, Is 2-dimethylaminoethanol (deanol) a precursor of acetylcholine? A neurochemical and behavioral investigation, Ph.D. thesis, University of Pittsburgh, Pittsburgh, PA.

Zahniser, N.R., Chou, D., and Hanin, I., 1977, Is 2-dimethylaminoethanol (deanol) indeed a precursor of brain acetylcholine? A gas chromatographic evaluation, *J. Pharmacol. Exp. Ther. 200:*545.

CHOLINE AVAILABILITY – CHOLINE HIGH AFFINITY TRANSPORT AND THE REGULATION OF ACETYLCHOLINE SYNTHESIS

L. A. Barker

Department of Pharmacology, Mt. Sinai School of Medicine,
City University of New York, New York, N.Y. 10029

INTRODUCTION

The use of precursor-loading with choline as a therapeutic modality raises the question of whether the plasma levels of choline directly regulate the synthesis of (ACh) in brain. In this chapter, the issues of choline availability and the transport of choline by cholinergic nerve endings in the regulation of (ACh) formation will be discussed. Data are presented which suggest that under normal physiological conditions brain ACh levels and turnover are not regulated by the levels of free choline in plasma and that the physiologic regulatory step in ACh synthesis is the high affinity uptake of choline by cholinergic nerve endings.

CHOLINE METABOLISM IN THE CNS

Most choline in brain tissue, in neurons as well as glia, is present as precursors, products and catabolites of phospholipid metabolism (Ansell and Spanner, 1978). In 1 gm of whole brain about 20 μmole of choline are present in the phospholipid pathway, in contrast, there are about 20 nmole present as (ACh) and 25 nmole present as free choline.

Brain tissue has little to no capacity for the *de novo* synthesis of choline. Compared to liver, the brain has less than 1% of the enzymatic activities responsible for the sequential methylation of phosphatidylethanolamine by S-adenosylmethionine to form phosphatidylcholine (Bremer and Greenberg, 1961). The lack of conversion of ethanolamine or its precursor, serine, to free choline or choline-containing lipids by brain tissue has been confirmed in several studies. Ansell and Spanner (1967, 1968a) demonstrated that the intracerebral injection of ^{14}C-ethanolamine leads to the labelling of phosphatidylethanolamine but not phospholipids containing choline. On the other hand, the intracerebral administration of labelled choline readily results in the labelling of ACh and choline containing lipids (Ansell and Spanner, 1968b; Barker *et al.*, 1972; Dowdall *et al.*, 1972). Using brain slices, Browning and Schulman (1968) studied the metabolism of serine and ethanolamine; both of which are precursors to phosphatidylcholine in the liver. No labelling of any choline-containing compounds could be demonstrated when the brain slices were incubated with labelled serine or ethanolamine and unlabelled methionine. The same was true when labelled methionine and unlabelled enanolamine or serine were used.

Although brain does not appear to synthesize choline *de novo*, free choline can be formed from the catabolism of choline containing lipids, e.g. phosphatidylcholine or lysophosphatidylcholine (Dross, 1975) and by the breakdown of phosphorylcholine (Ansell and Spanner, 1968b). It is known that in certain laboratory animals and man there is an efflux of choline from brain, as is demonstrated by higher choline levels on the venous side than the arterial side of the cerebral circulation (Choi *et al.*, 1975; Dross and Kewitz, 1972; Freeman *et al.*, 1975; Spanner *et al.*, 1976; Aquilonius *et al.*, 1975). The capacity of brain tissue to liberate choline from a bound form is further seen by postmortem increases in free choline at a rate of 20 nmole/gm/min following decapitation (Dross and Kewitz, 1972). In animals killed by microwave irradiation, postmortem increases in brain choline and decreases in brain ACh are not seen (Butcher and Butcher, 1974; Stavinoha *et al.*, 1973), presumably due to the rapid inactivation of enzymes that catalyze the breakdown of choline containing compounds.

The importance of free choline in brain derived from endogenous choline containing phospholipids for the synthesis of ACh is not clearly understood. An observation critical at this point is that choline used for the synthesis of ACh is free choline that arises from a source that is extracellular to the site of synthesis (Browning and Schulman, 1968; Collier and MacIntosh, 1969). Thus, the sources of brain free choline, and the routes by which it gains entry to the brain and to cholinergic nerve terminals are important considerations in the regulation of ACh synthesis.

Sources of Free Choline in Brain

In the preceding section, the formation of free choline in brain from the enzymatic breakdown of choline containing lipids was presented. The sources of brain free choline to be discussed in this section are free choline and lysophosphatidylcholine present in plasma.

Plasma Lysophosphatidylcholine

The possibility that plasma phosphatidylcholine or lysophosphatidylcholine are taken up by brain and subsequently broken down to yield free choline was initially proposed by Ansell and Spanner (for a recent review see Ansell and Spanner, 1978). Experimental confirmation for this notion came from the work of Illingworth and Portman (1972). Using squirrel monkeys, it was shown that doubly labelled lysophosphatidylcholine (prepared as a mixture of $1\text{-}^{14}C$ palmityl labelled and $[\text{Me-}^{3}\text{H}]$ choline labelled lysophosphatidylcholine) bound to albumin and injected intravenously is taken up intact and then metabolized by the brain. The plasma clearance of labelled lysophosphatidylcholine is rapid and peak accumulation in brain, about 1% of the injected dose, occurs in 20 min. Of the lysophosphatidylcholine taken up, about 30% is broken down to yield free choline. This free choline, in turn, is further metabolized to ACh, phosphorylcholine and betaine, labelled acetylcholine accounting for about 30-40% of the radioactivity present as water soluble metabolites of choline. Lysophosphatidylcholine constitutes 5-20% of the total plasma phospholipids (about 2 μmole/ml) or 100 to 400 nmole of lysophosphatidylcholine/ml. The findings of Illingworth and Portman (1972) suggest that every 20 min 1 ml of plasma can supply 1-4 nmole of lysophosphatidyl-choline and hence 0.3-1.2 nmole of free choline to brain.

The contribution of brain phosphatidylcholine or lysophosphatidylcholine to free choline is not known at this time. The results of one study suggest that the contribution of plasma and/or brain phosphatidylcholine and/or lysophosphatidylcholine to free choline in brain shows a species variation. For the rat, choline derived from a lipid form may provide almost 90%, for the rabbit about 50% and for mice about 20% of brain free choline. The remainder appears to be derived from free choline in plasma (Schuberth and Jenden, 1975).

Plasma Free Choline

Free choline in plasma arises from dietary sources as well as from the catabolism of choline containing lipids in the liver. Choline is removed from plasma into tissues by a saturable uptake process as well as by free diffusion (see Barker, 1976a, Freeman and Jenden, 1976, for reviews). The half life of intravenously injected choline is less than 1 min (Freeman *et al.*, 1975; Haubrich *et al.*, 1975), consequently elevated plasma levels are cleared in a short time. The ability of tissues to clear plasma free choline can be over-come and plasma levels can be elevated by continuous infusions (Eckernas, 1977; Choi, 1974; Freeman *et al.*, 1975; Gardiner and Paton, 1972; Gardiner and Gwee, 1974) or by the oral or parenteral administration of large doses of choline or phosphatidylcholine (Cohen and Wurtman, 1975; Wurtman *et al.*, 1977). Modest but significant increases above fasting levels are obtained at one hour after a meal (Eckernas, 1977). The tissue levels of choline appear to be related to plasma levels, but ACh synthesis does not correlate well with choline uptake into tissues (Haubrich *et al.*, 1974; 1975). Peripheral tissues are much more active than the CNS in clearing free choline from plasma. Nonetheless, it has been demonstrated in several laboratories that an elevation of plasma choline is followed by increase in brain choline levels (Choi *et al.*, 1975; Freeman *et al.*, 1975; Haubrich *et al.*, 1974, 1975; Racagni *et al.*, 1975).

Choline uptake into brain from plasma is mediated by a saturable process with a parallel diffusional component (Diamond, 1971; Pardridge and Oldendorf, 1977; Sparf, 1973). The uptake of choline into brain can be described by simple Michaelis-Menten kinetics plus a diffusional term.

$$v = \frac{V_{max} \cdot S}{K_T + S} + D \cdot S \qquad (1)$$

where v is the velocity of unidirectional flux; V_{max} the maximal flux seen at saturating concentrations of substrate, S; K_T the concentration of S which yields one-half V_{max}, and D, a constant for the non-saturable transport process. The apparent K_T for choline transport into rat brain is 360 μM, the V_{max} is 8.5 nmole/min/gm and D is 0.005 ml/min /gm (calculations based on data from Oldendorf and Braun, 1976). At a plasma con-centration of 10 μM, the predicted initial velocity of influx of free choline from plasma to brain is only about 0.6 nmole/min/gm. This is in contrast to the net efflux of choline from brain to plasma which in the rat occurs at a rate of about 6 nmole/min/gm (Ansell and Spanner, 1978; Dross and Kewitz, 1972).

Although there is a net efflux of choline from brain to plasma, free choline in brain and plasma readily exchange as has been demonstrated by the labelling of brain ACh following the intravenous administration of labelled choline (Aquilonius *et al.*, 1973; Choi *et al.*, 1975; Saelens *et al.*, 1973) or by the feeding of labelled choline (Hanin and Schuberth, 1974; Schuberth and Jenden, 1975). When labelled choline is administered in the diet, the specific activities of plasma and brain choline reach a steady state after a few days. In general, the steady state specific activity of brain free choline is less than that of plasma choline (Hanin and Schuberth, 1974) as would be expected from the generation of free choline in brain from a less highly labelled source, e.g. phosphatidyl-choline. Similarly, at steady state the specific activity of plasma choline is greater than that of cisternal CSF choline ([choline] = 2.3 μM) (Schuberth and Jenden, 1975). This suggested that the efflux of choline from brain is to both the plasma and the CSF.

The concentration of free choline in rat brain remains quite constant at about 30 μM throughout a 24-hr period when animals are fed *ad libitum* either a regular diet or a choline deficient diet from birth to 21 weeks (Haubrich *et al.*, 1976). Clearly, as the data of Pardridge and Oldendorf (1977) suggest, the steady state levels of brain free choline are maintained from sources other than free choline taken up from the plasma. As noted above, such sources may be plasma lysophosphatidylcholine as well as free choline generated from the enzymatic breakdown of choline containing phospholipids (Dross, 1975) or phosphate esters of choline (Ansell and Spanner, 1978) present in brain tissue.

Free Choline and ACh Levels in Brain

The steady state levels of ACh and choline in rat brain appear to be quite stable (see Table 1). Although the elevation of plasma choline in the rat by experimental means can be followed by marked increases, 200-300%, in the concentration of free choline in the brain, the subsequent changes in the content of ACh are small in comparison. For example, 15 min after maintaining plasma choline levels at 140 μM, the levels of choline in the cerebral cortex and striatum nearly double but no changes in cortical levels of ACh are seen and only a 10% increase in striatal ACh is observed (Eckernas, 1977).

TABLE 1

Choline and ACh Levels in Selected Brain Regions of the Rat[a]

Region	Choline (nmol/gm)	ACh (nmol/gm)
Cerebral Cortex	17.6	21.8
Striatum	24.9	88.3
Hippocampus	26.3	28.4
Hypothalamus	26.9	31.3
Cerebellum	17.1	6.5
Brain Stem	14.3	31.9

[a]Data taken from Butcher *et al.*, (1976).

In other studies, the administration of choline, 0.4 mmole/kg, i.p., to rats produces after 20 min a 2-3 fold increase in whole brain choline and only at 40 min is a significant increase, 1.2-1.3 fold, in ACh seen (Cohen and Wurtman, 1975). Comparable changes in choline and ACh levels at these times are also seen in the caudate nucleus and the hippocampus (Hirsch *et al.*, 1977). Large increases, 50-80%, have been seen following the intraventricular administration of choline in amounts 40-80 times the total brain content of free choline (Haubrich and Chippendale, 1976). Other investigators have found that the administration of choline, 0.2, 0.4 or 0.8 mmole/kg, i.p. to rats, produces no increase in ACh levels in either the caudate nucleus or the cerebral cortex at 20, 40 or 60 min after injection of choline (Pedata *et al.*, 1977). These findings are summarized in Table 2.

TABLE 2

Effect of Choline on Whole Brain and Brain Region Levels of ACh

Region	Dose (mMol/kg)	Route	ACh Levels (nanomol/gm)[a]		Ref
			Control	Treated	
Whole brain	0.4	i.p.	100%[b]	120-130%[b]	1
Cerebral Cortex	0.8	i.p.	20.6	18.7	2
Caudate nucleus	0.4	i.p.	48.7	63.1	3
	0.4	i.p.	29.3	31.6	3
	0.8	i.p.	66.2	65.0	2
	2500 nmoles (Total dose)	intraventricular	27.0[c]	45.0[c]	4
Hippocampus	0.4	i.p.	14.2	29.6	3
	0.4	i.p.	19.9	23.6	3
	5000 nmoles (Total dose)	intraventricular	13.0[c]	19.0[c]	4

[a] Values for 40 min after treatment, unless noted otherwise, (c), animals sacrificed by microwave irradiation.

[b] Absolute values not given.

[c] Because of cannulae used for intraventricular injection, the rats could not be sacrificed by microwave irradiation.

References: 1. Cohen and Wurtman, 1975; 2. Pedata *et al.*, 1977; 3. Hirsch *et al.*, 1977; 4. Haubrich and Chippendale, 1976.

The steady state levels of a neurotransmitter do not reveal the dynamic events that take place in synaptic transmission. It is therefore conceivable that the elevated brain choline levels produce an increase ACh turnover due to release and as a result, no marked changes in steady state levels are seen. This hypothesis has been tested (Eckernas, 1977) and it has been found that elevated levels of free choline in either the cerebral cortex or the striatum are not accompanied by an increase in the turnover of ACh. In the striatum, a small decrease in the turnover rate of ACh was observed (Eckernas, 1977). These effects of choline are qualitatively similar to those seen with more potent cholinomimetics such as oxotremorine or pilocarpine. In general, centrally acting cholinergic agonists produce a decrease in ACh turnover and/or an increase in tissue levels of ACh (Hanin and Costa, 1976). The direct actions of choline at ACh receptors must therefore be considered in any interpretation of experimental results showing changes in ACh levels following the administration of choline. Similarly, the known effects of choline administration on the levels of other putative neurotransmitters should be considered. Namely, choline, 0.7 mmole/kg, i.p., produces decreases in the whole brain content of norepinephrine, dopamine, aspartate, glutamate, glycine and GABA (Smith *et al.*, 1977).

In view of the small and variable changes in ACh levels that accompany rather large, 2-3 fold, increases in choline levels and the lack of an increased turnover of ACh under conditions where plasma and brain choline are elevated, one can conclude that under normal conditions the plasma and/or extracellular tissue levels of free choline are more than sufficient to support the synthesis of ACh. The rate limiting step(s) appears to be distal to the blood-brain transport of choline or one of its precursors.

Cellular Localization of Choline Used for ACh Synthesis

Within a cholinergic neuron, the highest content of ACh and choline acetyltransferase (CAT) are present at the nerve endings of the cell (Whittaker *et al.*, 1964). In many respects, the nerve ending is a metabolically independent unit of the neuron (Whittaker, 1969). In particular, it contains the enzymes for glycolysis as well as mitochondria for oxidative metabolism and thus can synthesize the acetyl-S CoA required for local metabolic needs, among which is the synthesis of ACh as shown below (Tucek, 1970).

Choline and Acetyl-S CoA CAT Acetylcholine + CoA-SH

As would be expected, the major site of ACh synthesis is at the nerve endings of a cholinergic neuron from where it is released during synaptic transmission.

The content of free choline in the nerve endings of cholinergic neurons is not known, but there is reason to believe it may be quite low and probably not participate in the synthesis of ACh under normal physiological conditions (See Barker, 1976a). That the choline used for the synthesis of ACh arises from sites extracellular to the loci of synthesis was shown by Browning and Schulman (1968) for brain slices and by Collier and MacIntosh (1969) for cholinergic nerve endings in the superior cervical ganglion. Using the potent inhibitor of choline transport, hemicholinium-3 (HC-3), Browning and Schulman demonstrated that the synthesis of labelled ACh from either labelled choline or labelled glucose was inhibited. Under the conditions of their experiments, it was shown that the synthesis of labelled ACh from labelled glucose was a direct measure of the total synthesis of ACh and not just a measure of label incorporation; thus the inhibition of synthesis by HC-3 strongly suggested that choline from an extracellular source is required. Collier and MacIntosh (1969) showed that the sustained synthesis and release of ACh by a superior cervical ganglion perfused *in situ* with physiological salts solution required the presence of choline in the perfusate. These observations clearly indicate that choline used for the synthesis of ACh arises from sites extracellular to the location of ACh synthesis and suggest an important role for choline transport at cholinergic nerve endings in the regulation of ACh synthesis.

CHOLINE UPTAKE AND ACh SYNTHESIS BY NERVE ENDINGS

The uptake of choline by nerve endings as a means of providing choline for the synthesis of ACh was first suggested by Birks and MacIntosh (1961) in their studies on ACh synthesis and release by the perfused superior cervical ganglion. With the advent of techniques for the isolation of intact, metabolically viable nerve endings from homogenates of brain tissue (Whittaker, 1959; Gray and Whittaker, 1962; Whittaker, 1969), it became possible to study the uptake and metabolism of choline by isolated nerve endings, synaptosomes, *in vitro*. The results of such studies, which will be presented below, have led to the conclusion that under normal physiological conditions the uptake of choline by a specific transport system present only at the membranes of cholinergic nerve endings is the primary regulatory step in the biosynthesis of ACh.

General Characteristics of Choline Uptake by Synaptosomes

The uptake of choline by nerve endings is mediated by two kinetically distinct and saturable processes, the so-called low affinity and high affinity transport systems (Dowdall and Simon, 1973; Haga and Noda, 1973; Yamamura and Snyder, 1973). Yamamura and Snyder (1973) showed that the synaptosomal uptake of choline can be described by the expression:

$$v = \frac{Vm_H * S}{K_{T_H} + S} + \frac{Vm_L * S}{K_{T_L} + S} \qquad (2)$$

where the subscripts H and L refer to the high and low affinity systems respectively and the other terms have the same definition as in equation (1).

The low affinity uptake for choline is found at the cell bodies as well as the nerve endings of virtually all neurons. The apparent Michaelis constant, K_T, for the synaptosomal low affinity carrier is in the order of 30-100 μM (see Table 3) and can mediate the influx as well as the efflux of choline from nerve endings (Diamond and Milfay, 1972; Barker, in press). It supplies choline for the synthesis of phosphorylcholine and does not appear to be associated with any appreciable synthesis of ACh (Haga and Noda, 1973; Kuhar *et al.*, 1973; Yamamura and Snyder, 1973; Barker *et al.*, 1978).

The high affinity uptake system for choline in brain tissue which has an apparent K_T between 0.9-8.0 μM (Table 3) is relatively unique in comparison to its low affinity counterpart. The high affinity transport process apparently is present only at the membranes of cholinergic neurons and here it seems to be restricted to the nerve endings (Dowdall and Zimmerman, 1977; Kuhar *et al.*, 1973; Suszkiw and Pilar, 1976; Yamamura *et al.*, 1974) and provides a good marker for cholinergic nerve endings (Carrol and Butterbaugh, 1975). The high affinity uptake of choline by synaptosomes, in contrast to the

TABLE 3

Apparent Kinetic Constants for the Synaptosomal Uptake of Choline

Synaptosomal Preparation	Apparent Michaelis Constants K_T (μM) H.A.	K_T (μM) L.A.	V_{max} (nmole/gm/min) H.A.	V_{max} (nmole/gm/min) L.A.	Ref
Rat fore-brain	4-8	40-50	1.7	5	1
Rat fore-brain	2.4	100	1.7	7	2
Rat Corpus Striatum*	4.0	n.d.	3	n.d.	3
Rat Corpus Striatum*	1.4	93.3	1.4	5.6	4
Rat Cerebral Cortex*	3.0	33.3	0.9	2.2	4
Rat Cerebellum*	n.d.	41.4	n.d.	1.0	4
Rat Hippocampus	0.9		2.0		5

*Data recalculated, assuming a protein value of 50 mg for the synaptosomal preparation isolated from 1 gm of tissue.

H.A. and L.A. are high affinity and low affinity respectively.

n.d. – not detected.

References. (1) Haga and Noda, 1973; (2) Barker and Mittag, 1975; (3) Guyenet *et al.*, 1973; (4) Yamamura and Snyder, 1973; (5) Simon and Kuhar, 1976.

low affinity, has a marked dependency upon sodium ions (Haga and Noda, 1973; Kuhar *et al.*, 1973; Simon and Kuhar, 1976; Yamamura and Snyder, 1973) as well as a requirement for chloride ions (Simon and Kuhar, 1976). The primary function of the sodium dependent high affinity uptake of choline by central nerve endings is to supply choline for the synthesis of ACh (Haga, 1971; Haga and Noda, 1973; Kuhar *et al.*, 1973; Yamamura and Snyder, 1973) and the uptake appears to be coupled to the synthesis of ACh (Barker and Mittag, 1975; Lefresene *et al.*, 1975) which also is preferentially released during synaptic transmission (Mulder *et al.*, 1974; Polak *et al.*, 1977).

Another distinguishing characteristic of the synaptosomal high affinity uptake of choline is its marked sensitivity to inhibition by the compound hemicholinium-3 (HC-3) (Guyenet *et al.*, 1973; Haga and Noda, 1973). The K_i value of HC-3 inhibition of high affinity transport is in the range of 25-60 nM (Barker and Mittag, 1975; Guyenet *et al.*, 1973; Haga and Noda, 1973; Yamamura and Snyder, 1973) in contrast to its K_i value for the inhibition in low affinity transport which is about 50 μM (Barker and Mittag, 1975; Haga and Noda, 1973).

Synaptosomal High Affinity Choline Transport and ACh Synthesis

Several investigators have shown that only choline transported by the high affinity carrier is used in the synaptosomal synthesis of ACh (Haga and Noda, 1973; Yamamura and Snyder, 1973; Guyenet *et al.*, 1973). This is evidenced by the Na^+ requirement for high affinity transport and ACh synthesis (Haga and Noda, 1973); the kinetic analysis of transport and synthesis which show that the K_T for high affinity transport is the K for acetylation (Haga and Noda, 1973; Barker and Mittag, 1975) and the demonstration that total inhibition of high affinity transport by HC-3 results in total inhibition of ACh synthesis as measured by the incorporation of ^3H-choline (Barker and Mittag, 1973) or 80% as measured by the incorporation of ^{14}C-glucose into ACh (Guyenet *et al.*, 1973). Similarly, HC-3 totally abolishes the stimulated uptake and acetylation of choline by brain slices previously depolarized by K^+ ions (Polak *et al.*, 1977).

The stoichiometry of high affinity choline transport and acetylation by intact synaptosomes provides further support for the notion that the synthesis of ACh is regulated by high affinity choline transport. In synaptosomes treated with an inhibitor of cholinesterase such as Soman or physostigmine, greater than 90% of the choline accumulated by the high affinity mechanism is converted to ACh (Yamamura and Snyder, 1973; Barker, unpublished). In the absence of an inhibitor of cholinesterases, some ACh is hydrolyzed during the extraction process and the observed conversion is about 65% (Barker and Mittag, 1975). Under the proper experimental conditions, a stoichiometry of almost 1 is obtained for the number of molecules of choline that are transported and acetylated. In kinetic terms, the V_{max} of transport = the V_{max} of acetylation of choline; and as noted above, the apparent Michaelis constant for the transport and acetylation of choline by synaptosomes are equal. There are also other properties expected from a coupled system (Barker and Mittag, 1975) i.e. the choline used for ACh synthesis appears to have no free existence in the nerve ending cytoplasm.

The ACh synthesized from choline taken up by the high affinity system is preferentially released during transmission; thus illustrating the fundamental role this transport system plays at central cholinergic nerve endings (Kuhar and Murrin, 1978). Much of the choline arising from the hydrolysis of released ACh is recaptured by cholinergic nerve endings for re-use in ACh synthesis and release. The exact proportions have not been measured for central endings, but have been estimated to be 50-60% for cholinergic nerve endings in a sympathetic ganglia (Collier and Katz, 1974) where virtually all of the recaptured choline is reconverted to ACh. The uptake and acetylation of choline by cholinergic nerve endings in the superior cervical ganglia *in situ* differs from that seen in isolated synaptosomes in that a kinetically defined high affinity system has not been demonstrated (see Kuhar and Murrin, 1978 for review) and that the specific uptake of choline leading to ACh synthesis is only seen under conditions of preganglionic stimulation (Collier and MacIntosh, 1969). These observations and those of others using brain minces depolarized by K^+ ions (Carrol and Goldberg, 1975) have led to the suggestion that under conditions of depolarization, the low affinity and not the high affinity uptake of choline supplies choline for ACh synthesis. However, it has been shown that a functional high affinity uptake mechanism for choline is necessary for the synthesis of ACh by synaptosomes depolarized by K^+ ions (Barker *et al.*, 1978). Namely, pretreatment of synaptosomes with the nitrogen mustard, N,N,N',N'-tetrakis-(2-choroethyl)-1-6-hexamediamine, $(ClCH_2CH_2)_2N(CH_2)_6N(CH_2CH_2Cl)_2$, (C6NM) results in a selective and irreversible inhibition of the high affinity uptake of choline. Synaptosomes so treated are capable of low affinity choline uptake. When they are incubated in the presence of depolarizing concentration of K^+ ions, the C6NM pretreated synaptosomes can release, but cannot synthesize ACh. The activity of CAT in synaptosomes pretreated with C6NM is not measurably reduced, thus the inhibition of ACh synthesis seen in this depolarized preparation appears to be due solely to the irreversible inhibition of the high affinity choline carrier.

The results of studies on the uptake and acetylation of choline by isolated nerve endings have demonstrated the fundamental role the high affinity uptake of choline plays in the regulation of ACh synthesis. The results of other investigators show that the same is true for nerve endings *in vivo*. Among the most interesting properties revealed in studies on intact animals is that the velocity of high affinity transport as measured *in vitro* and *in vivo* appears to be coupled to neuronal activity (Atweh *et al.*, 1975; Simon and Kuhar, 1975; Atweh and Kuhar, 1976; Jenden *et al.*, 1976; Simon *et al.*, 1976; Samoras and Contrera, 1977). It has been shown that pharmacological and physiological conditions which alter neuronal impulse-flow along a cholinergic pathway are accompanied by parallel changes in the velocity of choline uptake by the high affinity system. For example, electrical stimulation of the medial septal region which activates the septohippocampal cholinergic pathway results in an increase in the V_{max} of high affinity choline uptake and acetylation by hippocampal synaptosomes with no accompanying changes in the apparent K_T for uptake or the kinetics of CAT. Similarly, treatment of animals with drugs known to increase ACh turnover such as atropine or haloperidol results in an increased velocity of choline uptake and conversely for drugs known to decrease ACh turnover. Furthermore, the drug effects are region specific, i.e. barbiturates decrease ACh turnover and choline uptake in the hippocampus but not in the striatum, and thus are most likely due to drug effects on neuronal activity rather than a direct effect on the uptake system as has been shown (Atweh *et al.*, 1975). These results show that high affinity uptake of choline is not only a rate limiting step in the synthesis of ACh but is also a system which can accommodate the increased synthesis that is known to occur when ACh is released during synaptic transmission.

The results of studies on synaptosomes *in vitro* show that depolarization of the nerve ending *per se* is likely to be the basis for increased uptake and acetylation of choline (Barker, 1976b; Murrin and Kuhar, 1976). Although it is tempting to speculate that the increased uptake and acetylation of choline is directly related to a reduction in intraterminal ACh levels (Jenden *et al.*, 1976; Vaca and Pilar, 1977), this phenomenon can be demonstrated under conditions in which the release of ACh is blocked (Barker, 1976b; Collier and Ilson, 1977; Kuhar and Murrin, in press). Events that accompany depolarization other than transmitter release appear to be required for the activation of choline transport. Such events may be metabolic changes or Ca^{+2} influxes that are known to increase during depolarization. At this time it is not known whether the activation of uptake is due to an increase in the number of high affinity transport sites or due to an increased substrate turnover of extant sites (Barker, 1976b; Murrin and Kuhar, 1976).

The importance of the so-called high affinity uptake of choline by central cholinergic nerve endings as a necessary step in the synthesis of ACh, is now a well established experimental observation. This is demonstrated by its requirement for the synthesis of ACh under conditions of rest and depolarization; by the requirement for free extracellular choline for ACh synthesis; and by the changes that occur in the uptake and acetylation of choline by the high affinity system in response to changes in impulse flow along cholinergic pathways.

Synaptosomal Uptake and Acetylation of Choline Analogs

Several analogs of choline have been studied both as inhibitors and as substrates of the high affinity carrier. The object of these studies was to characterize the substrate recognition site of the transport system, to determine whether or not analogs of choline that possess hydroxyl groups will be acetylated and hence be precursors to false transmitters (Barker and Mittag, 1975; Simon *et al.*, 1975). The latter objective has obvious pharmacological implications in that such agents may be used to alter transmission at cholinergic synapses.

The minimal requirements for a choline analog to be recognized as a substrate by the high affinity site appear to be that it is a simple alkyl compound substituted at one end with a quaternary group, either an alkyl sulfonium (Frankenberg *et al.*, 1973) or an alkyl ammonium (Simon *et al.*, 1975) that it is no more than three methylene, ($-CH_2$) groups long and substituted on the other end by a hydroxyl or a group that is isoelectronic with a hydroxyl group such as an acetylenic, ($-C \equiv CH$), function (Barker, in press). ACh does not appear to be a substrate for the high affinity choline uptake system (Kuhar and Simon, 1974) but at low-micromolar concentrations can inhibit choline uptake (Yamamura and Snyder, 1973).

Analogs of choline that have been studied in detail as substrates for the synaptosomal high affinity choline uptake and acetylation system are monoethylcholine (N-ethyl-N,N-dimethyl-N-(2-hydroxyethyl) ammonium), homocholine (N,N,N-trimethyl-N-(3-hydroxypropyl) ammonium), and pyrrolidinocholine (N-methyl-N-(2-hydroxyethyl) pyrrolidinium (Barker and Mittag, 1975; 1976; Collier *et al.*, 1977). These three compounds were selected for detailed study because they represent the complete spectrum of substrates for CAT, and thus a study of their uptake and acetylation by synaptosomes would provide information concerning the relationship between the high affinity transport system and CAT. Of these three analogs, only monoethylcholine is a full substrate for CAT (Burgen *et al.*, 1956; Barker and Mittag, 1975). Pyrrolidinocholine is a partial substrate (Barker and Mittag, 1975) and homocholine is not a substrate for CAT (Burgen *et al.*, 1956; Dauterman and Mehrotra, 1963; Currier and Mautner, 1974; Collier *et al.*, 1977).

The uptake and degree of acetylation of these same analogs by intact synaptosomes is found to be nearly identical to that of choline; a finding totally unexpected from the results of studies on the acetylation mediated by CAT in a membrane free preparation. Based on these observations, it has been proposed that the apparent coupling seen between the high affinity transport and acetylation of choline may be physical rather than kinetic (Barker *et al.*, 1978). However, in the superior cervical ganglion, the uptake of homocholine can be temporally dissociated from its acetylation (Collier and Ilson, 1977) suggesting that the relationship between uptake and acetylation may not be the same for all cholinergic terminals (Barker *et al.*, 1975; and Barker *et al.*, 1978).

Regardless of the type of coupling seen between transport and acetylation, these results establish that choline analogs can be taken and acetylated by intact nerve endings. The results of other studies show that these three analogs of choline (Collier *et al.*,

1976; Collier *et al.*, 1977) as well as triethylcholine (Ilson and Collier, 1975; Ilson *et al.*, 1977) can be taken up and acetylated by preganglionic cholinergic nerve endings in a sympathetic ganglion and that the acetylated derivatives are released upon preganglionic stimulation by a Ca^{+2} dependent process. Thus these agents can act as precursors to false transmitter at cholinergic junctions. One of them, pyrrolidinocholine, has been shown to act presynaptically to produce an impairment in passive avoidance behavior in mice; presumably by virtue of its ability to act as a precursor to a cholinergic false transmitter (Glick *et al.*, 1975).

These observations clearly indicate that the substrate specificity of CAT *in vivo* is different from that in a membrane free environment. The bulk of CAT at nerve endings appears to be cytoplasmic (Fonnum, 1968) but a small proportion is membrane bound in a catalytically active form (Fonnum, 1968).

It may be that the membrane bound form of the enzyme is that which is important in the acetylation of choline and the choline analogs following (or during) high affinity transport (Barker *et al.*, 1978). At this point, it is also worth noting that CAT *per se* does not appear to be the site of the regulation of ACh synthesis. It is present in 9-10 fold excess above that required to support the turnover of ACh (Hebb, 1972). Also, the administration of potent inhibitors of CAT intraventricularly to mice (Glick *et al.*, 1973) or intraperitoneally to mice and guinea pigs (Krell and Goldberg, 1975) or rats (Carson *et al.*, 1972) causes an apparent inhibition of CAT but is not associated with any decrease in ACh levels. Thus the bulk of CAT may be a 'reserve' pool of enzyme.

IMPLICATIONS AND SPECULATIONS FOR
PRECURSOR LOADING THERAPY

The previous discussions have dealt with the results of basic research studies. The results of these studies permit one to say a great deal about the regulation of ACh synthesis at central cholinergic nerve endings in the non-pathological state. We have seen that the steady state levels and turnover of ACh are only slightly and variably altered by rather large changes in either plasma or brain regional levels of free choline. Further, it has been proposed and documented by experimental results that the major site for the regulation of ACh synthesis is at the so-called choline high affinity uptake step. At first approximation, these results from studies on choline transport and ACh synthesis are not compatible with the notion that the desirable effects seen with choline therapy are due to increased synthesis of ACh, i.e. a consequence of precursor loading. An alternative explanation is that the therapeutic effects of choline are due to its weak activity as a cholinergic agonist. However, caution must be applied in using the results of studies carried out on laboratory animals with no obvious neurological impairments to the results of clinical studies on patients with Huntington's chorea or tardive dyskinesia. Namely, it may well be that part of the biochemical pathology in such patients is a disturbance in the usual relationship that is seen between the high affinity uptake and acetylation of choline at nerve endings. In this hypothetical case, it may be necessary to elevate intracellular choline to a concentration near its apparent K_m value, 100 μM, for soluble CAT in order to maintain ACh synthesis and hence release. Were this the case, then precursor loading with choline may result in an increase of the formation and release of ACh.

ACKNOWLEDGEMENTS

The research carried out in the author's laboratory was supported by grants from NIMH (MH 24949), NINCDS (NS 08829), a Career Scientist Award from the Irma T. Hirschl Trust (1977-1978) and a NINCDS Career Development Award (1 K04-NS00274-01).

REFERENCES

Ansell, G.B., and Spanner, S., 1967, The metabolism of labelled ethanolamine in brain of the rat *in vivo, J. Neurochem. 14:*873.

Ansell, G.B., and Spanner, S., 1968a, The long-term metabolism of the ethanolamine moiety of rat brain myelin phospholipids, *J. Neurochem. 15:*1371.

Ansell, G.B., and Spanner, S., 1968b, The metabolism of [Me-^{14}C] choline in the brain of the rat *in vivo, Biochem. J. 110:*201.

Ansell, G.B., and Spanner, S., 1978, The sources of choline for acetylcholine synthesis, in *"Cholinergic Mechanisms and Psychopharmacology"* (D.J. Jenden, ed.), pp. 431-445, Plenum Press, New York.

Aquilonius, S.M., Flentge, F., Schuberth, J., Sparf, B., and Sundwall, A., 1973, Synthesis of acetylcholine in different compartments of brain nerve terminals *in vivo* as studied by the incorporation of choline from plasma and the effects of pentobarbital on this process, *J. Neurochem. 20:*1509.

Aquilonius, S.M., Ceder, G., Lying-Tunell, U., Malmlund, H.O., and Schuberth, J., 1975, The arteriovenous difference of choline across the brain of man, *Brain Res. 99:*430.

Atweh, S., and Kuhar, M.J., 1976, Effects of anesthetics and septal lesions and stimulation on ^{3}H-acetylcholine formation in rat hippocampus, *Eur. J. Pharmacol. 37:*311.

Atweh, S., Simon, J.R., and Kuhar, M.J., 1975, Utilization of sodium-dependent high affinity choline uptake *in vitro* as a measure of the activity of cholinergic neurons *in vivo, Life Sci. 17:*1535.

Barker, L.A., 1976a, Subcellular aspects of acetylcholine synthesis, in *"Biology of Cholinergic Function"* (A.M. Goldberg and I. Hanin, eds.), pp. 203-208, Raven Press, New York.

Barker, L.A., 1976b, Modulation of synaptosomal high affinity choline transport, *Life Sci. 18:*725.

Barker, L.A., (in press), The synaptosomal uptake of [^{3}H-N-Me]-N,N,N-trimethyl-N-propynyl-ammonium, *Fed. Proc. (Abs).*

Barker, L.A., and Mittag, T.W., 1973, Inhibition of synaptosomal choline uptake by naphthylvinylpyridiniums, *FEBS Lett. 35:*141.

Barker, L.A., and Mittag, T.W., 1975, Comparative studies of substrates and inhibitors of choline transport and choline acetyltransferase, *J. Pharmacol. Exp. Ther. 192:*86.

Barker, L.A., and Mittag, T.W., 1976, Synaptosomal transport and acetylation of 3-trimethylaminopropan-1-ol, *Biochem. Pharmacol. 25:*1931.

Barker, L.A., Dowdall, M.J., and Whittaker, V.P., 1972, Choline metabolism in the cerebral cortex of guinea pigs. Stable bound acetylcholine, *Biochem. J. 130:*1063.

Barker, L.A., Dowdall, M.J., and Mittag, T.W., 1975, Comparative studies on synaptosomes: high affinity uptake and acetylation of N-[Me-^{3}H] choline and N-[Me-^{3}H], N-hydroxyethylpyrrolidinium, *Brain Res. 86:*343.

Barker, L.A., Mittag, T.W., and Krespan, B., 1978, Studies on substrates, inhibitors and modifiers of the high affinity choline transport-acetylation system present in rat brain synaptosomes, in *"Cholinergic Mechanisms and Psychopharmacology"*, (D.J. Jenden ed.) pp. 465-480, Plenum Press, New York.

Birks, R., and MacIntosh, F.C., 1961, Acetylcholine metabolism in a sympathetic ganglion, *Can. J. Biochem. Physiol. 39:*787.

Bremer, I., and Greenberg, D.M., 1961, Methyl transferring enzyme system of microsomes in the biosynthesis of lecithin (phosphatidylcholine), *Biochem. Biophys. Acta 46:*205.

Browning, E.T., and Schulman, M.P., 1968, [^{14}C] Acetylcholine synthesis by cortex slices of rat brain, *J. Neurochem. 15:*1391.

Burgen, A.S.W., Burke, G., and Desbarats-Schonbaum, M.L., 1956, The specificity of brain choline acetylase, *Br. J. Pharmacol. 11:*308.

Butcher, S.H., and Butcher, L.L., 1974, Acetylcholine and choline levels in the rat corpus striatum after microwave irradiation, *Proc. West. Pharmacol. Soc. 17:*37.

Butcher, S.H., Butcher, L.L., Harms, M.S., and Jenden, D.J., 1976, Fast fixation of brain *in situ* by high intensity microwave irradiation: application to neurochemical studies, *J. Microwave Power 11:*61.

Carrol, P.T., and Butterbaugh, G.G., 1975, Regional differences in high affinity choline transport velocity in guinea pig brain, *J. Neurochem. 24:*929.

Carrol, P.T., and Goldberg, A.H., 1975, Relative importance of choline transport to spontaneous and potassium depolarized release of acetylcholine, *J. Neurochem. 25:*523.

Carson, U.G., Jenden, D.J., and Cho, A.K., 1972, The *in vivo* effects of some choline acetyltransferase inhibitors, *Proc. West. Pharmacol. Soc. 15:*127.

Choi, R.L., 1974, The distribution kinetics and turnover of choline and acetylcholine in plasma and brain of rats, Ph.D. Dissertation, University of California, Los Angeles (Xerox University Microfilms No. 75-9385).

Choi, R.L., Freeman, J.J., and Jenden, D.J., 1975, Kinetics of plasma choline in relation to turnover of brain choline and formation of brain acetylcholine, *J. Neurochem. 24:*735.

Cohen, E.L., and Wurtman, R., 1975, Brain acetylcholine: increase after systemic choline administration, *Life Sci. 16:*1095.

Collier, B., and Ilson, D., 1977, The effect of preganglionic nerve stimulation on the accumulation of certain analogues of choline by a sympathetic ganglion, *J. Physiol. (Lond.) 264:*489.

Collier, B., and Katz, H.S., 1974, Acetylcholine synthesis from recaptured choline by a sympathetic ganglion, *J. Physiol. 238:*639.

Collier, B., and MacIntosh, F.C., 1969, The source of choline for acetylcholine synthesis in a sympathetic ganglion, *Can. J. Physiol. Pharmacol. 47:*127.

Collier, B., Barker, L.A., and Mittag, T.W., 1976, The release of acetylated choline analogs by a sympathetic ganglion, *Mol. Pharmacol. 12:*340.

Collier, B., Lovat, S., Ilson, D., Barker, L.A., and Mittag, T.W., 1977, The uptake, metabolism and release of homocholine: studies with rat brain synaptosomes and cat superior cervical ganglion, *J. Neurochem. 28:*331.

Currier, S.F., and Mautner, H.G., 1974, On the mechanism of action of choline acetyltransferase, *Proc. Natl. Acad. Sci. USA 71:*3355.

Dauterman, W.C., and Mehrotra, K.N., 1963, The N-alkyl group specificity of choline acetylase from rat brain, *J. Neurochem. 10:*113.

Diamond, I., 1971, Choline metabolism in brain, *Arch. Neurol. 24:*333.

Diamond, I., and Milfay, D., 1972, Uptake of [^{3}H-methyl] choline by microsomal, synaptosomal, mitochondrial and synaptic vesicle fractions of rat brain. The effects of hemicholinium, *J. Neurochem. 19:*1899.

Dowdall, M.J., and Simon, E.J., 1973, Comparative studies on synaptosomes: uptake of [N-Me-^{3}H] choline by synaptosomes from squid optic lobes, *J. Neurochem. 21:* 969.

Dowdall, M.J., and Zimmerman, H., 1977, The isolation of pure cholinergic nerve terminal sacs (T-sacs) from the electric organ of juvenile *Torpedo, Neurosci. 2:*405.

Dowdall, M.J., Barker, L.A., and Whittaker, V.P., 1972, Choline metabolism in the cerebral cortex of the guinea pig: phosphorylcholine and lipid choline, *Biochem. J. 130:* 1081.

Dross, K., 1975, Effects of diisopropylfluorophosphate on the metabolism of choline and phosphatidylcholine in rat brain, *J. Neurochem. 24:*701.

Dross, K., and Kewitz, H., 1972, Concentration and origin of choline in the rat brain, *Naunyn Schmiedebergs Arch. Exp. Path. Pharmak. 274:*91.

Eckernas, S.A., 1977, Plasma choline and cholinergic mechanisms in the brain, *Acta Physiol. Scand. (Suppl.) 449:*1.

Fonnum, F., 1968, Choline acetyltransferase, binding to and release from membranes, *Biochem. J. 109:*389.

Frankenberg, L., Heimburger, G., Nilsson, C., and Sorbo, B., 1973, Biochemical and pharmacological studies on the sulfonium analogues of choline and acetylcholine, *Eur. J. Pharmacol. 23:*37.

Freeman, J.J., and Jenden, D.J., 1976, The source of choline for acetylcholine synthesis in brain, *Life Sci. 19:*949.

Freeman, J.J., Choi, R.L., and Jenden, D.J., 1975, Plasma choline: its turnover and exchange with brain choline, *J. Neurochem. 24:*729.

Gardiner, J.E., and Gwee, M.C.E., 1974, The distribution in the rabbit of choline administered by injection or infusion, *J. Physiol. (Lond.) 239:*459.

Gardiner, J.E., and Paton, W.D.M., 1972, The control of the plasma choline concentrations in the cat, *J. Physiol. (Lond.) 227:*71.

Glick, S.D., Mittag, T.W., and Green, J.P., 1973, Central cholinergic correlates of impaired learning, *Neuropharmacology 12:*291.

Glick, S.D., Crane, A.M., Barker, L.A., and Mittag, T.W., 1975, Effects of N-hydroxyethylpyrrolidinium methiodide, a choline analog, on passive avoidance behavior in mice, *Neuropharmacology 14:*561.

Gray, E.G., and Whittaker, V.P., 1962, The isolation of nerve endings from brain: An electron microscopic study of the cell fragments derived by homogenization and centrifugation, *J. Anat. 96:*79.

Guyenet, P., Lefresne, P., Rossier, J., Beaujouan, J.C., and Glowinski, J., 1973, Inhibition by hemicholinium-3 of [^{14}C] acetylcholine synthesis and [^{3}H] choline high affinity uptake in rat striatal synaptosomes, *Mol. Pharmacol. 9:*630.

Haga, T., 1971, Synthesis and release of [^{14}C] acetylcholine in synaptosomes, *J. Neurochem. 18:*781.

Haga, T., and Noda, H., 1973, Choline uptake systems of rat brain synaptosomes, *Biochem. Biophys. Acta 291:*564.

Hanin, I., and Costa, E., 1976, Brain acetylcholine turnover, in *"Biology of Cholinergic Function"*, (A.M. Goldberg, and I. Hanin, eds.), pp. 355-377, Raven Press, New York.

Hanin, I., and Schuberth, J., 1974, Labelling of acetylcholine in the brain of mice fed on a diet containing deuterium labelled choline: studies utilizing gas chromatography-mass spectrometry, *J. Neurochem. 23:*819.

Haubrich, D.R., and Chippendale, T.J., 1976, Regulation of acetylcholine synthesis in nervous tissue, *Life Sci. 20:*1465.

Haubrich, D.R., Wang, P.F.L., and Clody, D.E., 1974, Increase in tissue concentration of acetylcholine in guinea pigs *in vivo* induced by administration of choline, *Life Sci. 14:*921.

Haubrich, D.R., Wang, P.F.L., Clody, D.E., and Wedeking, W., 1975, Increase in rat brain acetylcholine induced by choline or deanol, *Life Sci. 17:*975.

Haubrich, D.R., Wang, P.F.L., Chippendale, T.J., Proctor, E., 1976, Choline and acetylcholine in rats: the effect of dietary choline, *J. Neurochem. 27:*1305.

Hebb, C.O., 1972, Biosynthesis of acetylcholine in nervous tissue, *Physiol. Rev. 52:* 918.

Hirsch, M.J., Growdon, J.H., and Wurtman, R.J., 1977, Increase in hippocampal acetylcholine after choline administration, *Brain Res. 125:*383.

Illingworth, D.R., and Portman, O.W., 1972, The uptake and metabolism of plasma lysophosphatidylcholine *in vivo* by the brain of squirrel monkeys, *Biochem. J. 130:* 557.

Ilson, D., and Collier, B., 1975, Triethylcholine as a precursor to a cholinergic false transmitter, *Nature 254:*618.

Ilson, D., Collier, B., and Boksa, P., 1977, Acetyltriethylcholine: a cholinergic false transmitter in cat superior cervical ganglion and rat cerebral cortex, *J. Neurochem. 28:*371.

Jenden, D.J., Jope, R.S., and Weiler, M.H., 1976, Regulation of acetylcholine synthesis: does cytoplasmic acetylcholine control high affinity choline uptake? *Science 194:* 635.

Krell, R.D., and Goldberg, A.M., 1975, Effect of choline acetyltransferase inhibitors on mouse and guinea pig brain choline and acetylcholine, *Biochem. Pharmacol. 24:* 391.

Kuhar, M.J., and Murrin, L.C., 1978, Sodium-dependent, high affinity choline uptake, *J. Neurochem. 30:*15.

Kuhar, M.J., and Simon, J.R., 1974, Acetylcholine uptake: lack of association with cholinergic neurons, *J. Neurochem. 22:*1135.

Kuhar, M.J., Sethy, V.H., Roth, R.H., and Aghajanian, K.K., 1973, Choline: selective accumulation by central cholinergic neurons, *J. Neurochem. 20:*581.

Lefresne, P., Guyenet, P., Beaujouan, J.C., and Glowinski, J., 1975, The subcellular localization of ACh synthesis in rat striatal synaptosomes investigated by the use of Triton X-100, *J. Neurochem. 25:*415.

Mulder, A.H., Yamamura, H.I., Kuhar, M.J., and Snyder, S.H., 1974, Release of acetylcholine from hippocampal slices by potassium depolarization: dependence on high affinity choline uptake, *Brain Res. 70:*372.

Murrin, L.C., and Kuhar, M.J., 1976, Activation of high-affinity choline uptake *in vitro* by depolarizing agents, *Mol. Pharmacol. 12:*1082.

Oldendorf, W.H., and Braun, L.D., 1976, [³H]Tryptamine and ³H-water as diffusible internal standards for measuring brain extraction of radio-labelled substances following carotid injection, *Brain Res. 113:*219.

Pardridge, W.M., and Oldendorf, W.H., 1977, Transport of metabolic substrates through the blood-brain barrier, *J. Neurochem. 28:*5.

Pedata, F., Wieraszko, A., and Pepeu, G., 1977, Effect of choline, phosphorylcholine, and dimethylaminoethanol on brain acetylcholine level in the rat, *Pharmacol. Res. Commun. 9:*755.

Polak, R.L., Molenaar, P.C., and van Gelder, M., 1977, Acetylcholine metabolism and choline uptake in cortical slices, *J. Neurochem. 29:*477.

Racagni, G., Trabucchi, M., and Cheney, D.L., 1975, Steady-state concentrations of choline and acetylcholine in rat brain parts during a constant rate infusion of deuterated choline, *Naunyn Schmiedebergs Arch. Pharmacol. 290:*99.

Saelens, J.K., Sinke, J.P., Allen, M.P., and Conroy, C.A., 1973, Some of the dynamics of choline and acetylcholine metabolism in rat brain, *Arch. Int. Pharmacodyn. Ther. 203:*305.

Samaras, G.M., and Contrera, J.T., 1977, Choline: high affinity uptake *in vivo* by rat hippocampus, *J. Neurochem. 28:*1373.

Schuberth, J., and Jenden, D.J., 1975, Transport of choline from plasma to cerebrospinal fluid in the rabbit with reference to the origin of choline and to acetylcholine metabolism in brain, *Brain Res. 84:*245.

Simon, J.R., and Kuhar, M.J., 1975, Impulse-flow regulation of high affinity choline uptake in brain cholinergic nerve terminals, *Nature 255:*162.

Simon, J.R., and Kuhar, M.J., 1976, High affinity choline uptake: ionic and energy requirements, *J. Neurochem. 27:*93.

Simon, J., Mittag, T.W., and Kuhar, M.J., 1975, Inhibition of synaptosomal uptake of choline by various choline analogs, *Biochem. Pharmacol. 24:*1139.

Simon, J.R., Atweh, S., and Kuhar, M.J., 1976, Sodium dependent high affinity choline uptake: a regulatory step in the synthesis of acetylcholine, *J. Neurochem. 26:*909.

Smith, J.E., Lane, J.D., Shea, P.A., and McBride, W.J., 1977, Neurochemical changes following administration of precursors of biogenic amines, *Life Sci. 21:*301.

Spanner, S., Hall, R.C., and Ansell, G.B., 1976, Arterio-venous differences of choline and choline lipids across the brain of rat and rabbit, *Biochem. J. 154:*133.

Sparf, B., 1973, On the turnover of acetylcholine in the brain, *Acta Physiol. Scand. (Suppl.) 397.*

Stavinoha, W.B., Weintraub, S.T., and Modak, A.T., 1973, The use of microwave heating to inactivate cholinesterase in rat brain prior to analysis for acetylcholine, *J. Neurochem. 20:*361.

Suszkiw, J.B., and Pilar, G., 1976, Selective localization of a high affinity choline uptake system and its role in ACh formation in cholinergic nerve terminals, *J. Neurochem. 26:*1133.

Tucek, S., 1970, The use of choline acetyltransferase for measuring the synthesis of acetyl-coenzyme A and its release from brain mitochondria, *Biochem. J. 104:*749.

Vaca, K., and Pilar, G., 1977, Mechanisms regulating acetylcholine synthesis at the neuromuscular junction, *Soc. Neurosci. Abs. III:*378, Abs. No. 1211.

Whittaker, V.P., 1959, The isolation and characterization of acetylcholine containing particles from brain, *Biochem. J. 72:*694.

Whittaker, V.P., 1969, The synaptosome, in *"Handbook of Neurochemistry"*, Vol. II, (A. Lajtha, ed.), pp. 327-364, Plenum Press, New York-London.

Whittaker, V.P., Michaelson, I.A., and Kirkland, R.J.A., 1964, The separation of synaptic vesicles from nerve ending particles (synaptosomes), *Biochem. J. 90:*293.

Wurtman, R.J., Hirsch, M.J., and Growdon, J.H., 1977, Lecithin consumption raises serum-free-choline levels, *Lancet 1:*68.

Yamamura, H.I., and Snyder, S., 1973, High affinity transport of choline into synaptosomes of rat brain, *J. Neurochem. 21:*1355.

Yamamura, H.I., Kuhar, M.J., Greenberg, D., and Snyder, S., 1974, Muscarinic cholinergic receptor binding: regional distribution in monkey brain, *Brain Res. 66:*541.

PHARMACOKINETIC STUDIES WITH CHOLINE CHLORIDE: A PRELIMINARY REPORT

L. E. Hollister[1,2], D. J. Jenden[4], J. R. DoAmaral[2,3], J. D. Barchas[2,3], K. L. Davis[1,2] and P. A. Berger[1,2]

[1]Veterans Administration Hospital, 3801 Miranda Avenue, Palo Alto, California 94304

[2]Department of Psychiatry and Behavioral Sciences, Stanford University School of Medicine, Stanford, California 94305

[3]Nancy Pritzker Laboratory of Behavioral Neurochemistry, Stanford University School of Medicine, Stanford, California 94305

[4]Department of Pharmacology, School of Medicine, University of California, Los Angeles, California 90024

INTRODUCTION

Choline chloride has been administered to human subjects in an attempt to increase brain acetylcholine (ACh) content and central cholinergic activity (Davis et al., 1975a; 1976; Eckernas, 1977; Growdon et al., 1977a; 1977b; Tamminga et al., 1977; Davis and Berger, 1978). In preclinical investigations choline chloride given orally or parenterally has been reported to increase ACh content in the rat brain (Haubrich et al., 1974; Cohen and Wurtman, 1976; Eckernas, 1977). Several human pathological conditions, including manic psychosis, tardive dyskinesia, and Huntington's disease have been transiently improved by intravenous administration of the cholinesterase inhibitor physostigmine (Davis et al., 1975b). This has led to trials of choline chloride in these conditions in an attempt to chronically increase central cholinergic activity (Davis et al., 1975b).

The possibility that administration of large oral doses of choline to man would increase brain ACh and central cholinergic activity has led to trials of the drug in a number of disorders beneficially affected by physostigmine (Haubrich et al., 1974; Cohen and Wurtman, 1975; Davis et al., 1975a; 1976; Eckernas, 1977; Growdon et al., 1977a; 1977b; Tamminga et al., 1977; Davis and Berger, 1978). These studies have found choline chloride to reduce the abnormal involuntary movements of some patients with Huntington's disease and tardive dyskinesia (Davis et al., 1975a; 1976; Eckernas, 1977;

533

Growdon *et al.*, 1977a; 1977b; Tamminga *et al.*, 1977; Davis and Berger, 1978). Consistent with these data are the findings that the subcutaneous administration of choline chloride diminishes the severity of apomorphine-induced stereotypy (Davis *et al.*, 1977). In addition, choline chloride has efficacy in the animal model of tardive dyskinesia (Davis *et al.*, 1977).

Preliminary reports are in general agreement that baseline choline levels are between 7.5 nmoles/ml and 15.2 nmoles/ml (Aquilonius and Eckernas, 1975; Growdon *et al.*, 1977c). Furthermore, these studies suggest that the half life of choline is long enough to make possible the sustained elevation of plasma choline.

In an attempt to determine the dosage of choline chloride that produced the highest sustained plasma choline concentration, we conducted a series of pharmacokinetic studies with choline chloride.

METHODS

Acute Studies

Nine patients received an oral dose of 5 g of choline chloride at 8:00 a.m. Plasma samples were taken immediately before drug administration and at 5 min, 30 min, 1 hr, 2, 4, 6, 8, 24 and 48 hr after choline chloride administration. Blood was drawn into heparinized tubes and immediately spun down in a cold room at $5^{\circ}C$ to separate the plasma. Plasma was stored at $-70^{\circ}C$ until it was analyzed. Identical samples were sent to two laboratories. Choline was analyzed by gas chromatography/mass spectrometry as previously described (Jenden *et al.*, 1974).

Chronic Studies

Eight patients receiving 4-20 g of choline chloride daily, in four equally divided doses, participated in this investigation. All patients initially received 1 g of choline chloride four times per day for a total of a 4 g per day increment, every 3 days, until a total dose of 20 g per day was reached. This 20 g per day dose was maintained for 4 weeks. Immediately before receiving their first dose of 1 g of choline chloride a blood sample was taken. Additional samples were taken at 8:00 a.m. on the morning before a patient's dose of choline chloride was increased. While taking 20 g per day of choline chloride, blood samples were taken on the third, sixth, ninth and twelfth day of this 20 g dosage. Following discontinuation of choline chloride, blood samples were drawn for the next 4 days at 8:00 a.m. All samples were drawn at 8:00 a.m. before the morning dose, and 11 hr after the previous dose. Blood samples were processed and analyzed as in the acute study.

RESULTS

Figure 1 describes the course of plasma choline after a single 5 g dose. Plasma levels rapidly rise reaching a peak after 2 hr. For the next 4 hr the level is fairly constant, and rapidly falls off from hours six to eight. After 8 hr the plasma choline level is close to the baseline, and changes very little over the next 40 hr.

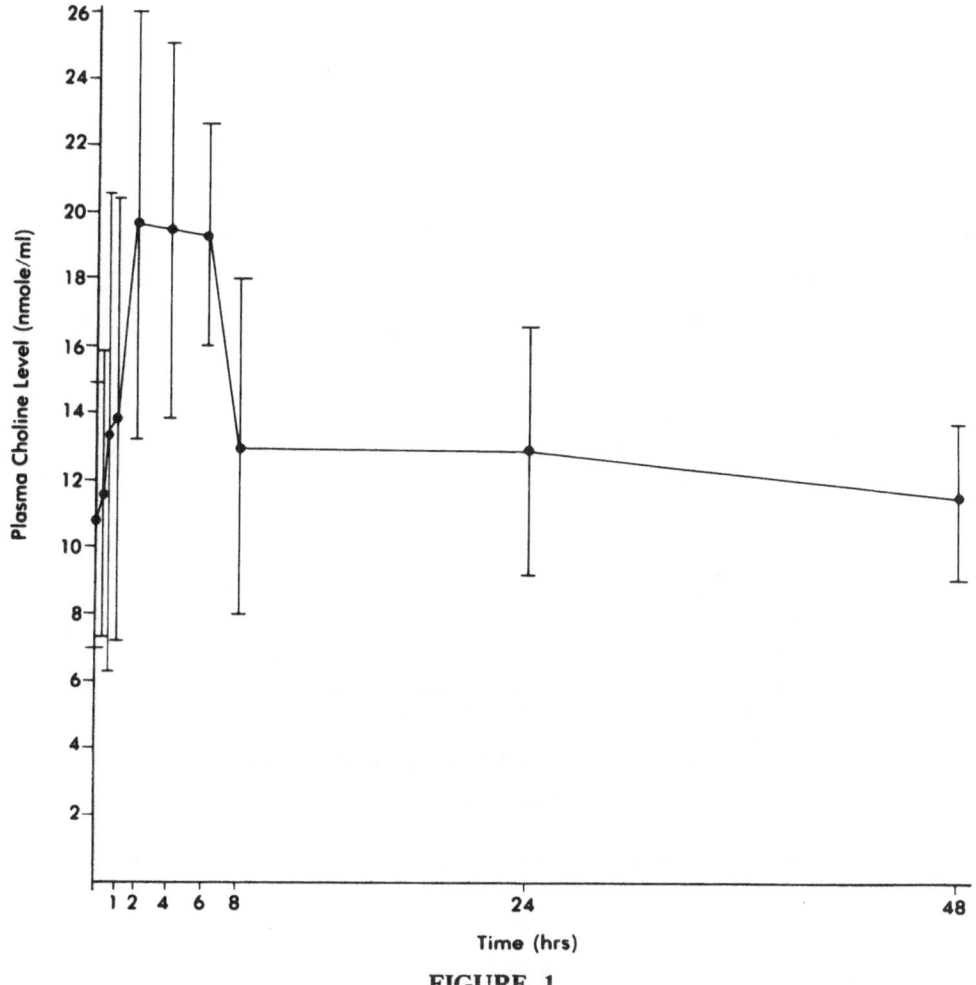

FIGURE 1

Plasma Choline Level After A Single 5 Gram Oral Dose

Figure 2 describes the plasma levels of choline as increasing doses of choline chloride were administered. Maximal levels are found when patients were receiving 20 g/day. A gradual dose dependent increase is apparent. However, the majority of the rise occurs after a dose of 4 g of choline chloride per day. On a daily dose of 20 g of choline per day in four divided doses, the plasma choline level shows little fluctuation (Table 1).

The disappearance of choline from the blood after the discontinuation of chronic choline chloride treatment is depicted in Figure 3. These patients had been receiving 20 g of choline daily for one month. As can be seen, baseline levels are closely approximated 72 hr after the last dose of choline chloride.

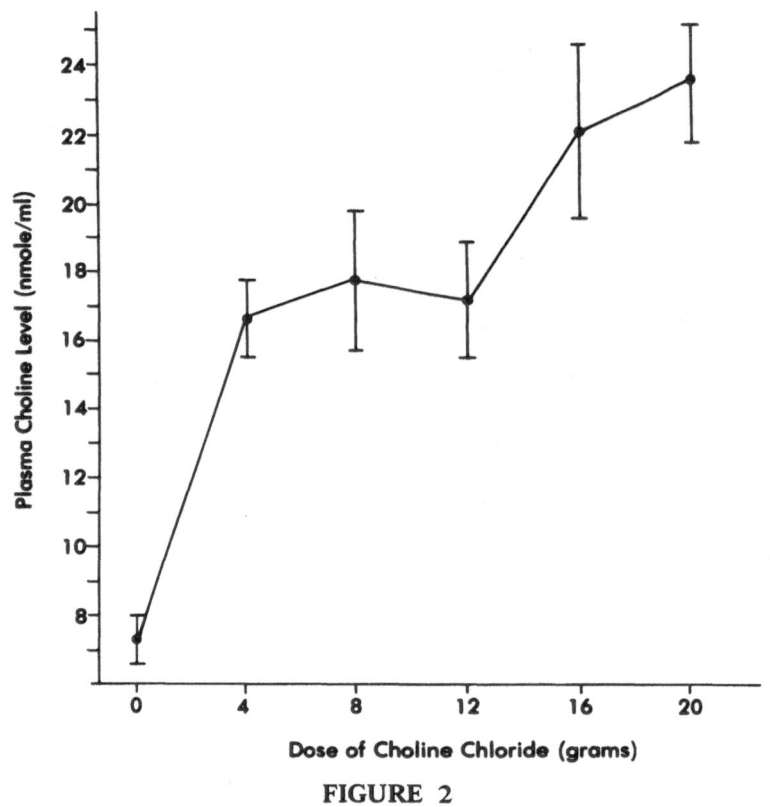

FIGURE 2

Plasma Choline Level After Increasing Doses of Choline Chloride

TABLE 1

Plasma Choline Levels After
Chronic Choline Chloride* Administration

Days on ChCl	Plasma Choline Level (nmoles/ml)
3	24.67 ± 1.58
6	21.4 ± 1.46
9	24.9 ± 1.23
12	23.9 ± 2.22

*20 grams p.o.

A Spearman correlation coefficient was calculated between plasma choline values determined from the same plasma sample, but in different laboratories (r = 0.821 p < .0001).

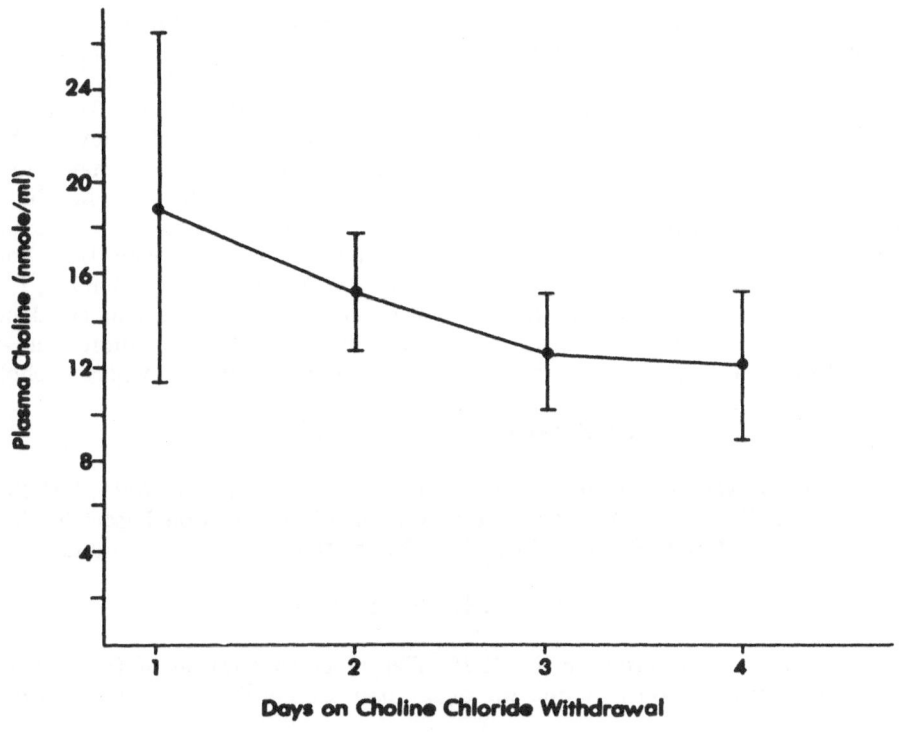

FIGURE 3

Plasma Choline Level After Discontinuation of Chronic Choline Chloride Treatment

DISCUSSION

These results indicate that the oral administration of choline chloride to man increases plasma choline levels in a dose dependent manner. Data from single dose studies suggest that plasma choline levels do not start to fall off until 6 hr after the administration of choline chloride. This offers some rationale for giving choline chloride in four divided oral doses. After chronic treatment, plasma choline levels diminished much more gradually than after the acute ingestion of a single 5 g dose. Thus, after a period of treatment longer intervals between choline chloride doses might be possible, and a sustained elevation in plasma choline maintained. These findings are in agreement with earlier reports (Aquilonius and Eckernas, 1975; Growdon et al., 1977c; Davis et al., 1978).

However, the choline levels determined in this study are somewhat lower than those obtained in previous reports, because blood samples were taken at a longer interval after the previous dose of choline chloride. Furthermore, this report is the first to employ the gas chromatography/mass spectrometry method of analysis. The high correlation found for determination of plasma choline levels from the same plasma sample in separate laboratories indicates the reliability of this method.

The relationship between the elevation in levels produced by choline ingestion and the therapeutic effect of choline is brought into question by the fact that there is a choline gradient from brain to blood (Dross and Kewutz, 1972; Choi *et al.*, 1975). The brain has approximately 13-20 nmole/ml more choline than the plasma. Thus, before elevations in plasma choline could be expected to increase brain choline levels, plasma levels need to be above approximately 28 nmoles/ml. It has been shown that a dose of intravenous choline rapidly is converted to phosphorylcholine, betaine, and phosphatidyl-choline with relatively little choline remaining as free choline (Rossiter and Strickland, 1970). Phosphatidylcholine can enter the brain and be hydrolized to yield free choline, which can be used for ACh synthesis (Jenden *et al.*, 1974; Freeman and Jenden, 1976). This route may be the source of the brain blood choline gradient (Freeman and Jenden, 1976). Hence the effect of choline ingestion on phosphatidylcholine may more accurately reflect its ultimate therapeutic action than the elevations produced in plasma choline.

ACKNOWLEDGEMENTS

This research was supported in part by Grants MH-03030, MH-17691, MH-23861, MH-24161, the Medical Research Service of the Veterans Administration, NIMH Specialized Research Center Grant MH-30854, and the Kate Pande Memorial Research Fund.

REFERENCES

Aquilonius, S.M., and Eckernas, S.A., 1975, Plasma concentration of free choline in patients with Huntington's chorea on high doses of choline chloride, *N. Engl. J. Med. 293:*1105.

Choi, R.L., Freeman, J.J., and Jenden, D.J., 1975, Kinetics of plasma choline in relation to turnover of brain choline and formation of acetylcholine, *J. Neurochem. 24:*735.

Cohen, E.L., and Wurtman, R.J., 1975, Brain acetylcholine: increase after systemic choline administration, *Life Sci. 16:*1095.

Cohen, E.L., and Wurtman, R.J., 1976, Brain acetylcholine control by dietary choline, *Science 191:*561.

Davis, K.L., and Berger, P.A., 1978, Pharmacological investigations of the cholinergic imbalance hypotheses of movement disorders and psychosis, *Biol. Psychiatry 13(1):* 23.

Davis, K.L., Berger, P.A., and Hollister, L.E., 1975a, Choline for tardive dyskinesia (a letter), *N. Engl. J. Med. 293:*152.

Davis, K.L., Hollister, L.E., Berger, P.A., and Barchas, J.D., 1975b, Cholinergic imbalance hypotheses of psychoses and movement disorders: strategies for evaluation, *Psychopharmacol. Comm. 1(5):*533.

Davis, K.L., Hollister, L.E., Barchas, J.D., and Berger, P.A., 1976, Choline in tardive dyskinesia and Huntington's disease, *Life Sci. 19:*1507.

Davis, K.L., Berger, P.A., Hollister, L.E., Simonton, S., and Barchas, J.D., 1977, Precursor loading with choline chloride, presented at the VI World Congress of Psychiatry, Honolulu, Hawaii, August 1977.

Davis, K.L., Berger, P.A., Hollister, L.E., DoAmaral, J.R., and Barchas, J.D., 1978, Cholinergic dysfunction in mania and movement disorders, in *"Cholinergic Mechanisms and Psychopharmacology"* (D.J. Jenden, ed.), pp. 755-779, Plenum Press, New York.

Dross, J., and Kewutz, H., 1972, Concentration and origin of choline in the rat brain, *Nauyn. Schmiedebergs Arch. Pharmacol. 274:*91.

Eckernas, S.A., 1977, Plasma choline and cholinergic mechanisms in the brain: methods, function and role in Huntington's chorea, *Acta Physiol. Scand. Suppl. 449:*1.

Freeman, J.J., and Jenden, D.J., 1976, The source of choline for acetylcholine synthesis in brain, *Life Sci. 19:*949.

Growdon, J.H., Hirsch, M.J., Wurtman, R.J., and Wiener, W., 1977a, Oral choline administration to patients with tardive dyskinesia, *N. Engl. J. Med. 297:*524.

Growdon, J.H., Cohen, E.L., and Wurtman, R.J., 1977b, Huntington's disease: clinical and chemical effects of choline administration, *Ann. Neurol. 1:*418.

Growdon, J.H., Cohen, E.L., and Wurtman, R.J., 1977c, Effects of oral choline administration of serum and CSF choline levels in patients with Huntington's disease, *J. Neurochem. 28:*229.

Haubrich, D.R., Wedeking, P.W., Wang, P.F.L., and Clody, D.E., 1974, Increase in tissue concentration of acetylcholine in guinea pigs *in vivo* induced by administration of choline, *Life Sci. 14:*921.

Jenden, D.J., Choi, L., Silverman, R.W., Steinborn, J.A., Roch, M., and Booth, R.A., 1974, Acetylcholine turnover estimation in brain by gas chromotography- mass spectrometry, *Life Sci. 14:*55.

Rossiter, R.J., and Strickland, K.P., 1970, Metabolism of phosphoglycerides, in *"Handbook of Neurochemistry, Vol. III"* (A. Lajtha, ed.), pp. 467-489, Plenum Press, New York.

Tamminga, C.A., Smith, R.C., Erickson, S.E., Chang, S., and Davis, J.M., 1977, Cholinergic influences in tardive dyskinesia, *Am. J. Psychiatry 134:*769.

CHOLINE CHLORIDE: EFFECT ON HYPERDOPAMINERGIC STATES IN ANIMALS

K. L. Davis[1,2], L. E. Hollister[1,2], A. L. Vento[1] and S. C. Simonton[1]

[1]Veterans Administration Hospital, 3801 Miranda Avenue,
Palo Alto, California 94304

[2]Department of Psychiatry and Behavioral Sciences, Stanford University
School of Medicine, Stanford, California 94305

INTRODUCTION

Although precursor loading with choline chloride or dimethylaminoethanol actually has been reported to increase brain acetylcholine (ACh) content, a concomitant increase in central cholinergic activity remains to be demonstrated (Haubrich *et al.*, 1974; Cohen and Wurtman, 1975; 1976; Eckernas, 1977; Hanin *et al.*, 1978).

Indirect evidence that choline chloride increases cholinergic activity comes from a number of sources. Clinical trials in patients with Huntington's disease, tardive dyskinesia and schizophrenia have compared the effects of choline chloride and physostigmine, an acetylcholinesterase inhibitor known to increase central cholinergic activity. In all cases there is a perfect correlation between a patient's response to physostigmine and choline chloride (Davis *et al.*, 1976). Electrophysiologic studies of choline chloride and physostigmine report similar effects for both drugs on peak alpha frequency (Pfefferbaum, 1978). Comparison of the clinical or electrophysiological effects of dimethylaminoethanol (deanol) and physostigmine have not been performed.

Agents that increase central cholinergic activity reverse apomorphine- or methyl-phenidate-induced stereotypy in rats (Janowsky *et al.*, 1972; Weiner *et al.*, 1976; Davis *et al.*, 1978). If choline chloride or deanol suppressed apomorphine- or methylphenidate-induced stereotypy this would indicate that these drugs increase central cholinergic activity. In one investigation neither acute nor chronic treatment of rats with deanol reversed apomorphine-induced stereotypy (Weiner *et al.*, 1976).

An animal model of tardive dyskinesia has been proposed (Schelkunov, 1967; Klawans and Rubovits, 1972; Tarsy and Baldessarini, 1973). When rats are chronically treated with neuroleptics, and these drugs are withdrawn, the animals have an exaggerated response to apomorphine. In this animal model it is conceivable that drugs which reduce the symptoms of tardive dyskinesia would only effect the increment in stereotypy produced by chronic exposure to neuroleptics.

Thus, choline chloride and deanol were given to animals previously treated with neuroleptics, as well as animals acutely challenged with apomorphine and methylphenidate. Both acute and chronic treatment with these potential cholinomimetics was tested. This chapter reports the results of these studies.

METHODS

Assessment of Stereotyped Behavior

In all experiments, stereotyped behavior was rated by two observers blind to the pretreatment regimen. Animals were rated for 45-sec periods beginning at 2 min and every 10 min thereafter for 60 min following apomorphine injection. Methylphenidate-induced stereotypy was assessed for 65-sec periods beginning 2 min after injection and continued every 10 min for 120 min. Stereotyped behavior was assessed according to a modification of a standard-point rating scale (Scheel-Kruger, 1971).

Drug Administration

Dosages of the following drugs administered were calculated as the salt: choline chloride, methylphenidate hydrochloride and apomorphine hydrochloride. Choline chloride was given subcutaneously (79 mg dissolved in 0.5 cc H_2O) or orally (375 mg dissolved in 0.5 cc H_2O). Control animals received 0.5 cc normal saline subcutaneously or 0.5 cc H_2O by gavage, respectively. Apomorphine and methylphenidate were given in dosages calculated for body weight of the animals.

Experiment 1

Effect of Subcutaneously Administered Choline Chloride on Apomorphine-Induced Stereotypy. Animals received a single subcutaneous injection of 79 mg of choline chloride followed 20 min later by a subcutaneous injection of apomorphine. Control animals received a subcutaneous injection of 0.5 cc normal saline. Three doses of apomorphine were tested, 0.25 mg/kg, 0.5 mg/kg, and 1.0 mg/kg. Naive animals were used for each dose of apomorphine.

Experiment 2

Effect of Acute Administration of Oral Choline Chloride on Apomorphine-Induced Stereotypy. A single dose of choline chloride (375 mg) was administered to naive animals by gavage. A control group of animals received 0.5 cc of H_2O by gavage. Twenty minutes later, they received one of three subcutaneous injections of apomorphine, 0.25 mg/kg, 0.5 mg/kg, or 1.0 mg/kg.

Experiment 3

Effect of Chronic Administration of Choline Chloride. Naive animals were given oral choline chloride daily for 5 weeks. Subcutaneous injections of 1.0 mg/kg apomorphine were administered on days 1, 8, 15, 22, 29 and 36. Apomorphine injections were given 20 min after choline chloride. Control animals in this study were gavaged daily with 0.5 cc H_2O.

Experiment 4

Effect of Acute and Chronic Administration of Choline Chloride on Methyl-phenidate-Induced Stereotypy. A group of naive rats were given 375 mg of choline chloride orally for 4 weeks. Another group of naive rats were gavaged daily with 0.5 cc H_2O. On days 1, 8 and 29 all animals were injected intraperitoneally with 30 mg/kg methylphenidate 20 min after choline chloride administration.

In experiments 5, 6 and 7 the effects of choline chloride were tested in animals with supersentitive dopamine receptors. In each experiment, animals received daily subcutaneous injections of 0.5 mg/kg haloperidol for 4 weeks. Haloperidol injections were then discontinued for 1 week. This was followed by four successive days of apomorphine injections. This protocol is presented in Table 1.

TABLE 1

	Treatment	Days of Administration
Haloperidol	0.5 mg/kg s.c.	1-28
Drug Free		29-35
Apomorphine	1.0 mg/kg s.c.	36
Apomorphine	0.5 mg/kg s.c.	37
Apomorphine	0.25 mg/kg s.c.	38
Apomorphine	0.125 mg/kg s.c.	39

Experiment 5

Effect of 4 Days of Choline Chloride on Apomorphine-Induced Stereotypy in Haloperidol Treated Animals. A group of haloperidol treated animals were given choline chloride by gavage only during the days of apomorphine challenges. Control animals were gavaged with 0.5 cc H_2O on the 4 days they received apomorphine injections. The order of apomorphine doses was 0.5 mg/kg, 0.25 mg/kg, and 0.125 mg/kg. The subcutaneous injections of apomorphine were given 20 min after choline chloride.

Experiment 6

Effect of 11 Days of Choline Chloride on Apomorphine-Induced Stereotypy in Haloperidol Treated Animals. A group of haloperidol treated animals received oral choline chloride during the period of haloperidol withdrawal and during apomorphine challenges. The four subcutaneous doses of apomorphine used were 1.0 mg/kg, 0.5 mg/kg, 0.25 mg/kg and 0.125 mg/kg. These injections were given 20 min after the choline chloride administration.

RESULTS

The effect of choline chloride, administered subcutaneously, on apomorphine-induced stereotypy is summarized in Figure 1. An analysis of variance indicates that animals receiving choline chloride had significantly less severe stereotypy than saline controls. In contrast, orally administered choline chloride given 20 min prior to a dose of apomorphine or methylphenidate did not significantly alter either apomorphine- or methylphenidate-induced stereotypy. There was still no significant effect of choline chloride on apomorphine-induced stereotypy. When choline chloride was administered 2½ hr and 20 min prior to the apomorphine challenge, chronic oral administration of choline chloride, for up to 5 weeks, also did not significantly modify either the severity or duration of apomorphine- or methylphenidate-induced stereotypy. This negative result occurred whether choline chloride was given 20 min or 2½ hr before apomorphine or methylphenidate. Thus, only when choline chloride was given subcutaneously did it significantly alter the stereotypy induced by increased dopaminergic activity.

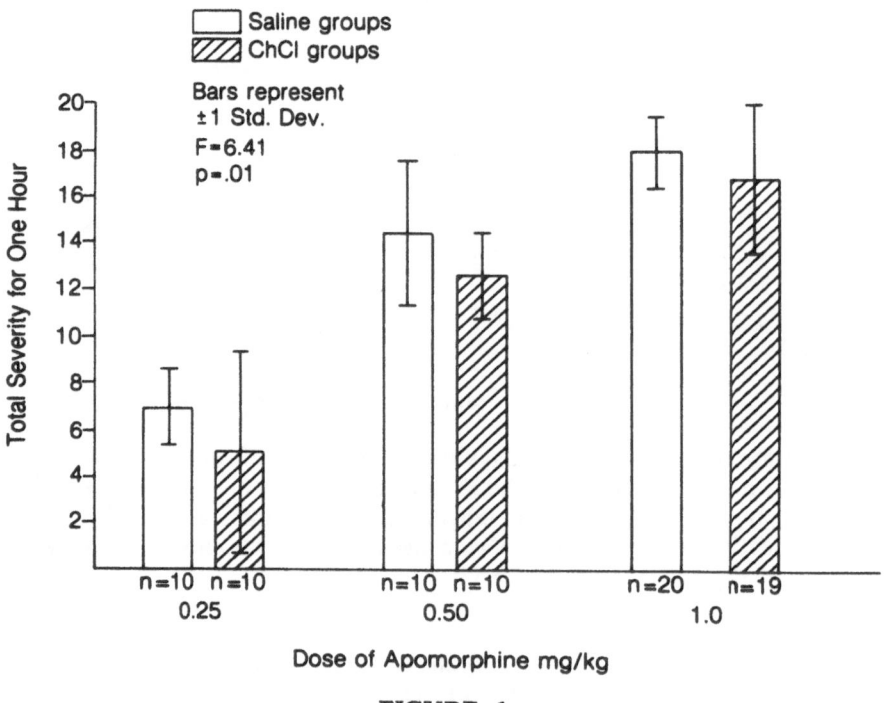

FIGURE 1

Effect of Choline Chloride (s.c.) on Apomorphine-Induced Stereotypy

Animals with a supersensitive dopamine receptor due to a 4 week exposure to neuroleptics were given choline chloride either acutely, chronically, or prophylactically. Both chronic (11 days) and prophylactic (39 days) administration of choline chloride significantly reduced apomorphine-induced stereotypy compared to saline control animals (Eckernas, 1977). Acute oral choline chloride administration on the 4 days of apomorphine administration did not significantly alter either the severity or duration of apomorphine-induced stereotypy compared to saline controls. All three groups are shown in Figure 2.

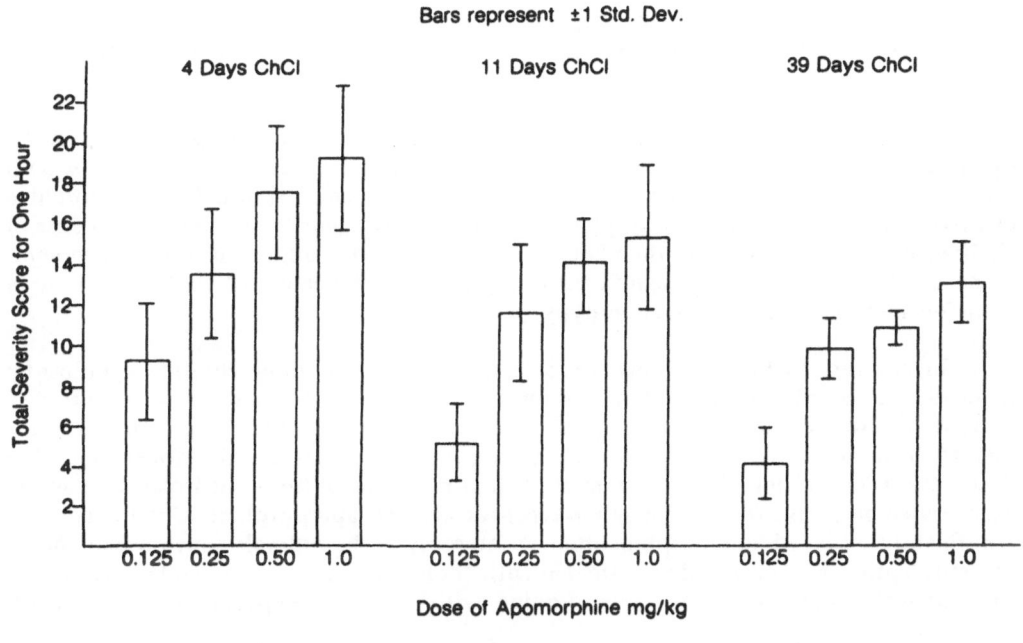

FIGURE 2

Effect of Duration of Choline Chloride Administration on Stereotypy Severity

DISCUSSION

These results indicate that when choline chloride is administered subcutaneously it diminishes the severity of apomorphine-induced stereotypy. This is consistent with the notion that central cholinergic activity can be increased by choline chloride administration. Furthermore, an effect of choline chloride on apomorphine-induced stereotypy was noted 20 min after choline chloride was given. This is consistent with the finding that brain acetylcholine (ACh) levels are elevated 20 min after the intraperitoneal administration of choline chloride to the rat (Cohen and Wurtman, 1975).

However, oral doses of choline chloride given acutely or for up to 5 weeks did not significantly decrease either methylphenidate- or apomorphine-induced stereotypy.

These results are not consistent with the report that supplementation of the diet of the rat with choline chloride significantly elevated brain ACh after 14 days (Cohen and Wurtman, 1976). This discrepancy suggests the elevation in brain ACh following chronic administration of choline is not associated with an increase in central cholinergic transmission.

Although choline chloride was administered orally in a variety of paradigms it never significantly diminished apomorphine- or methylphenidate-induced stereotypy. In both acute and chronic studies choline was given both 20 min and 2½ hr before apomorphine or methylphenidate. In man, peak plasma choline levels occur 2 hr after an oral dose of choline. However, varying the time between choline chloride administration and apomorphine challenge produced no significant changes in the efficiency of choline chloride in reducing apomorphine-induced stereotypy.

In contrast to these findings, chronic oral doses of choline chloride significantly reduced apomorphine-induced stereotypy in animals presumed to have a model of tardive dyskinesia. Production of a supersensitive postsynaptic dopamine receptor by exposing rats to high doses of neuroleptics has been suggested as an animal model of tardive dyskinesia (Schelkunov, 1967). Animals with a prior exposure to neuroleptics have an exaggerated response to the dopamine receptor agonist, apomorphine. Choline chloride significantly reduced apomorphine-induced stereotypy in animals previously exposed to neuroleptics. However, animals treated with choline chloride never had less stereotypy than animals challenged with apomorphine with no prior exposure to neuroleptics.

The results of these studies evaluating the efficacy of choline chloride in animal models of tardive dyskinesia are in agreement with a number of observations on the effects of choline chloride on patients with tardive dyskinesia. More than 4, but less than 11 days of high doses of choline chloride administration were necessary for the drug to significantly reduce apomorphine-induced stereotypy. In human studies significant improvement in the frequency of abnormal involuntary movements is also not seen until after 4 days of treatment. Choline chloride does not eliminate all abnormal involuntary movements in patients with tardive dyskinesia. Similarly choline chloride did not completely eliminate the increment in apomorphine-induced stereotypy caused by previous exposure to neuroleptics.

Thus, choline chloride has a complex series of effects. The route of administration profoundly influences its activity, as does the length of time it is administered. Furthermore, it may have effects on supersensitive receptors that it does not have on receptors with normal sensitivity. Additional studies are required to determine if the effects are the result of increased central cholinergic activity, and the effects that can be attributed to other neurochemical mechanisms.

ACKNOWLEDGEMENTS

This research was supported by the Medical Research Service of the Veterans Administration, the National Institute of Mental Health Specialized Research Center Grant MH-30854, U.S. Public Health Service Grant MH-03030 and the Kate Pande Memorial Research Fund.

REFERENCES

Cohen, E.L., and Wurtman, R.J., 1975, Brain acetylcholine: Increase after systemic choline administration, *Life Sci. 16:*1095.

Cohen, E.L., and Wurtman, R.J., 1976, Brain acetylcholine control by dietary choline, *Science 191:*561.

Davis, K.L., Hollister, L.E., Barchas, J.E., and Berger, P.A., 1976, Choline in tardive dyskinesia and Huntington's disease, *Life Sci. 19:*1507.

Davis, K.L., Hollister, L.E., and Tepper, J., 1978, Cholinergic inhibition of methylphenidate-induced stereotypy: Oxotremorine, *Psychopharmacology 56:*1.

Eckernas, S.A., 1977, Plasma choline and cholinergic mechanisms in the brain: Methods, function and role in Huntington's chorea, *Acta Physiologica Scand. Suppl. 449:*1.

Hanin, I., Kopp, U., Zahniser, N.R., Shih, T.M., Spiker, D.G., Merikangas, J.R., Kupfer, D.J., Foster, F.G., 1978, Acetylcholine and choline in human plasma and red blood cells: A gas chromatograph mass spectrometric evaluation, in *"Cholinergic Mechanisms and Psychopharmacology"* (D.J. Jenden, ed.), pp. 181-195, Plenum Press, New York.

Haubrich, D.R., Wedeking, P.W., Wang, P.F.L., and Clody, D.E., 1974, Increase in tissue concentration of acetylcholine in guinea pigs *in vivo* induced by administration of choline, *Life Sci. 14:*921.

Janowsky, D.S., El-Yousef, M.K., Davis, J.M., and Sekerke, H.J., 1972, Cholinergic antagonism of methylphenidate-induced stereotypy behavior, *Psychopharmacologia 27:*295.

Klawans, H.L., and Rubovits, R., 1972, An experimental model of tardive dyskinesia, *J. Neural. Transm. 33:*235.

Pfefferbaum, A., 1978, Electrophysiological effects of choline chloride and physostigmine. Presented at the Annual Meeting of the American Psychiatric Association, Atlanta, Georgia.

Scheel-Kruger, J., 1971, Comparative studies of various amphetamine analogues demonstrating different interactions with the metabolism of catecholamines in brain, *Eur. J. Pharmacol. 14:*47.

Schelkunov, E.L., 1967, Adrenergic effect of chronic administration of neuroleptics, *Nature 214:*1210.

Tarsy, D., and Baldessarini, R.J., 1973, Pharmacologically induced behavioral supersensitivity to apomorphine, *Nature 245:*262.

Weiner, W.J., Kanapa, D.J., Klawans, H.L., 1976, The effect of dimethylaminoethanol (DEANOL) on amphetamine-induced stereotyped behavior (AISB), *Life Sci. 19:*1371.

AUTHOR INDEX

SUBJECT INDEX
Abbreviations

ACh	acetylcholine
AChE	acetylcholinesterase
AChR	cholinergic receptor
ACTH	adrenocorticotropine hormone
AMP	adenosine monophosphate
AMPT	alpha-methyl-para-tyrosine
CAT	choline acetyltransferase
Ch	choline
ChE	cholinesterase
CNS	central nervous system
DA	dopamine
DFP	diisopropylfluorophosphate
DOPAC	dihydroxyphenylacetic acid
ECS	electroconvulsive shock
EEG	electroencephalogram
EKG	electrocardiogram
GABA	gamma aminobutyric acid
GAD	glutamic acid decarboxylase
HD	Huntington's disease
HVA	homovanillic acid
L-DOPA	levodopa
LTM	long-term memory
QNB	3-quinuclidinyl benzilate
RBC	red blood cell
STM	short-term memory
TD	tardive dyskinesia
TH	tyrosine hydroxylase

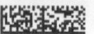